AORTIC DISSECTION

patients true stories and the innovations
that saved their lives

Germano Melissano • Roberto Chiesa
Editors

AORTIC DISSECTION

patients true stories and the innovations that saved their lives

edi·ermes

AORTIC DISSECTION patients true stories and the innovations that saved their lives
Germano Melissano • Roberto Chiesa (Editors)

ISBN 978-88-7051-565-7 - Paper edition

ISBN 978-88-7051-566-4 - Digital edition

Notices

Knowledge and best practice in this field are constantly changing. As new research and experience broaden our understanding, changes in research methods, professional practices, or medical treatment may become necessary.

Practitioners and researchers must always rely on their own experience and knowledge in evaluating and using any information, methods, compounds, or experiments described herein. In using such information or methods they should be mindful of their own safety and the safety of others, including parties for whom they have a professional responsibility.

With respect to any drug or pharmaceutical products identified, readers are advised to check the most current information provided (i) on procedures featured or (ii) by the manufacturer of each product to be administered, to verify the recommended dose or formula, the method and duration of administration, and contraindications.

It lies within the responsibility of practitioners, relying on their own experience and knowledge of their patients, to make diagnoses, to determine dosages and the best treatment for each individual patient and to take all appropriate safety precautions. To the fullest extent of the law, neither the Publisher nor the Authors, Contributors, or Editors, assume any liability for any injury and/or damage to persons or property as a matter of products liability, or arising from negligence or otherwise, or from any use or operation of any methods, products, instructions, or ideas contained in the material herein.

A book is the final product of a very complex series of operations that requires numerous tests on texts and images. It is almost impossible to publish a book with no errors. We will be grateful to those who find them and notify us. For enquiries or suggestions about this volume, please use the following address:

External relations - Edi.Ermes srl - Viale Enrico Forlanini, 65 - 20134 Milan (Italy)
Voice +39.02.70.21.121 - Fax +39.02.70.21.12.83

The Publisher is available for intellectual property owners with whom it was not possible to communicate, as well as for any inadvertent omissions and inaccuracies in the quotation of sources reproduced in this volume.

Paper edition printed in December 2016 by Aziende Grafiche Printing - Peschiera Borromeo, Milan, Italy
for Edi.Ermes - viale Enrico Forlanini, 65 - 20134 Milan, Italy
http://www.ediermes.it - Tel. +39.02.70.21.121 - Fax +39.02.70.21.12.83

This book is dedicated to the many people afflicted with aortic dissection,
to those who had the courage to undergo the operations described
and to the survivors who cope daily with the consequences of this disease.

Foreword

This gem of a book on aortic dissection brings together as authors all the superstars in the field and is edited by two of them, Germano Melissano and Roberto Chiesa. The volume contains the most thorough and up-to date information on this disease entity and its treatment. Interestingly it also includes two chapters which provide perspectives of patients suffering from this serious disease which is so often unrecognized and poorly treated. Accordingly this text is a "must have" for all specialists and generalists interested in the challenging disease process of aortic dissections.

This valuable text is published on the occasion of the highly esteemed "Aortic Surgery – How To Do It" international meeting, which has been running for 14 years and enjoys a superb international reputation. The meeting has a stellar faculty and has been endorsed by many scientific societies, as well as by the Marfan Foundation (a prominent U.S.-based patients association). It is attended annually by more than 1,000 delegates and is further described at www.aorticsurgery.it.

Books that were published for previous "How To Do It" meetings, such as Thoraco Abdominal Aorta: Surgical and Anesthetic Management (2012) and History of Aortic Surgery in the World (2014), were favorably reviewed and remain an important part of most libraries – especially ones that are used by vascular and cardiac surgeons and others interested in these difficult-to-treat entities. This volume is another in this outstanding series.

In the current exemplary volume, Drs. Melissano and Chiesa, have recruited as contributors all the world innovators and leaders who are advancing knowledge in the natural history and exciting new treatments of Types A and B aortic dissections. All the contributors are widely acknowledged to be world leaders and experts in the field. Their research and clinical excellence have led to the rapid advances in the treatment of these aortic dissection disease entities – advances which are slowly being adopted around the world. Clearly the achievements of these experts has been one of the most exciting developments in vascular disease treatment of the last 3 decades. All these achievements are beautifully summarized and illustrated in this outstanding book which is without equal and an indispensable addition to the library of anyone interested in the management of aortic dissections.

New York, December 2016

Frank J. Veith

Preface

Aortic Dissection is an exceptionally complex disease and remains one of the most misdiagnosed diseases across the globe. Although it is rare, doctors with an expertise in identifying and treating this disease are critical to our field. Diagnosis, even when correctly made, may bring ominous consequences for patients, especially when it is delayed. Treatment can also be extremely challenging, and correct timing is crucial.

Endovascular treatment of Aortic Dissection has been possible for more than 20 years, but can only be offered to select patients by skilled physicians. We must make do with inadequate tools since most endografts are not disease-specific, and an ideal graft to treat Aortic Dissection will not be available for many years. Open surgery can be very complex and challenging, and results are often unsatisfactory, especially for acute, complicated cases.

Most textbooks teach the clinical presentation of disease by simply listing symptoms, signs, and their relative frequency. However, a doctor becomes familiar with clinical presentation by actually observing cases in her clinical practice. Given the rarity of Aortic Dissection and its extremely variable presentations, it can be very difficult for an inexperienced doctor to make a correct diagnosis. It is, therefore, more important than ever for physicians to build their knowledge base of this area.

Aortic Dissection is a massive trauma for patients. In most cases, treated patients are not cured, they merely receive a palliation that takes care of the immediate risk of life and complications, but the more distal part of the aorta is still dissected, requiring the patient to submit to lifelong surveillance. This may cause a great deal of psychological distress, particularly when general practitioners are ill-equipped to handle their doubts, questions, and resulting psychological disorders. Surgeons often think their task is finished when a patient is dismissed from the hospital and a 6-month follow-up consultation is scheduled, but from the patient's perspective, the operation is not something that can be readily dismissed. Patients must live with the consequences of their illness every day. They want to know how their actions and their environment might affect the fate of their their bodies, and ultimately their lives.

Although the aorta is one organ and Aortic Dissection is one disease, Type A aortic dissection is usually treated by cardiac surgeons, and Type B aortic dissection, by vascular surgeons. This book discusses both types for the benefit of both specialists. Moreover, this book provides a unique glimpse into the lives of the patients who suffer with this disease. In addition to scientific chapters written by the most prominent experts in the field, we have included stories shared by Aortic Dissection survivors. All the stories are true, although they may have been slightly edited for length, language (they come from different parts of the world), and to make them anonymous. It is well known that facts are easily forgotten but stories and emotions stick in our minds, and our hope is that these stories will help readers remember and recognize Aortic Dissection when a similar case enters the ER. Maybe these stories will save a few lives.

We would like to gratefully acknowledge all the former patients who shared their aortic dissection stories and in particular our good friend Timo Söderlund who collected them and is hugely active in promoting awareness for this disease throughout the world. Many thanks also to all the very distinguished colleagues who took time from their extra-busy schedules to write their chapters and share their very valuable experience; special thanks to Martin Czerny who backed us up in this project from the very beginning. We would also like to thank Ms. Brittany Terwilliger for her assistance and expertise in the English language and Mrs. Adriana Lombardi who followed us patiently on behalf of the publisher Edi.Ermes.

Milan, December 2016

Germano Melissano *Roberto Chiesa*

THE MARFAN FOUNDATION

Know the signs. Fight for victory.

Professor Roberto Chiesa
Professor Germano Melissano
Ospedale San Raffaele, Milano
Universita Vita – Salute San Raffaele, Milano

Dear Professors Chiesa and Melissano,

I am writing in support of the 7th International Congress on the Aorta, which will highlight Aortic and Peripheral Surgery, scheduled for December 15-17, 2016. This meeting will bring global expertise to share new developments in clinical practice and research.

As the Chief Science Officer of The Marfan Foundation, a US based non-profit patient organization, it is extremely important to our patient population that cutting edge topics in aortic surgery and research are shared among physicians who care for patients that need these life-saving surgeries. I had the opportunity to attend a similar Congress in Milan in 2015 and the program was excellent. Inclusion of the leaders of patient organizations globally is needed so that we can bring our membership up-to-date and state-of-the-art information in life-saving aortic surgery.

I am happy to recommend this International Congress which has great potential and significance to the scientific and patient community.

Sincerely,

Josephine Grima

Josephine Grima, Ph.D.
Chief Science Officer

22 Manhasset Avenue, Port Washington, NY 11050
t 516 883 8712 f 516 883 8040 w Marfan.org

Center of Reference (CRMR) Marfan Syndrome and Related Disorders
Hôpital Bichat (secteur Cl Bernard) | AP-HP |
46 rue Henri Huchard, 75018 Paris
01.40.25.80.66

Paris, July 25th 2016,

To Prof. Chiesa and Prof. Melissano,

Subject : VASCern Support to the Aortic and Peripheral Surgery "HOW TO DO IT" Congress 2016

Dear Prof. Chiesa and Prof. Melissano,

European Reference Networks (ERNs) are part of an EU initiative to connect healthcare specialists across Europe to tackle complex or rare medical conditions that require highly specialised healthcare and a concentration of knowledge and resources. In line with this ambition, the VASCern network have applied to the ERN 2016 Call for proposal and submitted the VASCern Project Proposal for the ERN on Rare Multisystemic Vascular Diseases, together with 31 Healthcare Provider Member Applicants, including the SS Centro Malattie Rare – MarfanClinic represented by Dr. Alessandro Pini.

ERNs project proposals are currently under the European Commission's assessment, which will be followed by a technical assessment which should take place between September-November 2016. Afterwards, the first ERNs will obtain the label in January 2017.

I, Pr. Guillaume Jondeau, as the Network Coordinator of the ERN Project Proposal on Rare Multisystemic Vascular Diseases (VASCern), would like to support by this letter the world Congress on Aorta: Aortic and Peripheral Surgery "HOW TO DO IT" 2016, that you are organizing and which will take place in Milan between December 15-17th, 2016.

This 7th international Congress will tackle cutting-edge topics, explore new developments in clinical practice and relevant research, and access the latest information on aortic, peripheral, carotid and venous diseases. World-class speakers will discuss recent achievements in the vascular and endovascular field, industrial innovations and novel treatment approaches . An educational program will be proposed as well.

For these reasons, as VASCern Network Project Coordinator, I support the development of this Aorta Congress, and will communicate about it to our Network members as well as on our website.

Yours faithfully,

Pr. Guillaume Jondeau
VASCern project Network Coordinator
CRMR Marfan Syndrome and Related Disorders
FAVA-Multi, French Rare Multi-Systemic Vascular Diseases Network
AP-HP Hôpital Bichat-Claude Bernard, Paris

Contributors

Sthefano Atique Gabriel	Scientific Institute Ospedale San Raffaele, Milan, Italy
John G. Augoustides	University of Pennsylvania, Philadelphia, PA, USA
Ali Azizzadeh	McGovern Medical School at The University of Texas Health Science Center (UTHealth), Houston, TX, USA
Domenico Baccellieri	Scientific Institute Ospedale San Raffaele, Milan, Italy
Ramon Berguer	Trinidad Hospital Buenos Aires, Argentina, University of Michigan, Ann Arbor, MI, USA
Luca Bertoglio	Scientific Institute Ospedale San Raffaele, Milan, Italy
Guilherme Bicalho	SITE - Serviço Integrado de Técnicas Endovasculares, Rio de Janeiro, Brazil
James H. Black, III	The Johns Hopkins Hospital, Baltimore, MD, USA
Leo A. Bockeria	Bakulev Scientific Center for Cardiovascular Surgery, Ministry of Health of Russian Federation, Moscow, Russia
Adam J. Brownstein	Yale University School of Medicine, New Haven, CT, USA
Luciana Camacho-Lobato	ICVE - Instituto de Cirurgia Vascular e Endovascular, São Paulo, Brazil
Renata C. Castellano	Scientific Institute Ospedale San Raffaele, Milan, Italy
Nicholas J.W. Cheshire	Royal Brompton & Harefield Hospitals, London, United Kingdom
Laurent Chiche	Pitié-Salpêtrière Hôpital Universitaire, Paris, France
Roberto Chiesa	Vita-Salute San Raffaele University, Scientific Institute Ospedale San Raffaele, Milan, Italy
Guglielmo Cornero	Scientific Institute Ospedale San Raffaele, Milan, Italy
Joseph S. Coselli	Baylor College of Medicine, Houston, TX, USA
Thibault Couture	Pitié-Salpêtrière Hôpital Universitaire, Paris, France

Rodrigo Cunha	SITE - Serviço Integrado de Técnicas Endovasculares, Rio de Janeiro, Brazil
Martin Czerny	University Heart Center Freiburg-Bad Krozingen, Freiburg, Germany
Michael D. Dake	Stanford University School of Medicine, Stanford, CA, USA
Giuliano de A. Sandri	Mayo Clinic, Rochester, MN, USA
Hector W.L. de Beaufort	Policlinico San Donato IRCCS, University of Milan, Italy
Kim I. de la Cruz	Baylor College of Medicine, Houston, TX, USA
Monica De Luca	Scientific Institute Ospedale San Raffaele, Milan, Italy
Roberto Di Bartolomeo	S. Orsola-Malpighi Hospital, University of Bologna, Bologna, Italy
Luca Di Marco	S. Orsola-Malpighi Hospital, University of Bologna, Bologna, Italy
Bryan A. Ehlert	East Carolina University, Brody School of Medicine, Greenville, NC, USA
John A. Elefteriades	Yale University School of Medicine, New Haven, CT, USA
Benedetta Enrico	Stanford University School of Medicine, Stanford, CA, USA
Anthony L. Estrera	McGovern Medical School at The University of Texas Health Science Center (UTHealth), Houston, TX, USA
Christian D. Etz	Herzzentrum Leipzig-Universitätsklinik, Leipzig, Germany
Arturo Evangelista	Hospital Universitari Vall d´Hebron, Barcelona, Spain
Marissa Famularo	Cooper Medical School Rowan University, Camden, NJ, USA
Diego Ferreira	SITE - Serviço Integrado de Técnicas Endovasculares, Rio de Janeiro, Brazil
Marcelo Ferreira	SITE - Serviço Integrado de Técnicas Endovasculares, Rio de Janeiro, Brazil
Raffaella Gaetano	Rare Disease Center MarfanClinic®, ASST-Fatebenefratelli-Sacco, Milan, Italy
Julien Gaudric	Pitié-Salpêtrière Hôpital Universitaire, Paris, France

Alessandro Grandi	Scientific Institute Ospedale San Raffaele, Milan, Italy
Randall B. Griepp	Icahn School of Medicine, Mount Sinai Medical Center, New York, NY, USA
Josephina Haunschild	Herzzentrum Leipzig-Universitätsklinik, Leipzig, Germany
Hung-Lung Hsu	School of Medicine, National Yang-Ming University, Far Eastern Memorial Hospital, New Taipei City, Taiwan
Marine Hurard	VASCern Project, FAVA-Multi, AP-HP Hôpital Bichat-Claude Bernard, Paris, France
Michael J.H.M. Jacobs	Maastricht University Medical Center, Maastricht, The Netherlands
Teerawoot Jantarawan	Faculty of Medicine Siriraj Hospital, Mahidol University, Bangkok, Thailand
Guillaume Jondeau	Center of Reference Marfan Syndrome and Related Disorders, AP-HP Hôpital Bichat-Claude Bernard, Paris, France
Andrea L. Kahlberg	Vita-Salute San Raffaele University, Scientific Institute Ospedale San Raffaele, Milan, Italy
Arnoud V. Kamman	Policlinico San Donato IRCCS, University of Milan, Italy
Athanasios Katsargyris	Paracelsus Medical University, Nuremberg, Germany
Edouard Kieffer†	Hôpital Universitaire Pitié-Salpêtrière, Paris, France
Tilo Kölbel	University Hospital Hamburg-Eppendorf, Hamburg, Germany
Fabien Koskas	Hôpital Universitaire Pitié-Salpêtrière, Paris, France
George Kouvelos	Paracelsus Medical University, Nuremberg, Germany
Alessandro Leone	S. Orsola-Malpighi Hospital, University of Bologna, Bologna, Italy
Armando C. Lobato	ICVE - Instituto de Cirurgia Vascular e Endovascular, São Paulo, Brazil
Joseph V. Lombardi	Cooper Medical School Rowan University, Camden, NJ, USA
Silvio Magrin	Scientific Institute Ospedale San Raffaele, Milan, Italy

Daniele Mascia	Scientific Institute Ospedale San Raffaele, Milan, Italy
Tara M. Mastracci	The Royal Free London, NHS Foundation Trust, London, United Kingdom
Cristina Mattioli	Scientific Institute Ospedale San Raffaele, Milan, Italy
Barend Mees	Maastricht University Medical Center, Maastricht, The Netherlands
Germano Melissano	Vita-Salute San Raffaele University, Scientific Institute Ospedale San Raffaele, Milan, Italy
Vladimir A. Mironenko	Bakulev Scientific Center for Cardiovascular Surgery, Ministry of Health of Russian Federation, Moscow, Russia
Fabrizio Monaco	Scientific Institute Ospedale San Raffaele, Milan, Italy
Peter J. Mossop	St. Vincent's Hospital, Melbourne, Victoria, Australia
Hozan Mufty	Paracelsus Medical University, Nuremberg, Germany
Gustavo S. Oderich	Mayo Clinic, Rochester, MN, USA
Kyriakos Oikonomou	Paracelsus Medical University, Nuremberg, Germany
Davide Pacini	S. Orsola-Malpighi Hospital, University of Bologna, Bologna, Italy
Alessia Paglialonga	Italian National Research Council, Institute of Electronics, Computer and Telecommunication Engineering, Milan, Italy
Juan Carlos Parodi	Trinidad Hospital, Buenos Aires, Argentina University of Michigan, Ann Arbor, MI, USA
Benjamin O. Patterson	St George's Hospital, London, United Kingdom
Noud Peppelenbosch	Maastricht University Medical Center, Maastricht, The Netherlands
Marina Pieri	Scientific Institute Ospedale San Raffaele, Milan, Italy
Alessandro Pini	Rare Disease Center MarfanClinic®, ASST-Fatebenefratelli-Sacco, Milan, Italy
Wande B. Pratt	McGovern Medical School at The University of Texas Health Science Center (UTHealth), Houston, TX, USA
Ourania Preventza	Baylor College of Medicine, Houston, TX, USA

William J. Quinones-Baldrich UCLA Medical Center,
Los Angeles, CA, USA

Mauricio S. Ribeiro Mayo Clinic,
Rochester, MN, USA

Enrico Rinaldi Scientific Institute Ospedale San Raffaele,
Milan, Italy

Eduardo Rodrigues SITE - Serviço Integrado de Técnicas Endovasculares,
Rio de Janeiro, Brazil

Jose F. Rodríguez-Palomares Hospital Universitari Vall d´Hebron,
Barcelona, Spain

Fiona Rohlffs University Hospital Hamburg-Eppendorf,
Hamburg, Germany

Ulrich P. Rosendahl Royal Brompton & Harefield Hospitals,
London, United Kingdom

Sergey V. Rychin Bakulev Scientific Center for Cardiovascular Surgery,
Ministry of Health of Russian Federation, Moscow, Russia

Bartosz Rylski University Heart Center Freiburg-Bad Krozingen,
Freiburg, Germany

Hazim J. Safi McGovern Medical School at The University of Texas
Health Science Center (UTHealth), Houston, TX, USA

Taimur Saleem UCLA Medical Center,
Los Angeles, CA, USA

Salvatore Sardo University of Cagliari,
Cagliari, Italy

Geert Willem Schurink Maastricht University Medical Center,
Maastricht, The Netherlands

Chun-Che Shih Taipei Veterans General Hospital,
School of Medicine National Yang-Ming University,
Taipei, Taiwan

George Silvay Icahn School of Medicine, Mount Sinai Medical Center,
New York, NY, USA

Worawong Slisatkorn Faculty of Medicine Siriraj Hospital,
Mahidol University, Bangkok, Thailand

Timo Söderlund Sandared, Sweden

Alfred S. Song Baylor College of Medicine,
Houston, TX, USA

Sara Spelta Scientific Institute Ospedale San Raffaele,
Milan, Italy

Benjamin W. Starnes University of Washington,
Seattle, WA, USA

Akiko Tanaka McGovern Medical School at The University of Texas Health Science Center (UTHealth), Houston, TX, USA

Matt Thompson St. George's Hospital, London, United Kingdom

Gabriella Tognola Italian National Research Council, Institute of Electronics, Computer and Telecommunication Engineering, Milan, Italy

Philippe Tresson Pitié-Salpêtrière Hôpital Universitaire, Paris, France

Santi Trimarchi Policlinico San Donato IRCCS, University of Milan, Italy

Eric L.G. Verhoeven Paracelsus Medical University, Nuremberg, Germany

Wanchai Wongkornrat Faculty of Medicine Siriraj Hospital, Mahidol University, Bangkok, Thailand

Alberto Zangrillo Vita-Salute San Raffaele University, Scientific Institute Ospedale San Raffaele, Milan, Italy

Bulat A. Ziganshin Yale University School of Medicine, New Haven, CT, USA

Contents

1

Thoughts of an aortic dissection "survivor"

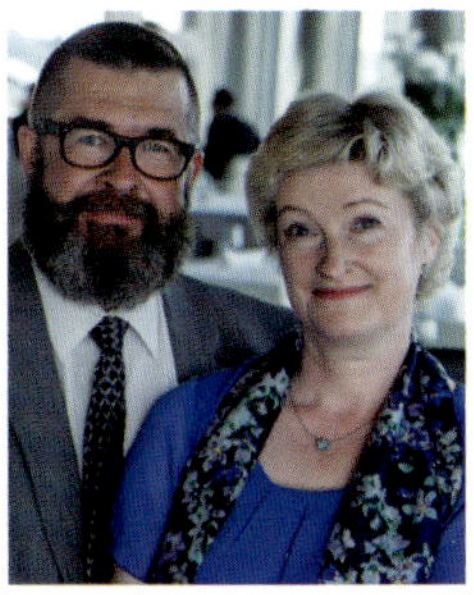

Timo Söderlund

Professor Germano Melissano asked me to write the opening chapter for this superb book. The dear Professor asked me to write down my thoughts on this rare aortic disease or condition from a patient's perspective. I am much honored to have been asked to do so, and have included also some personal background to explain why my family decided to get engaged in awareness about aortic dissection (AD) the way we did.

My aorta broke at 08:15 in the morning of October 1. The year was 2012, and I was 48 years old. Something ripped in my chest, and my immediate reaction was confusion, fear, and terror. As if a bomb had exploded right next to me. I did not understand what was happening, and my anxiety was at a level I had never felt before in my life. I wanted to run away and hide, escape. I thought I was going to die. But before we continue with the medical part of this story, let us go back in time, because the story started 48 years earlier.

1.1 The early years

I was born on May 27 in the year 1964 – my mother and father were immigrants to Sweden from Finland after World War II. Both came from poor families and had left their country to start a new life where work was to be found. Their marriage did not work out, and they divorced in 1967, so I grew up with my mother and sister, a rather poor little family, but we managed quite OK.

I was often beaten up in school, being called an immigrant. I was a quiet, shy child, and not hitting back resulted in a lot of beatings! I remember thinking "I hope I can become smart and change my life when I grow up". I also remember wanting to grow up fast and being disappointed that my brain did not work better, and I felt very limited by this. At the age of 11-12, I somehow decided to start reading lots of books. Up till then, my grades in school had not been good at all and my reading was limited to comics and adventure magazines for children. From the day I decided to start reading books, I did so with great enthusiasm. At the age of 15-16, I was reading quite fast and an endless stream of books passed before my eyes; the stories I read were about adventure, fantasy, science fiction, war and detective stories. I found an exciting life in the books I read. Somehow, the more I read, the faster I could read, and I started to get a bit smarter. My grades in school improved to slightly above average. From age 17 to 19, I was devoting all

---

Timo Söderlund (timo.soderlund@gmail.com)
Sandared, Sweden

G. Melissano - R. Chiesa (eds), Aortic Dissection patients true stories and the innovations that saved their lives

my spare time to school work and books. While my friends were chasing girls, I was "chasing" new books with fascinating stories and doing my homework. At 19, I completed the 12th grade in school as one of the top students of our school; my brain had started to work in a new way. A few weeks after graduation, I packed a few belongings in a bag and left home, never to return.

1.2 Ernest Hemmingway, Jack Kerouac, Charles Bukowski and University

The stream of books I read also included books by authors like Ernest Hemmingway, Jack Kerouac and Charles Bukowski. I got to know about these authors at the same time as I moved to Gothenburg in Sweden, where I began my university studies at Chalmers University of Technology in the field of Chemistry. The welcome to University life included many social parties. A few years passed and my results at university got progressively worse as my social adventures as a young student became more and more time consuming. Finally, I got to the point where I decided I had to leave campus, give up studying, since all the partying was beginning to ruin my study results. One day, I picked up a phone book and started calling companies in the west of Sweden in the field of organic chemistry, asking for a job. A few days later, I became employed in a plastic pipe factory.

1.3 Learning to handle projects

The process of maturing into a young man from the young boy who arrived on campus had come at the price of failed studies. This bothered me and, as I was now employed, I decided to try to refocus and to regain the determination I'd had when I first started to read books. This time I would try to use the same focus on my work, and the tasks I was assigned at work. I started my journey in the company on the factory floor, working on the production line and waiting for a place to open up in the engineering office. That opportunity came after a few months, and I joined the technical service department responsible for making technical drawings, keeping track of documentation of machinery, and introducing new technology in production machinery. I was the "young new guy" in a department of seven older engineers. My days were filled with an endless flow of short, simple projects that no one else wanted to do. For most people they would have seemed dull and boring. For me, it was a great way to learn new things and I tried to become more proficient at how to structure and organize these projects and do them as fast as possible.

After about a year, I got my own first big project. It was to introduce a brand new production-line in the production, involving state of the art technology and introducing computers for the first time to run the full production line of plastic pipes. This project taught me a lot. And the result was that people visited the company to see the new technological "miracle". During one of those visits, someone approached me and said "There is a company who is looking for a young man like you, and I think you should apply". I applied, got the job and changed companies at the age of 26, entering another field where my limited knowledge of organic chemistry again came to use. I joined the paint industry, which became my home base in business for well over 20 years.

1.4 Theory of becoming an expert in 10,000 hours

They say it takes 10,000 hours of focus and practice to become an expert on something. I would say it in a different way: it takes 3 years of hard work and focus to get to know a new job

– after 3 years you begin to know your stuff, and after 5 years you can become really good at it. So this is what I did. It took 3 years to get to know the paint industry from bottom up. I worked as a young engineer responsible for modernizing a paint factory by introducing new machinery controlled by computers to increase production output. Having done this, I was offered a post in the research and development department as manager of the laboratories and product development. As R&D manager, I was also invited to join the management team to run the company at the age of 28. This was the period when companies in Europe were focusing on quality management like ISO 9001. The quality management project in our company was given to me. Soon after we got our ISO 9001 certificate (1994) we decided to go for the environmental management systems EMAS and ISO 14001. In 1996, we got approval for both systems as one of the first paint producing companies in the world for these new standards. National television, newspaper and magazine reporters came in an endless flow to report on the paint company in Sweden that had gained these new approvals. The company (and I personally) got several environmental awards, and I was asked to speak at international conferences and on national television about environmental management, in practice, in the chemical industry.

At the age of 33, I knew a paint company from bottom up, and I was offered my first CEO position. This was a company about to embark on a large change of management, involving a merger of two fairly equal-sized companies into one company. We did that – and it was hard – but after this I knew a paint company not only from bottom up, but also from top down and side to side. And the skills I gained were acquired though an endless flow of projects. I was now 37 years old, and the year was 2001. There were still 11 years to go before the intima broke in my aorta, on the morning of October 1 in 2012.

1.5 Family, work, free time

At age 24, I had met Marianne, the love of my life. I was married and a father at the age of 25. Our first born was Oscar, followed by Erik and, finally, Elisabeth. Marianne was working in the local hospital, and had both feet firmly planted on the ground. She was never over concerned about advancing in her career, and had her focus on the family and children, while she let me venture in my line of work. Social interaction with friends like playing golf, going to the pub had no room in our life. To be honest, the sad part in all this was that I chose to devote almost all my time to business and work, and for long periods the family felt as though I was not there. Also when I was there, my mind was working on problems to solve in business. Knowing what I know today, I realize I should have devoted more time at home to the family and less to solving work problems. I now know today that that would also have made me much better at work.

1.6 Taking on harder assignments and increasing speed

At the age of 37, I got an offer to join a very big international group of companies. They had bought a small company in a new country for them (Sweden), and the company had gone downhill from the day they had bought it. Now it was facing bankruptcy and it either had to be closed down or changed rapidly so it could survive on its own. I said "Yes, please!" and thought that this was what I had been training for since the age of 26. I knew the business, I knew the market, I knew the products, I knew the production and distribution, and I knew many of the customers. It was a very hard turnaround, and we changed the company in a very tough way. We changed almost everything in a long string of small projects, many run side by side. It was a great success. The company was saved. From that day on, this line of work took me travelling all over the globe. I got a new assignment in the United Arab Emirates and basically did very much the same thing there. Later, these skills were used in other countries and companies around the world. I saw each assignment as a project that needed to be broken down into smaller projects to be executed in a specific order. At age 43, people (company owners and company CEOs) started to ask me for advice and I was invited to join a number of boards of directors as a senior advisor. I had done my 10,000 hours several times over, and I knew how to act in very demanding and critical situations in a company's history. My brain was fast, sharp, and was the tool I used. English, German, Swedish, Finnish and French were the languages I used.

1.7 Time stops – time to die

In September 2012, I was 48 years old, and had just said "yes" to a new assignment. The day I would start in my new role as one of the top managers of an international company was set for October 1, and I was preparing mentally for a positive but demanding challenge. At about 05:00am on October 1, I woke up and began going over the events of the day in my head, over and over again. I shaved, got dressed in suit and tie, and later headed off to the office, to begin in my new role. At 08:15am, sitting in an office talking to a senior executive of the company, time stopped as something exploded in my chest. The intima of my ascending aorta gave in and a dissection ripped its way through my bicuspid aortic valve. The dissection also chose to push its way in the media in the opposite direction of the aorta. It found its way up the left carotid artery causing extreme pain in the throat. It dissected the left subclavian artery, the whole length of the aorta, the left carotid artery (causing the kidneys to ache very badly on both sides of the back). Both iliac arteries were dissected, and on the right side the dissection travelled along the right femoral artery down to the foot.

Every breath I took when inhaling caused an extremely sharp ripping pain in my chest, so I tried to inhale as lightly and gently as possible. The left side of my throat hurt, my kidneys felt like they were going to explode and my chest felt like someone had bashed me with a baseball bat over and over again will full force and that there was a knife stuck in the heart that caused a ripping pain every time I inhaled. The pain was like having my head inside a church bell that was continuously ringing at 150 decibels. There was nowhere to run, nowhere to hide and I stumbled into another office saying "Call an ambulance – I'm going to die". Anxiety was all over me, and I really thought I was going to die.

The ambulance arrived and took me to the local hospital's Emergency Room where I was given morphine. The medical team on duty started to look for a heart attack; I tried to explain my pains, but the person listening had never met an acute aortic dissection patient before. So the main idea was that I must have had a heart attack. I was given more morphine for my pain, but no diagnosis could be found. I got gradually worse from pains, sedation and the condition of my heart and arteries. For six hours I was in a bad condition, no one having a clue what was wrong with me. I was given morphine and painkillers, and asked about the pain several times. The more morphine I got, the more it took the edge off the pain. My telling the doctors that the pain was less hard to endure, however, probably confused them a lot. I started to freeze, and was put under blankets. I got extremely thirsty but every drink of water felt like it was being poured into a desert, and each sip made me vomit ferociously. I felt like I could drink 100 liters of water and still remain thirsty. My wife was agitated shouting; "Help, please, help!", as we were left alone in a room in the ER.

At this point, fate decided that a new team of doctors came on shift in the emergency department of the hospital. One of the doctors immediately saw the signs no one else had seen and had an acute CT done. From that point on, not one second was spared to get my body to the nearest university hospital with a thoracic surgery team. Seven hours after my intima tore, I was again inside an ambulance taking me from the first hospital to the nearest university hospital equipped with a thoracic surgery department for immediate surgery. At this point my aortic valve was almost not functioning at all anymore; the aortic dissection had ripped it apart. In the ambulance, a paramedic gave me morphine against the pain and nitro to keep the heart beating. I asked him if I would die, and he answered truthfully "I don't know"; I asked him to call my wife, I spoke to her and said my goodbyes. I prepared to die. On arrival at the hospital, they wheeled me directly into surgery where a team was prepared and waiting for me. As they sedated me, I looked at the doors of the surgery theater, thinking, very sad and empty, "This is it. Now it's all over".

Around 16:40 in the afternoon, I closed my eyes from the sedation in the surgery department of Sahlgrenska University Hospital in Gothenburg, and the "magic" of a team of surgeons, nurses and anesthesiologist began that saved my life. Everything ended. There was no "old me" anymore. That person died on the table in the hands of the surgeons.

1.7.1 Control-Alt-Delete

I was floating in a black void. I could not see. I could not hear. But all of a sudden I was in this void. After an eternity I could hear something, but I did not understand what it was. Later there were colors but I did not understand those impressions either. My brain had had a reset, and things started all over for me. I had forgotten most names of friends, and I had to learn again, as if for the first time, to pee, poop, stand, talk and walk. During the 5 days I was kept in the ICU of the University Hospital I had several CTs. My heart valve was not perfect and I was told that the surgeons were considering redoing the aortic valve. The decision was made to leave the valve as it was, monitor it by regular check-ups and redo it, if necessary, at a later stage. My surgeon visited me every morning in the University Hospital to check on my progress. He told me about the aorta and aortic dissection – and I did not understand any more than that my main artery had broken and I had almost died. Death was very present for the coming weeks. And I was sent back to my home-town hospital. During surgery, which had gone very well as regards the aortic repair, I suffered some minor brain damage, probably from oxygen shortage or micro bleedings, that led to cognitive problems. For me, these problems unfortunately took away much of the brain capacity I had had before I got ill.

1.7.2 Recovery in the heart ward of a local hospital

I spent another 2 weeks in our local hospital getting ready to be sent home. Here I had training every day in order to learn to stand, walk, walk on stairs, etc. Lots of doctors passed my bed and one of them was most excited telling me that I had a very rare condition and had survived where most people die. He drew a picture of the aorta on a napkin and gave it to me. Some nurses came to my room just to look at me and said they had never met anyone with AD before. The only printed material given to me and my family was a general leaflet for open-heart surgery patients. There was no mention of aortic dissection in this leaflet. A few times during my stay, things happened that made me realize I had something that not all doctors knew so well. For instance, one morning a doctor said "OK, now you are better – so I will take away this medicine". From what I had been told before, this medicine was very important - I kept quiet but later the same day asked for the senior doctor in charge of the team to come to my bed. I asked about the change in medication, and was told "Oh no, we cannot take this away – I will put it back on your medicine list again". I still take the medicine today, almost 4 years later. From that moment, I decided to try and learn as much as possible about what had happened to me.

1.8 Cognitive brain damage – the way back – to what?

With no documentation from the hospital, diagnosed with "aortic dissection", I went home with access to Google and YouTube. The day I decided to have a look on internet to see what disease I had, I almost fainted. The first YouTube video I found was an instruction video made by a famous surgeon showing an open-heart procedure – it almost made me faint. My encounters with insurance companies and authorities taught me in a very abrupt way that I had something that was not listed in their indexes of diseases. To claim one of the insurances our family had paid for over 25 years, we had to fill in seven pages with small text and send it off to the insurance company. It was a task that took well over a month (something I could have handled in one hour before I got ill). For me this was so tough; I had enough difficulty just trying to handle my anxiety and cognitive problems. In contacts with the Swedish authorities who handle the social insurance system as part of Sweden's welfare, I was told they would have to undertake a special investigation into my disease since it was not in their official registers. I discovered that I had one of the 6,000 rare diseases listed in Orphanet, but not on the Swedish official list of 300 listed rare diseases.

1.9 It was not time to die - You probably survived for a purpose

Around the same time, my wife Marianne and I were asked to come for a visit to the university hospital that had saved my life (Sahlgrenska University Hospital in Gothenburg). The surgeon who was in charge of the team that had saved me met us. He explained what an aortic dissection is, and we discussed mortality and my future life prospects. He said two things which have stuck in my mind. First "Don't think too much about how long you will survive. Try to live here and now. Anyone can get cancer and die within three years from now, including me". Then he said "You probably wonder why you survived. No one knows why you survived, but it clearly wasn't your time to go yet. You are probably here for a reason".

1.9.1 Converting the new life to a project

So here I was, 48 years old, with a non-functioning brain, in a bad state physically and mentally. As a way to cope with this non-chosen new situation in life I gradually used what I had left of my brain's abilities in a way I was used to. I started to try and visualize some goals and then to break down the new reality into projects. This was what I had done for over 25 years before I got ill. Finally, it boiled down to a final goal: to survive as long as possible for my family, and to make this disease known as much as possible in order to help other future "victims" of the illness so they wouldn't have to go through the same things I had found so hard to cope with, e.g. by making contacts with authorities and others easier in the future. There was no patient organization for "Aortic Dissection" existing to be found anywhere in the world. I knew that making one's voice heard to authorities and big corporations and companies (also hospitals) would be impossible as a private person (unless one was very famous or wealthy) – so it had to be through a respected organization or association. So, together with 16 other survivors, we founded Aortadissektion Föreningen Skandinavien (Scandinavian Association for Aortic Dissection) on September 19 in 2014. To get the organization more established we immediately joined Rare Diseases Sweden and Eurordis in Europe. In the first 2 years, the organization grew from 17 to 109 members and it is today known by most of the University Hospitals in Scandinavia treating acute aortic dissection patients.

1.9.2 Trying to use the time given in the best way – the global approach

The first three years after the illness had struck were spent learning as much as possible about thoracic aortic dissections. Statistics, mortality rates, research projects, internet resources, organizations, foundations and hospital sites; trying to cover most aspects of this rare disease.

Back to the 10,000 hours approach again. But this time with a brain limited by cognitive problems, post-traumatic stress issues and a chemical "slowdown" due to beta-blockers and blood pressure medications. The whole process was also slowed down by my inability now to read long texts and my poor short-term memory.

The result of all the searching and reading was that I found two good approaches in the USA to helping people with our disease, through the family of the late US actor John Ritter who died of an acute aortic dissection. Amy Yasbeck, John Ritter's widow, and the Ritter family founded the "John Ritter Foundation for Aortic Health". Together with Dr Mileswicz at UT Health in Houston, Texas, they set up a research program for rare thoracic aortic diseases. One of the main objectives is to find genetic influence for thoracic aortic aneurysm and dissection (TAAD), so making it possible to identify the disease before it kills a person in an acute phase. To save lots of lives in the future, this is the way to go. And this research is worth supporting and talking about. It is groundbreaking, and can help save lives all over the planet. The second approach was a coalition set up in USA by the Ritter Foundation and other organizations to share information about aortic diseases, called the TAD Coalition. It consists of a group of US-based organizations and individuals who share a common mission of preventing premature deaths due to TAAD, by providing information to both the medical field and the general public. Unfortunately, the main initiatives are in USA, whereas I live in Sweden, Europe. So my approach had to be based on trying to share these good initiatives from USA with the rest of the world.

At the same time I was getting help for my limited brain functions from the Sahlgrenska University Hospital in Sweden through a research team working on memory problems and cognitive problems caused by dementia or brain damage. Having done a lot of tests, the theory was that my problems had been caused by either micro bleedings or oxygen shortage while I was in deep hypothermia during open-heart surgery. There were two main avenues proposed to help me get my brain back to a more functional state; the first was to start playing music, on an instrument of my choice. The second was to try to use the language skills I had had before I got ill. I tried music, and bought a nice new acoustic guitar, but that failed. I lost interest after about 20 seconds, since my fingers were numb (perhaps as a result of my medications) and I couldn't move them as fast or precisely as I needed to produce good music. So I turned to languages. And this, in combination with the idea to try to share awareness and join the forces of AD survivors globally, gave birth to the idea of a global Aortic Dissection Awareness Day.

1.10 The global Aortic Dissection Awareness Day – September 19 – the theory

The idea was to use a global day as a drawcard to try to find and unite people with our thoracic aortic diseases. Doing so, I decided to also include people with aortic diseases not in the thoracic aorta – to make all feel welcome and avoid excluding good people with resources from our project.

If I could help people to find each other not only in USA, but in countries all over the globe, perhaps we could get strong local initiatives going in multiple countries around the world. Initiatives that later could replicate the two good USA initiatives. If the number of hubs of research/awareness/patient groups increased globally, this would then boost the speed of research as these hubs could exchange information and results – and their collective intelligence and joint voice would perhaps be heard louder and clearer in the academic world, then in the university hospitals, and finally reach also the survivors and families.

The power of collective intelligence is also a factor that can boost development in an amazing way. If survivors revert from just feeling sorry for themselves and instead get organized in a collective manner, start using their ability to absorb information and filter it, to find the essential information from a survivor's perspective – at a global level – and then deliver this back to the researchers and hospitals doing the main research – this could help speed up research even more.

No more people waking up in a world where a doctor has to draw an aorta on a napkin to explain the disease, and then having to Google information about it at home. In this vision, there would be good written information given to the survivor and a way to find others through internet. Internet would shorten the process to get new resources active in the national hubs.

1.10.1 Aortic Dissection Awareness Day – September 19 – the practical breakdown of a big project

To make the vision real, things have to be done in the proper order – as always. First step (#1) is to locate all survivors around the globe. Second step (#2) is to bring them together so they can bond locally or nationally instead of just being in big global clusters where USA is dominant. Third step (#3) is to help them get organized nationally to build their local hub as a part of the global network of national hubs. Also to help the national hub build a relationship with national researchers investigating our diseases and to get known by University Hospitals, who can provide their hub with new members as more people are rescued from acute aortic dissections. Fourth step (#4) will be to help the national hubs get organized in their relations with the others. When this is done, my initial project will be completed.

To do all this, resources are needed but most of them are available for free. The communication platform to make this happen will be social media. Various channels will be used for various tasks. Facebook will be the main tool for letting people bond, globally, then nationally. LinkedIn is a great tool for building relations with researchers. Here, thoracic vascular surgeons can be easily identified, as well as the countries in which they are active. Twitter is a great tool for interacting with national media to help get the growing national hub better known. Wordpress is another great tool one can use to publish information on the internet. To help people get organized we can ask for the help of people in the rare disease organizations, who are working for all of us who have rare diseases. In Europe, for instance, we have Eurordis, which comprises over 700 patient organizations spread throughout more than 60 countries.

We also need to understand several things when we speak of a global approach that our friends in USA do not consider so much. The English language is a small language, globally speaking. Only 1 out of 20 people living on planet earth understand English. About 400,000,000 have English as their native language. To get my vision up and running, I want to address all seven billion people on the planet. That means another 6,600,000,000 people who do not have English as their native language. A global approach is a nice thought, but totally meaningless if we do not have local action and engagement. The work has to be done by real people, living in countries in Asia, Oceania, Middle East, Europe, Africa, South America and North America. So, the first thing is to find a toolbox that can be used on internet and in real life. We made an early estimation that perhaps only 1 out of 100 people with our disease are active on Facebook, for reasons related to age and the fact that Facebook reaches only a small portion of the people of the world.

The solution we found was to design a poster saying AORTIC DISSECTION and SEPTEMBER 19, possibly in all the languages of the globe. So far we have 24 languages corresponding to 40 countries. These languages/countries represent about 65% of the world's population since they include India, China, South America, Indonesia and other populated regions of our planet. Places where English is not used, and Facebook is sometimes not known at all. Then we produced a simple flyer that doctors can give patients in the hospital when they have come successfully through the operation. We have printed this flyer in seven languages so far: Spanish, Portuguese, Italian, German, Dutch, Swedish and English. To date, we have printed 2,000 posters and 20,000 flyers that we have sent by postal mail to over 750 addresses globally. Many of them are University Hospitals with thoracic aortic surgery departments around the globe.

1.11 Can aortic dissection awareness save lives in regions of the globe where there are no thoracic surgeons?

Life is not fair. Out of the 7 billion people on the globe, only a small share have access to thoracic surgery when they become ill from acute aortic dissections and need lifesaving surgery. In many parts of the world this kind of very advanced medical care is not present at all or is available for only a limited minority of the population who can afford it. To change this situation is beyond the capabilities of the Awareness Day project. But through the approach we have chosen - to share information about what causes the disease - I think also people in these regions of the world can be saved. But they have to be saved before they get ill, by understanding that the illness can be a familial illness, and that control of blood pressure is the first step to avoid falling ill acutely. And with this approach – by sharing information, measuring blood pressure and trying to control it either through medication or just by changing lifestyle and choice of food - perhaps many people can be saved also in regions of the world where there are no thoracic or vascular surgery departments available.

Most probably, people will have access to the social media much sooner than they will get university hospitals that can provide free of charge surgery for a whole population. Therefore, our approach is to target the entire planet, in as many local languages as possible, to find friends who believe as we do that sharing awareness save lives.

1.12 Final words

It all started through trying to make a real life change by making printed material available for the local hospitals in my region of Sweden. Then it grew to a patient organization in Scandinavia, and finally to a global movement to try and make a change and save the lives of people who today have no clue that they carry a hidden bomb inside their bodies, in the form of encoded mutations in their genes, that one day will make their main artery break down and probably will kill most of them.

So far the project has gone splendidly. We see growing local communities of survivors starting to meet in real life in many countries around the globe. We get a positive response from hospitals and surgeons, who think we are doing something good with our limited resources and understand why we do it – they say it makes a difference.

One saved life, anywhere on the planet, will justify this project. That life could be yours or mine. And I know that I was saved by a doctor who came on duty that particular Monday afternoon of October 1 2012 in Borås Sweden, who happened to know about my disease. He immediately could read the signs that a whole emergency team of junior and senior doctors had been unable to read for 6 hours prior. They had all read about it in medical school but had never encountered it in real life in their professional life.

Therefore, I firmly believe that also real life encounters are important to attain the goals we have set. We need to meet, hug and look each other in the eyes. To encounter people who can tell you how it really was.

This book is a fantastic step in this direction. The authors, who are world leaders in their fields of expertise, have chosen to take the views of the patients who survived and relay their experience to other doctors. This will give a new dimension to the disease. Readers of this book will find here not only "dry" text about intima, media, false lumens, and medical terms but, rather, the person in the emergency room on whom they are about to perform surgery and whose life they will be saving. Real people who have one of the most difficult diagnoses in the world, since it is so deadly and time is critical. Perhaps this book and the stories in it will bring to their mind "aortic dissection" when other options seem to be wrong. If so, this book could save lots of lives in the future thanks to its readers' awareness. I am sure it will.

"Thank you" to all the authors who contributed to this book. And "thank you" to all the readers of this book. It was a hero like you who saved my life. Thank you.

2

An introduction to Type B aortic dissection

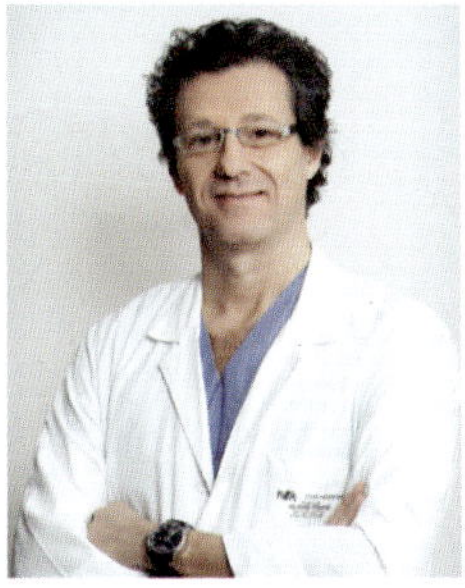

Germano Melissano

2.1 Introduction

Aortic dissection (AD) is a very complex disease. Its pathophysiology is not yet fully understood and the clinical presentation can be extremely variable and deceiving so that a straightforward diagnosis is not always the rule. Surgical therapy, both open and endovascular, is also challenging; the greatest challenge, however, may be life after AD and dissection survivors are to be commended for their ongoing efforts in coping with everyday life.

The complexity of the disease has its roots in the complexity of the structure of the aortic wall itself. The aortic wall structural characteristics are mostly related to the lamellar structure of the tunica media. In normal aortas, the lamellae consist of an orderly pattern of layers of elastic fibers alternated with layers of smooth muscle cells. The number of lamellae is highest (≈40) in the ascending aorta and decreases in the thoracic (≈30) and abdominal aorta (≈20); it should be noted that vasa vasorum within the tunica media are observed only when a larger number of lamellae are present; otherwise the aortic wall tissue is nourished directly from the lumen of the aorta [1].

Elastic fibers, unfortunately, are not produced after the first years of life and with age there is an ongoing tendency toward elastic fiber degeneration and loss, making the aorta a much stiffer structure (basically, the same loss of elasticity that we observe in the skin of aging persons occurs also in the aorta, but with more functional and less esthetic effects). Moreover, atherosclerotic changes with severe disarrangement of the medial lamellar structure and histological alterations such as cystic medionecrosis greatly alter the structural properties of the aortic tunica media [2].

It is important to realize that dissection affects the aorta within the layers of the tunica media (inner 1/3 – outer 2/3). Therefore, when terms such as "intimal tear" or "intimal lamella" are used, they do not actually refer to the histological tunica intima which is a mono-cellular layer (and, in spite of its great biological importance, has little or no structural significance); they refer, rather, to the tunica intima plus an important portion of the tunica media. Therefore, the outer wall of a dissected aorta is left with only the adventitia and part of the media and is clearly quite fragile [3]. This is responsible for frank ruptures of dissected aortas but also for ongoing aneurysmatic degeneration. It also explains the great technical difficulty with

---

G. Melissano (melissano.germano@hsr.it)
Vita-Salute San Raffaele University,
Scientific Institute Ospedale San Raffaele, Milan, Italy

G. Melissano - R. Chiesa (eds), Aortic Dissection patients true stories and the innovations that saved their lives

surgical suturing of acutely dissected aortas, and the higher risks of performing endovascular repair in the first hours or days of the acute phase.

2.2 Epidemiology

Type A AD is an uncommon disorder with an estimated annual incidence of between 2.9 and 4.5 per 100,000 [4, 5]; the incidence of the disease seems to have increased over time [6]. Type B AD accounts for 25 to 40% of all aortic dissections and the ratio of Type A to Type B was approximately 5:1 in different studies [7]. In the light of recent advances in diagnostics and medical management, and given the often more benign course of acute Type B AD with transition into a chronic form of disease [8], it is likely that the calculated annual incidence of 0.5-0.6/100,000 of Type B AD might be underestimated.

Approximately 75% of Type A AD occurs in people aged 40-70 years, with a peak in the 50-65 years range. In patients with Marfan syndrome or a bicuspid valve, the onset is earlier, usually in the third or fourth decades of life [9]. The male to female ratio in Type B AD patients varies among studies, ranging from 2 to 5:1 [10]. The highest incidence rates were found in men aged 65-74 years (14.6/100,000 person-years) and women aged 75-84 years (19.0/100,000 person-years) [11].

Limited information is available regarding the geographical, racial, and ethnic distribution of AD. However, different studies have stated that Type A AD is more common in the black than in the white population, and less common in Asians than in Caucasians [12]. Moreover, in the black population Type B AD is more common than Type A (52.4% vs. 47.6%, respectively) [13].

Different risk factors have been associated with AD:

- hypertension is the predominant cardiovascular risk factor in patients with aortic dissection, with 70–85% of individuals being affected. Whether hypertension is more common with Type B than Type A AD is unclear;
- tobacco use prevalence in patients with Type A AD is highly inconsistent, ranging from 38 to 70%. In addition, whether smoking is more common among patients with Type B than with Type A AD is still an open issue;
- several congenital cardiovascular disorders may be associated with Type A AD, most notably bicuspid valve and aortic coarctation. Bicuspid valve is found in 3% of patients with Type B AD. Similarly, 1% of individuals affected by aortic coarctation develop Type A AD;
- inflammatory diseases (giant cell arteritis, Takayasu's arteritis, rheumatoid arthritis, systemic lupus erythematosus, and Behçet disease) are considered a risk factor for Type A AD. Approximately 4% of individuals with Type A AD have aortitis, and Type A AD occurs in 1–5% of aortitis-affected individuals;
- syndromic conditions associated to Type A AD are Marfan syndrome, Loeys–Dietz syndrome, Ehlers-Danlos syndrome and Turner syndrome. Overall, about 5% of patients with Type A AD have Marfan syndrome and the syndrome is more common among those with Type A than with Type B AD. Conversely, up to 70% of patients with Marfan syndrome develop aortic dissection, which is Type A in 64–86% of cases and Type B in 14–36%;
- non-syndromic familial conditions have been associated to Type A AD. Approximately 16% of non-syndromic familial cases are Type A, while 11% are Type B AD; the remaining 73% have thoracic aneurysms without dissection;
- dilatation of the aorta is a well-established risk factor for thoracic dissection. For the descending thoracic aorta, the critical hinge point diameter at which there is an increased risk of either rupture or dissection is 7 cm [14];
- iatrogenic injuries can also cause AD, more commonly Type A. The most common procedures resulting in iatrogenic dissections are cardiac catheterization and cardiac surgery;
- use of drugs, particularly cocaine, appears to be temporally related to the development of Type A AD; the mean interval between cocaine use and onset of Type A AD is about 12 h.

2.3 Diagnosis

The cornerstone of AD treatment is a precise understanding of the specific anatomo-pathologic characteristics of each individual case. The best diagnostic tool to use depends on the type of dissection and the stage of the disease. Acute Type A dissection is usually diagnosed by ultrasound, preferably with transesophageal echocardiography (TEE, Fig. 2.1), and since the disease is highly lethal in the first hours, many patients undergo emergency surgery on the basis of TEE alone[15].

The management of Type B AD, on the other hand, requires a far more thorough assessment, which is usually obtained by means of computed tomography (CT) angiography (angio-CT) [16]. Magnetic resonance (MR) angiography is also an excellent diagnostic and research tool [17]; however, mainly due to logistic difficulties, it has limited clinical application in the acute setting.

When looking at the CT scan of a patient with Type B AD, there are several features that we need to consider:

- location and size of the primary proximal entry tear (Fig. 2.2): this is crucial to determine the type of dissection. The proximity to the supra-aortic trunks dictates the feasibility of thoracic endovascular aortic repair (TEVAR) with or without surgical de-branching or other means of revascularization;

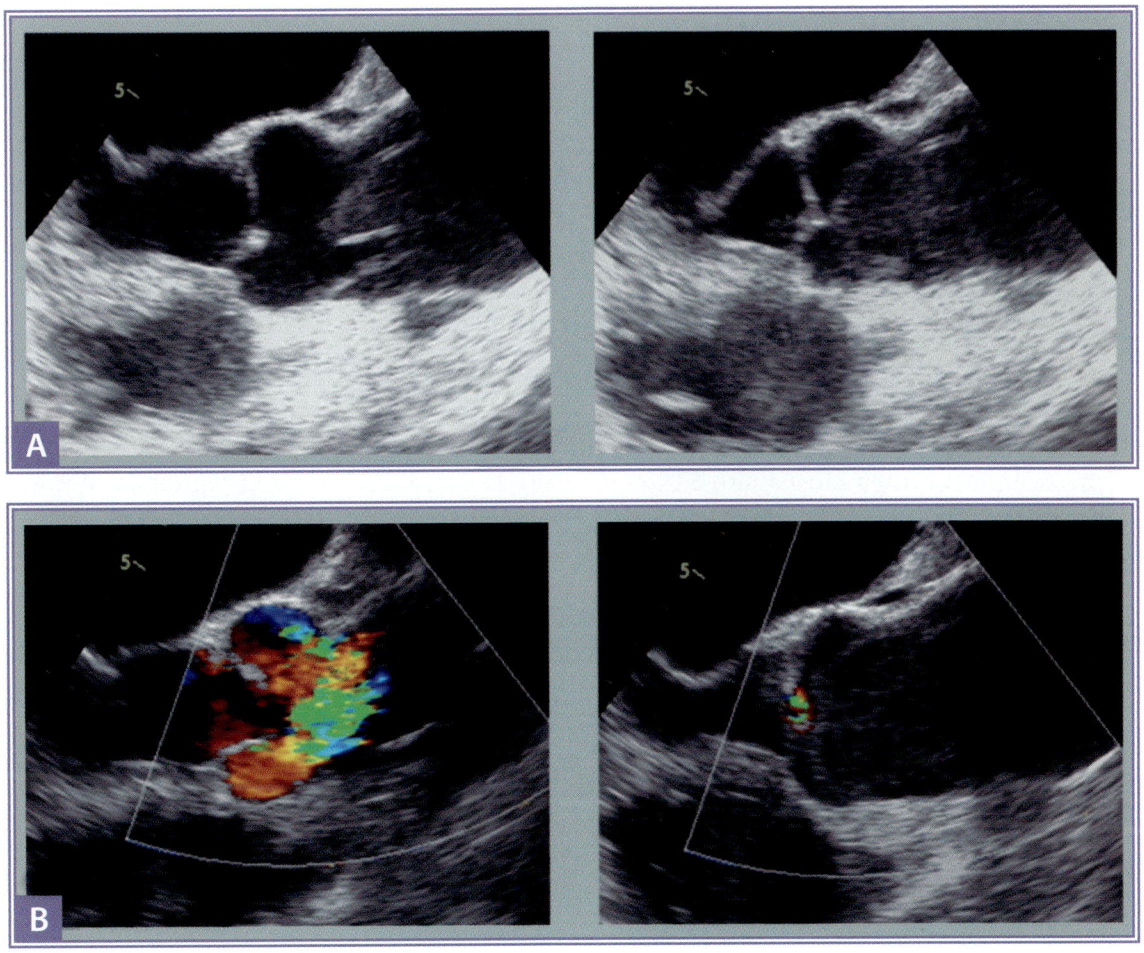

Fig. 2.1 Trans-esophageal long-axis image of a Type A AD. **A**, 2D-mode. The lamella is mobile in the ascending aorta. In the second picture, the false lumen compression reaches the valve and the coronary ostia. **B**, Color flow image of the same phases showing flow alteration.

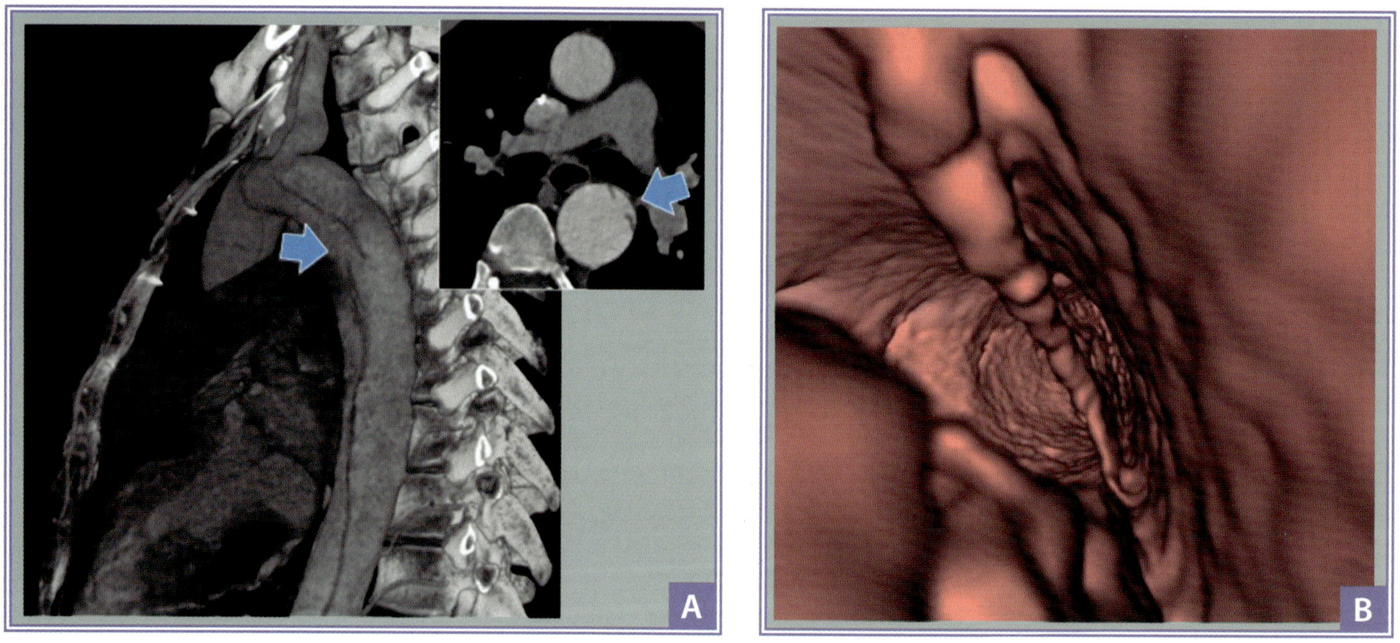

Fig. 2.2 Angio-CT scan of a Type B AD. **A**, Multi-planar reformatting with volume rendering. The proximal entry tear is located in the proximal part of the descending thoracic aorta (blue arrow). In the axial scan, the entry tear and the lamella are clearly visible (blue arrow) with compression of the true lumen. **B**, Virtual angioscopy enables one to determine the longitudinal extension of the entry tear and the two lumina.

- location and size of additional tears: these may be difficult to detect and intraoperative TEE (see Chapter 39), or intravascular ultrasound (IVUS, see Chapter 38) may be more helpful (Fig. 2.3);
- diameter of the non-dissected proximal landing zone: this will be used for sizing the stent-graft (Fig. 2.4);
- total diameter of the aorta and respective diameters of the true and false lumen: a tapered true lumen with significant mismatch between proximal and distal landing zones is common and requires an appropriate strategy (Fig. 2.5);

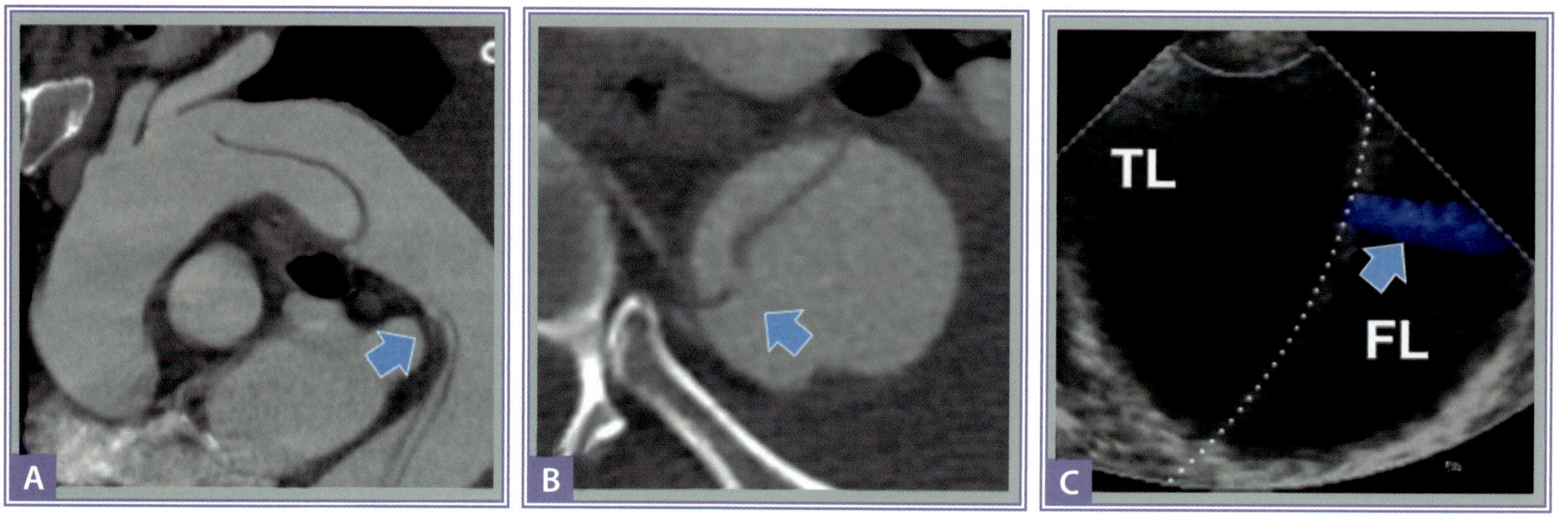

Fig. 2.3 **A**, Angio-CT- Multi-planar reformatting. In the descending aorta, the intimal tear typically originates within a few centimeters of the left subclavian artery because this segment of the aorta is subject to the greatest pressure fluctuations. However, additional tears (blue arrow) can be located anywhere in the thoracoabdominal aorta. **B**, Angio-CT – Axial scan. A small additional tear is visualized. **C**, Intra-operatively, small additional tears can be difficult to detect. TEE is very helpful to visualize them in the descending thoracic aorta.

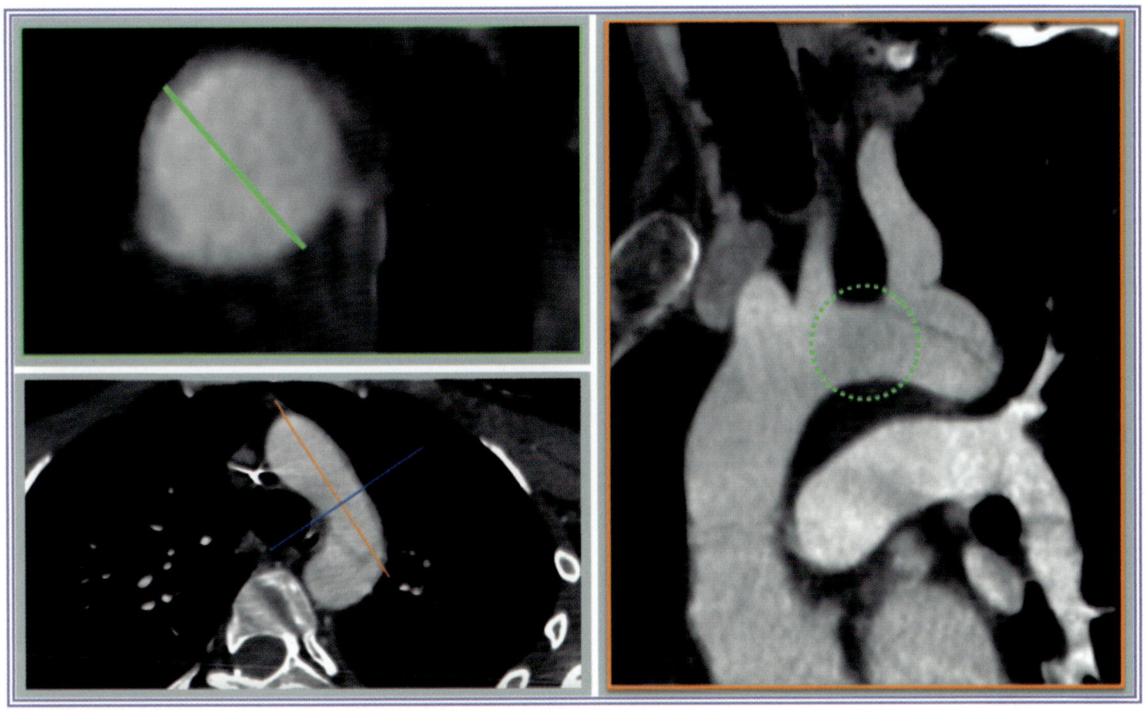

Fig. 2.4 Angio-CT – Multi-planar reformatting. The non-dissected proximal landing zone (green circle) is used for sizing the stent-graft.

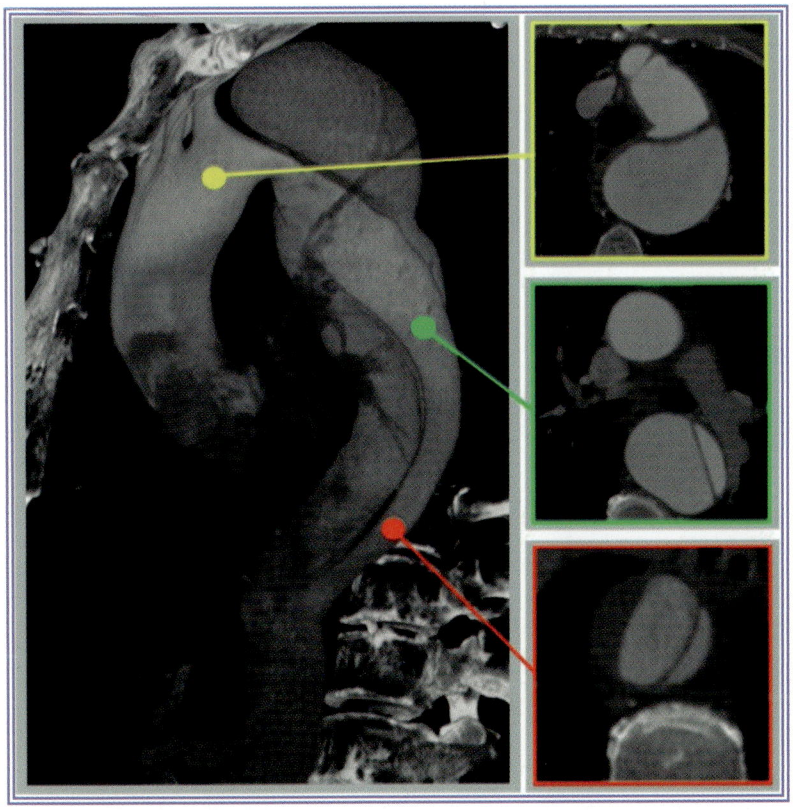

Fig. 2.5 Diameter of the entire aorta and of the true and false lumen in three different parts of the thoracic aorta: aortic arch (yellow), proximal (green) and distal (red) descending thoracic aorta. In the descending thoracic aorta, the true lumen is compressed by the dilated false lumen.

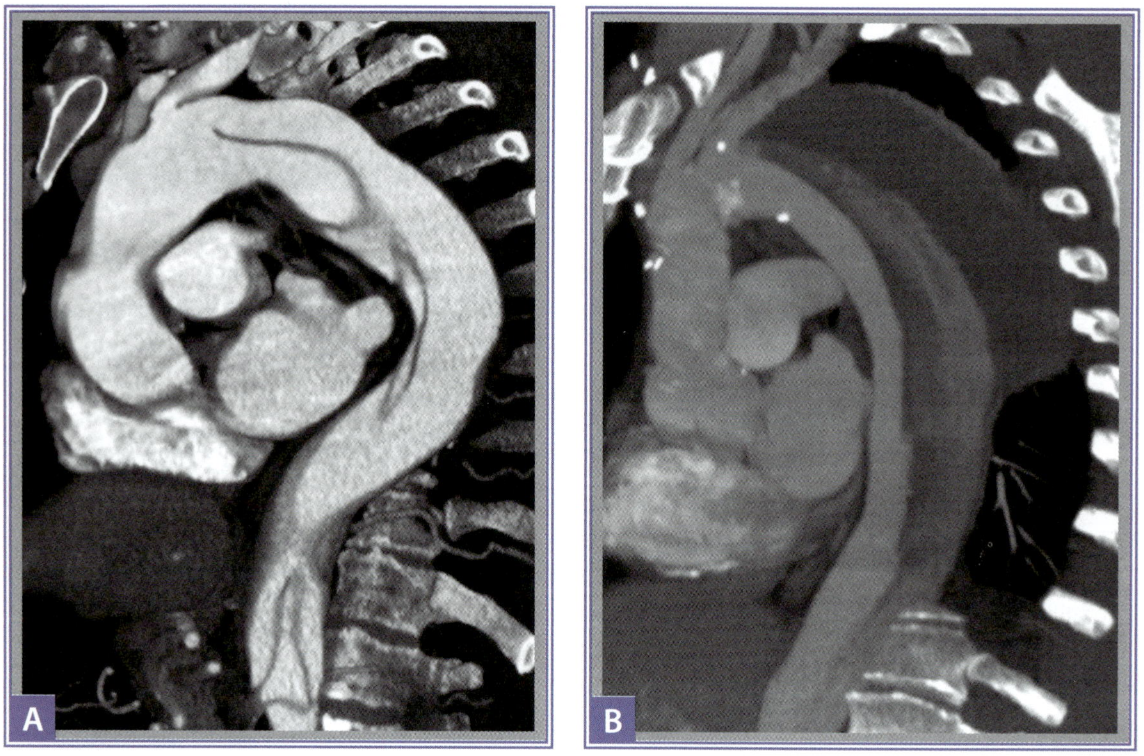

Fig. 2.6 **A**, Acute Type B AD with a thin mobile lamella and no significant thrombosis in the false lumen. **B**, Chronic Type B AD with thickened and stable lamella and aneurysmatic evolution of the partially thrombosed false lumen.

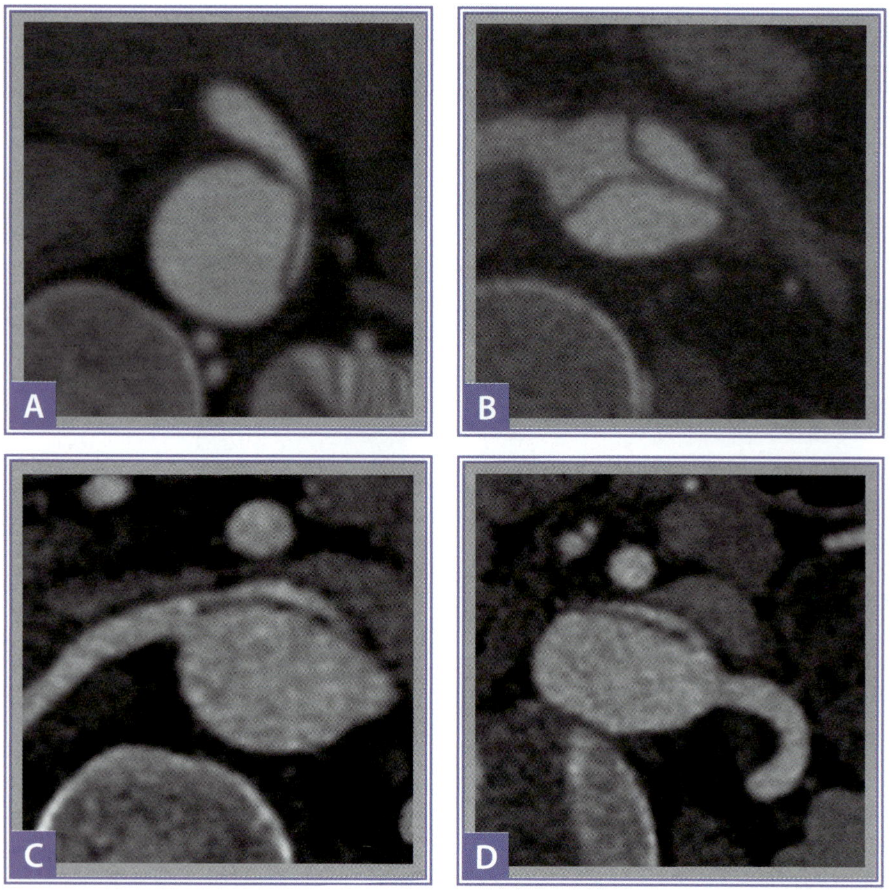

Fig. 2.7 Angio-CT - Axial scans. Various patterns of perfusion of splanchnic and renal arteries during Type B AD are shown. **A**, Dynamic malperfusion of the coeliac trunk. The true lumen is compressed by the false lumen with visceral malperfusion. **B**, Static malperfusion of the left renal artery. The dissection involves the vessel with compression of the true lumen and complete occlusion of the artery. **C**, The right renal artery is partially dissected and arises from both the true and false lumen. **D**, The left renal artery arises from the false lumen.

- degree of thrombosis of the false lumen (Fig. 2.6);
- patency (dissection) of splanchnic and renal arteries and origin from true/false lumen, organ perfusion (Fig. 2.7);
- diameter, patency, and dissection of the iliac arteries (Fig. 2.8);
- additional information is gathered regarding associated organ diseases and variant anatomy of the arteries (particularly the supra-aortic trunks, and the renal and splanchnic arteries), veins and kidneys (single, pelvic, horseshoe, etc.);
- in addition, electrocardiographic (EKG)-gated CT offers the opportunity to evaluate the coronary arteries; this is a crucial step before a thoracic aorta operative procedure, because treatment of critical coronary lesions helps prevent perioperative hemodynamic instability, which is one of the major causes of spinal cord ischemia [18].

Together with the axial scans, oblique multiplanar reconstructions (MPR) may be very useful due to the aortic tortuosity and the non-orthogonal path of the dissection plane. On the other hand, volumetric algorithms such as maximum intensity projections (MIP) should be used with caution since much of the intra-aortic detail, such as the intimal lamella or thrombus, could be lost.

In conclusion, Type B AD, even in an acute setting, requires a thorough CT diagnostic evaluation to disclose all the anatomic and pathologic details needed to plan the most appropriate treatment.

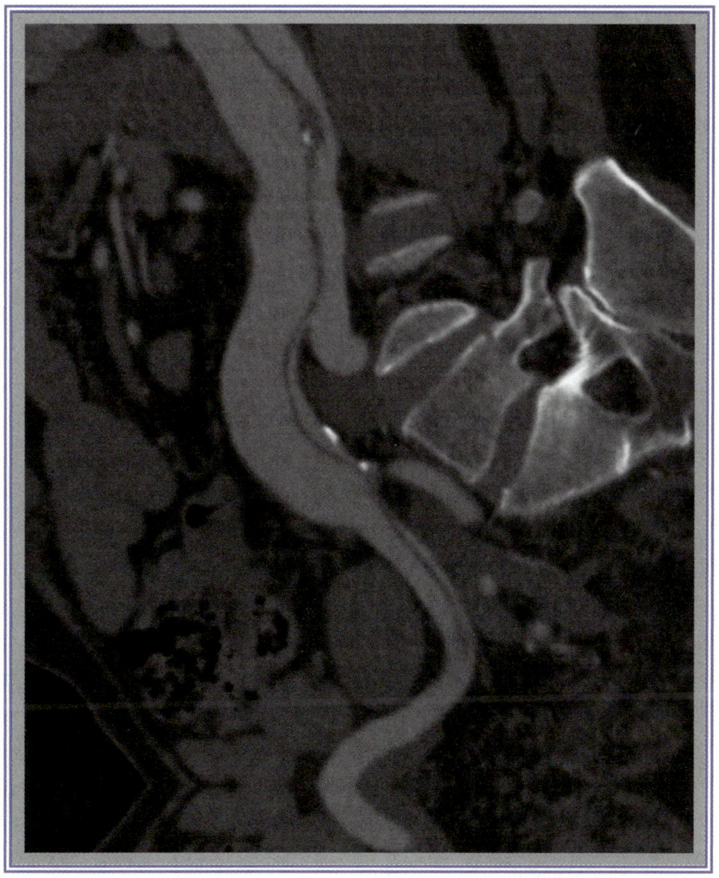

Fig. 2.8 Angio-CT – Multi-planar oblique reformatting showing involvement of the iliac arteries. This Type B AD involves the infra-renal aorta, the right common iliac artery and the proximal portion of the external iliac artery.

2.4 Pathophysiology and principles of therapy

Outcomes today regarding the stent-graft repair of aneurysms of the descending thoracic aorta are encouraging. Stent-grafts, in fact, were initially designed and approved for use in aneurysmal disease, where the technical and clinical goals are clear: to exclude the aneurysmal sac from arterial pressurization and thus reduce or, hopefully, abolish the risk of rupture. However, aneurysms currently represent only one-half or less of patients with indications for Thoracic EndoVascular Aortic Repair (TEVAR) [19]. Other indications include: traumatic injury, aorto-esophageal or aorto-bronchial *fistulae*, penetrating aortic ulcer (PAU), intramural hematoma (IMH) and, last but not least, complicated Type B AD. The goals of TEVAR for acute and sub-acute Type B AD are far less clear than for aneurysms. Remodeling and complete healing of the dissected aortic wall is certainly a desirable outcome but it is actually attained in only a fraction of cases [20].

The initial event of Type B AD is usually an intimal tear that allows blood to break into the aortic wall layers with creation of two lumina: a false lumen (FL) that frequently enlarges and a true lumen (TL) that may contract or even collapse. Blood flows in both lumina, as may be observed with TEE; however, malperfusion can occur as a consequence of static or dynamic events. Moreover, the reduced strength of the dissected aortic wall makes it more prone to progressive dilatation and eventually rupture (Fig. 2.9).

Endovascular treatment of acute and sub-acute Type B AD aims at excluding the FL from the circulation, avoiding malperfusion and preventing aortic enlargement and rupture. This may be obtained with both regular stent-grafts used to cover the intimal tears and with bare stents specifically designed to treat TL collapse and malperfusion (see Chapter 25).

From a technical point of view, this may be achieved by a stent-graft that:

1. obliterates the primary entry tear;
2. re-directs the blood flow into the TL; and
3. produces low turbulent flow in the FL and eventually promotes thrombosis of the FL (Fig. 2.10).

Another consequence of re-directing blood flow into the TL and decompressing the FL is that a compressed or collapsed TL may expand, thus preventing or relieving dynamic malperfusion.

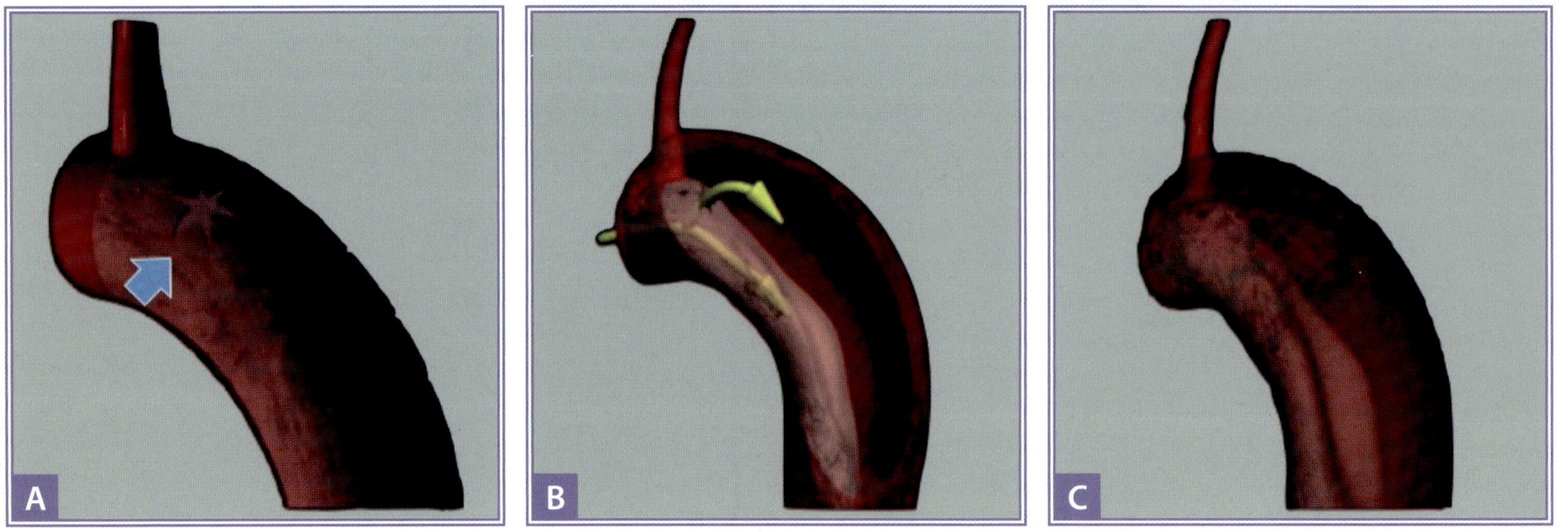

Fig. 2.9 Pathophysiology of Type B AD. **A**, The proximal entry tear (blue arrow) allows blood to break into the aortic wall layers with creation of two lumina. **B**-**C**, The false lumen enlarges and the true lumen collapses.

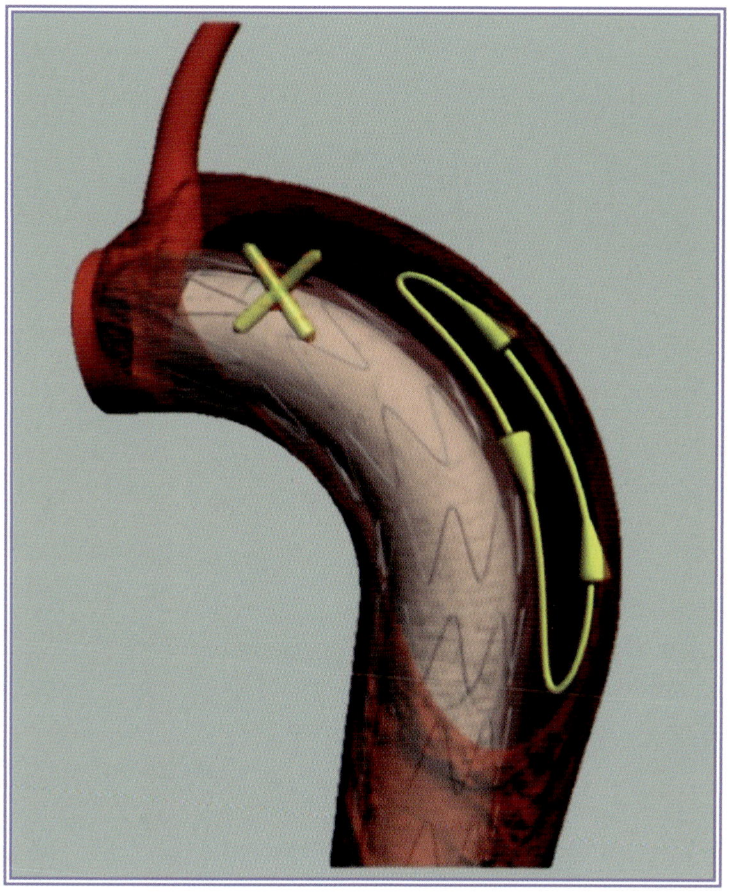

Fig. 2.10 Endovascular exclusion. The fabric covered stent-graft obliterates the primary entry tear, redirects the blood flow into the true lumen and produces low turbulent flow in the false lumen promoting thrombosis.

Possible additional problems include:

1. retrograde flow into the FL from the left subclavian artery; this may be treated percutaneously with a plug;
2. presence of high-flow secondary tears in the thoracic aorta; these are assessed intra-operatively with TEE, and may be treated with additional stent-grafts; this, however, has to be balanced against the increased risk of spinal cord ischemia;
3. additional secondary tears in the abdominal aorta (often adjacent to the splanchnic vessels) are commonplace and are usually left untreated;
4. flapping movements of the intimal lamella may prevent thrombosis of the FL;
5. a collapsed TL may fail to adequately expand with persistent distal malperfusion.

The two latter problems can be addressed by the Provisional Extension To Induce Complete Attachment (PETTICOAT) technique.

Other more complex techniques are nowadays available for specific problems and will be addressed later in dedicated chapters.

From a more clinical perspective, an endovascular approach is accepted by most authors for the treatment of acute and sub-acute Type B AD. However, for uncomplicated cases, optimal medical treatment is still considered the treatment of choice by most authors. This open issue will be discussed in Chapters 9.

In Type B AD, bowel malperfusion is one of the most difficult complications to interpret when only soft and non-specific symptoms are present; waiting for hard signs and symptoms,

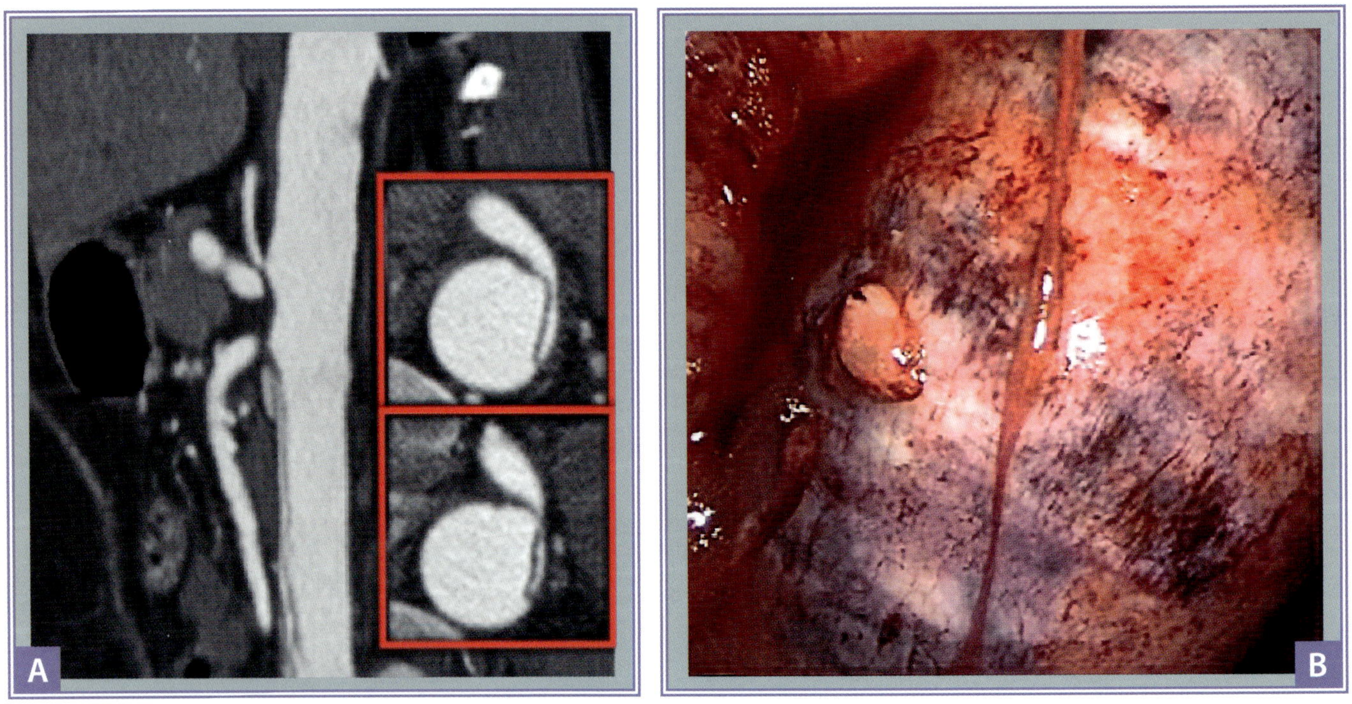

Fig. 2.11 **A**, Pre-operative Angio-CT showing dynamic malperfusion of both the coeliac trunk and superior mesenteric artery. **B**, Diagnostic laparoscopy demonstrates small bowel ischemia with sub-serosal hemorrhage and pallor.

however, may result in fatal bowel necrosis (Fig. 2.11). After an initial positive experience, in the last four years we have routinely used laparoscopy both preoperatively in patients with unclear abdominal symptoms and after TEVAR in all patients with unclear angiographic findings related to intestinal perfusion.

In conclusion, TEVAR has been shown to have a satisfactory degree of safety and efficacy in most acute and sub-acute complicated Type B AD cases, while the PETTICOAT technique may be used in selected cases to promote TL expansion and relieve malperfusion.

Chronic Type B AD with aneurysmal dilatation clearly requires treatment in reasonably fit subjects, when a critical diameter threshold is reached. Open surgery offers very good results when performed by experienced operators in high volume centers (see also Chapter 31). Recently, however, endovascular options that aim at total exclusion of the FL with complete sealing of the TL have also been proposed, and these will be discussed in Chapter 28.

REFERENCES

1) Levy B, Tedgui A. Biology of the arterial wall. Norwell, MA: Kluwer Academic, 1999.
2) O'Gara PT, DeSanctis RW. Acute aortic dissection and its variants. Toward a common diagnostic and therapeutic approach. Circulation 1995; 92: 1376-8.
3) Khan IA, Nair CK. Clinical, diagnostic, and management perspectives of aortic dissection. Chest 2002; 122: 311-28.
4) Clouse WD, Hallett JW Jr, Schaff HV, et al. Acute aortic dissection: population-based incidence compared with degenerative aortic aneurysm rupture Mayo Clin Proc 2004; 79: 176-80.
5) Mészáros I, Mórocz J, Szlávi J, et al. Epidemiology and clinicopathology of aortic dissection. Chest 2000; 117: 1271-8.
6) Olsson C, Thelin S, Ståhle E, Ekbom A, Granath F. Thoracic aortic aneurysm and dissection: increasing prevalence and improved outcomes reported in a nationwide population-based study of more than 14,000 cases from 1987 to 2002. Circulation 2006; 114: 2611-8.
7) Fattori R, Cao P, De Rango P, et al. Interdisciplinary expert consensus document on management of type B aortic dissection. J Am Coll Cardiol 2013; 61: 1661-78.

8) Fuster V, Halperin JL. Aortic dissection: a medical perspective. J Card Surg 1994; 9: 713-28.
9) Januzzi JL, Isselbacher EM, Fattori R, et al; International Registry of Aortic Dissection (IRAD). Characterizing the young patient with aortic dissection: results from the International Registry of Aortic Dissection (IRAD). J Am Coll Cardiol 2004; 43: 665-9.
10) Pacini D, Di Marco L, Fortuna D, et al. Acute aortic dissection: epidemiology and outcomes. Int J Cardiol 2013; 167: 2806-12.
11) Acosta S, Blomstrand D, Gottsäter A. Epidemiology and long-term prognostic factors in acute type B aortic dissection. Ann Vasc Surg 2007; 21: 415-22.
12) LeMaire SA, Russell L. Epidemiology of thoracic aortic dissection. Nat Rev Cardiol 2011; 8: 103-13.
13) Bossone E, Pyeritz RE, O'Gara P, Harris KM, Braverman AC, Pape L, Russo MJ, Hughes GC, Tsai TT, Montgomery DG, Nienaber CA, Isselbacher EM, Eagle KA; International Registry of Acute Aortic. Acute aortic dissection in blacks: insights from the International Registry of Acute Aortic Dissection. Am J Med 2013; 126(10): 909-15.
14) Elefteriades JA. Natural history of thoracic aortic aneurysms: indications for surgery, and surgical versus nonsurgical risks. Ann Thorac Surg 2002 ; 74: S1877-80.
15) Vignon P, Spencer KT, Rambaud G, et al. Differential transesophageal echocardiographic diagnosis between linear artifacts and intraluminal flap of aortic dissection or disruption. Chest 2001; 119: 1778-90.
16) Fisher ER, Stern EJ, Godwin JD 2nd, et al. Acute aortic dissection: typical and atypical imaging features. Radiographics 1994; 14:1263-71.
17) Prince MR, Narasimham DL, Jacoby WT, et al. Three-dimensional gadolinium-enhanced MR angiography of the thoracic aorta. AJR Am J Roentgenol 1996; 166:1387-97.
18) Spagnolo P, Giglio M. Role of cardiac CT in assessment of patients with thoraco-abdominal aortic aneurysm. R. Chiesa et al. (eds). Thoraco-abdominal aorta: surgical and anesthetic management. Milan: Springer-Verlag Italia, 2010
19) Hughes GC, Daneshmand MA, Swaminathan M,et al. "Real world" thoracic endografting: results with the Gore TAG device 2 years after U.S. FDA approval. Ann Thorac Surg. 2008; 86(5): 1530-7.
20) Criado FJ, Abul-Khoudoud O. Endograft repair of acute aortic dissection. Promises and challenges. J Cardiovasc Surg 2005; 46(2): 107 12.

3

The true stories of Type B aortic dissection

Edited by Daniele Mascia and Alessandro Grandi

In editing Type B AD patient's true stories we elected to leave them basically unchanged so as to better reflect the experience of the authors and their feelings. We did make them anonymous (names are fictitious, and reflect only the gender of the author) and sometimes we needed to slightly shorten them.

In boxes, we have added our comments that summarize what we ourselves have learned from the stories as we compared them with the classic information found in the textbooks. These comments are subjective and are meant purely as a "take home message" for readers with less clinical experience.

Please note that Type A AD patients' true stories, which can be found elsewhere in this book (see Chapter 5), have been edited differently. The editor of that section decided to extrapolate the key paragraphs from each story that he felt conveyed the strongest messages.

We are grateful to the patients for sharing their personal stories, and we hope that the experience for the reader will be as enriching and educating as it was for us to edit them.

Daniele Mascia (mascia.daniele@hsr.it)
Scientific Institute Ospedale San Raffaele, Milan, Italy

G. Melissano - R. Chiesa (eds), Aortic Dissection patients true stories and the innovations that saved their lives

Ron, 58 years old, Germany

A daughter's prospective on AD

My dad was an unlucky victim of a descending aortic dissection. I am telling his story, because he unfortunately died just a day after he was diagnosed with this.

Mortality of acute Type B AD can be as high as 10%

I will never forget that weekend. I feel like it was just yesterday. I was at work Friday night calling my dad a whole bunch of times to tell him that I got my keys to my new apartment. I was so excited to be finally moving in. He never answered but he soon called me back and left a message on my phone. He left me a voicemail and I soon called him back, and we talked about my new apartment and I told him that I would call him tomorrow, because I was at work. I wish that I knew that would be the last time I would ever talk to him on the phone.

He even drove himself to the hospital that night. I woke up to a text message from my brother to call him. I thought that was unusual because I never talk to him. I called him and he told me that there was something wrong with his aorta and that I shouldn't worry about it. That he has a 90% chance of survival. That he would be fine and not to make the drive down to the hospital. I was about 2 hours away and being studying in the health science field, I just knew something was not right and so of course I made the drive down there.

Although symptoms at presentation are often dramatic, milder cases are not uncommon

I woke up my whole family that was back where I lived and told them to get to the hospital. I told my mom what my brother told me and that something did not seem right. Of course I was right and my mom told me I needed to get there as soon as I could. Once I got to the hospital they pulled my sister and me aside and told us that he had a descending aorta dissection and that it was very serious. He was in the ICU when I finally got to see him. His left kidney was already gone from the lack of blood to it. They also could not perform surgery because it was so severe, if they had he would have died immediately. We were told to sit and wait and hopefully his blood pressure would stabilize. They sedated him that night.

Organ malperfusion often complicates Type B AD

The next morning which was Sunday changed my life forever. I got the worst phone call of my life. This time it was my sister calling me, telling me dad was doing really bad and I needed to get to the hospital. I was crying so hard at that point my sister put my mom on the phone. The first thing I asked her was "Is my father going to die?" and she replied back to me "I honestly don't know". When I got to the hospital the priest was already there. They gathered us in a room and explained to us what happened over night. Everything from his heart down was completely gone. He had no function anywhere.

Severe malperfusion of organs and limbs may be fatal in a matter of hours

As a family, we decided that he would not want to live as a vegetable and was going to die anyway. We took him off of everything and he passed within minutes.

Jody, 60 years old, USA

The importance of CT Scans

Pain at presentation is often excrutiating

Ongoing (or aggravating) chest pain in spite of normal cardiac findings is very suggestive of AD

I suffered a Type B aortic dissection. I felt a sudden sharp pain in the sternum region, which after two hours radiated to my flank; it was worse than childbirth labor (I have had three natural childbirths). This happened at 1:00am as I was preparing to go to bed. We called our GP; expecting a heart attack she took an EKG but it was quite normal. After an initial painkiller injection, the pain did not substantially subside and an hour later a second shot followed, which helped somewhat. Being at the maximum dose and for lack of a proper diagnosis our GP told us to go to the university hospital emergency department. We arrived there around 03:00 am.

CT scan is the gold standard imaging technique to diagnose Type B AD

A series of tests there did not produce any conclusive result, perhaps because I declined a CT scan of my chest because I had just two weeks earlier had one to control for the full recovery from pneumonia. The following two days I went through a few more tests; the gallbladder was not an option because it had been removed many years ago (at age 33), leaving the stomach as alternative suspect. A gastroscopy was planned but not carried out. Finally, I was CT scanned in the afternoon and I was diagnosed with Type B AD and told that I would stay in hospital for some time, to start conservative treatment.

'Some time' turned out to be 10 weeks! On the basis of several CT scans, which showed an aortic inner wall with a tear that over time had progressed all the way up to the aortic arch it was decided to schedule an operation to insert two endo-prostheses into the upper part of the aorta.

First-degree relatives should be tested and followed over time to check their aorta

I did not have a history of high blood pressure, high cholesterol or elevated blood sugar levels. I have smoked for 40 years, but my lungs were in 'amazingly' good shape. A genetic analysis concluded that there was no genetic predestination, although a far relative (a cousin of my mother) also suffered a dissection. My children were advised to keep an eye on their aorta.

Daniela, 32 year old, Italy

The false panic attack

Once a day I went to my local hospital saying I was having a panic attack. It had happened before, my chest would start to ache and hurt, and I would go in and they would give me a shot to help me relax, then send me home.

This time was different, the pain was as sharp as I never felt before. The doctor realized that something was wrong and asked me to get X-rays. When the results came back, he was worried, and asked me to get a CT scan done. I was worried at that point, because I know doctors don't just send patients out for extra tests "just because." He told me he suspected I was affected by the Marfan Syndrome. Come to find out, I had a Type B dissection with the aorta that was almost the size of a soda can. A pleural effusion was also present and they said that this was the cause of my breathing difficulty.

Pain may be accompanied by the feeling of impending doom

Pleural effusion may be only reactive, but it may also herald impending rupture

He immediately told me that I had to have emergency surgery, but there simply wasn't anyone qualified enough who could perform the operation. It took them a long time to get things in order, because none of the surgeons locally wanted to take my case, because everybody was certain I was going to die.

Eventually I had a consulting surgeon who signed on, as well as a cardiologist locally, and the next thing I knew my mom and I were on a private jet on our way to another hospital. After taking all the tests to make sure that my body was healthy enough to take the surgery, the doctor decided that everything was fine and we were ready to go.

Aortic dissection is uncommon, therefore most of the cases need to be transferred to a high volume specialized center in order to receive state-of-the-art treatment

The intervention passed without complications even if some time later, they told me that I had to have a second surgery, because my abdominal aorta was too big and there was the risk it would grow again. They told me they simply couldn't do it all in one surgery.

Staged interventions are often needed to reduce the surgical risk in very extensive disese

Carmen, 33 years old, USA

Dissection and pregnancy

The most common places in which a patient can feel pain are the chest, the back, mainly between the shoulders and the throat

I gave birth to my second baby girl. Twenty-two hours later, while nursing her around 8 pm, I had an aortic dissection. It was soon labeled an Type B AD. I was still in Labor and Delivery and felt a severe onset of pain. I was young, healthy and active, I was not pre-eclamptic, had no risk factors, delivery went smoothly.

The pain given by an aortic dissection is very sharp, almost impossible to compare it to any other

A ripping pain started from the base of my neck down my entire spine, then immediately a wave of pain across my stomach then hit me in the (left) chest and straight through my body to my back. I remember a doctor asking me my symptoms, I said "I feel like I'm having a heart attack or something" to which his response was "You're a little young for that". My obstetrician came fairly quickly but I felt my breathing weak and speaking was slow and quiet already. A chest X-ray and EKG were normal so the thought it was maybe something happened with the epidural, so I was sent for a CT scan. The radiologist diagnosed the aortic dissection.

I was sent to another hospital where a doctor thought the Type B dissection I had was manageable by medications but I continued to deteriorate. I had uncontrollable vomit/diarrhea, I could barely whisper and I felt my body shutting down. Thank God my husband asked for another opinion.

Referral to highly specialized centers is crucial to get appropriate treatment

A third hospital said I needed surgery. I underwent surgery there because it was Type B "complicated" meaning the dissection was involving the arteries arising from the aorta to the stomach and kidneys and there was no blood flow to my organs nor to my right leg.

Even for young and fit patients recovery after major procedures for Type B AD may be a struggle

Meanwhile they had told my family there was high chance I would not make it through surgery, I had not seen my baby (s) and I woke up not knowing where I was and then had to stay in the ICU for eleven days. Three-four of those days of admission and surgeries I have no memory of. I fortunately had no major complications after all this given the severity of what had happened. After finally somewhat lowering my blood pressure and stabilizing it with medications, they released me on tons of medications.

John, 41 years old, Netherland

Pain in renal failure

At 7.30 am whilst sitting on the sofa after a restful and peaceful night's sleep I felt a sharp burning sensation I thought it would pass, but after around 2 minutes I felt a "whooshing" sensation from my left arm down into my legs and back up again to my arm, this repeated itself four possibly five times. Then the pain started, and like no other pain I have ever felt or wish to again. It started in my chest and went right through to my back and in between my shoulder blades. It was at this time I called to my wife and said "something is seriously wrong; I need to go the hospital". The pain started to move downwards and was getting more severe and covering more of my upper torso.

Aortic dissection presentation is often in the early morning

The pain may be anticipated by various feelings that the patient has never experienced before

Pain may move downward as the dissection progresses

My brother went in and got a wheelchair whilst my wife informed the staff that I needed immediate attention. It seemed like I had half of the hospital staff surrounding me asking questions doing blood pressure and various tests plus putting a heart monitor on me. The readings from the monitor indicated that I wasn't have a heart attack and from that moment it seemed like there were no staff anymore the emergency was now over!

After cardiac problems have been excluded further testing is often delayed

The pain now was even more intense and had now travelled down into my abdomen. I was given Pethidine injected directly into my abdomen as well as morphine neither of which helped with relieving the pain. Eventually I was admitted to a ward where I was basically left in pain with no real urgency as to find out what was going on internally.

Pain may be refractory to treatment

On day 3, I told the staff that I had not been able to pass urine since being admitted, so they advised I drink more. Day 3 came and turned into day 4 with still no urine passing so they put me on a saline drip to increase the fluids to make me pee. Day 7, miraculously I was seen by a renal expert who informed the staff I was in acute renal failure. I was then transferred to another hospital. Within the hour they organized for me to have a catheter inserted into the femoral artery in my right groin area. For this to be placed *in situ* I had to be laid flat, it was at this moment the fluid in my body overtook my lungs and I went into respiratory failure. I fought and fought to stay alive and to breath but eventually stopped breathing. The doctors did whatever they needed to do to get me back and succeeded.

One of the possible complications of AD is organ malperfusion (static or dynamic)

I was transferred to a renal ward and put on dialysis. After four days my body settled and someone had the bright idea to send me down for an ultrasound. It was arranged that I would go down to theatre and have a renal stent placed which was very successful I passed urine the next morning. They also cut the dissection flap to release pressure from within the aorta which was also a great outcome.

In order to treat malperfusion syndrome, aortic fenestration and stent placement to restore renal perfusion may be performed

I had severe pain in my left shoulder for approximately six months prior to dissection and was diagnosed with having a frozen shoulder. After dissection and to this day I've had no problems regarding pain in the shoulder! I'm now scanned yearly next scan due February 2016. I have a renal stent *in situ*. I also have an abdominal aortic aneurysm that will need treatment.

I have also been through genetic testing and found to have the gene the *ACTA2* gene mutation.

Young patients who experienced AD should be investigated for genetic mutations or familial syndromes

Amy, 28 years old, USA

It runs in the family

I am a part-time reading teacher at an elementary school. One day, I got to school and found out that a substitute teacher did not show, and I would have to cover that classroom-no sweat! The day proceeded as normal, I ate lunch in the teacher's lounge, called my husband to see how his dentist appointment went, and walked down to the cafeteria to pick up "my" class. On the way up the steps (to get our coats for recess), I felt a terrible burning sensation in my chest and moderate pain. I thought it strange that a sandwich would cause such heartburn, but I tried to ignore it. With every step I took, the pain intensified. I felt as though someone had opened my chest with a chainsaw and lit a blowtorch and was aiming it directly into my abdomen and chest. I knew something was majorly wrong as I walked to the nurse's office and my left leg had gone numb. My father had a heart attack at the age of 41, and I assumed the same thing was happening to me, and I was only 28.

Aortic dissection may present with moderate pain which increases in a short time to became the worst pain the patient has ever felt. Sometimes it is described as a burning sensation, or a heartburn

The next thing I know, phone calls are being made to 911, my husband of only four months and my father at work. I was taken to a local hospital where at first they thought I was having an anxiety attack. This is where my story gets crazy.

Aortic dissection is still one of the most misdiagnosed diseases

Diagnosis however, can be straightforward after you have seen AD once

My father's sister had an aortic dissection in July of 2003. It took doctors two weeks to diagnose her, and after 14 surgeries, she is recovering slowly but surely. My father took one look at my symptoms and knew exactly what was happening to me. My father told the doctors to check me for aortic dissection, and the next thing you know, I was life-flighted to another clinic. If my aunt had not had an aortic dissection, I now truly believe that I would have died. I feel terrible that my aunt had to go through everything she did, but if she hadn't, I may not be here telling my story.

About ten hours into my whole ordeal, I finally had a stent placed in my descending aorta (endovascularly - I was very lucky to not have my chest opened up), and blood flow was re-established to my left leg (which I was told I almost lost). I thank my Vascular Surgeon and his team for saving my life. I'm told I was very close to death when I arrived at the clinic. I remained there for the next 2 weeks and then was sent back to spend 2 weeks at a local rehabilitation hospital. I am now on three medications daily to control my blood pressure and heart rate. I have also been placed on an antidepressant for depression-like symptoms. I have drop foot because of the lack of blood flow to my left leg and foot, and severe nerve damage, which is finally starting to regenerate (which is extremely uncomfortable and painful). I have completed physical therapy to try to regain my dorsiflection in my left foot and stimulate my nerves to regenerate quicker.

Arterial pressure control with medications is important in patients who suffered for an AD

Because of all of the stress on my body due to the dissection, I lost 30 pounds, my hair is fell out and I got acne. I returned to work for the the following school year. My next step was genetic testing at the clinic. They don't feel that I show characteristics of Marfan's, but they are going to test me for Ehlers-Danlos Syndrome (which I did not have). I will also most likely find out if I will ever be able to have children, which is a touchy area with me because children have always been my life and my husband and I haven't even been married two years and were thinking about starting a family.

Psychological disturbances are common after AD; they cannot be ignored and need to be dealt with appropriately

Since my dissection a year and a half ago, we've had four more dissections in my family, including my younger brother, who just turned 27. We are currently enrolled in a genetic study at the University due to the large number of dissections in our family. Luckily, everyone has survived due to our current knowledge on this subject which we never would have known if it weren't for all of the dissections in our family.

Relatives of patients who experienced AD should enter in a dedicated check-up program

Mary, 42 years old, UK

Genetic mutations

My brother and father had alredy had AD. I was scheduled to have tests in order to ensure my aorta was not dilated, and that there were no aneurysms present in my brain. All of my tests came back clear. In 2014 my life changed – I found out that I have a genetic mutation (*SMAD3* gene mutation). My brother also has this, and my father who passed away in 2008 also had it. Upon finding out this information, it was the belief that I was not high risk as I had never shown any symptoms. The last test I had as in May 2015, completely clear of anything.

Genetic counselling and cardiovascular consultations are important in familial aortic disease

One day, I got home at 9.30 pm. I had just sat down on the couch, when all of a sudden I had a sudden onset of back pain that cause me to scream out to my husband and fall to the ground. I did not know what was happening; I was trying to stand, but kept collapsing back on the ground. The pain was radiating around to my chest and down to my abdomen. The pain was unbelievable. I could literally feel the ripping.

The pain experienced during AD is very sharp, and may be associated with disorientation, neurological symptoms and syncope

The local hospital admitted me, and after me telling them twice I have a genetic disorder that causes dissections, they told me that it could just be food indigestion!! After two hours, they finally scanned me, and came to give me the news that I had a Type B AD. Within twenty minutes I was being flown by air ambulance to another hospital.

Referral to high volume centers is customary and useful to guarantee specialised treatment

The pain continued, even with pain relief. After 40 minutes, we arrived. I was admitted to hospital and was under close monitoring in the Intensive Care unit for five days, then approximately two weeks in vascular. For almost three weeks, I was managed with blood pressure medications. The surgeons did not want to operate because I am only 36 years old, the SMAD3 mutation carries many risks to operate, and it was a Type B. However, two days before going home, it was discovered that I had renal failure, and my left kidney was suffering from lack of blood flow. Due to the dissection creating a false lumen, true lumen was collapsing and was not able to provide enough blood flow. It was decided that I would have a stent inserted into my aorta. It was placed in my true lumen, allowing both of the true and false lumens to provide blood flow to my kidney. I have had follow up appointments with my cardiologist, where I was informed that there is no way of telling when this may happen again. The cardiologist showed me the results from May 2015, and informed me that since they were completely clear of any dilation, dissection or issues, this makes it obvious that my aortic dissection is not slow moving, or a gradual tear.

Organ malperfusion may manifest hours to days after the initial presentation of the disease

Lifelong follow up and appropriate pharmacologic management is very important after AD

My brother who is currently 38 years old had his dissection at 31, followed by a stroke a short time later. He had a full stent placed in his aorta. My father had two dissections, and also had a complete stent inserted. He had a brain aneurism a few years later, and died.

This entire ordeal was, and continues to be, the scariest time of my life. I have never experienced pain like this, and pray that I never have to ever again. I am currently on four different medications, three times a day, to ensure my blood pressure remains low.

Medical treatment by means of blood pressure control and pain relief is the first-line therapy after non-complicated Type B AD

Jane, 53 years old, Australia

Gallbladder surgery

A "Ripping" chest pain is a common presentation of AD

One night I got a feeling of a lump on my neck, I thought it was a disc problem so I kept going as usual. On my day off from work, I went out shopping, at around 10.00 am I felt like a huge rip on the torso I said "Oh no this is what a heart attack feels like". I got a pause between pain, and the pain was in contractions so I ran to the store and I told them "Call Emergency I just got a heart attack". The clerk held my hand and talked to the Emergency person on the phone.

The ambulance came 8 minutes after the call and they transported me to the hospital. While in the ambulance, they kept asking me my name, but the pain was so big that I didn't want to talk.

The pain experienced during acute AD is so very severe, it almost impossible to compare it to any other

They got my wallet thinking I didn't want to say my name for some reason other than the pain, then they got my identification. I was offered pain medicine, but I refused it because I wanted the doctor to check why the pain was happening. At the hospital, they put me in a room and offered me a bed, but I declined since I couldn't lie down, but only sit due to the pain. I got a morphine shot and started vomiting, and the nurse said they were going to send me home because it was not a heart attack. The nurse saw me vomiting and I told him that it might be my gallbladder, and they then took me to get an ultrasound. I went back to the room, having to take morphine every 4-5 hours.

Misdiagnosis is still very common with acute Type B AD

8:00 am the next morning gallbladder was removed, the nurse said everything ok but that blood pressure is weird. I was released to go home around 6 pm.

I came home with a pain every 4-6 hours, even with the medicine. I got a prescription for three days'worth of pain medicine, but the pain continued after the medicine ran out. I took some old medicine for two more days and then got better. Seven days after this, I got up, moved more, walked around, but I felt dizzy, and the pain started again: not as strong as before, but I had constant cramps in my back. It felt like it was going to start again, so I told my son "Let's go to the Emergency".

Pharmacologic therapy to control pain and hypertension are the cornerstone of best medical therapy for non-complicated AD

Back in the Emergency Room, I told the doctor that my back might have a broken disk. My blood pressure was very high, and the doctor ordered X-rays. After this, they then rushed me to an MRI, then to another room closer to the nurse office. The ER doctor then came and said that I had a dissection of the aorta and needed to go to another hospital. They then took me in the ambulance, blood pressure crazy, and at the other hospital a doctor was waiting, and the doctor said that I didn't need an operation, as it was a Type B dissection, and told me I needed blood pressure control therapy. I was in the ICU for about 2 days until the pressure got under control. I was moved to the second floor, and got released from the hospital 3 days afterwards.

Matt, 50 years old, Sweden

Emotional stress

Strong Emotional stress can occasionally initiate AD

Having had a disagreement with a colleague, I felt so upset and disappointed, because of some sad comments. I tried to control myself, felt my BP rising and there it was. I felt a strong "stabbing " in my upper back, from the inside out, and a painfully sweet tearing moving downward along my spine. It stopped on my waist below my kidneys. My breath shortened, painful 'cramps' on my kidneys, I couldn't swallow as if something had stuck in my esophagus. Sweating, unable to hold on to my feet. I was rushed to the nearest private clinic, after a few exams and blood test, heart doctors, couldn't figure out what it was wrong with me and released me, because it was not a heart problem.

The words "stab", "rip", "split" and "tear" are often used to describe the pain of AD acute phase

AD is often still not diagnosed or misdiagnosed

On my way home I went to another private doc because I was not feeling well. There he had me on the 'ultra sound' and taken the fitness test without seeing anything. I got worst and he assumed that I might have had a blocked artery. I was told that all my arteries were crystal clear. Due to the contrast medication my kidneys got worse, my BP rose and I nearly fainted. I was admitted there until they called a cardiovascular doctor to examine me. The next morning, after I was passed through CT he saw the AD right away. He emphasized that CT should have been done right away, since I had told them the symptoms.

Ongoing chest pain and migrant pain and hypertension when cardiac tests are negative are suggestive of AD

Organ malperfusion with renal involvement is a common complication of AD

My dissection was from top, all the way down to my iliac arteries, legs, and has affected and split my renal arteries. My kidneys were divided as well due to the formation of true and false lumens. My left kidney was held by the false lumen contributing 80% whereas my right kidney was held by the true lumen contributing 20%. There was a renal artery stenosis and the chances of keeping either kidney alive were slim. The strange thing about it was that they were also somehow interconnected. My right leg was in a bit of pain and the docs told me that it would continue to be like that due to a low blood circulation. Also I wouldn't be able to walk long distances from then onwards. I was medically managed with a lot of different medications, the major problem was to lower and stabilize my blood pressure and try to keep at least one kidney 'alive'. I stayed in the private clinic for about 20 days and at general hospital another 20 days.

Lower limb malperfusion may result in intermitting claudication but also critical limbs ischemia

When I got out I couldn't walk much, I was taking about nineteen pills a day and my psychological state was nearly below zero. I depended on others, couldn't lift any weight, scared of getting sick, every little tiny pain I thought it was AD related and didn't know what to do. One day I took the big decision to move on. I was very lucky because I had found very good doctors too (vascular who actually saved my life and became friends with, heart doctor who managed to cut my pills down to 3 per day, and a very good kidney doctor who I visit once every 2 months). I have my CT exams once every 6 months. Mostly due to the combination of good doctors and power of will I can walk long distances without any squeezed pain like it used to be, maintain fairly low BP and heart rate. I drink about 2.5 lt of fluids for my kidneys, go to work every day staying away from stressful environments and enjoy every moment with family who has been with me throughout.

Severe depression and reduction in the perceived quality of life is common after the acute phase

With appropriate support a good quality of life is achievable after AD, however continued follow-up is desirable

Connie, 53 years old, UK

Check-ups are necessary when dealing with AD

The most common symptom of AD is pain in the back, mainly between the shoulders. Neurologic symptoms in the lower limbs such as paraplegia or paraparesis are less usual

One day I drove in my car to pick up my daughter. I felt great. I do have the habit to drive until my tank is almost empty. This was one of these moments. I decided to go to fill up at the gas-station. This saved my life. I went into the gas-station to pay when I felt a terrible burning pain in my back. I had to sit down and after a few minutes I had to lay down on the ground because I lost all power in my body.

A lady came to me and yelled that they to had to call an ambulance. She also went to my car to get my phone and called my husband. In the mean time I lost the feeling in my legs, I couldn't move anymore and was scared to dead. In the ambulance they gave me lots of medications to reduce the terrible pain. It worked and I also got back the feeling in my legs.

My husband and children arrived. The ambulance brought me to the hospital where they made a scan (I can't remember that at all). I saw a lot of serious looking people, who told us what had happened. I had Type B AD. I had to stay in the hospital for at least 3 weeks. When I reacted well on the medications and my blood pressure would stay low, I could go home. If not, I would need a big operation with lot of possible complications. I heard the story but it didn't have any effect on me. Was it me they were talking about? Later my daughter told me that I was the only one who was completely calm. They brought me to the Intensive Care.

Lack of information to the patients and their family needs to be avoided as much as possible

I reacted great on the medications. They brought me to the nursing department. After 2 days the vascular surgeon came and told me that I could go home. I was very surprised because at that time I was in the hospital for just one week. I went home without any information from the doctors. After 6 weeks I came back to talk with the vascular surgeon about the second scan, which was made.

Doctor-patient communication is very important and much appreciated by the patients

The scans raided him. He had not seen them before. We saw that he was uncertain. He had to speak with his colleagues because the situation was complicated. He told us that I had to have an operation and to make a new appointment. For us the situation was so terrible that we decided never to go back to that man again. We went for a second opinion. There the vascular surgeon explained everything to us. I had a dissection Type B AD from my lungs up to my groin + two aneurysms, one in my chest and one in my belly. These aneurysms were growing. In my opinion there was no other way than to have an operation. The situation could only become worse. They decided to operate me.

During this period, I have had a lot of medical checkups. By giving me some time the wall of the aorta could become stronger what could reduce the risk of a rupture during the operation. The operation took 11 hours. They called my family that the operation went well but the next morning my family received the call that I wasn't doing very well. They had to operate again.

Patients need to know that paraplegia may complicate thoracic and thoraco-abdominal open and endovascular treatment, so they can give their consent to the procedure in an informed way

I could move my legs and everything inside was still working. I was frail but I felt pretty well. They brought me to the nursing department. There were ups-and-downs but after 3 weeks I was good enough to go home. YEAH. My condition was zero but every day I walked a little bit more. They gave me something again the pain in my back and ribs. The skin of my belly was ruptured, caused by the serial of operations. It felt heavy and made walking more difficult.

4

The clinical presentation of Type B aortic dissection

Germano Melissano, Daniele Mascia, Alessandro Grandi and Renata C. Castellano

The first historical report of an aortic dissection (AD) is the account written by King George II's physicians in 1760 [1], who vividly described the symptoms and catastrophic course of the disease. Even if today effective diagnostic tools are routinely available, Type B AD still remains the most frequently misdiagnosed pathology in Emergency departments [2]. Aortic dissection has a well-deserved reputation as a "great masquerader" and physicians perform a prompt and correct diagnosis in as few as 15 to 43% of patients [3]. The main cause for this is that patients suffering from Type B AD usually present a variety of symptoms and signs that mimic other far more common clinical conditions, and these are the first ones to be considered for diagnosis, especially in emergency. Few other conditions require such prompt diagnosis and treatment, since the mortality rate for complicated Type B AD approaches 10% during the first 48 hours if untreated. The rate for undiagnosed Type A AD is even higher.

The clinical presentation of Type B AD is largely the consequence of the blood creating a false channel within the aortic wall. The detachment of the aortic layers, which initiates distal to the left subclavian artery (LSA), rapidly propagates distally and may reach the abdominal aorta within a few heart beats. Three different (not mutually exclusive) clinical patterns can be distinguished that are characterized by:

- pain
- refractory hypertension, and
- malperfusion syndrome (visceral, lower limb and spinal cord ischemia).

4.1 Pain

Pain is usually the most common presenting symptom (in 84.8% of cases) [4] of Type B AD. It has a sudden onset and may be localized in the front or back of the chest, often in the interscapular region. Classically, the descriptions of the pain provided by patients include words such as "ripping," "burning," "splitting," "cutting," or "a hit in the chest", and the pain is also

G. Melissano (melissano.germano@hsr.it)
Vita-Salute San Raffaele University,
Scientific Institute Ospedale San Raffaele, Milan, Italy

G. Melissano - R. Chiesa (eds), Aortic Dissection patients true stories and the innovations that saved their lives

described as the worst they ever felt or that they could imagine [5]. Earlier studies highlighted the characteristics of ripping and tearing along with "migratory" as common terms used by patients to describe the quality of the pain [6]. Radiation of pain may extend to the neck, jaw, and one or both arms.

In some cases, the acute pain can subside after a few hours, being replaced by a deep ache. Then it can come back as strong as at the time of the acute event, and may even move further down if the dissection propagates. Refractory and migrant pain has been reported to be associated with the extension of the dissection and/or impending rupture [7]. The onset of the pain may follow energetic exercise or abrupt movements such as wood chopping, weight-lifting or playing any sport. Less commonly, minor trauma or an emotional stress may precede the event.

Another important finding is the prominent circadian and seasonal periodicity, e.g. aortic dissections present a primary morning peak (8 to 11 am) and a secondary evening peak (5 to 7 pm) [8]. The fact that aortic dissections frequently present in the early morning may be related to a surge in sympathetic activity leading to an increase in shear forces secondary to elevation of blood pressure and heart rate.

In all cases of chest pain, physicians usually have to exclude by appropriate tests other causes of chest discomfort such as myocardial ischemia, pulmonary embolism and pericarditis [9].1 Although, in patients with AD, the EKG findings may result abnormal and serum creatine kinase may be elevated, it has been found that ST-segment elevation occurs rarely in acute AD. However, ST-segment depression is a more common occurrence, and was noted in 16 of 50 (32%; C L 25-39%) patients analyzed by Weiss and coll. [10].

Syncope or loss of consciousness is often associated with the onset of pain, due to the pain itself or to a transient occlusion of the origin of the head vessels creating interferences with the aortic arch baroreceptors. In contrast to myocardial ischemia, patients with acute AD infrequently suffer from nausea or vomiting, and the pain is usually a crescendo in intensity. Other typical features include agitation, and patients can precisely recount the time of onset of the pain.

For this reason, particularly if other cardiac life-threatening conditions have been ruled out as the cause of pain, it is crucial to perform an imaging study of the aorta by means of CT scan. The most common features of acute AD that should alert the physician remain a history or presence of hypertension, sudden onset of pain, and subsequent caudal migration of the pain [11, 12]. Particular attention is necessary in young patients presenting with acute chest pain and a previously diagnosed connective tissue disorder (i.e. Marfan syndrome, Loeys-Dietz syndrome, Ehlers-Danlos syndrome), or in patients with a history of previous aortic or valve replacement.

Several blood tests have been proposed to help in diagnosis, such as D-Dimer or other circulating markers (activators and inhibitors of plasminogen, fibrinogen, elastin fragments and smooth-muscle myosin heavy chain proteins). The role of D-dimer is well established in the literature. Suzuki et al. reported a sensitivity of 97% among 220 patients with a clinical suspicion of aortic dissection [13]. D-dimer has near 100% sensitivity for acute aortic dissection, but very low specificity (the widely used cutoff level of 500 ng/mL for ruling out pulmonary embolism can also reliably rule out aortic dissection) [14]. A positive test should raise suspicion about aortic dissection. Conversely, the high negative predictive value of a negative D-dimer test renders the presence of aortic dissection disease very unlikely.

4.2 Refractory hypertension

Refractory hypertension (rHT) is quite common in patients with Type B AD, and is observed in nearly 70% of initial hospital presentations [6]. Patient demographics play an important role in this particular aspect. Patients younger than 40 years are more likely to present without hypertension. In contrast, elderly patients (aged ≥70 years) are more likely to be hypertensive at presentation, due to underlying atherosclerosis. The mechanism of rHT in patients with Type B AD is not clearly understood. Several hypotheses have been proposed:

- the formation of a "pseudo-coarctation" of the descending aorta due to reduction of flow in the true lumen by the dissection, with resultant upper extremity arterial hypertension
- the result of involvement of the aortic arch baroreceptors, release of catecholamines, and possible activation of the renin-angiotensin-aldosterone system (RAAS)
- renal artery malperfusion, causing renal ischemia, and the subsequent activation of the RAAS.

4.3 Malperfusion syndromes

Major branches of the aorta are commonly involved in the dissection, and the presenting clinical picture may be influenced by symptoms resulting from various degrees of ischemia of one or more of the affected organs. In the large autopsy study of Hirst and colleagues [15], dissection was observed in the celiac, mesenteric, or renal arteries in 28% of patients, in the iliac and femoral arteries in 26% and in the spinal arteries in 1.8% of cases. In large clinical studies of AD, symptomatic malperfusion of the major aortic branches was found in 15 to 33% of the patients [16-19].

As reported by White et al. [20], malperfusion in the setting of aortic dissection is defined as one or more of the following:

- visceral hypoperfusion with an acute abdomen
- abdominal pain out of proportion to physical examination findings in the setting of radiographic hypoperfusion of the mesenteric bed
- lactic acidosis attributed to visceral malperfusion
- need for bowel resection
- renal hypoperfusion, including oliguria or anuria in the setting of worsening renal function tests (creatinine or blood urea nitrogen) or radiographic evidence of impaired renal artery blood flow
- lower and/or upper left extremity hypoperfusion, indicated by abnormal pulse examination in conjunction with leg pain, pallor, paresthesia, or paralysis
- spinal cord hypoperfusion as noted by altered motor function of one or both legs attributed to a possible spinal cord source
- cerebral hypoperfusion as noted by focal neurological signs.

4.4 Conclusions

Type B AD poses considerable challenges to the treating physician in terms of diagnosis and treatment. The understanding of the pathophysiology and clinical presentation has matured in recent years and, nowadays, thanks to the proliferation of effective imaging modalities the diagnosis of this disease is constantly improving. Nevertheless, Type B AD remains the most misdiagnosed disease in the cardiovascular field. Because of its high mortality, especially in the acute phase, an early and correct diagnosis of Type B AD is crucial in patients presenting with acute chest pain, high blood pressure and signs of peripheral and visceral malperfusion, and could save many lives.

REFERENCES

1) Nicholls F. Observations concerning the body of his late majesty. F Philosoph Trans 1761; 52: 265-75.
2) Hansen MS, Nogareda GJ, Hutchison SJ. Frequency of and inappropriate treatment of misdiagnosis of acute aortic dissection. Am J Cardiol 2007; 99(6): 852-6.
3) Sullivan PR, Wolfson AB, Leckey RD, Burke JL. Diagnosis of acute thoracic aortic dissection in the emergency department. Am J Emerg Med 2000; 18: 46-50.
4) Tsai TT, Trimarchi S, Nienaber CA. Acute aortic dissection: perspectives from the International Registry of Acute Aortic Dissection (IRAD). Eur J Vasc Endovasc Surg. 2009; 37(2): 149-59.
5) Svensson LG, Crawford ES. Cardiovascular and vascular disease of the aorta. Philadelphia (PA): W.B. Saunders Company, 1997.
6) Pape LA, Awais M, Woznicki EM, et al. Presentation, diagnosis, and outcomes of acute aortic dissection: 17-year trends from the international registry of acute aortic dissection. J Am Coll Cardiol 2015; 66(4): 350-8.
7) Januzzi JL, Movsowitz HD, Choi J, Abernethy WB, Isselbacher EM. Significance of recurrent pain in acute type B aortic dissection. Am J Cardiol 2001; 87(7): 930-3.
8) Sumiyoshi M, Kojima S, Arima M, et al. Circadian weekly, and seasonal variation at the onset of acute aortic dissection. Am J Cardiol 2002; 89(5): 619-23.
9) Svensson L, Crawford E. Aortic dissection and aortic aneurysm surgery: clinical observations, experimental investigations, and statìstical analyses. Part II. Curr Probl Surg 1992; 29: 915-1057.
10) Weiss P, Weiss I, Zuber M, Ritz R. How many patients with acute dissection of the thoracic aorta would erroneously receive thrombolytic therapy based on the electrocardiographic findings on admission. Am J Cardiol 1993; 72(17): 1329-30.
11) Svensson L, Crawford E. Aortic dissection and aortic aneurysm surgery: clinical observations, experimental investigations, and statìstical analyses. Part II. Curr Probl Surg 1992; (29): 915-1057.
12) Eagle KA, Quertermous T, Kritzer GA, et al. Spectrum of conditions initially suggesting acute aortic dissection but with negative aortograms. Am J Cardiol 1986; 57(4): 322-6.
13) Suzuki T, Distante A, Zizza A, et al.; IRAD-Bio Investigators. Diagnosis of acute aortic dissection by D-dimer: the International Registry of Acute Aortic Dissection Substudy on Biomarkers (IRAD-Bio) experience. Circulation 2009; 119(20): 2702-7.
14) Trimarchi S, Sangiorgi G, Sang X, et al. In search of blood tests for thoracic aortic diseases. Ann Thorac Surg 2010; 90(5): 1735-42.
15) Hirst AE Jr, Johns VJ Jr, Kime SW Jr. Dissecting aneurysm of the aorta: a review of 505 cases. Medicine (Baltimore) 1958; 37(3): 217-79.
16) Borst H, Heinemann M, Stone C. Surgical treatment of aortic dissection. New York (NY): Churchill Livingstone, 1996.
17) Cambria R, Brewster D, Gertler J, et al. Vascular complications associated with spontaneous aortic dissection. J Vasc Surg 1988; 7: 199.
18) Fann JI, Sarris GE, Mitchell RS, et al. Treatment of patients with aortic dissection presenting with peripheral vascular complications. Ann Surg 1990; 212(6): 705-13.
19) Okita Y, Takamoto S, Ando M, Morota T, Kawashima Y. Surgical strategies in managing organ malperfusion as a complication of aortic dissection. Eur J Cardiothorac Surg 1995; 9(5): 242-6; discussion 247.
20) White RA, Miller DC, Criado FJ, et al.; Multidisciplinary Society for Vascular Surgery Outcomes Committee. Report on the results of thoracic endovascular aortic repair for acute, complicated, type B aortic dissection at 30 days and 1 year from a multidisciplinary subcommittee of the Society for Vascular Surgery Outcomes Committee. J Vasc Surg 2011; 53: 1082-90.

5

Introduction, true stories and clinical presentation of Type A aortic dissection

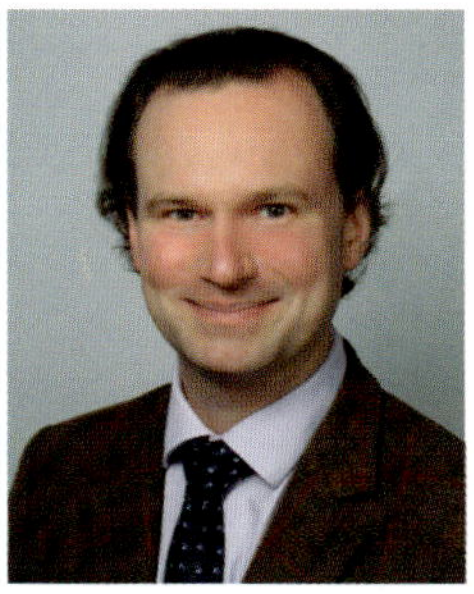

Martin Czerny and Bartosz Rylski

5.1 An introduction to Type A aortic dissection

5.1.1 Natural course

The natural course of acute Type A aortic dissection (AD) is fundamentally different from that of acute Type B AD, as the clinical development within the first week shows. In acute Type A AD, 9 out of 10 patients may die within one week if not treated. Conversely, in acute Type B AD, 9 out of 10 patients will survive in this initial period without access to treatment [1]. In a patient with acute Type A AD, the classical finding at CT scan is a dissection starting in the ascending aorta and propagating downstream (Fig. 5.1). Figure 5.2 shows the intraoperative view of an acute Type A AD before and after opening the aorta, with a view of the thin outer wall. The disease *per se* is rare, and aortas before they dissect have a regular shape and diameter, as can be seen from Figure 5.3 which compares a CT scan taken (by chance) one year before the dissection with the post-dissection CT - the diameter of the aorta prior to dissection was regular. In other words, to date it remains mostly unpredictable who will develop an acute Type A AD, apart from the few people who have connective tissue disease which carries a higher probability to develop the disease [2].

5.1.2 Understanding the disease

Recent work has suggested stratifying patients with acute Type A AD in the same mode as acute Type B AD, namely 'complicated' vs. 'uncomplicated', notwithstanding the fundamentally different impacts of an uncomplicated Type A and an uncomplicated Type B AD [3]. However, such a stratification enables an initial estimation of the complexity of the disease process that one is dealing with. Starting with the uncomplicated kind, an acute Type A AD is classified as uncomplicated in the absence of any kind of malperfusion where hemodynamic in-

Martin Czerny (martin.czerny@universitaets-herzzentrum.de)
University Heart Center Freiburg-Bad Krozingen,
Freiburg, Germany

G. Melissano - R. Chiesa (eds), Aortic Dissection patients true stories and the innovations that saved their lives

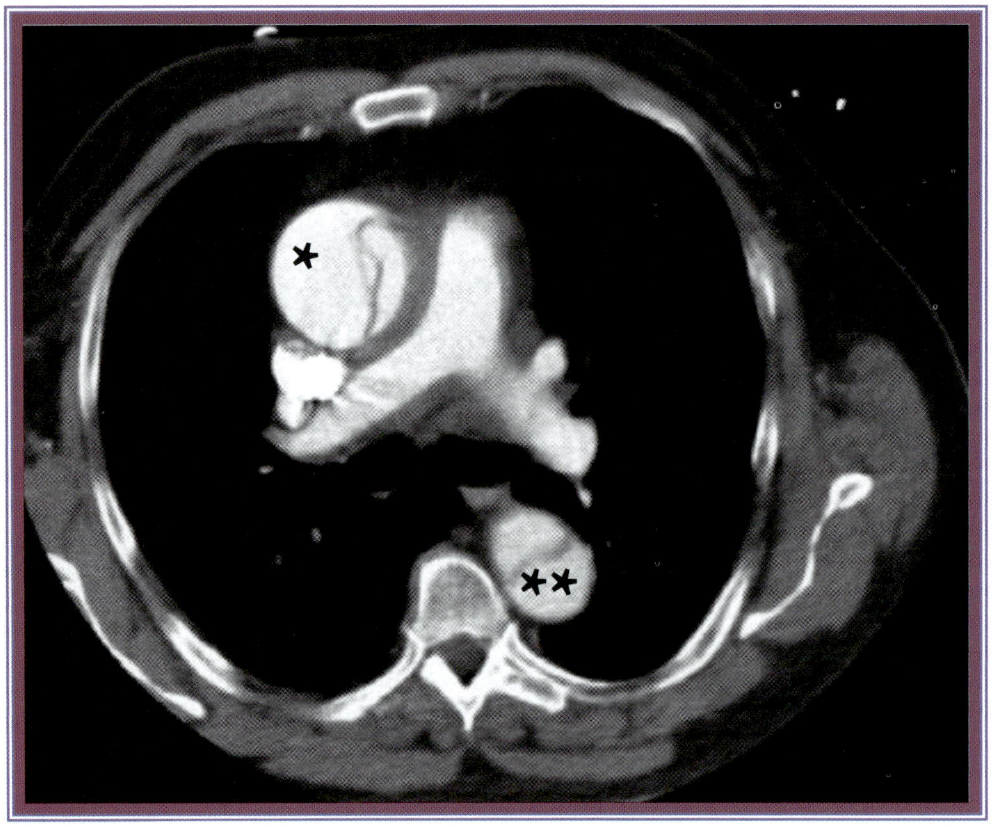

Fig. 5.1 CT scan with a classical finding in a patient with acute Type A AD depicting dissection starting in the ascending aorta (*) and extended to the descending aorta (**).

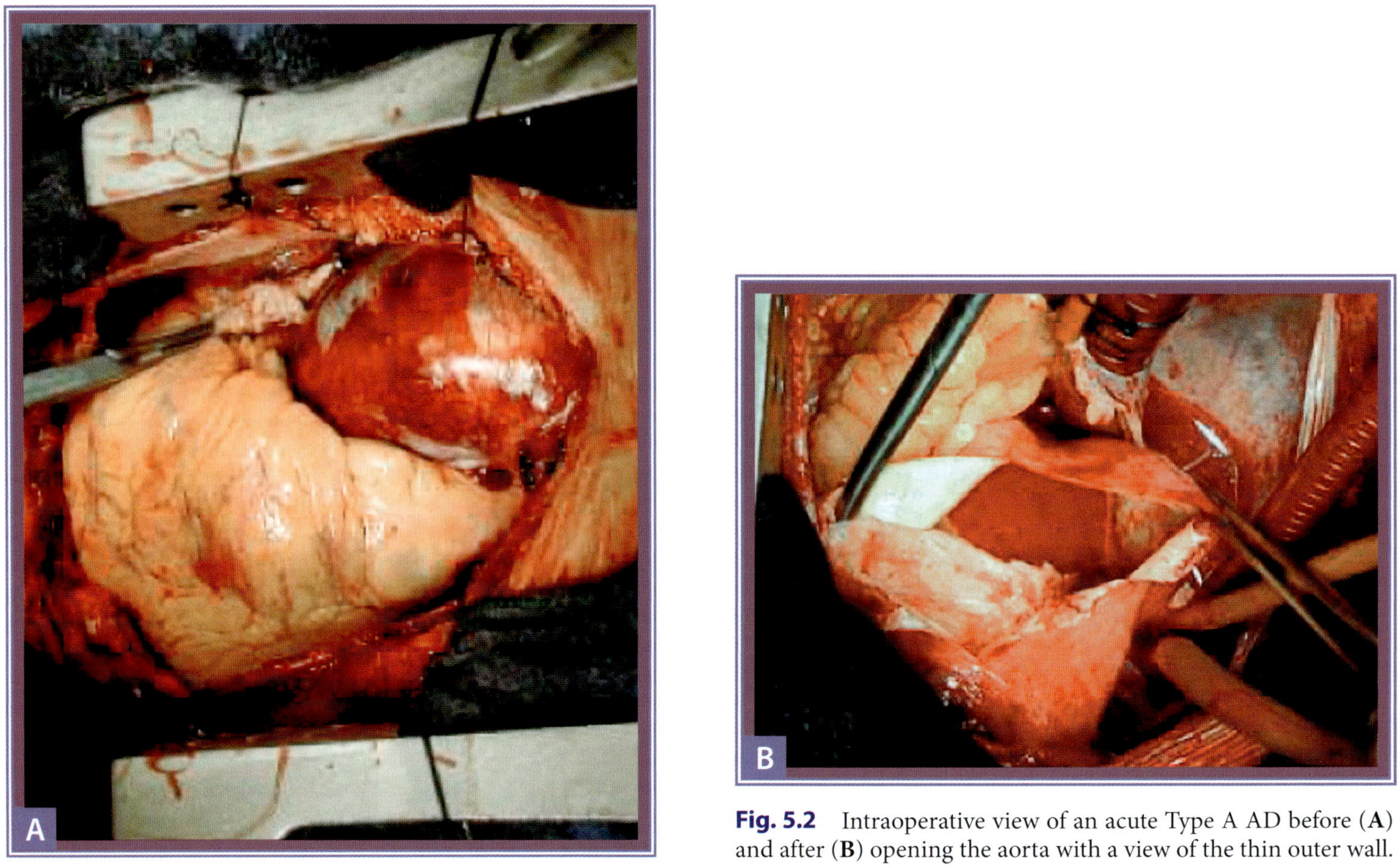

Fig. 5.2 Intraoperative view of an acute Type A AD before (**A**) and after (**B**) opening the aorta with a view of the thin outer wall.

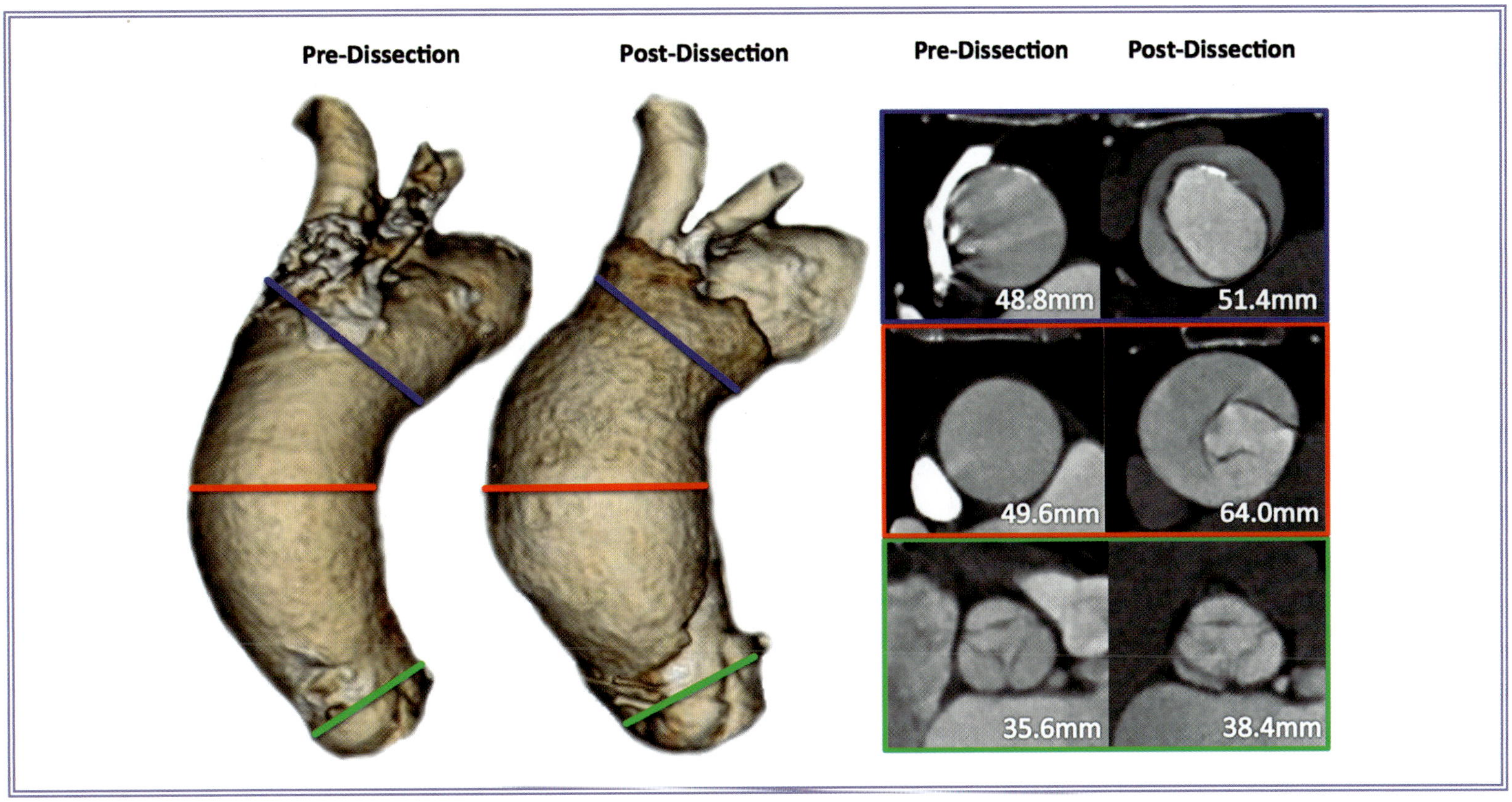

Fig. 5.3 Pre- and post-dissection CT angiography. Volume-rendered images of the ascending aorta and cross-sectional images at sinus of Valsalva (**green**), mid-ascending aorta (**red**), and area immediately proximal to the origin of the brochiocephalic artery (**blue**) with maximum diameters are provided. Reproduced from [2], with permission.

stability due to pericardial effusion is already regarded as malperfusion due to hemodynamic compromise. These so-called uncomplicated "Type A"s are highly likely to have their primary entry tear somewhere between the sinotubular junction and the brachiocephalic trunk, where replacement of the ascending aorta and hemiarch without extending the procedure either to the aortic root or arch is highly likely to solve the issue in more than 90% of cases.

The definition of complicated Type A AD, on the other hand, encompasses each and every clinical case with any kind of malperfusion. According to the specific organ system or systems involved in the malperfusion process, these patients will require a sophisticated modification of the surgical strategy to solve the issue. One example is coronary malperfusion. This is very rarely a cause of true atherosclerosis as AD and obliterative arteriopathy are mutually exclusive, but usually it is a consequence of the damage to the coronary ostia, very often requiring root replacement. Reattachment of a dissected coronary ostia can be very challenging and may sometimes require a change of strategy in order reestablish coronary perfusion [3, 4].

In the case of damage to the supraaortic branches, causing malperfusion associated with neurologic injury, classical ascending aorta and hemiarch replacement may not be sufficient to solve the problem and replacement of one or more supraaortic branches at different levels may be needed. In particular, if a primary entry tear is located in any other location than in the proximal thoracic aorta, extensive surgical correction is needed to fix the associated malperfusion [3, 4]. This clinical scenario is the classic situation for the application of a recent widely introduced surgical concept, i.e. frozen elephant trunk (FET) implantation. This approach permits the entire thoracic aortic pathology to be repaired by combining the best of both worlds, namely the deployment of a distal stent-graft portion in the proximal descending

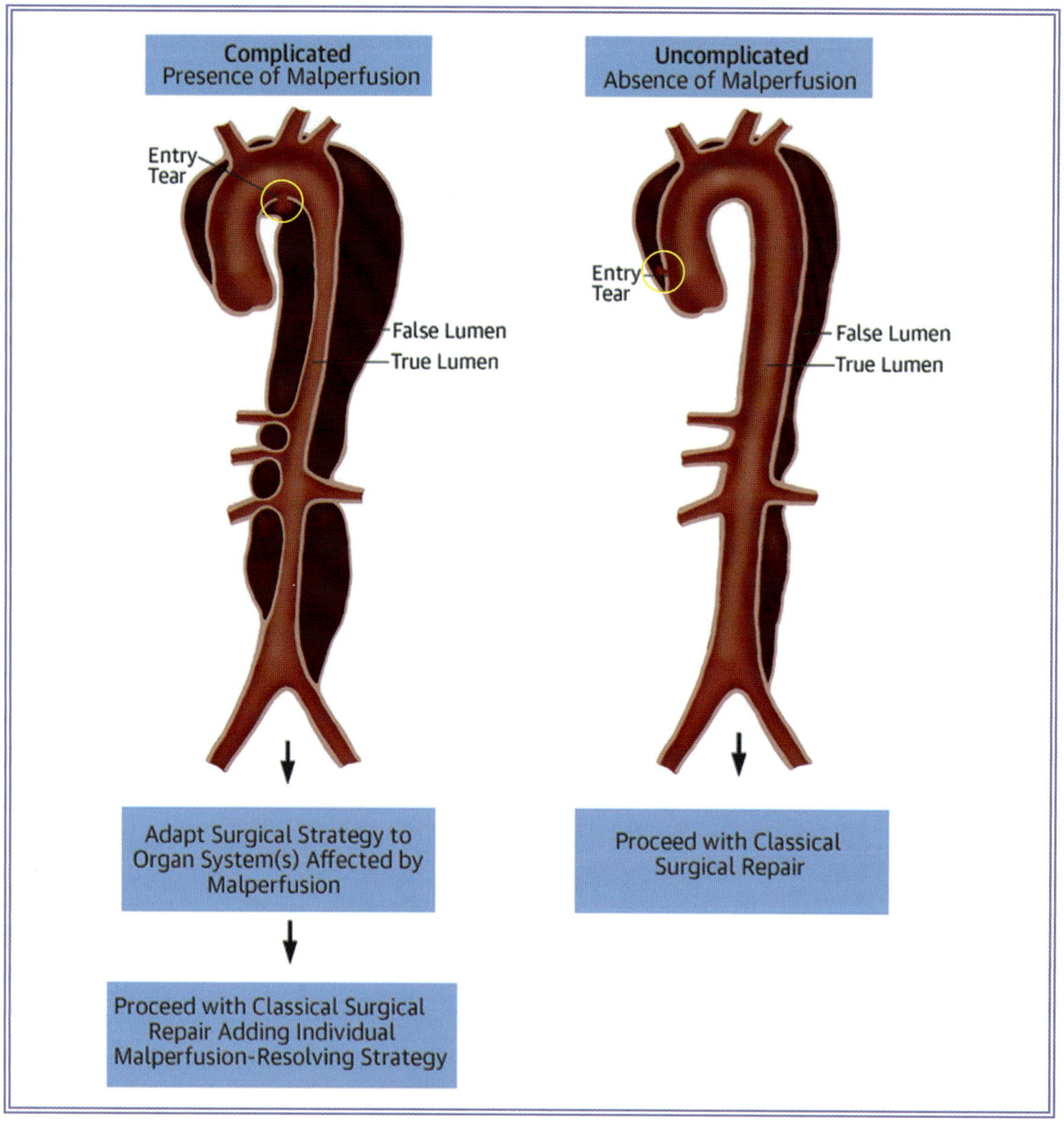

Fig. 5.4 Patients with a primary entry tear in the proximal descending aorta have a higher incidence of malperfusion compared to others. Reproduced from [3], with permission.

aorta for vessel stabilization and of a proximal classical Dacron portion for ascending aorta and arch replacement. Without doubt, this method represents a substantial amplification of the standard ascending aorta and hemiarch procedure and the current indication to apply this method should be followed very strictly [5].

Hence, as with acute Type B AD, the key issue is to appropriately address the primary entry tear, since effective treatment of the very segment where the primary entry tear is located can promote patient survival by preventing progression and eventual rupture, will resolve malperfusion if present, and very often will prevent progression of the disease, in particular as regards diameter increase in the long term [6]. The importance of the location of the primary entry tear in determining whether a dissection will be complicated or uncomplicated is highlighted in the schematic representation in Figure 5.4, i.e. patients with a primary entry tear in the proximal descending aorta have a higher incidence of malperfusion compared to others.

5.1.3 The past

Forty years ago, surgery for acute Type A AD was regarded as a "warm autopsy". The groundbreaking work by Griepp et al. who introduced the concept of deep hypothermia to enable extensive proximal thoracic aortic surgery through a lowered metabolism paved the way for a standardized approach to surgically correct the underlying pathology [7].

However, until the early 1990s, clinical results were impossible to achieve on account of neurologic injury associated to the hypothermic circulatory arrest time needed to fix the pathology.

5.1.4 The present

The major step forward that led to current standards was the introduction of the selective antegrade cerebral perfusion concept during hypothermic circulatory arrest, the credit for which is shared equally between Daniel Guilmet, Jean Bachet and Teruhisa Kazui [8, 9]. In addition, routine cannulation of the right subclavian artery as inflow for arterial return during acute and chronic thoracic aortic surgery provided a major boost for improved results [10]. These two modifications, which cut mortality and morbidity in half, have led to the excellent results that are reported today. It should also be mentioned that the best results are achieved by centers of excellence with a respectively high caseload, as this is decisive for success in each and every specialty [11].

5.1.5 The future

Endovascular therapy has been rapidly embraced by the medical community in various acute and chronic thoracic and abdominal aortic pathologies, and has changed current medical practice [12-14].

However, its application in the proximal thoracic aorta has confronted physicians with unforeseen challenges, given that the composition of the aortic wall is fundamentally different in the aortic root and the ascending aorta with an extremely high degree of elasticity which cannot be adequately addressed by any current self-expanding technology.

In addition, the propagation of the dissection process in many cases also has a retrograde component against the bloodstream, which can very often affect the non-coronary sinus. As a consequence, the concept of a landing zone had to be converted into the concept of a sealing zone with all its inherent limitations. This has led to the proposal of a new pioneering concept, namely the introduction of a valve-carrying endovascular conduit, the "Endo-Bentall", as the aortic annulus is the only component of the entire proximal thoracic aortic functional unit which will remain unaffected by the dissection disease process. The future will show if this concept is the right way to advance the field in acute Type A AD [15].

5.1.6 Follow-up

After having survived surgery for the acute situation, the story continues as many patients will experience the sequelae of the chronic disease process in the years to come. Remaining dissection of downstream aortic segments predisposes to chronic dilation, leading to aneurysm formation, which eventually will warrant treatment.

This fact highlights the need for aortic centers where the aorta is seen, followed and treated as an organ and patients are subject to a strict follow-up protocol, as this is the only means to anticipate, treat or prevent.

5.2 The true stories of Type A dissection

The aim of this section is to share the personal experience of patients who suffered an acute Type A AD. We aimed at synthesizing the pattern according to the following components: the description of pain which generally has an abrupt onset but still may be missed by ER physicians, since only 4 out of 1000 patients with chest pain actually have acute AD; the migrant nature of the pain, which is a consequence of the propagation of the dissection; and the clinical appearance of any kind of malperfusion (per se defined as complicated Type A AD).

5.2.1 Description of the pain

Björn, 48 years old, Sweden

Inside a church bell

I got ill sitting at a desk in an office of a colleague at 08:40 in the morning, stretching for a cup of coffee. It started by me getting confused: I got an enormous feeling of anxiety and panic. I didn't feel the pain in the beginning. I rose, excused myself and said "I'm going to the toilet". In that moment the pain hit me in the chest, throat and back. It was like my head was inside a church bell. The pain was sharp, and penetrated everything. I thought I was going to die.

Alanis, 43 years old, England

You've got mail

It happened at 12.15 pm. I was sitting down sending an email. I felt a huge pressure around my chest and back which also felt like an achy pain, my thighs and upper arms went numb and I had pains in my neck and jaw. I had to stop what I was doing and take deep breaths but the pain wasn't excruciating. After a few minutes the feeling came back in my arms and thighs and the pain in my neck and jaw went, I still had the pressure/pain on my chest and back.

Alisha, 60 years old, USA

An intense workout

One of my goals for my 60th birthday was to complete an unassisted pull-up to go along with the full push-ups I had managed to accomplish a few months before. After completing a set of lunges with shoulder presses and a set of pull-ups, I felt a tearing pain go across my chest, and I went to the floor. My trainer asked if I was okay and I said "No", as my mind was telling me "cardiac insufficiency". My shoulder blades began to hurt. Staff elevated my feet and gave me some water. The ambulance was quick to arrive, noted that I had a drop in blood pressure, and took me to the nearest ER.

Mackenzie, 30 years old, New Zealand

Out cycling

After a routine check, I was out cycling with a friend when I felt a pop in the center of my chest. I decided I might hop off my bike as I didn't feel quite right and didn't want to alarm my friend. Then, major pain.

Ingrid, 51 years old, Sweden

Lovely family reunion. Or was it?

One day in August, my life changed with the notion a little click in my chest. It felt like the first lash of a little fetus in the womb, the very first time. Or like the wig of a fish-tail. The time was approximately 20:30 on a beautiful Saturday night. A lovely family reunion with barbecue was over and I had just picked two fine bouquets of garden flowers and was about to only attach the rubber band around them, when it happened. I told my husband "Something's happened right now, here in my chest, and it's causing strong pain".

Chan, 34 years old, China

The day two people were born

On a Saturday I was chatting with my parents when I felt a throbbing pain in between my chest. We panicked and thought of options to get medical help. My belief in the quotation "A friend in need is a friend indeed" became stronger with this experience. My husband called our close friends for support as we headed to the hospital and they were by our side until the entire ordeal was over. We were attended by the doctor on call at the hospital who diagnosed it to be acid reflux and prescribed paracetamol to relieve the pain.

Through the night the pain subsided and I woke up on Sunday to a cheerful me in good spirits to wish my sister a happy birthday! Sunday was great, spent the entire day with no pain at all. The pain started again the next day and stopped only two days later, Tuesday, the day two people were born – my second life and my baby girl, my life. I had piercing pain in the middle of my chest and at the very same point behind my back.

At 5:30 am the pain really intensified and we decided to page my obstetrician and rush to the hospital again. He made a call and I was immediately rushed to one of the best teaching/public hospitals. Initially things moved slowly and they monitored my baby's heartbeat, who was doing great.

The pain subsided through the day with the blood pressure medication. By evening they had narrowed down on what was wrong with me. My aorta had ruptured and needed to be fixed immediately. They would do a Caesarian section first and get the baby out and after that the aortic surgery would be done.

Josh, 35 years old, USA

Painless dissection

I survived five weeks with an untreated ascending aortic dissection in 1998. I was 35 at the time. The main reason in my case for delaying in the diagnosis was that I never really had a lot of pain – other than briefly – and that I didn't really feel much worse than "usual". It all started on my 35th birthday. I got ready to go to bed, sat down on the edge of the bed, stretched, and the pain in the chest hit me, hard. It kind of "popped" in my chest, just on the left edge of the breastbone and then hurt. A lot.

I thought "Heart attack?". I called the doctor's office my company used for regular health care. I was given an appointment before lunch the next day. When I got there the nurse first took an EKG. It showed nothing out of the ordinary. Then I met the doctor, and told him about the sudden pain the night before, how it "popped" in my chest and came. He made a physical exam, including listening to my heart. He couldn't find anything wrong with me. He didn't hear anything strange listening to my heart. He told me he thought it might have been a muscle in the chest jumping in place.

On the evening of the third day I started feeling ill, and then became bedfast for five days in what I assumed was the 'flu. But there weren't the typical flu symptoms; it just felt like high fever. I noticed that I had less and less energy, and hardly could do anything without getting tired.

Kimberly, 52 years old, USA

Electric shocks

At 5:00 am, excruciating pain that was radiating throughout my entire body awakened me. I was suddenly seized by what felt like hundreds of electrical shocks throughout my chest and abdomen. Surely, this is what it must feel like to be electrocuted, I remember thinking. While others have documented a “tearing sensation” as the first, telltale sign of an ascending aortic dissection, my symptoms were more like a series of intense electrical shocks. I lay in bed for about ten minutes, waiting for the pain to subside.

Norina, 64 years old, Germany

Saturday morning storm

On a Saturday morning I awoke in the morning at the usual time around 7.00 am, feeling generally unwell and I had a stomach upset but expected to just get on with the day. I went downstairs just after 08.30 and started my usual routine of tidying up where my dog had slept in her crate. At about 08.45 as I bent forward I felt something like a pop in the left side of my chest about mid-point just under my heart, almost immediately followed by a loud whoosh-ing noise in my head as if I was in a plane and all the windows had been blown out. It was so loud and frightening. But I managed to get myself to stand upright by leaning on to the dog crate.

5.2.2 The migrant pain

Björn, 48 years old, Sweden

The pain was in my back, my chest, my throat (left side of throat). All of a sudden it felt like someone pulled down a zipper inside my stomach. From up towards down. It did not hurt. Then my kidneys started hurting. When I breathed in, the pain culminated.

Alisha, 60 years old, USA

The ambulance was quick to arrive, noted that I had a drop in blood pressure, and took me to the nearest ER. Based on my description of what had happened and my vitals , the doctors there in the ER did an immediate CT scan and discovered the dissection. I had never heard of an aortic dissection; all I knew was that something seriously bad was happening.

Philippa, 54 years old, Sweden

I wonder whose hand is lying on my lap and realize it’s my own. I have pain but not very strong at this point. The pain is slowly moving down into the stomach.

Maria, 64 years old, Italy

Shortly after my return home on bending down to a cupboard I had an uncomfortable taught/pulling vibration sensation down the left side of my face from the temple and down the jaw accompanied by an extremely loud high-pitched noise in my left ear – much louder than the normal tinnitus whistle. I thought I was having a stroke but this only lasted a short time – no more than a few minutes.

Mackenzie, 30 years old, New Zealand

I fell to my knees as with every heart beat the pain went down and I couldn't breathe. Everything hurt. Back, chest, abdomen.

5.2.3 The clinical appearance of any kind of malperfusion

Ann Mary, 66 years old, USA

I was camping in Colorado and getting ready to go to bed for the night when the pain struck. It was the worst I had ever experienced and my right leg became paralyzed. I could not reach for my cell but I realized my car keys were in my hand. So I hit the emergency button to sound the alarm on my car several times and someone came to see what was wrong. I asked him to call 911 - I thought I was having a heart attack. The ambulance arrived. Still in so much pain and with my leg still paralyzed they got me on the stretcher and took me to a clinic in a small town. In the ambulance, my leg began to regain strength and when I arrived I was able to walk normally.

Brenda, 47 years old, England

I could hear my son was still about in the house and I shouted his name and within a few seconds he came to find me. The strange sensation in my legs was getting rapidly worse - to say they were numb is not right - the sensation was that of a cold ballooning sensation. It was as if this part of me was being transformed, as if the lower part of my body and both legs were being blown up with something cold making it feel as if I was sitting on this cold squidgy cushion which was my body. I had lost all normal sensation in this part of my body and it was extremely unpleasant and worse on the left side. At times it eased off a little but then returned worse than before.

"Or better- the ability of the physician to listen to what the patient is saying"

5.3 The clinical presentation of Type A aortic dissection

5.3.1 Initial clinical presentation

Pain may be the best biomarker available in acute AD, be it Type A or B. It is all about asking the right questions, listening to the answers, and then doing the right things. Acute chest pain during the course of an AD is unique, as we have seen in the previous section. And also the propagation of pain is a perfect surrogate of the dynamics of the disease, which is incomparable to any other thoracic pathology whether it be related to pulmonary parenchyma (e.g. pneumothorax) or the vertebral column (e.g. disc prolapse).

5.3.2 Diagnosis

Only 4 out of 1000 patients referred with acute chest pain to an Emergency department will finally be diagnosed with acute AD. In other words, it is a rare disease. Therefore, the only way to increase the percentage of correct diagnoses is by raising awareness about the disease so that the signs prompt its suspicion. If the physician listens closely, patients will describe perfectly the development of pain and thereby will enable the treating physician to distinguish between unspecific chest pain for any reason and classical dissection pain, e.g. "the pain started in my anterior chest, moved towards the back in between my shoulders and went downwards" or "the pain started in between my shoulders, went upwards and moved across to the anterior chest". This is what patients tell you when they have sustained an acute Type A AD, but you have to ask the right questions and you have to listen closely. Then, after the suspicion has been raised, the next question is whether to perform or not a CT scan, and what the threshold is for making the decision. Another variable entering the clinical arena are weather conditions, as increasing evidence suggests that there is a clear correlation between seasons as well as altering weather conditions, suggesting a peak in spring and autumn as well as a peak during temperature changes, in particular from warmer to colder temperatures. Similar observations have been made in patients with acute coronary syndromes [16]. As a consequence, raised suspicion of Emergency Room physicians during the above-mentioned changes in weather conditions may also help in identifying individuals with acute AD.

REFERENCES

1) Mészáros I, Mórocz J, Szlávi J, et al. Epidemiology and clinicopathology of aortic dissection. Chest 2000; 117: 1271-8.
2) Rylski B, Blanke P, Beyersdorf F, et al. How does the ascending aorta geometry change when it dissects? J Am Coll Cardiol 2014; 63: 1311-9.
3) Czerny M, Schoenhoff F, Etz C, et al. The Impact of pre-operative malperfusion on outcome in acute Type A aortic dissection: results from the GERAADA registry. J Am Coll Cardiol 2015; 65: 2628-35.
4) Pacini D, Leone A, Belotti LM, et al.; RERIC (Emilia Romagna Cardiac Surgery Registry) Investigators. Acute type A aortic dissection: significance of multiorgan malperfusion. Eur J Cardiothorac Surg 2013; 43(4): 820-6.
5) Shrestha M, Bachet J, Bavaria J, et al. Current status and recommendations for use of the frozen elephant trunk technique: a position paper by the Vascular Domain of EACTS. Eur J Cardiothorac Surg 2015; 47: 759-69.
6) Krähenbühl E, Maksimovic S, Sodeck G, et al. What makes the difference between the natural course of a remaining type B dissection after type A repair and a primary type B aortic dissection? Eur J Cardiothorac Surg 2012;41: e110-5.
7) Griepp RB, Stinson EB, Hollingsworth JF, Buehler D. Prosthetic replacement of the aortic arch. J Thorac Cardiovasc Surg 1975; 70: 1051-63.
8) Guilmet D, Roux PM, Bachet J, et al. A new technic of cerebral protection. Surgery of the aortic arch. Presse Med 1986; 15: 1096-8.
9) Kazui T, Inoue N, Ito T, et al. Clinical study on surgical treatment of aortic arch aneurysm using selective cerebral perfusion or hypothermic circulatory arrest. Nihon Kyobu Geka Gakkai Zasshi 1989; 37: 44-8.
10) Sabik JF, Lytle BW, McCarthy PM, Cosgrove DM. Axillary artery: an alternative site of arterial cannulation for patients with extensive aortic and peripheral vascular disease. J Thorac Cardiovasc Surg 1995; 109: 885-90.
11) Lenos A, Bougioukakis P, Irimie V, et al. Impact of surgical experience on outcome in surgery of acute type A aortic dissection. Eur J Cardiothorac Surg 2015; 48: 491-6.
12) Nienaber CA, Kische S, Rousseau H, et al.; INSTEAD-XL trial. Endovascular repair of type B aortic dissection: long-term results of the randomized investigation of stent grafts in aortic dissection trial. Circ Cardiovasc Interv 2013; 6(4): 407-16.
13) Czerny M, Funovics M, Sodeck G, et al. Results after thoracic endovascular aortic repair in penetrating atherosclerotic ulcers. Ann Thorac Surg 2011; 92: 562-6.
14) Gottardi R, Funovics M, Eggers N, et al. M. Supra-aortic transposition for combined vascular and endovascular repair of aortic arch pathology. Ann Thorac Surg 2008; 86: 1524-9. Erratum in: Ann Thorac Surg 2014; 97: 739.
15) Rylski B, Szeto WY, Bavaria JE, et al. Development of a single endovascular device for aortic valve replacement and ascending aortic repair. J Card Surg 2014; 29: 371-6.
16) Vencloviene J, Babarskiene R, Dobozinskas P, Siurkaite V. Effects of weather conditions on emergency ambulance calls for acute coronary syndromes. Int J Biometeorol 2015; 59: 1083-93.

6

Clinical and molecular genetics of thoracic aortic aneurysm and dissection

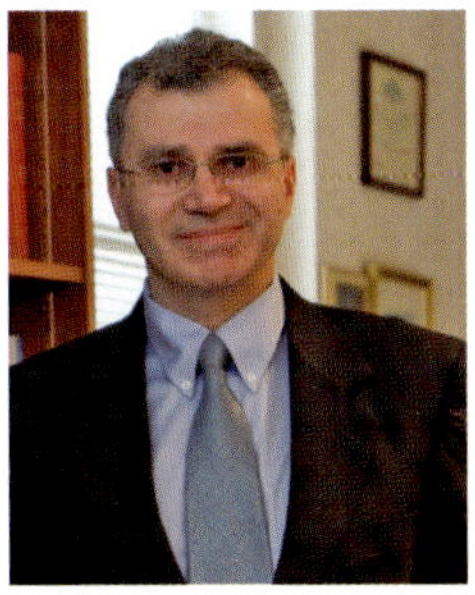

John A. Elefteriades, Adam J. Brownstein and Bulat A. Ziganshin

6.1 Introduction

The development of an ascending thoracic aortic aneurysm (TAA) is a silent but potentially fatal disease, as it can lead to dissection or rupture. The annual incidences of aortic dissection (AD) and rupture are both estimated to be 3.5 per 100,000 patients [1]. However, the actual incidence of dissection is most likely underestimated given that these patients are misdiagnosed up to 30% of the time [2], often with myocardial infarctions [3]. Given that the natural history of TAAs is to enlarge progressively until dissection or rupture occurs, treatment is targeted at preventing such complications through surgery [4].

However, studies have shown that nearly 60% of patients with Type A dissections have aortic diameters <5.5 cm, the commonly used cutoff for surgical intervention, and 40% of patients have diameters <5 cm [5]. Despite these disheartening results, AD are inextricably linked to TAAs, as patients with an aorta ≥4.5 cm are 6.3 thousand times more likely to have an AD than those with aortas ≤3.4 cm [6]. Given the potential lethality of complications associated with TAAs (the most devastating being a dissection [7] which primarily determines life expectancy) [8], it is imperative for clinicians to better understand which patients are at risk of developing thoracic aortic aneurysm and dissection (TAAD).

The concept that inherited conditions can manifest with the formation of TAAs began with the discovery of Marfan Syndrome in 1896 and with the recognition in 1912 that aortic disease is an important clinical manifestation [7]. Since then, more than 30 heritable conditions have been described that can potentially manifest with aortic and arterial aneurysms [9]. However, the familial nature of non-syndromic TAAD was not determined until the late 1990s [10, 11]. At Yale, the discovery of a family with 3 generations of AD, including a 12-year-old girl, who was the youngest individual to die from an AD at Yale-New Haven Hospital [12], incited a search for the genetic underpinnings of TAAD. Ever since this search began, there has been an explosion in the discovery of new genes that underlie TAAD.

Currently, the genetic nature of TAAD is well established, and multiple genes have been shown to cause TAAD [7, 8, 12-14]. To date, there are at least 30 genes that are known to contribute to TAAD (Table 6.1), with new candidate genes being discovered regularly. The major-

John A. Elefteriades (john.elefteriades@yale.edu)
Yale University School of Medicine,
New Haven, CT, USA

G. Melissano - R. Chiesa (eds), Aortic Dissection patients true stories and the innovations that saved their lives

Table 6.1 Genes causative of syndromic and non-syndromic thoracic aortic aneurysm and dissection

Gene	Location	Protein	Syndromic TAAD	Non-syndromic FTAAD	Associated disease/syndrome	Inheritance	OMIM No. (phenotype)
ACTA2	10q23.31	Smooth muscle α-actin	+	+	FTAA 6 + multisystemic smooth muscle dysfunction	AD	611788 + 613834
BGN	Xq28	Biglycan	+	–	Unidentified CTD	X-linked	301870 (gene)
COL1A1	17q21.33	Collagen 1 α1 chain	+	–	Ehlers-Danlos syndrome, arthrochalasia type (VIIa) + classic type	AD	130060 + 130000
COL1A2	7q21.3	Collagen 1 α2 chain	+	–	Ehlers-Danlos syndrome, arthrochalasia type (VIIb) + cardiac valvular type	AD	130060 + 225320
COL3A1	2q23.2	Collagen 3 α1 chain	+	–	Ehlers-Danlos syndrome, vascular type (IV)	AD	130050
COL4A5	Xq22.3	Collagen 4 α5 chain	+	–	Alport syndrome	XLD	301050
COL5A1	9q34.3	Collagen 5 α1 chain	+	–	Ehlers-Danlos syndrome, classic type (I)	AD	130000
COL5A2	2q23.2	Collagen 5 α2 chain	+	–	Ehlers-Danlos syndrome, classic type (II)	AD	130000
EFEMP2	11q13.1	Fibulin-4	+	–	Cutis laxa, AR type Ib	AR	614437
ELN	7q11.23	Elastin	+	–	Cutis laxa, AD	AD	123700
EMILIN1	2p23.3	Elastin microfibril interfacer 1	+	–	Unidentified CTD	AD	130660 (gene)
FBN1	15q21.1	Fibrillin-1	+	+	Marfan syndrome	AD	154700
FBN2	5q23.3	Fibrillin-2	+	–	Contractural arachnodactyly	AD	121050
FLNA	Xq28	Filamin A	+	–	Periventricular heterotopia	XLD	300049
FOXE3	1p33	Forkhead box 3	-	+	FTAA	AD	601094 (gene)
LOX	5q23.1	Lysyl oxidase	-	+	FTAA	AD	153455 (gene)
MAT2A	2p11.2	Methionine adenosyltransferase II alpha	-	+	FTAA	AD	601468 (gene)
MFAP5	12p13.31	Microfibril-associated glycoprotein 2	-	+	FTAA 9	AD	616166
MYH11	16p13.11	Smooth muscle myosin heavy chain	-	+	FTAA 4	AD	132900
MYLK	3q21.1	Myosin light chain kinase	-	+	FTAA 7	AD	613780
NOTCH1	9q34.3	NOTCH1	-	+	FTAA with BAV	AD	109730
PRKG1	10q11.2-q21.1	Type 1 cGMP-dependent protein kinase	-	+	FTAA 8	AD	615436
SKI	1p36.33-p36.32	Sloan Kettering proto-oncoprotein	+	–	Shprintzen-Goldberg syndrome	AD	182212
SLC2A10	20q13.12	Glucose transporter 10	+	–	Arterial tortuosity syndrome	AR	208050
SMAD2	18q21.1	SMAD2	+	–	Unidentified CTD with arterial aneurysms/dissections	AD	601366 (gene)

Table 6.1 *(Continued)*

Gene	Location	Protein	Syndromic TAAD	Non-syndromic FTAAD	Associated disease/syndrome	Inheritance	OMIM No. (phenotype)
SMAD3	15q22.33	SMAD3	+	+	Loeys-Dietz syndrome Type 3	AD	613795
SMAD4	18q21.2	SMAD4	+	–	JP/HHT syndrome	AD	175050
TGFB2	1q41	TGF-β2	+	+	Loeys-Dietz syndrome Type 4	AD	614816
TGFB3	14q24.3	TGF-β3	+	-	Loeys-Dietz syndrome Type 5	AD	615582
TGFBR1	9q22.33	TGF-β receptor type 1	+	+	Loeys-Dietz syndrome Type 1	AD	609192
TGFBR2	3p24.1	TGF-β receptor type 2	+	+	Loeys-Dietz syndrome Type 2	AD	610168

A "+" symbol in the syndromic TAAD column indicates that the gene is causative of syndromic TAAD (same for the non-syndromic TAAD column). A "– " symbol in the syndromic TAAD column indicates that the gene is not known to cause syndromic TAAD (same for the non-syndromic TAAD column).
AD indicates autosomal dominant; AR, autosomal recessive; BAV, bicuspid aortic valve; CTD, connective tissue disease; FTAA, familial thoracic aortic aneurysm; FTAAD, familial thoracic aortic aneurysm and dissection; HHT, hereditary hemorrhagic telangiectasia; JP, juvenile polyposis; OMIM, Online Mendelian Inheritance in Man; TGF, transforming growth factor; TAAD, thoracic aortic aneurysm and dissection; *TGFBR*, TGF-β receptor; XLD, X-linked dominant.

ity of these genes encode proteins involved in the extracellular matrix (FBN1, FBN2, COL3A1, EFEMP2), the smooth muscle cell contractile unit (*ACTA2, MYH11, MYLK, FLNA, PRKG1*), or the TGF-β signaling pathway (*TGFβ2, TGFβ3, TGFBR1, TGFBR2, SMAD3, SLC2A10*).

The clinical impact of these exciting discoveries has been significant, since the specific mutated gene can be used to detect those at risk for dissection at aortic diameters <5.0 cm [15]. For example, the *MYLK* gene is exclusively involved in AD [16], while the *ACTA2* gene causes AD at small sizes [17, 18]. Furthermore, the 2010 U.S. Guidelines for the Diagnosis and Management of Patients with Thoracic Aortic Disease [19] reflect the significant contribution of genetics to TAAD. These Guidelines recommend: aortic imaging for first-degree relatives of patients with TAA and/or dissection to identify those with asymptomatic disease (Class I, Level of Evidence: B), and aortic imaging for second-degree relatives if one or more first-degree relatives are found to have thoracic aortic dilatation, aneurysm, or dissection (Class IIa, Level of Evidence: B).

While this relatively new genetic information poses potential challenges in terms of counseling patients regarding the appropriate time for surgical intervention, it also opens up a window of opportunity to offer more personalized care to patients based on their underlying genetics. This chapter will address the current understanding of the genetics of thoracic aortic aneurysm and dissection and will offer clinical implications specific for each causative gene.

6.2 Genetic nature of thoracic aortic aneurysm and dissection

While Marfan syndrome represents the most well studied disease that contributes to TAAD, studies have demonstrated that it accounts for less than 5% of all cases of TAAD [12, 13]. As previously mentioned, our discovery of a family with three generations of AD led us to believe that there must be other unidentified genes that contribute to TAAD. Therefore, our team at the Aortic Institute at Yale began investigating hundreds of families and constructing pedigrees to determine if patients have other affected family members. Among the first 100 families that were investigated, we found that 21% of patients had an affected family member [11] (Fig. 6.1), which was the exact same percentage that Dr. Diana Milewicz and colleagues had also reported [10]. This percentage is undoubtedly a marked underestimate, as it represents only those family members who have been imaged and found positive for aneurysm. Routine imaging of all family members would yield a much higher percentage.

With this newfound knowledge of a familial predisposition for TAAD, we sought to investigate the mechanism of inheritance among these families. We discovered that the predomi-

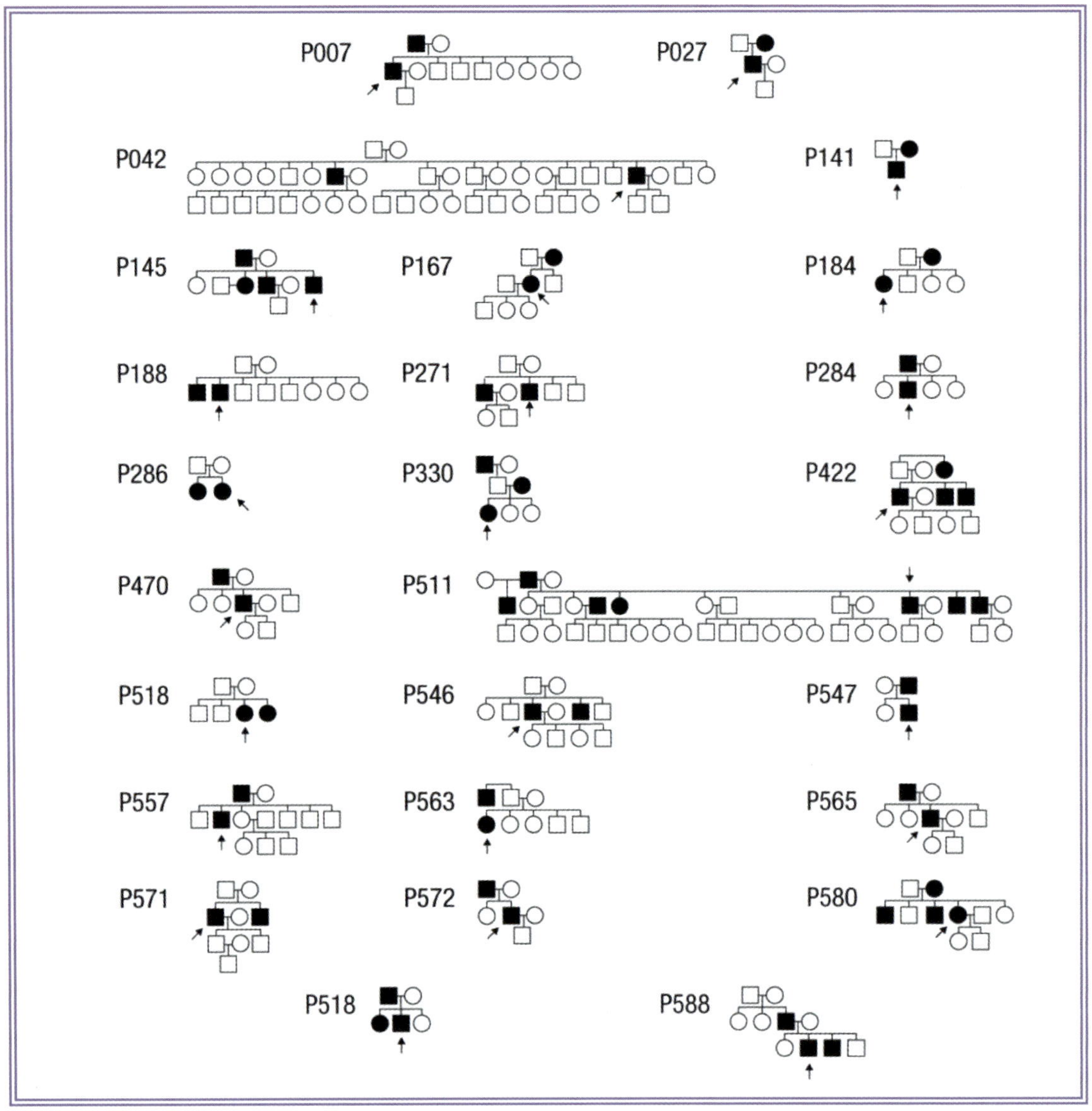

Fig. 6.1 21 out of 100 of the first probands investigated by the authors with TAAD had a positive family history. These 21 positive pedigrees are displayed here. Reproduced from [11], with permission.

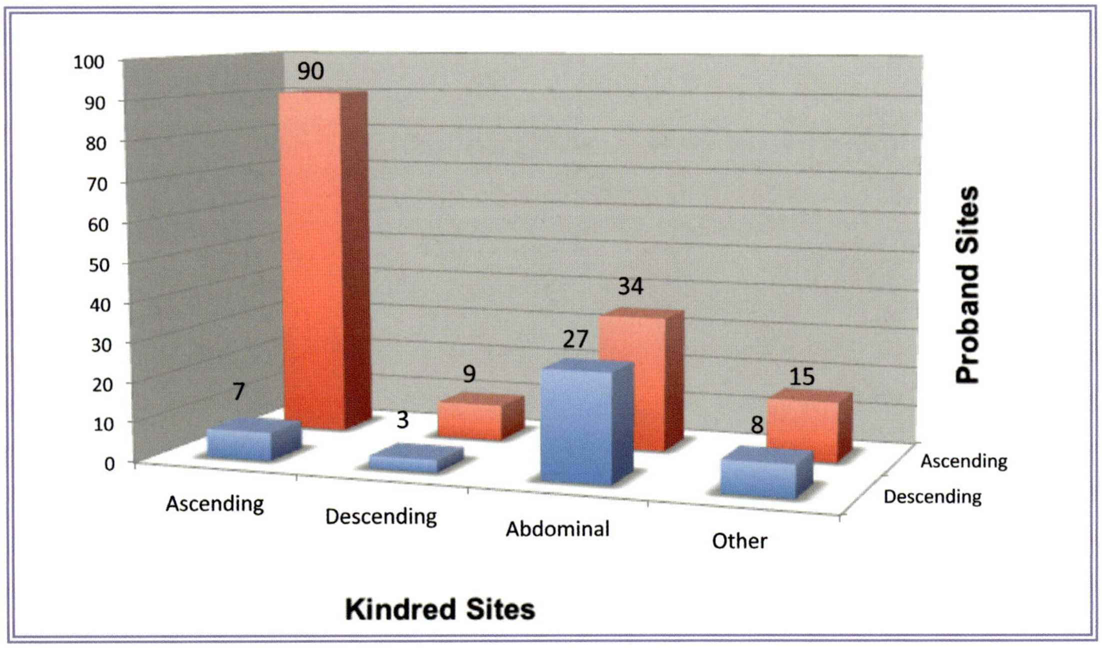

Fig. 6.2 Distribution of sites of arterial aneurysms and dissections in kindred of familial probands. Reproduced from [20], with permission.

nant mechanism of inheritance was autosomal dominant (38.5%), indicating that members within each generation of families are likely to be affected [20]. This study, along with a prior study from Dr. Milewicz [21], demonstrated that TAAD is inherited with reduced penetrance and variable expressivity, indicating that a single gene is the most likely culprit for some familial aneurysms [22]. Other modes of inheritance were identified as well, including autosomal recessive in 26.9% of patients and autosomal dominant or X-linked in 23.1% of patients [20]. 11.5% of patients exhibited other modes of inheritance.

As we continued to investigate the family histories of our patients, we observed that those patients with ascending aortic disease were more likely to have family members with ascending aortic disease as well [20] (Fig. 6.2). On the contrary, those with descending aortic disease were most likely to have family members with abdominal aortic aneurysms [20]. These observations led us to conclude that ascending aortic aneurysms represent a different disease from descending and abdominal aortic aneurysms [12], possibly related to the different embryological origin of the ascending aorta (neural crest) vs. the descending and abdominal aorta (mesoderm) [23-26]. While ascending aneurysms are highly familial, non-calcified, and non-atherosclerotic, descending and abdominal aortic aneurysms are highly associated with atherosclerosis and are often calcified and irregular with clot formation [12] (Fig. 6.3).

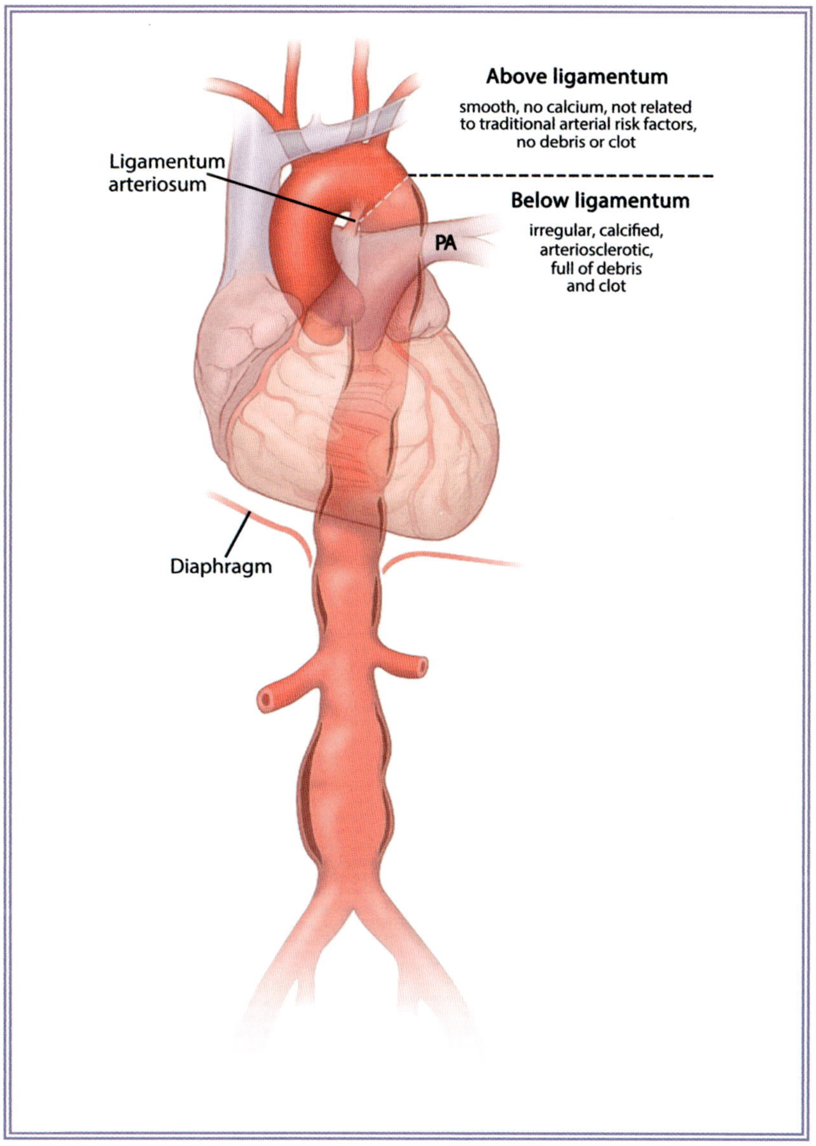

Fig. 6.3 Aortic aneurysm is really two diseases: ascending/arch disease differs markedly from descending/abdominal disease. Reproduced from [148], with permission.

6.3 Syndromic versus non-syndromic thoracic aortic aneurysm and dissection

Currently, TAAD can be classified into 2 main categories: syndromic (associated with abnormalities of other organ systems) and non-syndromic (manifestations restricted to the aorta) [13, 27]. Patients with syndromic TAAD suffer from Marfan syndrome (MFS), Ehlers-Danlos syndrome (EDS), Loeys-Dietz syndrome (LDS), arterial tortuosity syndrome (ATS), aneurysm-osteoarthritis syndrome (AOS), or other *TGFB* mutations [9, 13, 27], among several other syndromes. In addition to disease of the thoracic aorta and the cardiovascular system in general, these patients may also suffer from abnormalities in the integumental, musculoskeletal, ocular, and/or craniofacial systems [28]. Patients with non-syndromic TAAD can be grouped into two distinct categories: familial (more than one family member affected) and sporadic (no affected family members) [13]. Taken together, non-syndromic TAAD accounts for 95% of all cases of TAAD.

The next section will explore the clinical manifestations, especially as they pertain to AD, of these syndromic causes of TAAD, followed by a detailed look at the molecular genetics underlying TAAD.

6.3.1 Marfan syndrome

MFS is a multisystemic disease that affects the sexes equally and has an incidence of 2-3 cases per 10,000 individuals [29]. It is characterized by changes to the skeletal system (disproportionate overgrowth, joint laxity, vertebral column deformity), the ocular system (ectopia lentis), and the cardiovascular system (TAAD, mitral/aortic valve disease) [8]. Its diagnosis

Table 6.2 2010 Revised Ghent nosology for Marfan syndrome*

In the absence of FHx: • Ao (Z ≥2) and EL = MFS • Ao (Z ≥2) and FBN1 mutation = MFS • Ao (Z ≥2) and Syst (≥7 pts) = MFS • EL and *FBN1* mutation with known Ao enlargement = MFS
In the presence of FHx • EL and FH of MFS = MFS • Syst (≥7 pts) and FHx of MFS = MFS • Ao (Z ≥2 above 20, ≥3 below 20 yrs) + FHx of MFS = MFS
Systemic score: 7 or higher is considered positive • Wrist and thumb sign: 3 points • Wrist or thumb sign: 1 • Pectus carinatum: 2 • Pectus excavatum: 1 • Hindfoot deformity: 2 (med rotation of med malleolus) • Pes planus: 1 • Pneumothorax: 2 • Dural ectasia: 2 • Reduced upper/lower segment and increased armspan/height and no severe scoliosis: 1 • Scoliosis or kyphosis: 1 • Reduced elbow extension: 1 • 3 of 5 facial features†: 1 • Skin striae: 1 • Myopia: 1 • Mitral valve prolapse: 1

† Facial features: dolichocephaly, downward slanting palpebral fissures, enophthalmos, retrognathia, and malar hypoplasia. Ao, aortic diameter at sinus of Valsalva; EL, ectopia lentis; FHx, family history; med, medial; MFS, Marfan syndrome; syst, systemic score; Z, z-score.

* Data derived from [30].

is based on the revised Ghent nosology, which utilizes clinical criteria, family history, and genetic testing of the *FBN1* gene [30] (Table 6.2). MFS is primarily caused by heterozygous mutations in the *FBN1* gene, and to this date, more than 1,800 mutations have been identified as causative of the disease [31]. MFS follows an autosomal dominant pattern of inheritance with high penetrance and variable inter/intra familial expressivity [13].

The primary cardiovascular manifestation is aneurysm of the aortic root (annuloaortic ectasia), which can extend to the ascending aorta [28]. This places patients at increased risk for dissection, as the two most important risk factors for dissection are aortic size and a family history of dissection [29]. Not only are MFS patients at increased risk for Type A AD as a result of annuloaortic ectasia, but they also are at increased risk of Type B AD even among patients with prophylactic ascending aortic surgery and only a mildly dilated descending aorta [32]. Generally, AD or the requirement for prophylactic aortic root surgery do not occur until the third or fourth decade of life, but can occur earlier [9].

6.3.2 Ehlers-Danlos syndrome

Ehlers-Danlos syndrome (EDS) Type IV, otherwise known as the vascular subtype of EDS, is an autosomal dominant disease caused by highly penetrant mutations in *COL3A1* [13]. All Ehlers-Danlos syndromes together have an estimated prevalence of 1:10,000-1:25,000, with the vascular subtype accounting for 5-10% of all cases [33]. The 4 major clinical diagnostic criteria are (1) thin, translucent skin, (2) extensive bruising, (3) characteristic facial appearance, and (4) arterial, digestive, or uterine fragility or rupture [33]. The majority of initial clinical presentations attributable to arterial or gastrointestinal complications and occur at an average age of 23 years [13]. Arterial ruptures or dissections account for the majority of deaths [33], with the mean age of death being 48 years [34].

6.3.3 Loeys-Dietz syndrome

Loeys-Dietz syndrome (LDS), which was originally described in 2005 [35, 36], is an autosomal dominant disorder with 3 characteristic features: (1) arterial tortuosity/aortic aneurysms, (2) bifid/broad uvula or cleft palate, and (3) hypertelorism [36]. Patients can also and often do exhibit features that overlap with MFS, including cardiovascular, craniofacial, and skeletal abnormalities [8]. Originally, LDS was classified based on the severity of craniofacial (type 1 – typical dysmorphic features of hypertelorism, craniosynostoses, cleft palate) or cutaneous features (type 2 – mild dysmorphic features with velvety, translucent skin and easy bruising) [37]. However, regardless of the severity of systemic features, LDS patients are at significantly increased risk of AD and aneurysm rupture at relatively young ages and small aortic diameters [37]. Therefore, a revised nosology has been proposed based on the causative gene: Type 1 (*TGFBR1* mutations); Type 2 (*TGFBR2* mutations); Type 3 (*SMAD3* mutations) – previously known as aneurysm-osteoarthritis syndrome (see below); Type 4 (*TGFB2* mutations) – cerebral and aortic aneurysms with arterial tortuosity and skeletal manifestations [13, 37]. This revised nosology indicates that a mutation in any of the genes above plus presentation with an aortic aneurysm or dissection is sufficient for diagnosis regardless of the severity of systemic features [37].

Initial reports indicated that the natural history of LDS involves early onset and rapid progression of thoracic aortic aneurysms with a mean age of death of 26.1 years, with AD being a major cause of death [35, 37]. However, when compared to patients with MFS, LDS Type 2 patients in one study had similar rates of aortic dilatation (80%) and AD and similar rates of death once the disease had been diagnosed [38]. However, patients with LDS 1,2, and 3 have been shown to dissect at aortic diameters of 3.9-4.0 cm, in sharp contrast to the increased risk of dissection in MFS patients at aortic diameters >5.0 cm [35, 37].

6.3.4 Arterial tortuosity syndrome

Arterial tortuosity syndrome (ATS), which was originally described in 2006, is a rare autosomal recessive disorder characterized by tortuosity of the aorta and medium-sized arteries with increased risk of aneurysm and dissection of the aorta and focal stenosis of the aorta and pulmonary artery [9, 39]. The disease is also characterized by increased risk for ischemic vascular events, craniofacial abnormalities (high palate with dental crowding), musculoskeletal abnormalities (arachnodactyly, joint laxity, and pectus excavatum, hypotonia), hernias, and ocular involvement [9, 40]. ATS has only been described in approximately 100 patients and is caused by mutations in *SLC2A10*, which encodes the facilitative glucose transporter GLUT10 [39, 41]. In contrast to prior studies, which indicated severe disease with a mortality rate of 40% by 5 years of age [42], more recent cohorts indicate that patients live longer than previously thought [41, 43]. One cohort of 3 families shows that 11 patients are alive with a mean age of 23 years [41]. Interestingly, in this same cohort, only 3 patients have aortic aneurysms and there have been no reported AD.

6.3.5 Aneurysm-osteoarthritis syndrome

Aneurysm-osteoarthritis syndrome (AOS), which was originally described in 2011 and is now classified as LDS Type 3, is an autosomal dominant disorder caused by mutations in the *SMAD3* gene, which encodes a key regulator in the TGF-β pathway [44]. It is characterized by arterial aneurysms, dissections, and tortuosity associated with mild craniofacial, skeletal, and cutaneous anomalies as well as early onset osteoarthritis [44]. In one cohort of patients, cardiovascular abnormalities were found in 89% of patients, including primarily TAAD as well as aneurysms of other arteries, left ventricular hypertrophy (in the absence of hypertension), atrial fibrillation, and congenital cardiac anomalies [45]. 72% of these patients had aortic aneurysms mainly at the level of the sinuses of Valsalva, and 33% suffered from AD at aortic diameters ranging from 4.0-6.3 cm.

6.4 Molecular genetics of thoracic aortic aneurysm and dissection

As mentioned earlier, familial TAAD (FTAAD) represents an inherited form of the disease without the systemic manifestations of the syndromic forms of TAAD listed above. The evidence indicates that FTAAD is a more virulent disease than sporadic TAAD (STAAD), as FTAAD patients present at an earlier age (58.2 vs. 65.7) and have aneurysms that grow at faster rates (0.21 cm/yr vs. 0.16 cm/yr) [20]. Additionally, FTAAD is not associated with traditional risk factors for arterial disease, including coronary artery disease and dyslipidemia [11, 20].

When considering the genetics of TAAD, it is important to emphasize that mutations in the same gene can cause both syndromic and non-syndromic forms of TAAD [9]. This may partially be explained by the significant intrafamilial variability in many of the syndromic forms of TAAD, which can cause systemic manifestations in certain family members that are absent in others [9]. Furthermore, the variability in clinical presentations among individuals with identical mutations could possibly be explained by unidentified genetic modifiers [46].

As previously stated, the majority of genes causative of TAAD encode proteins involved in the extracellular matrix, the smooth muscle cell contractile unit, or the TGF-β signaling pathway. We will present these causative genes based on this categorization and will also provide practical clinical implications for each of the genes (Fig. 6.4 and Table 6.3).

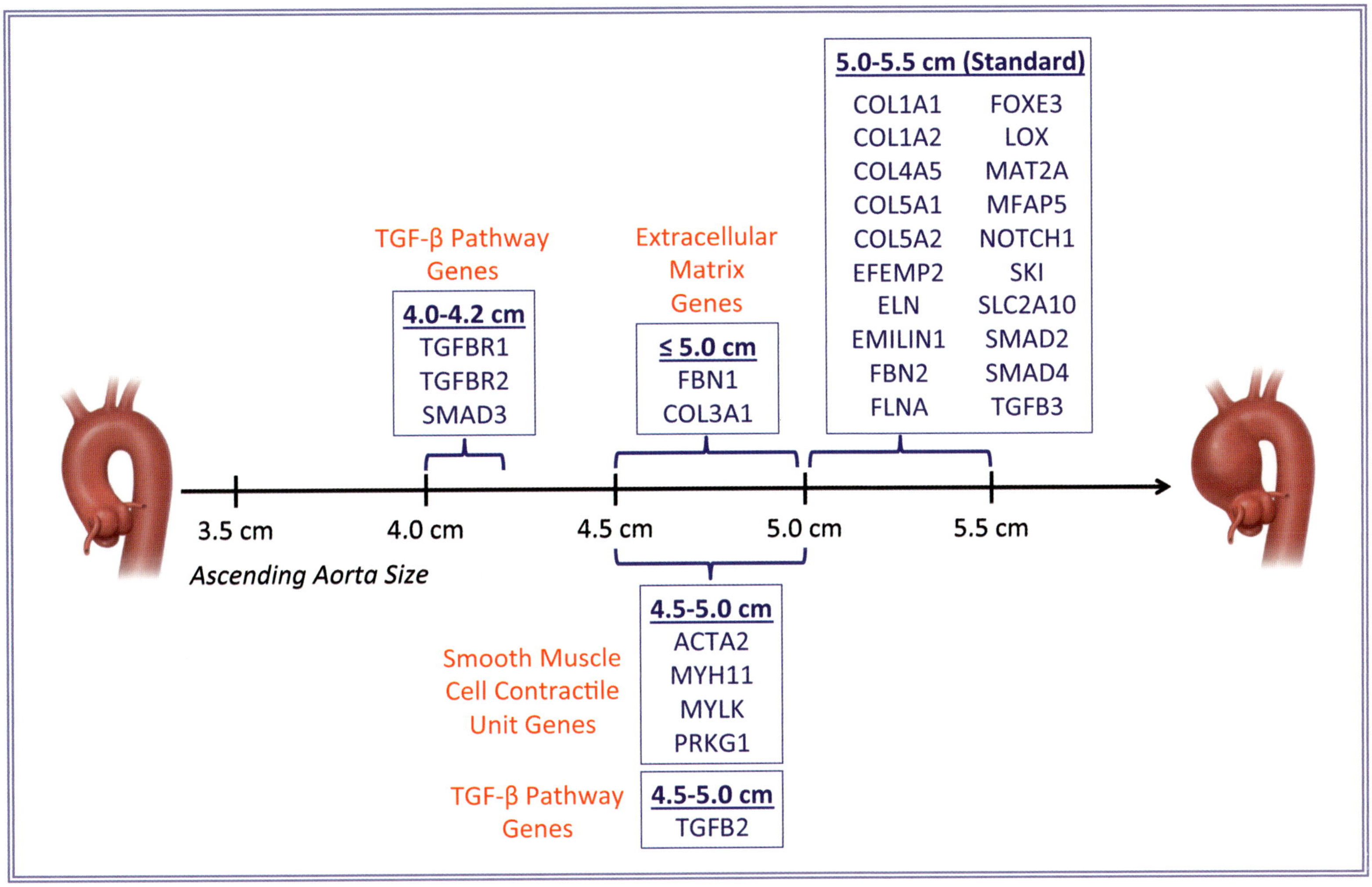

Fig. 6.4 Ascending aorta dimensions for prophylactic surgical intervention.

Table 6.3 Associated vascular characteristics and size criteria for elective surgical intervention for each gene causative of thoracic aortic aneurysm and dissection

Gene	Associated disease/syndrome	Associated clinical characteristics of the vasculature	Ascending aorta size (cm) for surgical intervention
ACTA2	FTAA 6 + multisystemic smooth muscle dysfunction	TAAD, early aortic dissection*, CAD, stroke (Moyamoya disease), BAV	4.5-5.0[b] [7, 98]
BGN	Unidentified CTD	ARD, TAAD, pulmonary artery aneurysm, cerebral aneurysm, arterial tortuosity	Standard
COL1A1	Ehlers-Danlos syndrome, arthrochalasia type (VIIa)	Dissection of infrarenal aorta, iliac, and femoral arteries	Standard
COL1A2	Ehlers-Danlos syndrome, arthrochalasia type (VIIb)	Borderline aortic root enlargement	Standard
COL3A1	Ehlers-Danlos syndrome, vascular type (IV)	TAAD, early aortic dissection*, dissection of visceral arteries, vessel fragility	5.0[a] [115]
COL4A5	Alport syndrome	Onset of aortic disease at young ages (ages 25-32) with XLAS	Standard
COL5A1	Ehlers-Danlos syndrome, classic type (I)	ARD, rupture/dissection of medium sized arteries	Standard
COL5A2	Ehlers-Danlos syndrome, classic type (II)	ARD	Standard
EFEMP2	Cutis laxa, AR type Ib	Ascending aortic aneurysms, arterial tortuosity and stenosis	Standard
ELN	Cutis laxa, AD	ARD, ascending aneurysms, BAV	Standard
EMILIN1	Unidentified CTD	Ascending and descending aortic aneurysms	Standard

Table 6.3 (*Continued*)

Gene	Associated disease/syndrome	Associated clinical characteristics of the vasculature	Ascending aorta size (cm) for surgical intervention
FBN1	Marfan syndrome	ARD, TAAD, AAA/dissection, pulmonary artery dilatation, arterial tortuosity	5.0 [7, 19]
FBN2	Contractural arachnodactyly	Rare ARD and aortic dissection	Standard
FLNA	Periventricular heterotopia	Aortic aneurysms, peripheral arterial dilatation, PDA, cerebral aneurysm	Standard
FOXE3	FTAA	TAAD (primarily Type A dissection)	Standard
LOX	FTAA	TAAD, possibly associated with BAV	Standard
MAT2A	FTAA	Thoracic aortic aneurysms	Standard
MFAP5	FTAA 9	Aortic root dilatation, TAAD	Standard
MYH11	FTAA 4	TAAD, early aortic dissection*, PDA, possibly occlusive vascular disease	4.5-5.0 [7, 91]
MYLK	FTAA 7	Early thoracic aortic dissections, enlarged descending thoracic/abdominal/other arteries, coronary artery aneurysm/dissection, aortic tortuosity	4.5-5.0[b] [7, 16]
NOTCH1	FTAA with BAV	TAAD, bicuspid aortic valve	Standard
PRKG1	FTAA 8	TAAD, early aortic dissection*, enlarged descending thoracic/abdominal/other arteries, coronary artery aneurysm/dissection, aortic tortuosity	4.5-5.0 [100]
SKI	Shprintzen-Goldberg syndrome	ARD, arterial tortuosity, other (splenic) arterial aneurysms	Standard
SLC2A10	Arterial tortuosity syndrome	ARD, ascending aortic aneurysms, arterial tortuosity	Standard
SMAD2	Unidentified CTD with arterial aneurysms/dissections	ARD, ascending aortic aneurysms, vertebral/carotid aneurysms and dissections	Standard
SMAD3	Loeys-Dietz syndrome Type 3	ARD, TAAD, early aortic dissection*, AAA/dissection, arterial tortuosity, other arterial aneurysms, BAV	4.0-4.2 [7, 19]
SMAD4	JP/HHT syndrome	ARD, aortic dissection, AVMs, cerebral aneurysms	Standard
TGFB2	Loeys-Dietz syndrome Type 4	ARD, TAAD, arterial tortuosity, BAV	4.5-5.0[c] [118]
TGFB3	Loeys-Dietz syndrome Type 5	ARD, TAAD, AAA/dissection, other arterial aneurysms	Standard
TGFBR1	Loeys-Dietz syndrome Type 1	ARD, TAAD, early aortic dissection*, AAA/dissection, arterial tortuosity, other arterial aneurysms, BAV	4.0-4.2 [7, 19]
TGFBR2	Loeys-Dietz syndrome Type 2	ARD, TAAD, early aortic dissection*, AAA/dissection, arterial tortuosity, other arterial aneurysms, BAV	4.0-4.2 [7, 19]

It is important to note that since mutations in many of these genes are rare and have only recently been implicated in TAAD, there is a lack of adequate prospective clinical studies of individuals affected by mutations in the majority of these genes. Therefore, it is difficult to establish threshold diameters for intervention for TAAs. One must consider each individual on a case by case basis, taking into account the rate of change in aneurysm size (>0.5 cm per year is considered rapid) and any family history of aortic dissection.
AAA indicates abdominal aortic aneurysm; AD, autosomal dominant; AR, autosomal recessive; ARD, aortic root dilatation; AVM, arteriovenous malformation; BAV, bicuspid aortic valve; CAD, coronary artery disease; CTD, connective tissue disease; FTAA, familial thoracic aortic aneurysm; HHT, hereditary hemorrhagic telangiectasia; JP, juvenile polyposis; PDA, patent ductus arteriosus; TAAD, thoracic aortic aneurysm and dissection; XLAS, X-linked Alport syndrome.
Standard = surgical intervention at 5.0-5.5 cm
Early aortic dissection* = dissection at aortic diameters <5.0 cm
[a] There is no data to set threshold diameters for surgical intervention for Ehlers-Danlos Syndrome Type IV [115].
[b] Individuals with *MYLK* and *ACTA2* mutations have been shown to have aortic dissections at diameter ≤4.0 cm [16, 96].
[c] There is limited data concerning the timing of surgical intervention for Loeys-Dietz Syndrome Type 4. However, there has been a case of Type A aortic dissection at aortic diameters <5.0 cm [118], hence the recommended threshold range of 4.5-5.0 cm.

6.4.1 Extracellular matrix genes

The pathophysiology of AD, which occurs when there is a tear in the intima of the aortic wall that then extends into the media, is linked to medial degeneration [47]. Medial degeneration is characterized by smooth muscle cell (SMC) loss, fragmentation and depletion of elastic fibers, and accumulation of proteoglycans and glycosaminoglycans within cell depleted areas of the aortic media [47]. However, medial degeneration is not the root cause of dissection but rather a pathological consequence of a primary process [8]. Nevertheless, mutations that alter the structure of the aortic media are directly linked to the formation of TAAD.

The aortic media is composed of >50 alternating layers of elastic lamellae and SMCs [48]. Elastin fibers are composed of elastin surrounded by microfibrils and associated proteins. These microfibrils attach to the surface of SMCs via focal adhesions, which are also where the contractile unit within the SMC attaches [48]. Disruption of this elastin-contractile unit is thought to underlie TAAD [48].

FBN1

FBN1, the causative gene of MFS, encodes the protein fibrillin-1, an important component of microfibrils [48]. The majority of mutations causing MFS are missense, though frameshift mutations, nonsense mutations, splicing errors, and complete deletion of the *FBN1* gene have also been shown to cause MFS [48]. By either altering the deposition of fibrillin-1 within microfibrils or by reducing the amount of fibrillin-1 capable of forming microfibrils via haploinsufficiency, these mutations are thought to disrupt the elastin-contractile unit [48]. Furthermore, through the interaction of fibrillin-1 with latent TGF-β binding protein (LTBP), deficiency of the protein is thought to alter the sequestration of the TGF-β latent complex, leading to an increase in the release of TGF-β [8]. It is now well established that increased TGF-β signaling is the inciting event for TAA formation in MFS and is a chief characteristic of syndromic and non-syndromic TAAD [7].

The specific mutations identified within the *FBN1* gene of patients who undergo genetic testing have important clinical ramifications. One study of over 1,000 MFS patients identified that mutations in exons 24-32 caused a more severe and complete phenotype, including earlier age of diagnosis and increased probability of ascending aortic dilatation [49]. These patients, however, did not have higher rates of AD, which can possibly be explained by their higher rate of pre-emptive aortic surgery [49]. Additionally, truncating and splicing mutations in *FBN1* have been shown to be associated with higher rates of aortic events (dissection/surgery) that occur at younger ages (29 years vs. 51 years for missense mutations) among patients who satisfy the revised Ghent criteria [50]. This study also demonstrated that nearly all patients who presented with an aortic event before age 40 had a truncating or splicing mutation. Furthermore, in a recent prospective study, patients with haploinsufficient mutations (deficient fibrillin-1 production solely by the non-mutated allele) had a 2.5-fold increased risk of cardiovascular death and a 2.4-fold increased risk of the combined endpoint of death or dissection than patients with dominant-negative mutations (abnormal fibrillin-1 interacts with normal fibrillin-1) [51]. Though the majority of *FBN1* mutations are associated with MFS, one recent study found that 3% of familial TAAD patients had mutations in *FBN1* [52].

In terms of the clinical diagnosis of MFS, a recent study illustrated that 27% of patients with a pathogenic or likely pathogenic variant did not fulfill the revised Ghent criteria [53]. The authors therefore suggest that utilizing genetic testing as opposed to purely clinical features for diagnosing MFS is quite beneficial. Once patients are identified, an aortic diameter threshold of 5.0 cm for prophylactic aortic surgery is acceptable given the low rate of complications at smaller diameters [7] unless the aorta dilates rapidly (>0.5 cm/year) [19]. However, given that some patients do experience AD at diameters <5.0 cm [54], a family history of AD may justify prophylactic surgery at smaller aortic sizes [7].

FBN2

FBN2, the causative gene in congenital contractural arachnodactyly, a rare autosomal dominant syndromic condition, encodes fibrillin-2, another component of microfibrils [55]. Studies have shown that the majority of mutations occur between exons 24 and 35 of the gene [56] and are occasionally associated with aortic root dilatation [57, 58]. Though rare, Type A AD has been reported in a patient with a variant that resulted in deletion of exon 32 of the *FBN2* gene [59]. Given the rare nature of this disorder and the even rarer occurrence of TAAD, prospective studies are needed to assess risk of AD [57]. However, patients with *FBN2* mutations should be regularly screened for aortic dilatation via cardiac imaging [9].

COL3A1 and other collagen genes

COL3A1, the causative gene in EDS Type IV (vascular type), encodes the pro-α1 chain of type III collagen [60], which is an essential component, along with type I collagen, of the aortic media [48]. It is believed that mutations in *COL3A1* alter the triple helix structure of type III collagen, thereby predisposing patients to arterial tears or dissections [33]. The triple helix amino acid structure consists of repeated glycine-X-Y sequences [33], with the majority of mutations being missense mutations that lead to glycine substitutions [61]. More than 600 *COL3A1* mutations have been identified to cause EDS Type IV, with 50% being *de novo* and 50% being inherited mutations [61].

Just as with MFS, the specific mutations within the *COL3A1* gene have important clinical implications. One study, which categorized patients into two groups based on mutations that led to the production of either 10-15% (MIN) or 50% (haploinsufficiency) normal collagen, found that patients in the haploinsufficiency group had significantly increased rates of aortic pathology, including dissection, though they presented at an older age than those in the MIN group [61]. Patients within the MIN group included those with glycine substitution mutations, the most common type of mutation identified. This difference in aortic pathology was corroborated by another study demonstrating that patients with haploinsufficiency had higher rates of aortic complications compared to those with glycine substitutions and splice-site mutations [62]. Despite the increased rates of aortic complications in those with haploinsufficiency, these patients, along with those with variants in the N- or C-terminal region of the protein, were shown to have milder disease than those with glycine substitutions and splice-site mutations [62].

In a natural history study of over 1,200 individuals (630 index cases and 601 relatives) with EDS 4, Pepin et al. found that disease of the aorta (aneurysm, dissection, rupture), which occurred at a mean age of 35.7 years and was the leading vascular complication (22%), led to death in 68% of cases [63]. They also found that over 90% of identified mutations in the *COL3A1* gene were missense or splice site variants and that the type of mutation was associated with differing survival rates. The median survival rates for splice site acceptor, splice site donor, and glycine substitution mutations were 52, 37, and 51 years, respectively. All 3 mutations types had a significantly higher hazard ratio compared to those with null mutations (loss of stable mRNA transcript from one allele) with donor site mutations having the highest hazard ratio. Furthermore, among those with glycine substitution mutations, the specific amino acid that replaced glycine was important for survival, with valine substitutions having the highest hazard ratio [63].

As AD have been shown to occur even without significant development of an aortic aneurysm [8] in EDS Type IV patients, it is challenging to counsel patients regarding prophylactic aortic surgery. Furthermore, surgery can be quite dangerous in these patients as they have excess vessel fragility [13].

COL1A1 and *COL1A2*, the causative genes in EDS arthrochalasia type and osteogenesis imperfecta, encode pro-α1 and 2 chains of type I collagen, respectively [64]. Mutations of *COL1A1* have been associated with dissection of the infrarenal aorta as well as the iliac and femoral arteries [64]. Mutations in *COL1A2* are involved in the development of cardiac valvular disease and borderline aortic root enlargement [9, 65]. Mutations in *COL5A1* and *COL5A2*, which encode components of type V collagen, cause the classical type of EDS [66]. Aortic root dilation was diagnosed in classical EDS in 33% of patients at a mean age of 23.4 in one study [67], but progression to AD is rare [19]. While mutations in *COL5A1* have been shown to cause similar clinical presentations to the vascular type of EDS caused by *COL3A1* mutations, including arterial rupture and dissection of medium sized arteries [68, 69], variants in *COL5A2* have not been associated with AD [70]. However, one mutation that resulted in deletion of both the *COL3A1* and *COL5A2* genes causing haploinsufficiency of both genes was associated with AD [70]. The authors attributed this clinical presentation primarily to deletion of the *COL3A1* gene. Nonsense mutations in *COL4A5*, which encodes a component of type IV collagen and is the causative gene in X-linked Alport syndrome, have been associated with aortic aneurysm and dissection [71, 72]. Despite the rarity of aortic and other arterial dissection/rupture in patients with mutations in collagen genes other than *COL3A1*, it may be prudent to consider screening these patients via baseline echocardiogram to assess for aortic dilatation.

EFEMP2

EFEMP2 (*FBLN4*), the causative gene of autosomal recessive cutis laxa type IB, encodes fibulin-4, an ECM protein that plays an important role in the assembly and function of elastic fibers [73]. Mutations in *EFEMP2* lead to ascending aortic aneurysms, arterial tortuosity and stenosis, and cutis laxa [73-75]. Not only is fibulin-4 critical for elastogenesis but mouse studies have shown it plays an important role in collagen maturation [76, 77] and mutations in the gene have been associated with increased TGF-β signaling in aortic tissue of affected patients [73]. As far as we are aware, there are no reported cases of AD, though most patients present in infancy or at very young ages.

ELN

Heterozygous mutations in *ELN*, which encodes the protein tropoelastin, are the cause of autosomal dominant cutis laxa [78]. Several studies have shown that mutations within *ELN* are associated with aortic dilatation and aneurysm formation [78, 79]. In one of these studies, one of the probands' uncles suffered from an AD at age 26, though he did not exhibit skin laxity while alive [78]. In both of these studies, affected patients had dilatation of the aortic root. Culturing of patients' fibroblasts in one of the studies demonstrated increased TGF-β signaling, which the authors speculated is due to disorganized elastic fibers [79]. Furthermore, a study involving patients with a 7q11.23 microduplication and another involving patients with a 7q11.23 triplication, a region of the chromosome that encompasses the *ELN* gene, found that almost all patients had aortic dilation or an ascending aortic aneurysm [80, 81]. Therefore, though longitudinal studies are lacking, regular aortic imaging in these patients is required to prevent the development of complications from aortic dilatation and aneurysm formation [78].

EMILIN1

The elastin microfibril interface 1 (*EMILIN1*) gene encodes an ECM protein that associates with microfibrils and elastic fibers and is involved in elastogenesis, vessel assembly, and regulation of TGF-β1 [82]. A recent study identified a proband with one ascending and one descending aortic aneurysm. He was found to have a mutation in the signal peptide cleavage site of *EMILIN1*, which led to abnormal accumulation of the protein in the endoplasmic reticulum and subsequent cellular apoptosis and altered ECM integrity [82]. Further studies are needed to confirm the role of *EMILIN1* in the formation of thoracic aortic aneurysms, as this is the first reported case involving this gene [48].

MFAP5

MFAP5 encodes microfibril-associated glycoprotein 2 (MAGP-2), a structural constituent of the ECM that has been shown to interact with other components of the ECM, including fibrillin-1 and tropoelastin, and can also bind to both TGF-β1 and β2 [83]. A recent study utilizing whole exome sequencing identified 2 distinct mutations (one nonsense and one missense) within *MFAP5* that caused TAAD in 2 separate families, with one of the probands presenting with a Type A AD at 58 years of age [83]. Moreover, the affected family members had dilations of the aortic root and aortic tissue collected from the proband with the AD showed enhanced TGF-β signaling. Both of these findings are consistent with what is seen in patients with mutations in other genes linked to TAAD [84]. Interestingly, atrial fibrillation was also present in multiple affected members of one of the two families studied. Given the clear possibility for AD in affected patients, regular cardiac imaging to prevent such complications would be prudent.

LOX

LOX encodes a member of the lysyl oxidase protein family, which are a group of extracellular copper enzymes that cross-link collagens and elastin [85]. Two recent reports show that mutations in *LOX* resulted in thoracic aortic aneurysms leading to AD, with one patient presenting at age 11 with an ascending aortic aneurysm and several patients with AD in their 50s and 60s [85, 86]. Multiple variants were identified, with mutations resulting either in haploinsufficiency or alteration of a highly conserved catalytic domain [85]. Since *LOX* encodes the enzyme primarily responsible for the cross-linking of collagen and elastin in the aorta, without the enzyme's activity, it is thought that the result is abnormal aortic development with decreased and fragmented elastic fibers [85]. Furthermore, through its amine oxidase activity, LOX has been shown to bind to and inactivate free TGF-β [87, 88]. Since fibulin-4 is crucial for recruiting LOX to fibrillin microfibrils, decreased enzymatic inactivation of TGF-β by LOX as a result of fibulin-4 deficiency may also contribute to the predisposition towards aortic aneurysms in individuals with *FBLN4* mutations [88]. Interestingly, 3 of 20 *LOX* mutation carriers in one of the studies had bicuspid aortic valves [85]. More clinical data is needed to determine the risk of AD in LOX-mediated TAAD.

BGN

BGN, an X-linked gene, encodes the biglycan protein, which is a leucine-rich proteoglycan involved in the maintenance and assembly of the ECM [89]. Biglycan has been shown to interact with components of the ECM, including collagens and elastin, and with growth factors, including TGF-β [89]. Loss-of-function mutations in *BGN* were recently identified in individuals with syndromic TAAD from 5 separate families. These individuals presented with TAAD at young ages (earliest cases of aortic aneurysm and AD were at age 1 and 15, respectively), along with several MFS and LDS-like extracardiovascular characteristics, including hypertelorism, pectus deformity, and joint hypermobility, among others [89]. Furthermore, the aortic walls of affected individuals demonstrated increased TGF-β signaling, especially within the adventitia, which is the aortic wall layer where biglycan is mostly found [89]. *BGN*, along with *FLNA*, are the only genes shown thus far to be causative of X-linked TAAD.

6.4.2 Smooth muscle cell genes

The smooth muscle cell plays a vital role in the function and maintenance of the aortic media. The contractile unit of the SMC is comprised of actin thin filaments and myosin thick filaments, which interact to generate the force of contraction [48]. Actin filaments are not only attached to the cell surface via focal adhesions but also to the nuclear membrane, allowing SMCs to convert mechanical stimuli into resultant biochemical activity [48]. It is thought that mutations in genes that disrupt these linkages lead to impaired sensation of mechanical stress in the aortic wall by SMCs, thereby altering their ability to adequately regulate and remodel the ECM [48].

MYH11

MYH11 encodes the smooth muscle myosin heavy chain, an essential contractile protein within SMCs [90]. In 2006, two families with FTAAD and patent ductus arteriosus (PDA) were found to have mutations in *MYH11*, which affected the C-terminal coiled-coil region of the SMC myosin heavy chain [90]. Another study confirmed the role of *MYH11* in FTAAD by identifying novel mutations in family members affected by TAAD and PDA, though there was variable expressivity of both as well as decreased penetrance of the mutation [91]. Interestingly, pathology from two affected patients revealed SMC disarray and focal hyperplasia of SMCs with evidence of dysregulation of insulin-like growth factor 1 and angiotensin II, as opposed to TGF-β [91]. This pathology is distinct from typical TAAD pathology and may contribute to the increased rates of vascular occlusive disease in these patients [91].

In two other studies [92, 93], the same deletion variant in *MYH11* was identified in a Dutch family and two Japanese families, though this variant and a missense variant did not segregate with disease in the Dutch families. It is therefore possible that unidentified genes are somehow contributing to the clinical phenotype observed in these Dutch families, which included a case of Type A dissection in a 24-year-old [92]. Prophylactic aortic surgery is warranted at ascending aortic diameters of 4.5-5.0 cm for patients with *MYH11* mutations [7], yet as the authors of the Dutch study maintain, family members of affected patients without *MYH11* mutations should still participate in regular cardiac imaging given that the mutation has been shown not to segregate with disease [92].

Finally, a duplication of 16p13.11, a chromosomal region that contains *MYH11*, has been shown to occur at higher rates among patients with STAAD [94] and is estimated to impart an eightfold higher risk for development of TAAD [46]. However, further studies are needed to determine if *MYH11* is the culprit gene in this chromosomal duplication.

ACTA2

ACTA2 encodes the smooth muscle α-actin, which polymerizes to form thin filaments that are crucial for SMC contraction [48]. Mutations in *ACTA2* that cause TAAD were originally described in 2007, with several studies showing that *ACTA2* mutations account for 12-21% of FTAAD [17, 95, 96]. The majority of identified mutations are missense mutations that result in a dominant negative mechanism that decreases actin filament assembly [17], though nonsense mutations have been identified as well [97]. Interestingly, in contrast to a prior study that did not demonstrate altered TGF-β signaling in the aortas of patients with *MYH11* mutations [91], Renaud et al. found increased TGF-β signaling in the aortas of patients affected with *ACTA2* mutations as well as those with *MYH11* [97]. Specific mutations in *ACTA2* have also been linked to early-onset coronary artery disease, stroke, iris flocculi, and livido reticularis [18, 96]. Additionally, a heterozygous de novo missense mutation, R179H, was associated with severe multisystemic smooth muscle dysfunction, with all 5 patients presenting with ascending aortic aneurysms at ages ranging from 11 to 26 years [98].

Among family members with *ACTA2* mutations, the most common presentation is thoracic AD, though the penetrance is approximately 50% [46]. A study of 277 patients with various *ACTA2* mutations demonstrated a lifetime cumulative risk of aortic events (dissection or repair) of 76% by age 85 [99]. The majority of patients presented with thoracic AD (88%) at a median age of 35 years with more Type A than Type B dissections (54 vs. 21%). However, patients with Type B dissections presented at significantly younger ages (27 vs. 36 years). Interestingly, the p.R179 and p.R258 substitution mutations were associated with increased risk for aortic events and at younger ages (100% by age 25 and 90% by age 63, respectively). In prior studies, these variants have been associated with increased severity of vascular disease, including PDA, early onset stroke, and tortuosity of small arteries of the retina [99]. On the contrary, p.R185Q and p.R118Q mutations were associated with a significantly decreased risk for aortic events relative to other *ACTA2* mutations. In fact, p.R185Q mutation carriers had a cumulative risk of aortic events of only 57% by age 77. Importantly, AD occurred at aortic diameters <5.0 cm in 1/3 of patients who suffered from Type A dissections. Moreover, in another study, for 3 out of 8 women with *ACTA2* mutations who had peripartum AD, the aortic diameters at the time of dissection ranged from 3.8 to 4.7 cm [100]. Therefore, patients with *ACTA2* mutations warrant surgical intervention at aortic diameters between 4.5 and 5.0 cm [7] to hopefully stave off their increased risk for dissection.

MYLK

MYLK encodes myosin light chain kinase, a ubiquitously expressed kinase that phosphorylates regulatory light chain (RLC), thereby initiating SMC contraction [16]. In a candidate gene approach using DNA from 193 probands and involving multiple genes regulating SMC contraction, 5 variants in *MYLK* were identified, with 2 that were shown to segregate with AD in two families [16]. These two mutations (p.R1480X and p.S1759P) were found to result in decreased kinase activity and, therefore, decreased SMC contraction [16]. Importantly, affected patients were found to have AD at aortic diameters that were minimally dilated (even at 4.0 cm) [16]. A recent study by Hannuksela et al., which identified a novel 2-bp deletion variant leading to a premature stop codon, also found that affected individuals suffered AD at diameters <5.0 cm [101]. Though patients with *MYLK* mutations should receive prophylactic surgery at ascending aortic diameters between 4.5 and 5.0 cm [7], these findings make it extremely difficult to counsel patients regarding the appropriate time to intervene surgically, as they can dissect at even smaller diameters.

PRKG1

PRKG1 encodes type I cGMP-dependent protein kinase (PKG-1), which is activated upon binding of cGMP and leads to SMC relaxation via activation of the phosphatase that dephosphorylates myosin RLC [48]. Only one variant (c.530G>A), which was identified in 4 families, has been shown to cause FTAAD [102]. By altering the cGMP binding site of PKG-1, this gain of function mutation leads to constitutive activation of the kinase, leading to decreased phosphorylation of the myosin RLC, promoting SMC relaxation [102]. In this report, 63% of patients presented with AD at an average of 31 years, with the youngest being 17 years old. Only 2 patients with AD had aortic measurements available, with one having an ascending aortic diameter of 4.3 cm and the other having an aortic root diameter of 5.7 cm at the time of dissection. Affected family members also exhibited other vascular abnormalities, including enlargement of the descending thoracic aorta, abdominal aorta, and other arteries, including the coronaries [102]. Though there is limited data on *PRKG1* mutations, affected patients most likely should receive prophylactic surgeries at the same diameter as patients affected by other SMC genes, namely 4.5-5.0 cm.

FLNA

FLNA encodes filamin A, an important anchoring protein that links actin filaments in SMCs to the transmembrane integrin receptors in focal adhesions of the cell membrane, and thereby plays a prominent role in maintaining cell shape and cell signaling [48]. *FLNA* mutations are the cause of X-linked dominant periventricular heterotopia (PH), which is a neuronal migration disorder that primarily affects females and can lead to seizures, aortic aneurysms, PDA, and EDS-like features, including hyperextensible joints and skin laxity [103]. In a recent study examining a cohort of 47 individuals with the X-linked disorder, the majority of mutations identified were truncating and only 1 out of 34 patients had aortic dilation [104]. However, the estimated incidence of aortic dilation in X-linked PH is unknown, as there have been several patients in other cohorts identified with aortic dilation/aneurysms [103, 105]. As far as we are aware, no cases of AD have been reported. Given the variable expressivity of vascular features, cardiac imaging in these patients is warranted to screen for aortic and pulmonary dilatation [105].

MAT2A

MAT2A encodes methionine adenosyltransferase II alpha (MAT-IIα), which catalyzes the production of S-adenosylmethionine (SAM), a critical enzyme involved in cellular metabolism [106]. Two mutations in *MAT2A*, c.10131A>C (p.Glu344Ala) and c.1067G>A (p.Arg356His), were recently implicated in FTAAD and are thought to disrupt the enzyme activity of MAT-IIα [106]. While the exact mechanism by which *MAT2A* mutations lead to TAAD is unclear, it is thought that decreased enzymatic activity of MAT-IIα alters SMC metabolism, perhaps by increasing oxidative stress or decreasing methylation activity within SMCs [106]. In this study, 8 out of 18 (44%) of mutation carriers had dilatation of the ascending aorta and/or aortic root at a median age of 50 years. Though there were no reported cases of AD, one obligate carrier died suddenly at the age of 32 from unknown causes [106]. While there is limited data on the clinical phenotypes of *MAT2A* mutation carriers, the data suggests that affected patients may have a more benign presentation than other FTAAD patients (i.e. no episodes of AD and youngest presentation with TAA at age 37). Therefore, the authors of this study postulate that a second environmental or genetic factor may be possibly required for patients to develop TAAD [106].

FOXE3

FOXE3, which encodes the forkhead transcription factor FOXE3, was just recently implicated in FTAAD in a large family with 8 identified cases of acute AD [107]. Seven out of eight family members presented with Type A AD at an average age of 45.6 years, with one family member having prior normal aortic imaging. Through exome and Sanger sequencing of this family and 564 unrelated FTAAD probands, 8 *FOXE3* variants were identified, which were all missense mutations that changed amino acids at the C-terminal end of the DNA-binding domain [107]. Through knockout mouse studies, Kuang et al. demonstrated that FOXE3 is crucial for populating the ascending aorta with differentiated SMCs during development and for SMC response to aortic wall stress [107]. Further clinical studies are necessary for determining the risk of AD in these patients and the timing of prophylactic aortic surgery to prevent such complications.

6.4.3 TGF-β pathway genes

Studies have consistently shown that increased TGF-β signaling is a feature of both syndromic and non-syndromic TAAD [7]. TGF-β exerts its effect on cells through both the canonical and non-canonical pathways (Fig. 6.5). The canonical pathway involves activation of the TGF-β receptor, phosphorylation of regulatory SMADs (SMAD 2 and 3), recruitment of SMAD4 to form a SMAD2/3-SMAD4 complex, importation into the nucleus, and activation of gene transcription [7, 47]. Normally, there is an autoregulatory feedback loop on TGF-β signaling provided by the canonical pathway [108]. However, it is believed that loss-of-function mutations in TGF-β pathway genes lead to an upregulation of TGF-β signaling, especially through the non-canonical pathways due to loss of this feedback inhibition [7, 108]. The resulting upregulation in TGF-β is thought to be a crucial element in the formation of TAAD.

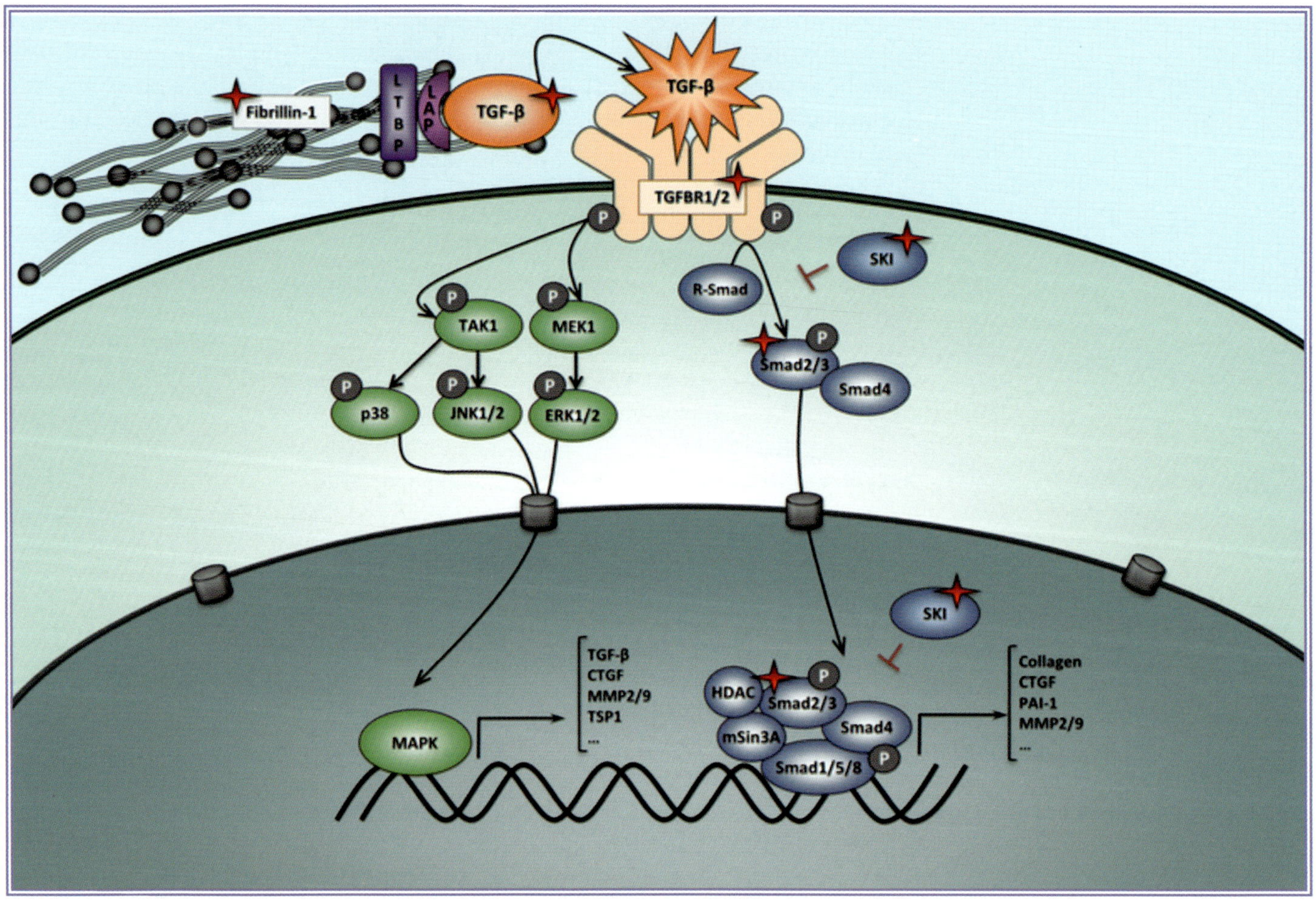

Fig. 6.5 Overview of canonical and non-canonical TGF-β signaling. Reproduced from [149], with permission. By interacting with the large latent complex of TGF-β, comprised of the latent TGF-β binding protein (LTBP) and the latency-associated protein (LAP) [7], microfibrils composed of fibrillin-1 help sequester TGF-β, preventing it from exerting its effect on cells. Once TGF-β is released, it can activate both the canonical (blue) and non-canonical (green) pathways. The canonical pathway involves activation of the TGF-β receptor, phosphorylation of regulatory SMADs (SMAD 2 and 3), recruitment of SMAD4 to form a SMAD2/3-SMAD4 complex, importation into the nucleus, and activation of gene transcription. SKI, which is a negative regulator of the canonical signaling pathway, acts by hindering many of these processes. TGF-β receptors also activate the noncanonical pathway, which involve multiple different SMAD-independent cascades. Upregulation of the non-canonical pathway is believed to be crucial to the development of aortic aneurysms [7]. As depicted by the red stars, mutations only in the genes that encode components of the canonical signaling pathway have been shown to be causative of thoracic aortic aneurysms and dissections.

TGFBR1 and TGFBR2

TGFBR1 and *2*, the causative genes in LDS Type 1 and 2, respectively, encode the 2 major human TGF-β receptor subunits [28]. Thus far, mutations in *TGFBR1* and *TGFBR2* have been almost exclusively missense and usually occur in the kinase domain of the receptors [28]. Studies have clearly demonstrated that mutations in both *TGFBR1* and *2* not only cause LDS but also non-syndromic FTAAD [109, 110], illustrating the wide range of clinical phenotypes seen with mutations in these genes [46]. In fact, identical *TGFBR2* mutations have been reported in FTAAD patients and LDS patients displaying the typical characteristics of the syndrome [46].

Though initial reports did not show a difference in clinical presentation between LDS patients with *TGBR1* vs. *TGFBR2* mutations [35], a study of multigenerational TAAD families with *TGFBR1* or *2* mutations did find differences in clinical presentations [110]. In this study, the average age of presentation with vascular disease, including aortic aneurysms and dissections, was significantly younger in the *TGFBR1* cohort than *TGFBR2* cohort (31.4 vs. 45.6 years) [110]. Interestingly, men with *TGFBR1* mutations presented primarily with ascending aortic disease, whereas women with *TGFBR1* mutations often presented with aneurysms and dissections of other arteries. This led to lower rates of survival in men with *TGFBR1* mutations than women with *TGFBR1* mutations, which was not seen in the *TGFBR2* cohort. Finally, no individuals presented with AD at aortic diameters <5.0 cm with *TGFBR1* mutations, but 3 individuals did with *TGFBR2* mutations. Based on these results, the authors suggest that individuals with *TGFBR1* mutations may not require prophylactic surgery for ascending aortic aneurysms at aortic diameters <5.0 cm due to their low risk of dissection at small diameters, though further data is required [110].

However, a recent cohort evaluating 33 genetically confirmed LDS adults over time found that those with *TGFBR2* mutations had a fivefold higher risk of needing aortic surgery than those with *TGFBR1* mutations with the surgeries tending to occur at younger ages [111]. While initial studies indicated that LDS leads to more severe aortic disease than MFS, in this study, the aortic dilation rate was calculated over a median period of 2 years and was found to be similar to previously calculated values for those with MFS (0.67 mm/yr in LDS vs. 0.49 mm/yr in MFS) [111, 112]. Furthermore, the authors of this study observed a relatively milder aortic phenotype with a median age of first clinical presentation (surgery, death, dissection) of 50 as compared to the initial report describing a median age of 26 [35]. These differences could possibly be explained by the inclusion of only adults in this recent study and the fact that the majority of patients had *TGFBR1* mutations [111]. These results also indicate the remarkable heterogeneity in clinical severity among LDS patients, who exhibit considerable intra- and interfamilial differences [111].

The current guidelines indicate that those with LDS and mutations in *TGFBR1* or *TGFBR2* should probably receive prophylactic surgery at ascending aortic diameters between 4.0 and 4.2 cm [7, 19, 113]. However, as Milewicz et al. argue, these guidelines may be overly aggressive, particularly for medically treated adult patients [114]. As the European guidelines state, more research is required to establish definitive criteria for surgical intervention [115].

TGFB2 and TGFB3

TGFB2, which encodes the TGF-β2 ligand, is the causative gene in LDS 4 [37]. In 2012, Boileau et al. identified two mutations (frameshift mutation in exon 6 and nonsense mutation in exon 4) in two large unrelated families with FTAAD along with intracranial aneurysms and subarachnoid hemorrhage [116]. These mutations are thought to lead to haploinsufficiency of *TGFB2*. They found that the youngest case of AD occurred at age 31 (mean of 35 years) and no dissections occurred at minimal aortic enlargement [116]. Further heterozygous mutations or deletions were detected in eight families with autosomal dominant TAAD and variable clinical expression, along with the finding of increased TGF-β signaling in the aorta of affected patients [117]. In another cohort of 146 TAAD patients, 6 were found to harbor mutations in *TFGB2*, including premature truncating mutations and missense mutations, with two cases of Type A AD and four cases of significant mitral valve disease [118]. One of the cases of AD occurred at an aortic diameter <5.0 cm. Multiple other reports have found novel *TGFB2* mutations in patients affected by FTAAD with variable expressivity of extracardiovascular manifestations, including skeletal and craniofacial abnormalities [119-121].

TGFB3, which encodes the TGF-β3 ligand, has recently been implicated in syndromic TAAD (known as LDS 5) with associated craniofacial, skeletal, and cutaneous anomalies [122]. Recently, several mutations were identified in *TGFB3*, including truncating mutations and in-frame splice site mutations, which the authors hypothesize cause a loss of function of *TGFB3* [122]. Missense mutations in regions critical for TGF-β3 activation by integrins and TGF-β3 processing were also identified. In this study of 43 patients with *TGFB3* mutations from 11 families, multiple family members had vascular abnormalities, including 4 patients with Type A and 6 patients with Type B AD, which occurred at median ages of 51 and 44.5, respectively [122]. No cases of AD at small diameters were found. Other cases of *TGFB3* mutations have been reported in pubertal age children presenting with characteristics of both MFS and LDS [123, 124], with one of the patients presenting with a mildly dilated aortic root [125]. Given the risk for aortic aneurysm and dissection, it is recommended that patients affected with *TGFB3* mutations receive yearly echocardiograms to evaluate the aortic root as well as baseline imaging of the entire aorta plus side branches [122].

SMAD3 and other SMAD genes

SMAD3, the causative gene in LDS 3, also known as aneurysm-osteoarthritis syndrome (AOS), encodes a protein involved in the canonical TGF-β signaling pathway [126]. The majority of *SMAD3* mutations identified to date involve the MH2 domain of the protein [127], a well-conserved region that is important for forming a complex with SMAD4 [44]. This interaction is critical for translocation of the SMAD complex into the nucleus, where it can alter gene transcription [44]. As these mutations cause a premature stop of translation through a frameshift or a substitution of highly conserved amino acids, it is believed this leads to a loss of function of SMAD3 [127].

In the initial description of AOS, 60% of affected individuals had an aortic aneurysm or dissection, with some of the dissections occurring at minimally dilated ascending aortas (4.0-4.5 cm) [44]. In another cohort of 44 patients with AOS, 71% of patients had an aortic root aneurysm and 15 deaths occurred at a mean age of 54 years [128]. AD accounted for 60% of deaths in this cohort, with some occurring at mildly enlarged ascending aortas. Cerebrovascular abnormalities were diagnosed in 56% of patients and aneurysms of other arteries in the thorax and abdomen were diagnosed in 33% [128]. In an exome sequencing study of 181 probands with FTAAD, it was determined that *SMAD3* mutations account for 2% of FTAAD [126]. In this study of 42 affected individuals, 50% presented with TAAD, with several others presenting with intracranial aneurysms and abdominal aortic aneurysms. There is clearly a wide spectrum of clinical phenotypes as some mutation carriers exhibited the characteristic extracardiovascular features of MFS, LDS, and AOS [126].

Importantly, in another study, one patient with a *SMAD3* mutation underwent prophylactic ascending aortic surgery for a progressively enlarging aorta at the age of only 12 months [127]. This patient's maternal aunt was discovered to have died suddenly from AD at the age of 18. Remarkably, this family exhibited a wide range of age of onset of TAAD (ranging from 1 to 54 years), which the authors attribute to unidentified genetic or environmental factors [127]. Patients with *SMAD3* mutations warrant extensive cardiovascular imaging via echocardiogram plus imaging of the cerebral, abdominal, and thoracic vasculature regularly to determine the rate of growth of any aneurysms [128]. Given that cases of dissection have been reported at minimally enlarged aortic diameters, patients with *SMAD3* mutations would benefit from prophylactic surgery at diameters between 4.0 and 4.2 cm, just as is the case with *TGBR1/2* mutations [7].

In addition to *SMAD3*, *SMAD4*, which also encodes a key player in the TGF-β signaling pathway, has been linked to TAAD [129]. Patients with both juvenile polyposis syndrome and hereditary hemorrhagic telangiectasia (JPS-HHT), which are associated with heterozygous loss-of-function mutations in *SMAD4*, were recently examined for aortic disease in two chart review studies [130, 131]. Both studies reported cases of AD in middle-aged individuals and several cases of aortic dilatation. Therefore, individuals with *SMAD4* mutations and JPS-HHT should undergo screening for aortic aneurysms and regular imaging via echocardiography [129].

Furthermore, *SMAD2*, which encodes another important SMAD protein that forms a complex with SMAD3 after its phosphorylation by the TGF-β receptor, has recently been associated with TAAD [132]. In this study, 4 individuals from 3 families were found to have *SMAD2* missense mutations located in the MH2 domain, which is the same evolutionarily conserved region where mutations are found that cause *SMAD3* related TAAD [132]. One of the probands, who developed a de novo *SMAD2* mutation, was a 17-year-old woman who was suspected of having MFS and presented with aortic root dilatation. Another proband presented with an ascending aortic aneurysm of 5.0 cm at age 46, while a third was found to have vertebral/carotid aneurysms and dissections and a brother who died from an abdominal AD at age 50 [132].

SKI

SKI encodes the Sloan Kettering proto-oncoprotein (SKI), which functions as a negative regulator of the canonical TGF-β signaling pathway by hindering SMAD2 and SMAD3 activation, preventing translocation of the activated SMAD2/3-SMAD4 complex into the nucleus, and by inhibiting transcription of TGF-β target genes [133]. Mutations in *SKI* have been shown to underlie Shprintzen-Goldberg syndrome (SGS), which is characterized by similar craniofacial, skin, skeletal, and cardiovascular features as MFS and LDS, along with intellectual disability and skeletal muscle hypotonia [133-135]. Thus far, 17 different mutations in SGS patients have been identified, with all of them occurring in either the SMAD2/3 binding domain or the Dachshund-homology domain (DHD), which is crucial for binding to transcriptional corepressors [136]. Interestingly, all mutations occur in exon 1 and 73% of all affected patients have mutations affecting 5 SKI amino acid residues [136]. Many of the affected patients have aortic root dilatation [133], though, as far as we are aware, no cases of dissection have been reported. Though aneurysmal disease appears to be more benign and less penetrant in SGS as compared to MFS and LDS, baseline echocardiography is recommended with yearly screening in children followed by every 2-3 years in adults [136].

SLC2A10

SLC2A10, the causative gene in ATS, encodes GLUT10, a facilitative glucose transporter [39]. Since decorin, a natural inhibitor of TGF-β signaling, is regulated by a glucose response element in its promoter, it is believed that loss-of-function mutations in *SLC2A10* will lead to upregulation of TGF-β signaling via downregulation of decorin [13, 39]. A total of 23 mutations have been identified to cause ATS, including 12 missense mutations, 5 nonsense mutations, 5 deletions leading to premature termination of translation, and 1 splice site mutation [41]. Ritelli at al. observed that 2 out of 12 patients had ascending/aortic root aneurysms [41], while Callewaert et al. found that 2 adults (aged 23 and 35) out of 16 total patients had rapidly progressive aortic root dilation [43]. However, given that the mean ages of these cohorts were 15 and 12.9 years, respectively, these patients may generally be too young to manifest with aortic root dilatation, a complication that occurs more frequently in adulthood [41]. Affected patients require baseline full body vascular imaging with follow-up imaging depending on the results and any family history of progressive aneurysmal disease, and possibly also regular echocardiograms to determine aortic root diameters [43, 137].

6.4.4 Bicuspid aortic valve and thoracic aortic aneurysm and dissection

Bicuspid aortic valve (BAV) is the most common congenital heart defect, affecting 1-2% of the general population [46]. Though only 5% of patients with BAV will develop an AD, BAV still causes significantly more cases of AD than MFS despite the fact that there is a 40% risk of dissection in MFS patients [12]. This can be explained by the low prevalence (1/10,000 people) of MFS. Furthermore, AD associated with BAV occurs long before the aortic valve becomes significantly stenotic [12]. The risk of AD in BAV patients is ninefold higher compared to patients with a normal tricuspid aortic valve [46].

Unfortunately, however, the molecular genetics underlying BAV and associated TAAD is currently unclear. *NOTCH1*, which encodes a transmembrane protein that functions as a transcriptional cofactor, has been associated with BAV/TAAD [138-140]. NOTCH1, which activates the NOTCH signaling pathway, plays a role in cardiac embryogenesis and maintenance of the aorta [139]. Yet, mutations in *NOTCH1* are only estimated to contribute to 4% of BAV with or without TAAD [7]. As Andelfinger et al. suggest, there may be several factors that could explain why it has been so challenging to understand the genetic basis of BAV/TAAD, including the fact that BAV/TAAD exhibits significant genetic heterogeneity with reduced penetrance and that several genes may interact to contribute to this phenotype [7].

6.4.5 New dissection genes

Recently, two new "dissection genes" (as we like to call them) have been identified that increase the risk of AD among carriers.

Among patients who suffer from sporadic TAAD, variants in *FBN1* have been linked to AD. In particular, the rs2118181 SNP, which was first identified by a research team led by Dr. Milewicz [141], was found to be highly associated with sporadic TAAD. In an independent patient population, our group found that carriers of the rs2118181 SNP had a 76% increased risk of thoracic AD as compared to noncarriers [142] (Fig. 6.6 A).

The second gene we identified that predisposes to AD is *KIF6*. The protein product of this gene is a kinesin, a group of motor proteins that play a role in intracellular transport along microtubules [143]. *KIF6* entered the clinical arena when the Trp719Arg variant in the gene was found to be associated with myocardial infarctions and coronary heart disease [143]. This variant may alter the ability of KIF6 to transport its cargo by disrupting protein-protein interactions [143]. Interestingly, our group found that patients with this same variant have a twofold higher risk of developing an AD than noncarriers [144] (Fig. 6.6 B).

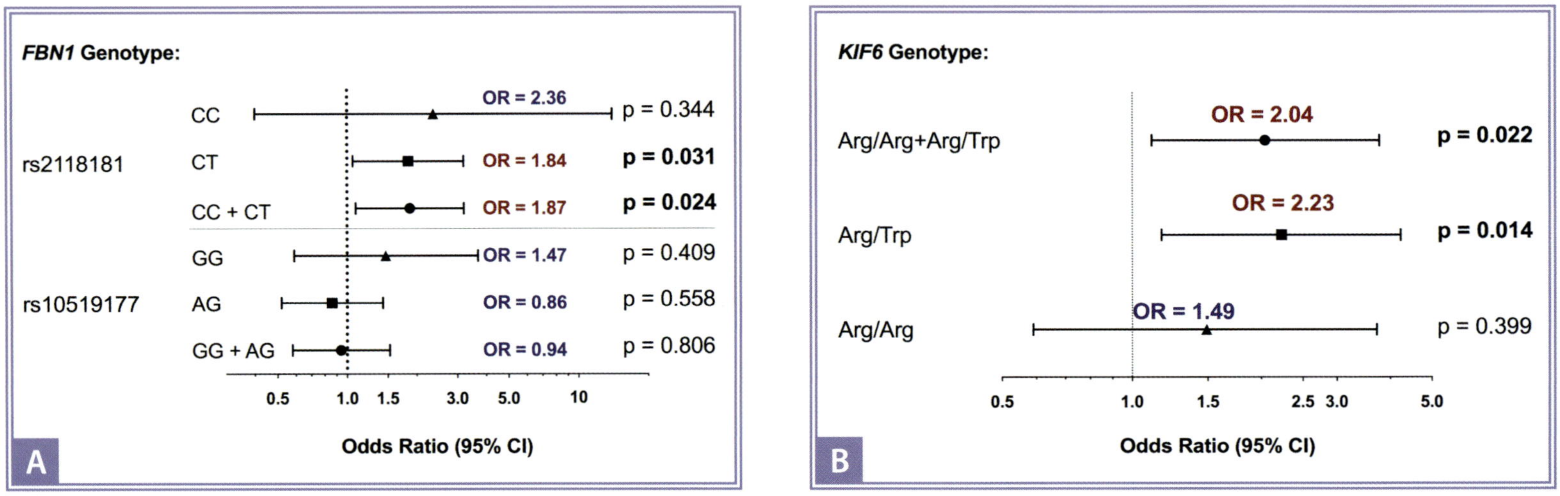

Fig. 6.6 A substitution mutation at the rs2118181 locus on the *FBN1* gene predisposes two-fold toward the development of AD (**A**). The presence of the Arg/Trp and Arg/Arg + Arg/Trp alleles in the *KIF6* gene predisposes toward the development of AD (**B**). (Panel A based on data from [142]; Panel B based on data from [150]).

Furthermore, a recent study discovered that the intronic SNP rs11172113 of the *LRP1* gene, which encodes low-density lipoprotein receptor-related protein 1, was associated with a decreased risk for sporadic thoracic aortic dissection (STAD) [145]. On the other hand, this study found that the rs2272007 SNP of the *ULK4* gene, which encodes unc-51-like kinase 4, was associated with an increased risk for STAD and that *ULK4* genomic deletions were associated with TAAD [145].

These findings illustrate the promise that genetics holds for identifying which patients are specifically at increased risk for AD.

6.5 Genetic testing for thoracic aortic aneurysm and dissection

6.5.1 Whole exome sequencing

While it is well-established that approximately 20% of TAAD individuals have a positive family history, only one-quarter to one-third of FTAAD can be explained by our current genetic understanding [46]. It is estimated that syndromic genes, including *FBN1* and TGF-β pathway genes (*TGFBR1*, *TGFBR2*, *SMAD3*, *TGFB2*), account for 10% of FTAAD, *ACTA2* accounts for 12-21%, and other FTAAD genes previously mentioned in this chapter collectively account for 1-2% [114]. Therefore, there is clearly a significant degree of genetic heterogeneity underlying TAAD, with many more mutations and genes yet to be discovered.

Given the importance of genetic testing in TAAD patients, in 2012, we at the Aortic Institute at Yale initiated a clinical program of routine genetic testing of these patients via comprehensive whole exome sequencing (WES) (DNA sequencing the exons (coding regions) of all genes in the genome [146]). This concept of comprehensive genetic testing for thoracic aortic disease is very new, and we believe it has multiple advantages: (1) WES is comprehensive and tests for all known TAAD genes, (2) the entire exome is sequenced so that we can reanalyze the data once new genes are discovered, (3) WES is becoming more cost-effective than conducting single gene tests, and (4) WES provides genome-wide data that can be "mined" for new variants and genes.

To date, we have completed WES for 211 patients with TAAD (mean age 56.5 ± 14.2 years, range 15-83). Twenty-three specific genes known to cause TAAD underwent focused analysis: *ACTA2*, *ADAMTS10*, *COL1A1*, *COL1A2*, *COL3A1*, *COL5A1*, *COL5A2*, *ELN*, *FBLN4*, *FBN1*, *FBN2*, *FLNA*, *MAT2A*, *MYH11*, *MYLK*, *NOTCH1*, *PRKG1*, *SKI*, *SLC2A10*, *SMAD3*, *TGFBR1*, *TGFBR2*, *TGFB2*. Of the 211 patients, 150 (71.1%) were found to carry no mutations in this panel of genes. Of the remaining 61 individuals, 68 variants were identified as potentially causative of TAAD with 65 of these variants occurring in the panel of tested genes. Three deleterious variants occurred in other genes, namely *TGFB3* (n=1) and *MIB1* (n=2). Among the 65 variants in TAAD-related genes, 7 were found to be deleterious (*FBN1*, n=3; *TGFBR2*, n=2; *FLNA*, n=1; *MYLK*, n=1), while 58 were classified as variants of unknown significance (VUS). Variants in *FBN1*, *NOTCH1*, and *MYH11* were most commonly seen (17%, 15%, and 14%, respectively) (Fig. 6.7). These findings differ from prior reports that identified *ACTA2* as the most commonly affected gene in FTAAD.

Through the use of WES, it will be possible to identify both unreported variants in TAAD-related genes as well as novel genes that underlie this disease. These results will permit construction of a comprehensive library of genetic variants that are associated with TAAD.

6.5.2 Single site Sanger sequencing

Sanger sequencing is a method of DNA sequencing during which DNA polymerases copy single-stranded DNA templates by adding nucleotides to a growing chain [146, 147]. Once a

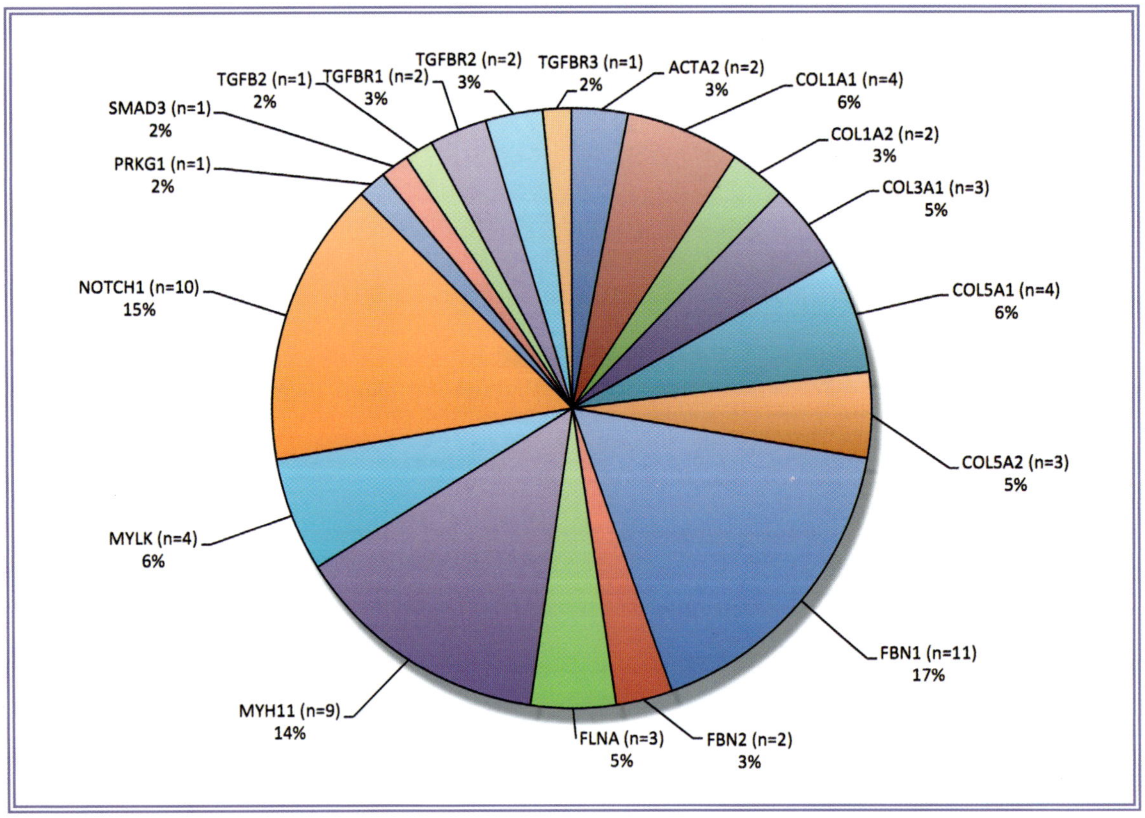

Fig. 6.7 Frequency distribution of genetic defects in TAAD-related genes based on the Yale Aortic Institute routine genetic testing program.

proband is identified via WES, Sanger sequencing is a very effective tool for screening family members by specifically targeting the gene in which an abnormal variant was identified in the proband.

Examples of the substantial clinical benefits of single site Sanger sequencing of family members are depicted in two families (see pedigrees A and B in Fig. 6.8). In the family shown in pedigree A, a pathogenic missense mutation was identified via WES in the proband (red arrow) in the *MYLK* gene (S175P). Sanger sequencing was then conducted in 9 first-degree relatives, three of whom (including the proband) had suffered from Type A AD, which occurred at aortic diameters of 4.0 cm or less. The proband's son (shown with an asterisk), who was having his aortic root measured regularly since the age of 16 and was being treated with beta blockers, was found to be a carrier of the deleterious mutation at the age of 31. Since his aortic root was 3.9 cm, approaching the early danger zone for AD, the decision was made to proceed with elective surgery on the ascending aorta. The proband's niece and nephew (shown with a # sign) were also found to harbor the pathogenic mutation at the ages of 19 and 15, respectively, and have been receiving regular aortic imaging to monitor for aneurysmal growth.

In the family presented in Panel B of Figure 6.8, a variant of unknown significance in the *TGFBR1* gene was found to segregate with disease, as it was identified in all living family members with TAAD. The proband's niece (shown with an asterisk), was found to harbor the variant, and has thus been receiving regular aortic imaging along with angiotensin-receptor blocker therapy to discourage aneurysmal growth.

These two families demonstrate how critical genetic testing is for providing appropriate preventative care for patients with TAAD. Since the underlying causative gene in any given

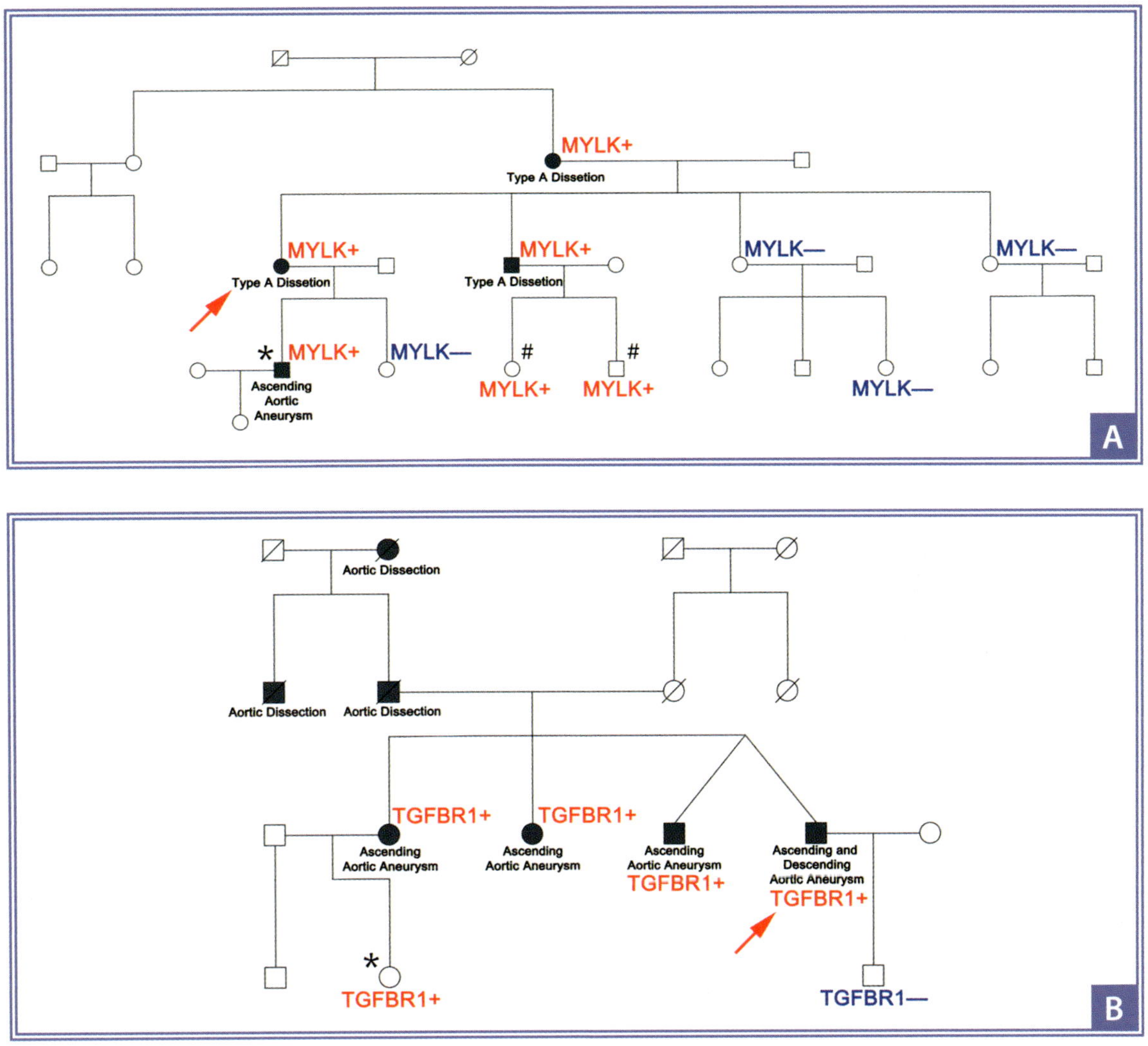

Fig. 6.8 Pedigrees of 2 families who underwent comprehensive genetic testing. A deleterious *MYLK* mutation was found in 6 out of 10 tested family members (**A**). A variant of unknown significance was identified in the *TGFBR1* gene, which segregated with disease (**B**). Reproduced from [14], with permission.

family can predict who is at risk for TAAD, how their aortic disease will manifest, and their risk for dissection at different sized aortas [114], personalized treatment can be provided depending on the specific gene mutation identified.

6.6 Conclusion

Over the past two decades, we have witnessed an explosion in our understanding of the genetics of thoracic aortic aneurysms and dissection. We have gone from first appreciating the familial nature of TAAD to now identifying multiple genes that fundamentally alter the extracellular matrix, smooth muscle cell function, or the TGF-β signaling pathway, thereby predisposing to this disease. We anticipate that, in the coming years, we will be able to provide personalized care for patients depending on the underlying genetic mutation that they harbor. As genetic testing becomes more widespread, we will be able to identify even more individuals at risk and thus provide regular cardiovascular imaging and timely prophylactic surgery to prevent the devastating complication of AD. Although, as surgeons, we emphasize the elegance and effectiveness of surgical therapies for thoracic aortic aneurysm and dissection, we recognize that the most important breakthrough in combating this fatal disease is currently, and will continue to be, on the genetic front.

REFERENCES

1) Clouse WD, Hallett JW Jr, Schaff HV, et al. Acute aortic dissection: population-based incidence compared with degenerative aortic aneurysm rupture. Mayo Clin Proc 2004; 79(2): 176-80.
2) Ramanath VS, Oh JK, Sundt TM 3rd, Eagle KA. Acute aortic syndromes and thoracic aortic aneurysm. Mayo Clin Proc 2009; 84(5): 465-81.
3) Ziganshin BA, Elefteriades JA. Guilt by association: a paradigm for detection of silent aortic disease. Ann Cardiothorac Surg 2016; 5(3): 174-87.
4) Chau KH, Elefteriades JA. Natural history of thoracic aortic aneurysms: size matters, plus moving beyond size. Prog Cardiovasc Dis 2013; 56(1): 74-80.
5) Pape LA, Tsai TT, Isselbacher EM, et al. Aortic diameter >or = 5.5 cm is not a good predictor of type A aortic dissection: observations from the International Registry of Acute Aortic Dissection (IRAD). Circulation 2007; 116(10): 1120-7.
6) Elefteriades JA, Ziganshin BA, Rizzo JA, et al. Indications and imaging for aortic surgery: size and other matters. J Thorac Cardiovasc Surg 2015; 149 (2 Suppl): S10-3.
7) Andelfinger G, Loeys B, Dietz H. A decade of discovery in the genetic understanding of thoracic aortic disease. Can J Cardiol 2016; 32 (1): 13-25.
8) Gillis E, Van Laer L, Loeys BL. Genetics of thoracic aortic aneurysm: at the crossroad of transforming growth factor-beta signaling and vascular smooth muscle cell contractility. Circ Res 2013; 113(3): 327-40.
9) Bradley TJ, Bowdin SC, Morel CF, Pyeritz RE. The expanding clinical spectrum of extracardiovascular and cardiovascular manifestations of heritable thoracic aortic aneurysm and dissection. Can J Cardiol 2016; 32(1): 86-99.
10) Biddinger A, Rocklin M, Coselli J, Milewicz DM. Familial thoracic aortic dilatations and dissections: a case control study. J Vasc Surg 1997; 25 (3): 506-11.
11) Coady MA, Davies RR, Roberts M, et al. Familial patterns of thoracic aortic aneurysms. Arch Surg 1999; 134 (4): 361-7.
12) Elefteriades JA, Pomianowski P. Practical genetics of thoracic aortic aneurysm. Prog Cardiovasc Dis 2013; 56(1): 57-67.
13) Pomianowski P, Elefteriades JA. The genetics and genomics of thoracic aortic disease. Ann Cardiothorac Surg 2013; 2(3): 271-9.
14) Ziganshin BA, Bailey AE, Coons C, et al. Routine genetic testing for thoracic aortic aneurysm and dissection in a clinical setting. Ann Thorac Surg 2015; 100(5): 1604-11.
15) Milewicz DM, Regalado ES. Use of genetics for personalized management of heritable thoracic aortic disease: how do we get there? J Thorac Cardiovasc Surg 2015; 149 (2 Suppl): S3-5.
16) Wang L, Guo DC, Cao J, et al. Mutations in myosin light chain kinase cause familial aortic dissections. Am J Hum Genet 2010; 87 (5): 701-7.
17) Guo DC, Pannu H, Tran-Fadulu V, et al. Mutations in smooth muscle alpha-actin (ACTA2) lead to thoracic aortic aneurysms and dissections. Nat Genet 2007; 39 (12): 1488-93.
18) Guo DC, Papke CL, Tran-Fadulu V, et al. Mutations in smooth muscle alpha-actin (ACTA2) cause coronary artery disease, stroke, and Moyamoya disease, along with thoracic aortic disease. Am J Hum Genet 2009; 84 (5): 617-27.
19) Hiratzka LF, Bakris GL, Beckman JA, et al. 2010 ACCF/AHA/AATS/ACR/ASA/SCA/SCAI/SIR/STS/SVM Guidelines for the diagnosis and management of patients with thoracic aortic disease. A Report of the American College of Cardiology Foundation/American Heart Association Task Force on Practice Guidelines, American Association for Thoracic Surgery, American College of Radiology, American Stroke Association, Society of Cardiovascular Anesthesiologists, Society for Cardiovascular Angiography and Interventions, Society of Interventional Radiology, Society of Thoracic Surgeons, and Society for Vascular Medicine. Journal of the American College of Cardiology 2010; 55(14): e27-e129.
20) Albornoz G, Coady MA, Roberts M, et al. Familial thoracic aortic aneurysms and dissections - Incidence, modes of inheritance, and phenotypic patterns. Annals of Thoracic Surgery 2006; 82(4): 1400-6.
21) Milewicz DM, Chen H, Park ES, et al. Reduced penetrance and variable expressivity of familial thoracic aortic aneurysms/dissections. Am J Cardiol 1998; 82(4): 474-9.
22) Milewicz DM, Regalado ES, Shendure J, Nickerson DA, Guo DC. Successes and challenges of using whole exome sequencing to identify novel genes underlying an inherited predisposition for thoracic aortic aneurysms and acute aortic dissections. Trends Cardiovasc Med 2014; 24(2): 53-60.

23) Liu W, Zhao N, Li XF, et al. A novel FBN2 mutation in a Chinese family with congenital contractural arachnodactyly. FEBS Open Bio 2015; 5: 163-6.
24) Cheung C, Bernardo AS, Trotter MW, Pedersen RA, Sinha S. Generation of human vascular smooth muscle subtypes provides insight into embryological origin-dependent disease susceptibility. Nat Biotechnol 2012; 30(2): 165-73.
25) Gittenberger-de Groot AC, DeRuiter MC, Bergwerff M, Poelmann RE. Smooth muscle cell origin and its relation to heterogeneity in development and disease. Arterioscler Thromb Vasc Biol 1999; 19(7): 1589-94.
26) Ruddy JM, Jones JA, Ikonomidis JS. Pathophysiology of thoracic aortic aneurysm (TAA): is it not one uniform aorta? Role of embryologic origin. Prog Cardiovasc Dis 2013; 56 (1): 68-73.
27) El-Hamamsy I, Yacoub MH. Cellular and molecular mechanisms of thoracic aortic aneurysms. Nat Rev Cardiol 2009; 6(12): 771-86.
28) Isselbacher EM, Lino Cardenas CL, Lindsay ME. Hereditary influence in thoracic aortic aneurysm and dissection. Circulation 2016; 133 (24): 2516-28.
29) Judge DP, Dietz HC. Marfan's syndrome. Lancet 2005; 366 (9501): 1965-76.
30) Loeys BL, Dietz HC, Braverman AC, et al. The revised Ghent nosology for the Marfan syndrome. J Med Genet 2010; 47(7): 476-85.
31) Collod-Beroud G, Le Bourdelles S, Ades L, et al. Update of the UMD-FBN1 mutation database and creation of an FBN1 polymorphism database. Hum Mutat 2003 22 (3): 199-208.
32) den Hartog AW, Franken R, Zwinderman AH, et al. The risk for type B aortic dissection in Marfan syndrome. J Am Coll Cardiol 2015; 65(3): 246-54.
33) Germain DP. Ehlers-Danlos syndrome type IV. Orphanet J Rare Dis 2007; 2:32.
34) Pepin M, Schwarze U, Superti-Furga A, Byers PH. Clinical and genetic features of Ehlers-Danlos syndrome type IV, the vascular type. New Engl J Med 2000; 342 (10): 673-80.
35) Loeys BL, Schwarze U, Holm T, et al. Aneurysm syndromes caused by mutations in the TGF-beta receptor. New Engl J Med 2006; 355 (8): 788-98.
36) Loeys BL, Chen J, Neptune ER, et al. A syndrome of altered cardiovascular, craniofacial, neurocognitive and skeletal development caused by mutations in TGFBR1 or TGFBR2. Nat Genet 2005; 37(3): 275-81.
37) MacCarrick G, Black JH 3rd, Bowdin S, et al. Loeys-Dietz syndrome: a primer for diagnosis and management. Genet Med 2014; 16 (8): 576-87.
38) Attias D, Stheneur C, Roy C, et al. Comparison of clinical presentations and outcomes between patients with TGFBR2 and FBN1 mutations in Marfan syndrome and related disorders. Circulation 2009; 120 (25): 2541-9.
39) Coucke PJ, Willaert A, Wessels MW, et al. Mutations in the facilitative glucose transporter GLUT10 alter angiogenesis and cause arterial tortuosity syndrome. Nat Genet 2006; 38(4): 452-7.
40) Callewaert B, De Paepe A, Coucke P. Arterial tortuosity syndrome. In: Pagon RA, Adam MP, Ardinger HH, et al. (Eds). Seattle (WA): GeneReviews (R), 1993.
41) Ritelli M, Chiarelli N, Dordoni C, et al. Arterial tortuosity syndrome: homozygosity for two novel and one recurrent SLC2A10 missense mutations in three families with severe cardiopulmonary complications in infancy and a literature review. BMC Med Genet 2014; 15: 122.
42) Wessels MW, Catsman-Berrevoets CE, Mancini GM, et al. Three new families with arterial tortuosity syndrome. Am J Med Genet A 2004; 131 (2): 134-43.
43) Callewaert BL, Willaert A, Kerstjens-Frederikse WS, et al. Arterial tortuosity syndrome: clinical and molecular findings in 12 newly identified families. Hum Mutat 2008; 29(1): 150-8.
44) van de Laar IM, Oldenburg RA, Pals G, et al. Mutations in SMAD3 cause a syndromic form of aortic aneurysms and dissections with early-onset osteoarthritis. Nat Genet 2011; 43(2): 121-6.
45) van de Laar IM, van der Linde D, Oei EH, et al. Phenotypic spectrum of the SMAD3-related aneurysms-osteoarthritis syndrome. J Med Genet 2012; 49(1): 47-57.
46) Luyckx I, Loeys BL, Curriculum topic: Disease of the aorta, trauma to the aorta and heart. The genetic architecture of non-syndromic thoracic aortic aneurysm. Heart 2015; 101(20): 1678-84.
47) Wu D, Shen YH, Russell L, Coselli JS, LeMaire SA. Molecular mechanisms of thoracic aortic dissection. J Surg Res 2013; 184 (2): 907-24.
48) Karimi A, Milewicz DM. Structure of the elastin-contractile units in the thoracic aorta and how genes that cause thoracic aortic aneurysms and dissections disrupt this structure. Can J Cardiol 2016; 32 (1): 26-34.
49) Faivre L, Collod-Beroud G, Loeys BL, et al. Effect of mutation type and location on clinical outcome in 1,013 probands with Marfan syndrome or related phenotypes and FBN1 mutations: an international study. Am J Hum Genet 2007; 81 (3): 454-66.
50) Baudhuin LM, Kotzer KE, Lagerstedt SA. Increased frequency of FBN1 truncating and splicing variants in Marfan syndrome patients with aortic events. Genet Med 2015; 17(3): 177-87.
51) Franken R, Groenink M, de Waard V, et al. Genotype impacts survival in Marfan syndrome. Eur Heart J 2016 [Epub ahead of print].

52) Regalado ES, Guo DC, Santos-Cortez RL, et al. Pathogenic FBN1 variants in familial thoracic aortic aneurysms and dissections. Clin Genet. 2016; 89(6): 719-23.
53) Baudhuin LM, Kotzer KE, Lagerstedt SA. Decreased frequency of FBN1 missense variants in Ghent criteria-positive Marfan syndrome and characterization of novel FBN1 variants. J Hum Genet 2015; 60(5): 241-52.
54) Gott VL, Greene PS, Alejo DE, et al. Replacement of the aortic root in patients with Marfan's syndrome. The New England journal of medicine. 1999; 340(17): 1307-13.
55) Putnam EA, Zhang H, Ramirez F, Milewicz DM. Fibrillin-2 (FBN2) mutations result in the Marfan-like disorder, congenital contractural arachnodactyly. Nat Genet 1995; 11(4): 456-8.
56) Frederic MY, Monino C, Marschall C, et al. The FBN2 gene: new mutations, locus-specific database (Universal Mutation Database FBN2), and genotype-phenotype correlations. Hum Mutat 2009; 30(2): 181-90.
57) Callewaert BL, Loeys BL, Ficcadenti A, et al. Comprehensive clinical and molecular assessment of 32 probands with congenital contractural arachnodactyly: report of 14 novel mutations and review of the literature. Hum Mutat 2009; 30(3): 334-41.
58) Gupta PA, Putnam EA, Carmical SG, et al. Ten novel FBN2 mutations in congenital contractural arachnodactyly: delineation of the molecular pathogenesis and clinical phenotype. Hum Mutat 2002; 19(1): 39-48.
59) Takeda N, Morita H, Fujita D, et al. Congenital contractural arachnodactyly complicated with aortic dilatation and dissection: Case report and review of literature. Am J Med Genet A 2015; 167A(10): 2382-7.
60) Smith LB, Hadoke PW, Dyer E, et al. Haploinsufficiency of the murine Col3a1 locus causes aortic dissection: a novel model of the vascular type of Ehlers-Danlos syndrome. Cardiovasc Res 2011; 90(1): 182-90.
61) Shalhub S, Black JH 3rd, Cecchi AC, et al. Molecular diagnosis in vascular Ehlers-Danlos syndrome predicts pattern of arterial involvement and outcomes. J Vasc Surg 2014; 60(1): 160-9.
62) Frank M, Albuisson J, Ranque B, et al. The type of variants at the COL3A1 gene associates with the phenotype and severity of vascular Ehlers-Danlos syndrome. Eur J Hum Gene. 2015; 23(12): 1657-64.
63) Pepin MG, Schwarze U, Rice KM, Liu M, Leistritz D, Byers PH. Survival is affected by mutation type and molecular mechanism in vascular Ehlers-Danlos syndrome (EDS type IV). Genet Med 2014; 16(12): 881-8.
64) Malfait F, Symoens S, De Backer J, et al. Three arginine to cysteine substitutions in the pro-alpha (I)-collagen chain cause Ehlers-Danlos syndrome with a propensity to arterial rupture in early adulthood. Hum Mutat 2007; 28(4): 387-95.
65) Schwarze U, Hata R, McKusick VA, et al. Rare autosomal recessive cardiac valvular form of Ehlers-Danlos syndrome results from mutations in the COL1A2 gene that activate the nonsense-mediated RNA decay pathway. Am J Hum Genet 2004; 74 (5): 917-30.
66) De Paepe A, Malfait F. The Ehlers-Danlos syndrome, a disorder with many faces. Clin Genet 2012; 82(1): 1-11.
67) Wenstrup RJ, Meyer RA, Lyle JS, et al. Prevalence of aortic root dilation in the Ehlers-Danlos syndrome. Genet Med 2002; 4(3): 112-7.
68) Mehta S, Dhar SU, Birnbaum Y. Common iliac artery aneurysm and spontaneous dissection with contralateral iatrogenic common iliac artery dissection in classic ehlers-danlos syndrome. Int J Angiol 2012; 21(3): 167-70.
69) Monroe GR, Harakalova M, van der Crabben SN, et al. Familial Ehlers-Danlos syndrome with lethal arterial events caused by a mutation in COL5A1. Am J Med Genet A 2015; 167 (6): 1196-203.
70) Meienberg J, Rohrbach M, Neuenschwander S, et al. Hemizygous deletion of COL3A1, COL5A2, and MSTN causes a complex phenotype with aortic dissection: a lesson for and from true haploinsufficiency. Eur J Hum Genet 2010; 18 (12): 1315-21.
71) Kashtan CE, Segal Y, Flinter F, Makanjuola D, Gan JS, Watnick T. Aortic abnormalities in males with Alport syndrome. Nephrol Dial Transplant 2010; 25 (11): 3554-60.
72) Earl TJ, Khan L, Hagau D, Fernandez AB. The spectrum of aortic pathology in alport syndrome: a case report and review of the literature. Am J Kidney Dis 2012; 60 (5): 821-2.
73) Renard M, Holm T, Veith R, et al. Altered TGFbeta signaling and cardiovascular manifestations in patients with autosomal recessive cutis laxa type I caused by fibulin-4 deficiency. Eur J Hum Genet 2010; 18(8): 895-901.
74) Hucthagowder V, Sausgruber N, Kim KH, Angle B, Marmorstein LY, Urban Z. Fibulin-4: a novel gene for an autosomal recessive cutis laxa syndrome. Am J Hum Genet 2006; 78(6): 1075-80.
75) Hebson C, Coleman K, Clabby M, et al. Severe aortopathy due to fibulin-4 deficiency: molecular insights, surgical strategy, and a review of the literature. Eur J Pediatr 2014; 173(5): 671-5.
76) Papke CL, Tsunezumi J, Ringuette LJ, et al. Loss of fibulin-4 disrupts collagen synthesis and maturation: implications for pathology resulting from EFEMP2 mutations. Hum Mol Genet 2015; 24 (20): 5867-79.
77) Igoucheva O, Alexeev V, Halabi CM, et al. Fibulin-4 E57K knock-in mice recapitulate cutaneous, vascular and skeletal defects of recessive cutis laxa 1b with both elastic fiber and collagen fibril abnormalities. J Biol Chem 2015; 290 (35): 21443-59.

78) Szabo Z, Crepeau MW, Mitchell AL, et al. Aortic aneurysmal disease and cutis laxa caused by defects in the elastin gene. J Med Genet 2006; 43 (3): 255-8.
79) Callewaert B, Renard M, Hucthagowder V, et al. New insights into the pathogenesis of autosomal-dominant cutis laxa with report of five ELN mutations. Hum Mutat 2011; 32(4): 445-55.
80) Parrott A, James J, Goldenberg P, et al. Aortopathy in the 7q11.23 microduplication syndrome. Am J Med Genet A 2015; 167A(2): 363-70.
81) Guemann AS, Andrieux J, Petit F, et al. ELN gene triplication responsible for familial supravalvular aortic aneurysm. Cardiol Young 2015; 25 (4): 712-7.
82) Capuano A, Bucciotti F, Farwell KD, et al. Diagnostic exome sequencing identifies a novel gene, emilin1, associated with autosomal-dominant hereditary connective tissue disease. Hum Mutat 2016; 37(1): 84-97.
83) Barbier M, Gross MS, Aubart M, et al. MFAP5 loss-of-function mutations underscore the involvement of matrix alteration in the pathogenesis of familial thoracic aortic aneurysms and dissections. Am J Hum Genet 2014; 95(6): 736-43.
84) Mohamed SA, Sievers HH, Hanke T, et al. Pathway analysis of differentially expressed genes in patients with acute aortic dissection. Biomark Insights 2009; 4: 81-90.
85) Guo DC, Regalado ES, Gong L, et al. LOX mutations predispose to thoracic aortic aneurysms and dissections. Circ Res 2016; 118(6): 928-34.
86) Lee VS, Halabi CM, Hoffman EP, et al. Loss of function mutation in LOX causes thoracic aortic aneurysm and dissection in humans. Proc Natl Acad Sci U S A. 2016; 113(31): 8759-64.
87) Atsawasuwan P, Mochida Y, Katafuchi M, et al. Lysyl oxidase binds transforming growth factor-beta and regulates its signaling via amine oxidase activity. J BIOL CHEM 2008; 283(49): 34229-40.
88) Lindsay ME, Dietz HC. The genetic basis of aortic aneurysm. Cold Spring Harb Perspect Med 2014; 4(9): a015909.
89) Meester JA, Vandeweyer G, Pintelon I, et al. Loss-of-function mutations in the X-linked biglycan gene cause a severe syndromic form of thoracic aortic aneurysms and dissections. Genet Med 2016; [Epub ahead of print].
90) Zhu L, Vranckx R, Khau Van Kien P, et al. Mutations in myosin heavy chain 11 cause a syndrome associating thoracic aortic aneurysm/aortic dissection and patent ductus arteriosus. Nat Genet 2006; 38(3): 343-9.
91) Pannu H, Tran-Fadulu V, Papke CL, et al. MYH11 mutations result in a distinct vascular pathology driven by insulin-like growth factor 1 and angiotensin II. Hum Mol Genet 2007; 16(20): 2453-62.
92) Harakalova M, van der Smagt J, de Kovel CG, et al. Incomplete segregation of MYH11 variants with thoracic aortic aneurysms and dissections and patent ductus arteriosus. Eur J Hum Genet 2013; 21(5): 487-93.
93) Imai Y, Morita H, Takeda N, et al. A deletion mutation in myosin heavy chain 11 causing familial thoracic aortic dissection in two Japanese pedigrees. Int J Cardiol 2015; 195: 290-2.
94) Kuang SQ, Guo DC, Prakash SK, et al. Recurrent chromosome 16p13.1 duplications are a risk factor for aortic dissections. PLoS Genet 2011; 7(6): e1002118.
95) Morisaki H, Akutsu K, Ogino H, et al. Mutation of ACTA2 gene as an important cause of familial and nonfamilial nonsyndromatic thoracic aortic aneurysm and/or dissection (TAAD). Hum Mutat 2009; 30(10): 1406-11.
96) Disabella E, Grasso M, Gambarin FI, et al. Risk of dissection in thoracic aneurysms associated with mutations of smooth muscle alpha-actin 2 (ACTA2). Heart 2011; 97(4): 321-6.
97) Renard M, Callewaert B, Baetens M, et al. Novel MYH11 and ACTA2 mutations reveal a role for enhanced TGFbeta signaling in FTAAD. Int J Cardiol 2013; 165(2): 314-21.
98) Milewicz DM, Ostergaard JR, Ala-Kokko LM, et al. De novo ACTA2 mutation causes a novel syndrome of multisystemic smooth muscle dysfunction. Am J Med Genet A 2010; 152A(10): 2437-43.
99) Regalado ES, Guo DC, Prakash S, et al. Aortic disease presentation and outcome associated with ACTA2 mutations. Circ Cardiovasc Genet 2015; 8(3): 457-64.
100) Regalado ES, Guo DC, Estrera AL, Buja LM, Milewicz DM. Acute aortic dissections with pregnancy in women with ACTA2 mutations. Am J Med Genet A 2014; 164A (1): 106-12.
101) Hannuksela M, Stattin EL, Klar J, et al. A novel variant in MYLK causes thoracic aortic dissections: genotypic and phenotypic description. BMC Med Genet 2016; 17(1): 61.
102) Guo DC, Regalado E, Casteel DE, et al. Recurrent gain-of-function mutation in PRKG1 causes thoracic aortic aneurysms and acute aortic dissections. Am J Hum Genet 2013; 93(2): 398-404.
103) Sheen VL, Jansen A, Chen MH, et al. Filamin A mutations cause periventricular heterotopia with Ehlers-Danlos syndrome. Neurol 2005; 64(2): 254-62.
104) Lange M, Kasper B, Bohring A, et al. 47 patients with FLNA associated periventricular nodular heterotopia. Orphanet J Rare Dis 2015; 10: 134.
105) Reinstein E, Frentz S, Morgan T, et al. Vascular and connective tissue anomalies associated with X-linked periventricular heterotopia due to mutations in Filamin A. Eur J Hum Genet 2013; 21(5): 494-502.

106) Guo DC, Gong L, Regalado ES, et al. MAT2A mutations predispose individuals to thoracic aortic aneurysms. Am J Hum Genet 2015; 96(1): 170-7.
107) Kuang SQ, Medina-Martinez O, Guo DC, et al. FOXE3 mutations predispose to thoracic aortic aneurysms and dissections. J Clin Invest 2016; 126(3): 948-61.
108) Lindsay ME, Dietz HC. Lessons on the pathogenesis of aneurysm from heritable conditions. Nature 2011; 473(7347): 308-16.
109) Pannu H, Fadulu VT, Chang J, et al. Mutations in transforming growth factor-beta receptor type II cause familial thoracic aortic aneurysms and dissections. Circulation 2005; 112(4): 513-20.
110) Tran-Fadulu V, Pannu H, Kim DH, et al. Analysis of multigenerational families with thoracic aortic aneurysms and dissections due to TGFBR1 or TGFBR2 mutations. J Med Genet 2009; 46(9): 607-13.
111) Teixido-Tura G, Franken R, Galuppo V, et al. Heterogeneity of aortic disease severity in patients with Loeys-Dietz syndrome. Heart 2016; 102(8): 626-32.
112) Detaint D, Michelena HI, Nkomo VT, et al. Aortic dilatation patterns and rates in adults with bicuspid aortic valves: a comparative study with Marfan syndrome and degenerative aortopathy. Heart 2014; 100(2): 126-34.
113) Boodhwani M, Andelfinger G, Leipsic J, et al. Canadian Cardiovascular Society position statement on the management of thoracic aortic disease. Can J Cardiol 2014; 30(6): 577-89.
114) Milewicz D, Hostetler E, Wallace S, et al. Precision medical and surgical management for thoracic aortic aneurysms and acute aortic dissections based on the causative mutant gene. J Cardiovasc Surg (Torino) 2016; 57(2): 172-7.
115) Erbel R, Aboyans V, Boileau C, et al. 2014 ESC Guidelines on the diagnosis and treatment of aortic diseases: Document covering acute and chronic aortic diseases of the thoracic and abdominal aorta of the adult. The Task Force for the Diagnosis and Treatment of Aortic Diseases of the European Society of Cardiology (ESC). Eur Heart J 2014; 35(41): 2873-926.
116) Boileau C, Guo DC, Hanna N, et al. TGFB2 mutations cause familial thoracic aortic aneurysms and dissections associated with mild systemic features of Marfan syndrome. Nat Genet 2012; 44(8): 916-21.
117) Lindsay ME, Schepers D, Bolar NA, et al. Loss-of-function mutations in TGFB2 cause a syndromic presentation of thoracic aortic aneurysm. Nat Genet 2012; 44(8): 922-7.
118) Renard M, Callewaert B, Malfait F, et al. Thoracic aortic-aneurysm and dissection in association with significant mitral valve disease caused by mutations in TGFB2. Int J Cardiol 2013; 165(3): 584-7.
119) Gago-Diaz M, Blanco-Verea A, Teixido-Tura G, et al. Whole exome sequencing for the identification of a new mutation in TGFB2 involved in a familial case of non-syndromic aortic disease. Clin Chim Acta 2014; 437: 88-92.
120) Leutermann R, Sheikhzadeh S, Brockstadt L, et al. A 1-bp duplication in TGFB2 in three family members with a syndromic form of thoracic aortic aneurysm. Eur J Hum Genet 2014; 22(7): 944-8.
121) Ritelli M, Chiarelli N, Dordoni C, et al. Further delineation of Loeys-Dietz syndrome type 4 in a family with mild vascular involvement and a TGFB2 splicing mutation. BMC Med Genet 2014; 15: 91.
122) Bertoli-Avella AM, Gillis E, Morisaki H, et al. Mutations in a TGF-beta ligand, TGFB3, cause syndromic aortic aneurysms and dissections. J Am Coll Cardiol 2015; 65(13): 1324-36.
123) Rienhoff HY Jr, Yeo CY, Morissette R, et al. A mutation in TGFB3 associated with a syndrome of low muscle mass, growth retardation, distal arthrogryposis and clinical features overlapping with Marfan and Loeys-Dietz syndrome. Am J Med Genet A 2013; 161A(8): 2040-6.
124) Kuechler A, Altmuller J, Nurnberg P, et al. Exome sequencing identifies a novel heterozygous TGFB3 mutation in a disorder overlapping with Marfan and Loeys-Dietz syndrome. Mol Cell Probes 2015; 29(5): 330-4.
125) Matyas G, Naef P, Tollens M, Oexle K. De novo mutation of the latency-associated peptide domain of TGFB3 in a patient with overgrowth and Loeys-Dietz syndrome features. Am J Med Genet A 2014; 164A(8): 2141-3.
126) Regalado ES, Guo DC, Villamizar C, et al. Exome sequencing identifies SMAD3 mutations as a cause of familial thoracic aortic aneurysm and dissection with intracranial and other arterial aneurysms. Circ Res 2011; 109(6): 680-6.
127) Wischmeijer A, Van Laer L, Tortora G, et al. Thoracic aortic aneurysm in infancy in aneurysms-osteoarthritis syndrome due to a novel SMAD3 mutation: further delineation of the phenotype. Am J Med Genet A 2013; 161A(5): 1028-35.
128) van der Linde D, van de Laar IM, Bertoli-Avella AM, et al. Aggressive cardiovascular phenotype of aneurysms-osteoarthritis syndrome caused by pathogenic SMAD3 variants. J Am Coll Cardio 2012; 60(5): 397-403.
129) Teekakirikul P, Milewicz DM, Miller DT, et al. Thoracic aortic disease in two patients with juvenile polyposis syndrome and SMAD4 mutations. Am J Med Genet A 2013; 161A(1): 185-91.
130) Wain KE, Ellingson MS, McDonald J, et al. Appreciating the broad clinical features of SMAD4 mutation carriers: a multicenter chart review. Genet Med 2014; 16(8): 588-93.

131) Heald B, Rigelsky C, Moran R, et al. Prevalence of thoracic aortopathy in patients with juvenile polyposis syndrome-hereditary hemorrhagic telangiectasia due to SMAD4. Am J Med Genet A 2015; 167A(8): 1758-62.
132) Micha D, Guo DC, Hilhorst-Hofstee Y, et al. SMAD2 Mutations are associated with arterial aneurysms and dissections. Hum Mutat 2015; 36(12): 1145-9.
133) Doyle AJ, Doyle JJ, Bessling SL, et al. Mutations in the TGF-beta repressor SKI cause Shprintzen-Goldberg syndrome with aortic aneurysm. Nat Genet 2012; 44(11): 1249-54.
134) Shprintzen RJ, Goldberg RB. A recurrent pattern syndrome of craniosynostosis associated with arachnodactyly and abdominal hernias. J Craniofac Genet Dev Biol. 1982; 2(1): 65-74.
135) Robinson PN, Neumann LM, Demuth S, et al. Shprintzen-Goldberg syndrome: fourteen new patients and a clinical analysis. Am J Med Genet A 2005; 135(3): 251-62.
136) Schepers D, Doyle AJ, Oswald G, et al. The SMAD-binding domain of SKI: a hotspot for de novo mutations causing Shprintzen-Goldberg syndrome. Eur J Hum Genet 2015; 23(2): 224-8.
137) Castori M, Ritelli M, Zoppi N, et al. Adult presentation of arterial tortuosity syndrome in a 51-year-old woman with a novel homozygous c.1411+1G>A mutation in the SLC2A10 gene. Am J Med Genet A 2012; 158A(5): 1164-9.
138) Garg V, Muth AN, Ransom JF, et al. Mutations in NOTCH1 cause aortic valve disease. Nature 2005; 437(7056): 270-4.
139) McKellar SH, Tester DJ, Yagubyan M, et al. Novel NOTCH1 mutations in patients with bicuspid aortic valve disease and thoracic aortic aneurysms. J Thorac Cardiovasc Surg 2007; 134(2): 290-6.
140) Proost D, Vandeweyer G, Meester JA, et al. Performant mutation identification using targeted next-generation sequencing of 14 thoracic aortic aneurysm genes. Hum Mutat 2015; 36(8): 808-14.
141) LeMaire SA, McDonald ML, Guo DC, et al. Genome-wide association study identifies a susceptibility locus for thoracic aortic aneurysms and aortic dissections spanning FBN1 at 15q21.1. Nat Genet 2011; 43(10): 996-1000.
142) Iakoubova OA, Tong CH, Rowland CM, et al. Genetic variants in FBN-1 and risk for thoracic aortic aneurysm and dissection. PloS one 2014; 9(4): e91437.
143) Iakoubova OA, Tong CH, Rowland CM, et al. Association of the Trp719Arg polymorphism in kinesin-like protein 6 with myocardial infarction and coronary heart disease in 2 prospective trials: the CARE and WOSCOPS trials. J Am Coll Cardiol 2008; 51 (4): 435-43.
144) Iakoubova OA, Tong CH., Catanese J, et al. KIF6 719Arg Genetic Variant and Risk for Thoracic Aortic Dissection. Aorta (Stamford) 2016; [in press].
145) Guo DC, Grove ML, Prakash SK, et al. Genetic Variants in LRP1 and ULK4 Are Associated with Acute Aortic Dissections. Am J Hum Genet 2016; 99(3): 762-9.
146) Biesecker LG, Green RC. Diagnostic clinical genome and exome sequencing. New Engl J Med 2014; 370(25): 2418-25.
147) Sanger F, Coulson AR. A rapid method for determining sequences in DNA by primed synthesis with DNA polymerase. J Mol Biol 1975; 94(3): 441-8.
148) Elefteriades JA, Farkas EA. Thoracic aortic aneurysm clinically pertinent controversies and uncertainties. J Am Coll Cardiol 2010; 55(9): 841-57.
149) Verstraeten A, Alaerts M, Van Laer L, Loeys B. Marfan syndrome and related disorders: 25 years of gene discovery. Hum Mutat 2016; 37(6): 524-31.
150) Iakoubova OA, Tong CH, Catanese J, et al. KIF6 719Arg genetic variant and risk for thoracic aortic dissection. Aorta (Stanford). DOI: 10.12945/j.aorta.2015.16.003 [In Press]).

7

DISSECT: a new nomenclature to help facilitate the assessment of aortic dissection in the endovascular era

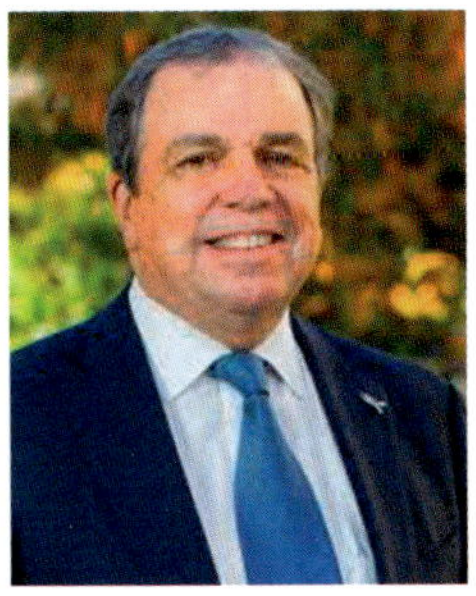

Michael D. Dake and Benedetta Enrico

7.1 Introduction

Aortic dissection (AD) is a catastrophic event responsible for a wide range of clinical manifestations. In any individual, the particular effects experienced are related to the pattern and extent of aortic and branch vessel involvement that occurs as a consequence of the dissection, and, in the longer term, the ability of the aorta to resist the dilating forces of the circulation.

Originally described by Morgagni in 1761 [1], AD remained a highly lethal disease for which no effective therapy, including medical treatment, was available until 1955, when surgical repair was introduced [2].

From the early experience gained with operative management, it became apparent that there are distinct differences between patients with dissection involving the ascending aorta, who have a worse immediate prognosis, and those with descending AD [3-6]. The importance of this differentiation was initially recognized by Hume and Porter [7], and later emphasized in the two most commonly referenced classification systems – the DeBakey [4] and Stanford [8] systems – proposed in 1965 and 1970, respectively. These two most commonly adopted classification schemes for dissection are both in widespread use and generally well understood. They both work extremely well in the context of patients requiring a decision regarding open surgical repair or conservative medical therapy.

Although both the DeBakey and Stanford classifications have been established for more than 40 years, there is no consensus regarding which is preferred; they were developed prior to the use of sophisticated diagnostic imaging modalities during an era of limited surgical options when the intent was simply to group patients into categories based on the advisability of surgery or medical treatment, and not to explore the full extent of disease characteristics that may critically influence both immediate- and longer-term outcomes. Both are not particularly well-suited to adapt to the increasing practice of endovascular repair because neither precisely encompasses primary entry tears located in the aortic arch, allows for definition of an inter-

Michael D. Dake (mddake@stanford.edu)
Stanford University School of Medicine,
Stanford, CA, USA

G. Melissano - R. Chiesa (eds), Aortic Dissection patients true stories and the innovations that saved their lives

mediate period from onset of symptoms that is between acute and chronic groups (i.e. a subacute group), assesses the direction of dissection extension (antegrade, retrograde, mixed), takes into account distal complications secondary to acute or chronic branch vessel occlusion, nor discriminates based upon patency of the aortic false lumen.

The goal of the DISSECT classification system is to provide an easy to assimilate and memorable method of accounting for the critically important factors that influence contemporary decision-making for the management of AD.

7.2 DISSECT classification

The intent of the DISSECT categorization system is to provide a framework that facilitates communication regarding the key aspects of AD that influence its contemporary management. It is hoped that it will supplement the traditional DeBakey and Stanford classification schemes by encompassing the critical anatomical factors these two systems consider, while also recognizing key clinical manifestations and additional imaging data that now inform and influence contemporary management considerations.

Additionally, the system might be used to promote standardization of morphologic and pathophysiologic parameters used to report treatment outcomes. The premise of the categorization is based on the determination of six factors.

7.2.1 D – Duration of dissection

Duration of dissection is defined as time from onset of symptoms:

- acute: <2 weeks from initial onset of symptoms;
- subacute: 2 weeks to 3 months after symptom onset;
- chronic: >3 months from initial symptoms.

The duration of dissection has significance with respect to prognosis, treatment, and response totherapy. Acute dissection of the ascending aorta has poor prognosis when treated medically, with approximately 60% of patients dying in the short term owing to complications of the disease, while the outcome for acute dissection of the descending thoracic aorta is less poor, with an initial hospital mortality rate of about 13% [9].

By contrast, the natural history of chronic dissections is relatively benign in comparison to the acute state. The lower incidence of life-threatening complications in the chronic state is reflected in treatment patterns. Chronic dissections are more likely to be treated non-urgently than acute dissections, and recent series have suggested that endovascular therapy for chronic Type B AD has a lower mortality and complication rate than therapy for acute Type B AD [10, 11].

The chronicity of the dissection also has relevance with regard to aortic remodeling after endovascular therapy, which is significantly greater in patients with acute dissection. There is evidence that aortic remodeling is associated with improved survival in the midterm, and that persistence of false lumen (FL) perfusion is associated with disease progression [12-14].

Endovascular repair of acute dissection is associated with rapid expansion of the true lumen and a reduction in the false lumen. In contrast, endovascular treatment for chronic dissection can induce false lumen thrombosis in the treated segment, but is not associated with major change in true and false lumen diameters. Favorable aortic remodeling was seen in patients undergoing TEVAR for acute AD in the form of significant reduction in FL diameter (and volume) and corresponding increase in TL diameter (and volume) after intervention. This was associated with a lower incidence of endoleak or distal reperfusion and resultant re-intervention [15].

In contradistinction to patients with acute disease, patients with chronic dissection had a greater variation in the degree of luminal remodeling after TEVAR. It has been postulated that the thicker, fixed septum with multiple fenestrations commonly seen in patients with chronic dissections makes the aorta less susceptible to remodeling than what is observed in patients with acute dissection. In addition, chronic patients exhibited a wide range, between 38% and 91.3%, of complete FL thrombosis post stent-graft placement [12].

The explanation for the variable rate of aortic remodeling observed in chronic patients may lie in differing perioperative practices over time or between centers. One procedural issue that has evolved over the last 20 years involves the consideration of the optimal length of aortic stent-graft coverage in AD. Those who advocate longer device coverage have proposed many arguments to support their position. For example, one study showed that a short length of aortic coverage (<162 mm) was less likely than longer coverage to result in favorable aortic remodeling at an average follow-up of 36 months [16]. Others, who advocate longer coverage, were concerned that the distal end of the stent may damage the friable aorta tissue due to movement with the cardiac cycle if coverage was too short [17].

In addition, a longer length of coverage causes a greater proportion of the FL to be physically compressed, and minor fenestrations, or even a large reentry tear, are more likely to be covered. It has been shown that AD with infrarenal extension (DeBakey IIIb) displays less tendency to remodel than disease that stops above the abdomen (DeBakey IIIa) because standard TEVAR of the segment of aorta only above the diaphragm will often not address major distal reentry tears in the abdomen [14].

Furthermore, the chronicity of the disease at the time of TEVAR has been shown to influence the frequency of complete FL thrombosis. The INSTEAD (Investigation of STEnt Grafts in Aortic Dissection) [18] Trial intervention arm reported a rate of 92.6% for total FL thrombosis at 1 year after TEVAR. Patients were recruited into the TEVAR cohort at a median of 3.5 weeks and a mean of 7.5 weeks after the diagnosis of AD. In comparison, the study with the lowest rate of FL thrombosis post TEVAR treated patients at a mean of 100 weeks post diagnosis and achieved FL thrombosis in only 39% of patients, even with 3-year follow-up. The proportion of patients with thoraco-abdominal extension of the dissection was similar in both groups. The difference noted between these two reports suggests that the classification of AD into simply "acute" and "chronic" is insufficient, and that the "sub-acute" classification used in the VIRTUE study of the endovascular treatment of Type B AD to describe TEVAR when it is performed 2 to 4 weeks after the acute event may be more clinically relevant.

7.2.2 I – Intimal tear (primary) location in the aorta

Traditionally, the location of the primary entry tear commonly defines the indication for emergency surgical intervention. Similarly, in many cases the location of the entry tear defines the anatomic suitability for TEVAR. Crucial information includes not only the exact location of the tear but also the location of the tear relative to the greater curve (convexity) or inner curve (concavity) of the aorta.

Phantom studies have also demonstrated that the larger the intimal tear in the proximal aorta, the greater the tendency to exacerbate true lumen collapse. Furthermore, it has been showed that systolic pressure in the false lumen, in comparison with the true lumen, falls with decreasing tear size. Therefore, increased pressure with greater tear size will result in higher wall stress and risk of dilatation.

It has been additionally suggested that proximal location of the entry tear was shown to cause a rise in false lumen diastolic pressure, thereby influencing the tendency toward dilatation. Recent advances in imaging have confirmed that entry tears are often identified in the aortic arch and in the abdominal aorta as well as in the ascending and descending thoracic aorta [19, 20].

Entry tears in the aortic arch and abdominal aorta are not specifically characterized in previous classification systems – DeBakey and Stanford classifications.

7.2.3 S – Size of the dissected aorta

This data is based on the maximum trans-aortic diameter measured in an orthogonal plane to the aorta centerline display.

7.2.4 SE – Segment of extension

The segmental extent of the AD defines the longitudinal involvement of the dissected aorta and also defines the terminal location of secondary fenestrations or re-entry tears in the aortic lamella. The distal extent of the AD influences presentation, treatment, prognosis, and efficacy of treatment. Clearly, the distal extent of the dissection may influence presentation through complications affecting distal branch vessels or lower limb arterial supply. The DeBakey and Stanford systems pay more attention to the primary entry tear than the extent of the dissection, although the modified DeBakey classification does differentiate between dissections with limited (II and IIIa) and more extensive (I and IIIb) aortic involvement [21]. With greater follow-up of AD patients, it has become apparent that even after successful surgical intervention in the ascending aorta, there remains a significant incidence of distal false lumen expansion and chronic aneurysm formation [22, 23].

Indeed, the distal extent of the dissection and the patency of the false lumen influence the likelihood of late complications. In terms of endovascular therapy, the segmental extent of the dissection has been shown to influence response to treatment. Rodriguez et al. [24] demonstrated that complete thoracic false lumen thrombosis occurred in 64% of patients with a DeBakey IIIa dissection compared with just 45% in patients with more extensive distal dissection (IIIb) following thoracic endograft placement.

7.2.5 C – Complications related to the dissection

Traditionally, dissections are classified as complicated or uncomplicated. The major complications include:

- aortic valve involvement;
- cardiac tamponade;
  - rupture;
  - branch vessel malperfusion or symptomatic branch vessel involvement defined as anatomic and clinical manifestations of branch vessel compromise (e.g., static and/or dynamic branch involvement with accompanying stroke, paraplegia, coronary, mesenteric, visceral, renal, and/or extremity symptoms);
- progression of aortic involvement with proximal or distal extension of dissection;
- uncontrollable hypertension;
- persistent, difficult to manage pain;
- rapid false lumen dilation and/or overall trans-aortic enlargement of >10 mm within the first 2 weeks of initial diagnosis.

The differentiation between complicated and uncomplicated dissection has significance with regard to prognosis in Type B AD. Estrera et al. [25] reported the outcomes of 159 patients with Type B AD. Complicated dissection occurred in 47% of patients and was associated with a hospital mortality of 18%. This was compared with uncomplicated dissection that was diagnosed in 53% of patients and had a mortality of 1.2%.

7.2.6 T – Thrombus formation

The status of thrombosis within the aortic false lumen (evaluation of patency within the dissected aortic segments as imaged by computed tomography, magnetic resonance, ultrasound, or transesophageal echocardiography) has been shown to affect progression of disease and prognosis for dissection patients. In this regard, three distinct categories are used to describe thrombus within the aortic FL.

These include:

- P – patent aortic false lumen: evidence of flow or contrast opacification within the false lumen throughout the length of the dissected aorta without associated thrombus.
- CT – complete thrombosis of the aortic false lumen: no evidence of flow or contrast opacification within dissected segments of the aorta.
- PT – partial thrombosis of the aortic false lumen: longitudinal thrombosis of a segmental portion of the aortic false lumen or circumferential thrombus that partially fills the false lumen constitute partial or incomplete thrombosis within the dissected aorta.

The most frequently quoted study that details the importance of false lumen thrombosis was reported by Tsai et al. [26] who studied patients with Type B AD and demonstrated that those with partial thrombosis of the FL at any aortic level had a worse prognosis and an increased mortality relative to those with a completely thrombosed false channel.

7.3 Management strategies

In terms of clinical management, traditional strategies of surgical intervention and medical therapy dictate a strict distinction in the approaches to complicated and uncomplicated acute Type B AD.

The emergence of endovascular alternatives, including TEVAR, have stimulated a re-consideration and debate regarding what constitutes "uncomplicated" dissection, which patients are initially "uncomplicated", but at increased risk of early complications, and the advisability of a more aggressive early interventional approach to prevent disease progression.

Rupture, malperfusion, hemorrhagic pleural effusion, periaortic hematoma, refractory pain, and uncontrollable hypertension constitute the major complications of acute Type B AD. If the patient is experiencing aortic rupture, the immediate consideration when evaluating management options is whether the aortic anatomy is suitable for TEVAR. Does the aortic morphology meet the anatomical requirements for TEVAR to completely cover the primary entry tear and depressurize the false lumen?

Similarly, clinically relevant branch vessel malperfusion is a dangerous complication. In fact, up to 30% of patients with AD exhibit some level of branch artery malperfusion with clinical symptoms, blood chemistry abnormalities and/or hemodynamic or physiological deficits that correspond to imaging findings of branch vessel compromise. As with aortic rupture, a focused imaging evaluation of the dissected aorta with special focus on the mechanism of branch vessel involvement is a prerequisite to determining the appropriateness of TEVAR management. In both cases – rupture and malperfusion – a step by step treatment approach is preferred. For example, in cases of malperfusion syndrome caused by branch vessel involvement, it is critical to re-assess the adequacy of branch vessel perfusion post TEVAR by carefully evaluating the flow within the aortic lumens as well as the involved branch/branches after endograft placement. If the branch vessel compromise is not corrected by the initial TEVAR, further diagnostic attention must be directed to determine the cause of ongoing ischemia before undertaking further intervention.

Particular attention should be paid to patients who have sustained pain or in whom hypertension is refractory to aggressive medical therapy, in the absence of other complications. Early intervention with TEVAR should be considered in these patients because both these conditions are known to foreshadow rapid disease progression and/or impending rupture.

Traditionally, and according to current international guidelines, stable patients with an initially uncomplicated acute Type B AD should receive optimal medical treatment exclusively as the primary management strategy for their disease. Despite adequate antihypertensive therapy, the long-term prognosis of patients with "uncomplicated" Type B AD is characterized by progression of disease with aortic aneurysm formation in 25-30% within four years, and survival rates from 50 to 80% at five years and 30 to 60% at 10 years. Occasionally, re-dissection, new septal tears or extension of the FL may occur with or without adequate management of hypertension and cause organ malperfusion or ischemic events.

In a prospective randomized trial comparing endograft placement and medical therapy with medical therapy exclusively in patients with uncomplicated Type B AD, TEVAR was associated with a greater early mortality, often in the peri-procedural period. After two years however, TEVAR showed a marked benefit relative to medical therapy alone with a dramatic reduction in late aortic-specific mortality at five years of follow-up. Because of the inherent risk of peri-procedural adverse events including stroke, paraparesis, and death, as well as the possible complications induced directly by the device (i.e., retrograde Type A dissection, new entry tears, et cetera) it is important to critically evaluate the risks and benefits of early TEVAR in order to justify its use in patients with uncomplicated acute Type B AD.

Timely selection of those patients at high risk for developing complications and progression of disease may influence the use of early TEVAR intervention, preferably in the sub-acute (between 14 days and 3 months after diagnosis) or early chronic phase, which offers a potential to improve the overall long-term outcomes for this vulnerable group. Indeed, the early identification of reliable prognostic factors for adverse events may prove essential to facilitate the successful triage of patients and determine those who can be managed medically and those who will benefit from close imaging surveillance in the near-term, and in the long-term from timely and even prophylactic TEVAR.

In this regard, the identification of sub-groups of patients with disease features proven to be associated with early disease progression is a logical approach to stratifying a management strategy that selects patients who may benefit most from early TEVAR.

To date, a variety of clinical features, anatomic dimensions and morphologic characteristics have been proposed as prognostic factors that can predict the risk of disease progression in patients with initially "uncomplicated" Type B AD. Refining the list of factors and better understanding the predictive power of each consideration is an important challenge currently facing all interested parties.

Similarly, accurately defining the anatomic and morphologic features of acute Type B AD that may place patients at increased risk for a procedural complication or untoward TEVAR result is critical to establishing a patient safety profile that may support more assertive endovascular intervention in patients at low risk of procedural adverse events.

REFERENCES

1) Morgagni GB. De Sedibus et Causis Morborum per Anatomen Indigatis [The sites and causes of disease demonstrated by autopsy]. Bologna; 1761 (Translated by Benjamin Alexander, London 1769).
2) DeBakey ME, Cooley DA, Creech O Jr. Surgical considerations of dissecting aneurysm of the aorta. Ann Surg 1955; 142: 586-612.
3) Austen WG, DeSanctis RW. Surgical treatment of dissecting aneurysm of the thoracic aorta. N Engl J Med 1965; 272: 1314-7.
4) DeBakey ME, Henley WS, Cooley DA, Morris GC, Crawford ES, Beall AC. Surgical management of dissecting aneurysms of the aorta. J Thorac Cardiovasc Surg 1965; 49: 130-49.
5) Warren WD, Beckwith J, Muller Jr WH. Problems in the surgical management of acute dissecting aneurysm of the aorta. Ann Surg 1956; 144: 530-48.
6) Wheat Jr MW, Palmer RF, Bartley TD, Seelman RC. Treatment of dissecting aneurysms of the aorta without surgery. J Thorac Cardiovasc Surg 1965; 50: 364-73.
7) Hume DM, Porter RR. Acute dissecting aortic aneurysms. Surgery 1963; 53: 122-54.
8) Daily PO, Trueblood HW, Stinson EB, Wuerflein RD, Shumway NE. Management of acute aortic dissections. Ann Thorac Surg 1970; 10: 237-47.
9) Suzuki T, Mehta RH, Ince H, et al. Clinical profiles and outcomes of acute type B aortic dissection in the current era: lessons from the International Registry of Aortic Dissection (IRAD). Circulation 2003; 108(Suppl. 1): II312-7.
10) Winnerkvist A, Lockowandt U, Rasmussen E, Radegran K. A prospective study of medically treated acute type B aortic dissection. Eur J Vasc Endovasc Surg 2006; 32: 349-55.
11) Tsai TT, Fattori R, Trimarchi S, et al. Long-term survival in patients presenting with type B acute aortic dissection: insights from the International Registry of Acute Aortic Dissection. Circulation 2006; 114: 2226-31.
12) Yang CP, Hsu CP, Chen WY, et al. Aortic remodeling after endovascular repair with stainless steel-based stent graft in acute and chronic type B aortic dissection. J Vasc Surg 2012; 55: 1600-10.
13) Mani K, Clough RE, Lyons OT, et al. Predictors of outcome after endovascular repair for chronic type B dissection. Eur J Vasc Endovasc Surg 2012; 43 386-91.
14) Andacheh ID, Donayre C, Othman F, Walot I, Kopchok G, White R. Patient outcomes and thoracic aortic volume and morphologic changes following thoracic endovascular aortic repair in patients with complicated chronic type B aortic dissection. J Vasc Surg 2012; 56: 644-50.
15) Kim KM, Donayre CE, Reynolds TS, et al. Aortic remodeling, volumetric analysis, and clinical outcomes of endoluminal exclusion of acute complicated type B thoracic aortic dissections. J Vasc Surg 2011; 54: 316-24.
16) Qing KX, Yiu WK, Cheng SW. A morphologic study of chronic type B aortic dissections and aneurysms after thoracic endovascular stent grafting. J Vasc Surg 2012; 55: 1268-75.
17) Manning BJ, Dias N, Manno M, et al. Endovascular treatment of acute complicated type B dissection: morphological changes at midterm follow-up. J Endovasc Ther 2009; 16: 466-74.
18) Nienaber C, Rousseau H, Eggebrecht H, et al. Randomized Comparison of Strategies for Type B Aortic Dissection The INvestigation of STEnt Grafts in Aortic Dissection (INSTEAD) Trial; Circulation. 2009; 120: 2519-28.
19) Tsai TT, Isselbacher EM, Trimarchi S, et al. Acute type B aortic dissection: does aortic arch involvement affect management and outcomes? Insights from the International Registry of Acute Aortic Dissection (IRAD). Circulation 2007; 116(Suppl. 11): 150-6.
20) Mantelas M, Antonitsis P, Kaitzis D, Hatzibaloglou A, Moros I. Spontaneous isolated dissection of the abdominal aorta: single center experience. Interact Cardiovasc Thorac Surg 2009; 8: 398-401.
21) Reul GJ, Cooley DA, Hallman GL, Reddy SB, Kyger ER 3rd, Wukasch DC. Dissecting aneurysm of the descending aorta. Improved surgical results in 91 patients. Arch Surg 1975; 110: 632-40.
22) Park KH, Lim C, Choi JH, et al. Midterm change of descending aortic false lumen after repair of acute type I dissection. Ann Thorac Surg 2009; 87: 103-8.
23) Fattouch K, Sampognaro R, Navarra E, et al. Long-term results after repair of type A acute aortic dissection according to false lumen patency. Ann Thorac Surg 2009; 88: 1244-50.
24) Rodriguez J, Olsen D, Lucas L, Wheatley G, Ramaiah V, Diethrich EB. Aortic remodeling after endografting of thoraco abdominal aortic dissection. J Vasc Surg 2008; 47: 1188-94.
25) Estrera AL, Miller CC 3rd, Safi HJ, et al. Outcomes of medical management of acute type B aortic dissection. Circulation 2006; 114(Suppl. 1): I384-9.
26) Tsai TT, Evangelista A, Nienaber CA, et al. Partial thrombosis of the false lumen in patients with acute type B aortic dissection. N Engl J Med 2007; 357:349-59.

8

The European Reference Network in the field of the vascular rare diseases

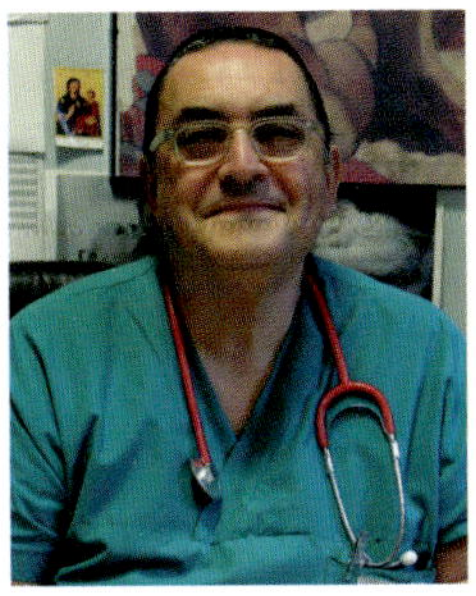

Alessandro Pini, Gabriella Tognola, Alessia Paglialonga, Marine Hurard, Raffaella Gaetano and Guillaume Jondeau

8.1 Background

Rare diseases (RD) are defined in the European Union as life-threatening and/or chronically debilitating conditions that affect less than 5 per 10,000 people. Therefore, these small numbers of patients and their geographic dispersion are an obstacle to the diagnosis, access to care, research and improvement of medical expertise. European Reference Networks (ERNs) for rare diseases have been advocate for years to overcome these obstacles, by linking research and knowledge centres, updating and contributing to the latest scientific findings and ensuring the availability of subsequent treatment facilities where necessary. The main goal is to assure the equity in access to prevention, diagnosis and care for patients with a RD throughout the European Union. By 2011 the European Directive on the application of patient's rights in cross-border healthcare was adopted and established a legal framework for cross-border healthcare within the European Union (EU). One of the aims of the directive is to promote cooperation between the health systems of Member States including the establishment of European Reference Networks (ERNs). ERNs are an excellent model to overcome some of the specific problems of rare diseases: scarcity of patients, resources and expertise.

8.2 Problems, solutions and benefits related to the European Reference Network organization

Many problems have been identified at first in defining objectives, tools and strategies. The overview of centres of reference in the different Member States shows that:

- very few countries have official centres of reference;
- only very few countries have a national centre for the coordination of the activities of the regional centres and the creation of a national clinical database for each rare disease or homogeneous group of diseases;
- the official centres of reference cover very different types of centres;

Alessandro Pini (pini.alessandro@asst-fbf-sacco.it)
Rare Disease Center MarfanClinic®, ASST-Fatebenefratelli-Sacco,
Milan, Italy

G. Melissano - R. Chiesa (eds), Aortic Dissection patients true stories and the innovations that saved their lives

- the concept of the centre of reference is not used by some Member States with a regionally-organised health care system and a low level of coordination between regions;
- many centres of expertise, acting as centres of reference, are not labelled as such but are well established by reputation.

On 24 October 2011, during the third meeting of the European Union Committee of Experts on Rare Diseases (EUCERD), the Recommendations on Quality Criteria for Centres of Expertise for Rare Diseases in Member States were unanimously adopted. Developing Centres of Expertise and European Reference Networks in the field of rare diseases has been proposed in the Council Recommendation on an Action in the Field of Rare Diseases and more recently in the Cross-Border Healthcare Directive as a means of organising care for the thousands of heterogeneous rare conditions affecting scattered patient populations across Europe. In order to share knowledge and expertise more efficiently, the EUCERD recommendations seek to introduce harmonious standards of quality practices by elaborating criteria for the Member States to incorporate into their process to designate Centres of Expertise. The 45 Recommendations build upon this work already achieved and assist the Member States to develop their healthcare pathways at both the national and EU levels in the field of rare diseases. The recommendations cover the Mission and Scope of the Centres of Expertise; the Criteria for Designating Centres of Expertise; the Process of Designating and Evaluating National Centres of Expertise; and the European Dimension of Centres of Expertise.

ERN status should represent a clear added-value in terms of:

- easier adoption and spread of innovations in medical science and health technologies;
- facilitation of medical training; faster dissemination of agreed standards of care and general knowledge in the area of expertise;
- increased profile and recognition of the participants.

Inasmuch, ERNs will attract the best experts and a higher number of patients and, although they are supposed to facilitate cross-border health care, it is expected that the pooling of resources and the e-Health solutions will decrease the burden of travelling for the patients.

Another expected though not explicit benefit is that the Networks and their members will be in a better position to apply for research funding and further develop and accelerate basic and translational research. Existing networks in the R&D field have arisen "ad hoc" in response to specific funding calls either from DG Santé or from DG research.

Rare disease estimate number is 6-8000 and it should have been impossible to select individual ERNs from a clinical and organizational perspective. Therefore, each rare disease has been grouped into homogeneous cohorts by considering the clinical area, the underlying disease mechanism or pathway, the clinical group and the intervention areas. The Orphanet classification of rare diseases, which is structured around 116 groups of diseases, has been grouped thematically into 31 RD categories; however, when dealing with ERNs there are some overlaps and some redundant groups. At present 23 official networks were created. The *Filières de santé maladies rares* were adequately based on what was already in place in the French health system. The main problem stays when we try to extrapolate these country-specific pathways to a broader coverage.

8.3 VASCern – A future perspective for rare multisystemic vascular disease patients

From November 2015 to June 2016 a close collaboration between more than 35 European Centres dedicated to multisystemic vascular rare diseases have been created in order to organize a Vascular ERN. By now this ERN project, which is coordinated by the French Centre of Reference for Marfan Syndrome and Related Disorders, went through the first eligibility check by the European Commission and is now under evaluation by a Quality Certification Agency to assess the performances of the Network and each participating Centre (Healthcare Providers).

The Vascular RD have been sub grouped by clinical, pathogenetic and therapeutic characteristics. For each subgroup of vascular RD (Rare Diseases Working Group, RDWG), a chairman and 1 co-chairman have been identified to overlook and coordinate more strictly the implementation of the initiatives. Inasmuch, transversal working groups (WG) have been created for the e-Health projects, communication, databases, ethics, as well as training and education. A specific patient WG has been also created. In particular, we will be concerned about medium sized arteries RD. At first a number of common gaps have been identified in order to evaluate the possible strategies which could have been offered. Clinical guidelines, imaging, diagnostic pathways, predictors of disease severity, threshold for/timely surgery among subgroups, medical treatment, non-pharmacologic treatment, pregnancy management, guidelines for sport activities, counselling, appropriate follow-up have been identified as main goals to achieve. The standardisation of care is one of the major aims, as well as sharing of experience and definition of clinical outcomes.

8.4 The e-Health role in the European Reference Network

Information and Communication Technologies (ICT) applied to health and healthcare systems can increase their efficiency, improve quality of life and unlock innovation in health markets. The introduction of e-health services – digitally-based, networked, Internet-aided – and the rapid transfer of medical and scientific information for clinical, research and convenience purposes is already under way. E-health services and tools are at first web-enabled and are built for routinely use on personal computers or laptops and, in a rapid increase, for mobile devices, smartphones and tablets. The wellbeing market enabled by digital technologies (mobile applications and mobile devices) is rapidly growing. The convergence between wireless communication technologies and healthcare devices and between health and social care is creating new frontiers in business. Redesigning the delivery of care and the 'silver economy' are highly promising markets.

e-Health can provide benefit to citizens, patients, health and care professionals but also to health organisations and public authorities. e-Health – when applied effectively – delivers more personalised "citizen-centric" healthcare, which is more targeted, effective and efficient and can help to reduce errors, as well as the length and costs of hospitalisation. It facilitates socio-economic inclusion and equality, quality of life and patient empowerment through greater transparency, access to services and information and the use of social media for health.

The e-Health Network set up by Directive 2011/24/EU is the main strategic and governance body at EU level to work towards interoperability of cross-border e-Health services. It is essential to establish safeguards to allow citizens to use health and well being applications with confidence and awareness and subsequently ensure "the integration of user-generated data with official medical data so that care can be more integrated, personalised and useful for patients" (Toomas Hendrik Ilves).

Effective data protection is vital for building trust in e-Health. It is also a key driver for its successful cross-border deployment, in which harmonisation of rules concerning cross border exchange of health data is essential.

During the period 2014-2020, research and innovation is supported under "Health, demographic change and wellbeing" of Horizon 2020, in the areas of:

- ICT and computational science and engineering framework for digital, personalised, and predictive medicine, including advanced modelling and simulation;
- innovative instruments, tools and methods for unlocking the value of data and for advanced analytics, diagnostics and decision making;
- new digital media, web and mobile technologies and applications, as well as digital instru-

ments that integrate healthcare and social care systems and support health promotion and prevention;
- e-Health systems and services with strong user involvement, focusing on interoperability and the integration of emerging patient-centric technologies for cost-effective healthcare.

Since 2012, the Commission is encouraging Member States to develop and share their national (including regional) e-Health strategies, taking into account international recommendations, and deploying promising solutions for active and healthy ageing at a larger scale. Since 2014, sets of common indicators have been made available to measure the added value and benefit of e-Health solutions, based on work funded by the Commission in partnership with stakeholders.

Among other objectives, the Connecting Europe Facility (CEF) sets out to facilitate the deployment of cross-border interoperable ICT services of general interest such as e-Health by overcoming the barriers of the high initial investment costs and risks associated with this deployment.

The e-Health WG and the ERN priorities on the ICT side are fully in line with the priorities set in e-Health at European level. Our objectives and activities follow the belief that e-Health has already gained a central role within the objectives of any health policy and in the future of patients health and wellbeing. This WG will harmonize the needs in ICT and e-Health across Centres and develop key guiding principles, technical specifications, cross-border platforms to take full advantage of the impressive potential of e-Health tools in this ERN and, in general, for the management of Rare Diseases.

8.5 e-Health – Connecting people and connecting health systems in Europe

There is a general call for a change in the way of organizing and managing the delivery of health services. Therefore we have updated the hypotheses of solutions for the Rare Multisystemic Vascular Diseases ERN in line with the objectives indicated by EC on e-Health.

The general aims at European level, that we follow in the development of this WG, are:
- empower patients and caregivers;
- optimize health resources availability;
- get a greater access to personal health data;
- increase sustainability and efficiency of health systems;
- support for patients' access in healthcare services across Europe.

The proposals reported in Table 8.1 has to be considered as general hypothesis towards the novel, essential opportunities offered by e-Health applied to an ERN and, in particular for the Rare Multisystemic Vascular Disease ERN.

Among all these proposals a priority ranking will be set based upon the following criteria:
- objective need (classified as: urgent, of medium relevance and of minor relevance);
- feasibility (time to realization and temporal resources, internal resources, and financial support).

A priority ranking will be discussed and set at the beginning of the ERN activities and a temptative schedule will be set up in order to allocate the resources.

Regarding to "financial pressure on health systems", e-Health represents one of the main solutions to fit the increasing need for health services and better health quality with the actual decreasing financial availability.

Each of the proposed solutions must be also evaluated in considering their potential impact in terms of:
- better access to health services (easier, ubiquitous, faster, less time consuming, less km/miles,

Table 8.1 e-Health applied to an ERN

e-Health – Challenges (as set by the EC)	ERN general proposals	Empowered target group
Changes in the national health systems (e.g. digitalization, integrated care, new medical techno/services)	Mobile (and web-based) APP (derived from "Explo-Rare®") to optimize the search for the most appropriate HCP for a specific Rare Disease*	Patients Caregivers and families GPs - Nurses Specialists
	E-Cloud system to collect and share medical data in order to allow a Patient to access to her/his data from everywhere and 7d/24h*	Patients GPs Specialists
	E-Cloud system to share medical databases for clinic and research 7d/24h	Specialists Researchers
	Mobile and web-based APP to share and update diagnostic and therapeutic guidelines flow-charts, workflow and best practices, and simplify decision making processes*	GPs Nurses Specialists MD students
	Patient registry for a common subgrouping of Patients based on OrphaCode and for a shared datasets	Specialists Researchers
	Shared e-cloud digital medical records to homogenize data collection*	HCPs Researchers
	Telemedicine (a 7d/24h service at EU level offered by the Network HCPs) based on the e-cloud shared digital Medical Records *	HCPs Patients
Paradigm shift from doctor-centered healthcare to patient-centered healthcare	Mobile and Web-based APP to maximise infos about the ERN and about rare diseases (to a better knowledge and to solve the daily problems) – This APP could be addressed within the clinical records by the HCPs A social network infos zone as well as a YouTube Channel could be used and shared to share information and knowlegde	Patients Caregivers and families GPs Nurses School personnel
Demand for more patient engagement	Mobile (and web-based) APP (derived from "Explo-Rare®") to optimize the search for the most appropriate HCP for a specific Rare Disease*	Patients Caregivers and families GPs - Nurses Specialists
	E-Cloud system to collect and share medical data in order to allow a Pt to access to his data from everywhere and 7d/24h*	Patients GPs Specialists
	E-Cloud system to share medical databases for clinic and research 7d/24h	Inter-specialist consulting
	Telemedicine (a 7d/24h service at EU level offered by the Network HCPs) based on the e-cloud shared digital Medical Records*	HCPs Patients
	ERN website with forums for Pts and different target groups	Patients Caregivers and families
Shortages and uneven distribution of health professionals	Telemedicine (a 7d/24h service at EU level offered by the Network HCPs) based on the e-cloud shared digital Medical Records *	HCPs Patients
	E-Cloud system to share medical databases for clinic and research purpose, available 7d/24h	Inter-specialist consulting
	Mobile and web-based APP to share and update diagnostic and therapeutic guidelines flow-charts, workflow and best practices, and semplify decision making processes*	GPs Nurses Specialists MD students
	Mobile and Web-based APP for monitoring of health parameters and a common HCPs's Centre to healthcare surveillance	Patients Caregivers and families

Table 8.1 (*Continued*)

e-Health – Challenges (as set by the EC)	ERN general proposals	Empowered target group
Health inequalities and inequities in access to healthcare	Mobile and web-based and/or YouTube structured e-Learning program (theory and practice) Different tone of voice to adapt to the target courses	GPs Nurses Specialists HCPs
	e-Learning platform to evaluate and certificate the updating knowledge – (theory and practice) courses – Different tone of voice to adapt to the target	GPs Nurses Specialists HCPs
	Webinars to share infos and knowledge (different tone of voice related to target)	HCPs Specialists GPs Patients Caregivers and families
	Create a quality benchmark and a system for rating each HCP performance (based on self assessment and regular online evaluation) in order to guarantee a high quality standardization	HCPs

All proposals signed with * might be shared with other ERNs with common needs in order to reduce the costs and resources needed for the developments so to share common platforms, tools, and technical specifications.

Many proposals tackle more than one of the main challenges as they are multi-purpose and multi-domain and, also, different proposals and activities share common structures and overlapping targets as well as methodologies.

less need for face-to-face encounters, more shared opinions and information/knowledge…);
- optimizing the waiting lists for clinical evaluation;
- general and specific benefits (clinical, diagnostic, …), i.e. better care, faster diagnosis, integrated services, improved outcomes;
- prevention and reduction of emergecies and related costs (due to more effective monitoring system), significant saving of money for healthcare systems;
- Key Performance Indicators (KPI) and quality monitoring related to each item;
- additional benefits related to better healh and wellbeing, in terms e.g. of better family and social participation, improved productivity on the workplace, and overall economic growth;
- lowering of caregiver's commitment (time, efforts, reduced productivity, impact on individual lives) and related costs.

Talking abouth technologies, it is important to say that the technology we need is 'ready' as most of the ICT infrastructures, technologies, and platforms are already affordable and ready to be developed and adapted to the specific needs of the ERN and HCPs; efforts have to be directed to widen the internet/internet mobile access and to improve the speed of the data transfer and the quality of apps and web services.

8.6 Information and communication technologies could unlock innovation in health markets

The potential impact in terms of innovation and business opportunities is relevant. The development and improvement of e-Health services could open novel opportunities for SMEs, industries and healthcare systems across several domains.

SMEs and industries (not related to drug development in this case) might benefit thanks to the creation of new markets for e-Health services, platforms, issues (e.g., data security and privacy) and the growth of new customers' needs. We could hypothise partnerships with companies involved in:

- health/wellness promotion;
- consumer and health related retail (including related needs, e.g. in food industry as relevant to the specific disease; sport industries; leisure activities and wellbeing);
- general communication among the different actors;
- insurance companies and banks.

The innovative e-health services could be part of merging program in developing opportunities for patients/clients associated with standard service offers (i.e. e-Health APP offered free of charge with affiliation, subscription of standard services). These could be part of the financial support to develop the e-Health programs of the ERN.

The need to share infos and data about the patients related to the ERN and their needs could stimulate the development of new medical instruments and managing systems by SMEs and industries as well the identification of new customers and new services (e.g., automated monitoring system to identify abnormalities of a particular parameter and to manage to alarm automatically the HCP personnel who follows the patient – a kind of a Smart Clinical Decision Assistant System).

8.7 e-Managing support

In order to get these targets and optimizing the management of resources, a management platform could also be developed in accordance with experts in management engineering. A central coordination system (centered in Paris) with a peripheral control will be established to improve the control of financial flows and resources allocation and automatically rate and rank a project or activity (clinical or research) based upon urgency of need, financial sustainability, HCPs' characteristics, feasibility.

8.8 Data platform for patient registry

Data registry platform must be compatible with the local/regional/national data registries and should allow dynamic and query-based extraction of data. Privacy should be guaranteed as well as intellectual property and data protection. It can provide and manage the sharing of digital data between health professionals in the same country or across countries (a key EU target to cross-border health assistance). The platform should:

- be active and responsive 24h/7d;
- be reachable from everywhere (e-cloud) and with every ICT system (PC/mobile);
- respect patient privacy (PW and consensus, etc) as set by deep collaboration with the ethics WG;
- collect data and information according to homogeneous minimum requirements, as shared and discussed among the ERN Centres;
- include modules and data processing algorithms developed for specific extraction of data for research purposes (i.e. genotype/phenotype correlation, patient cohorts, and so on);
- allow a continuous updating and implementation to increase and simplify data use and analysis;
- respect intellectual properties and data protection via automatic trackability and alert systems while consulting or downloading data.

In collaboration with patient WG and ethics WG this platform could help to define safety and quality of care based on data quality, data transmission standards or clinical competence criteria. Treatment quality survey could be another target point to reach.

We should also consider the possibility to develop a scalable data registry (platform and related services and interfaces) so that every patient could consult his own data set as well as download the information he/she needs (e.g. in case of emergency, the data should be shared to clinicians involved in the cure of the patient by means of specific consensus and a specific individual PW, for example, and the data should be reacheable via PC or mobile). The individual electronic access to their own health-related data is a main target of EU. This part have to be set in collaboration with ethics WG, too. All kind of data search and use should be trackable in order to have a record of them and define properly the effective value of the system/service.

8.9 Specific m-Health tools – mobile app

To share the information about the ERN Centres characteristics, the services offered and the way to contact and reach each Centre is within the targets of the EU plans for the health promotion and for e-Health. Each patient should be able to choose the right clinical centre for his/her needs and this is a key principle within the EU. In Italy, in Lombardy, the Centre that chairs this WG (Rare Disease Center – Luigi Sacco Hospital) has developed a specific mobile (smartphone IOS & Android) APP which is named "Explo-Rare") to this purpose. It has been developed for the Expo2015 (available from 1st of May 2015) and it is currently available in 6 languages, in order to help as many people as possible (Italian, English, Spanish, Chinese, Russian and Arabic). The language is automatically selected by the language set up for the smart-phone.

The App is free of charge and this WG will adapt this program to be implemented on wider scale and in a larger set of languages so to cover the whole ERN. The App will be further developed by including additional data from the whole ERN (a specific form will be distribuited to all the participating Centres to recall the informations). The data will be translated/completed in the languages of the participants of the network and a new name will be defined for the App.

Decision support systems could be a part of mobile App development which can well be inserted within the objectives and tools of the Training/learning WG.

8.10 Telehealth

Telemedicine programs are another target of the EU for the health. Within the ERN a novel integrated platform could be developed, including e.g. services for teleradiology (this part could be included within the data registry), remote patient monitoring, 24 hous/7days call centres. It could also be useful to launch a call within the ERN to get infos about existing ones to share or adapt (the launch of calls is another item described below).

8.11 Training/Learning

e-Health provides platforms to implement the learning strategies indicated by the Training/Learning WG and make them easier to use and more effective compared to conventional, face-to-face meetings or academic lectures. We could distinguish different targets of these actions and, accordingly, different levels of strategies and different technologies/settings, as follows:

- medicine student -pre-service – nurse;
- in service GPs and not-RD specialists;
- in service professionals related to ERN Centres;
- patients and caregivers.

A specific ERN YouTube® Channel shall be designed in order to share scientific meetings held by each centre or congressual events or single traditional lessons for professionals.

8.12 Webinars

The term "webinar" is a portmanteau of web and seminar, meaning a presentation, lecture, or workshop that is transmitted over the web. During webinars there is the possibility of interactive participation between participants. Web conferencing may be used for various types of online collaborative services including web seminars ("webinars"), webcasts, and peer-to-peer web meetings. It may also be used in a more narrow sense to refer only to the peer-to-peer web meeting context, in an attempt to disambiguate it from the other types of collaborative sessions.

In general, web conferencing is made possible by TCP/IP connections. Services may allow real-time and point-to-point communications as well as multicast communications from one sender to many receivers.

REFERENCES

- European Commission 2nd Conference on ERN (Report), Lisbon, October 2015.
- EUCERD Recommendations on Rare Disease European Reference Networks (RD ERNs).
- Evangelista T, Hedley V, Atalaia A, et al. The context for the thematic grouping of rare diseases to facilitate the establishment of European Reference Networks. Orphanet Journal of Rare Diseases 2016; 11: 17.
- Palm W, Glinos IA, Rechel B, et al. Building European Reference Networks in health care. European Observatory on Health Systems and Policies a partnership hosted by WHO, 2013.
- Pini A, Tognola G, Paglialonga A, Gaetano R. VASCern - E-Health WG plan, 2016.

9

Pharmacological treatment of aortic dissection

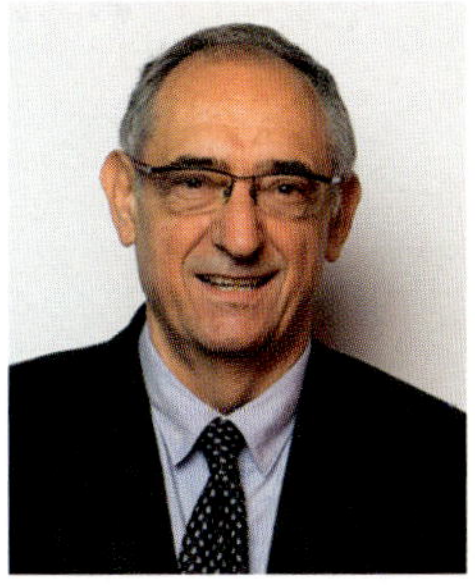

Arturo Evangelista and Jose F. Rodríguez-Palomares

Acute aortic syndrome (AAS) is an acute lesion of the aortic wall involving the aortic media. The term covers aortic dissection (AD), intramural haematoma (IMH), and penetrating atherosclerotic ulcer (PAU). Acute dissection is defined as that occurring within 2 weeks of onset of the initial pain; subacute, between 2 and 12 weeks from the onset of pain; and chronic, more than 12 weeks from the onset of pain [1].

9.1 Diagnosis

Early diagnosis of AAS is crucial for reducing mortality in acute phase and improving prognosis. Focused cardiac ultrasound can be useful in the diagnosis for time-sensitive rapid assessment of aortic root size, left ventricular function, aortic regurgitation, pericardial effusion or tamponade [2] and presence of intimal flap in the aortic root, proximal ascending aorta, aortic arch or abdominal aorta [3]. However, should AD be clearly suspected, prompt and competent interpretation of diagnostic contrast-enhanced CT or other imaging is mandatory for undelayed triaging and proper treatment [4]. In several circumstances such as unstable haemodynamic patients with a clear diagnosis of Type A AD, the best strategy could be early transfer to the operating theatre and to perform a TOE under general anaesthesia before beginning surgical treatment.

9.2 Management

On admission, all AAS patients undergo a standardised protocol management including transfer to intensive care unit, continuous arterial pressure monitoring, central venous access for administration of intravenous antihypertensive agents, and urine output monitoring via catheter. The initial goals are to halt progression of the dissection by decreasing impulse force (of systolic pressure) and control pain; beta-blocking agents (labetalol, metoprolol), calcium channel blockers, nitroglycerine and sodium nitroprusside are used in that order to ensure anti-impulse management with the aim of maintaining blood pressure <120 mmHg [5]. Patients

Arturo Evangelista (aevangel@vhebron.net)
Hospital Universitari Vall d'Hebron,
Barcelona, Spain

G. Melissano - R. Chiesa (eds), Aortic Dissection patients true stories and the innovations that saved their lives

Table 9.1 Management of patients with suspected aortic dissection

1) **General measures**
   a) Establish two large bore (>18 gauge) IV's
   b) Administer supplemental oxygen by nasal cannula or nonrebreather mask
   c) Put patient on cardiac monitor
   d) Get an EKG, portable chest X-ray, place a Foley catheter
   e) Obtain CBC, chemistry panel, coagulation panel, UA, CK, Troponin, d-dimer
   f) Type and cross 10 units packed red blood cells (PRBC's)
   g) Set up an arterial line

2) **Early cardiothoracic surgical consultation**

3) **Definitive imaging**
   a) Computed tomography angiogram
   b) Transoesphageal echocardiogram

4) **Blood pressure, heart rate, and pain management**
   Systolic blood pressure <120 mmHg
   Heart rate <60 beats/min
   Morphine (for pain relief)

   a) First line: β-blockers
      - Labetalol, bolus (15 mg) ± a drip (5 mg/hour),
      - In patients with obstructive pulmonary disease, blood pressure lowering with calcium channel blockers
   b) If hypertension persists:
      - Additional vasodilator (i.v. sodium nitroprusside to titrate blood pressure to 100-120 mmHg)
   c) If tachycardia persists, add:
      - Esmolol (loading 0.5 mg/kg over 2-5 min, followed by a drip of 10-20 μg/kg/min)
      - Diltiazem drip (loading 0.25 mg/kg over 2-5 min, followed by a drip of 5mg/h)

5) **Haemodynamically unstable patients**
   a) Tracheal intubation, mechanical ventilation
   b) Blood pressure support with crystalloid and colloid (PRBCs if rupture is suspected)
   c) TOE at bedside in the Emergency Department or in the Operating Room

remain in cardiovascular intensive care until blood pressure and pain are well controlled and medication can be administered orally (Table 9.1).

Drug therapy to control pain and the haemodynamic state is essential. Initial management of AAS, particularly dissection, is directed at limiting the propagation of dissected wall components by control of the blood pressure and lowering dP/dt (pressure development). In general, the aim is to maintain systolic pressure of 100-120 mmHg and heart rate of 60-80 bpm to pro-

Table 9.2 Medical management of AAS

The initial management of AAS is directed to clinically stabilize the patient and prevent propagation of the dissection and aortic rupture.

A – Immediate invasive haemodynamic monitoring is advised, through an intra-arterial catheter and urinary catheter.
B – Pain should be treated promptly with intravenous opiates. Persisting pain may indicate progression of the dissection or an impending rupture.
C – In patients with hypertension at presentation, medical therapy is administered to decrease aortic wall stress. Blood pressure should be <120 mmHg systolic and ≤70 mmHg diastolic, and the heart rate <70 beats/ minute.
D – In patients presenting with refractory hypotension, rapid volume expansion should be administered in combination with vasopressors such as norepinephrine or phenylepinephrine to maintain organ perfusion, before the patient receives definitive surgical repair.

vide sufficient end-organ perfusion, with the use of intravenous beta-blockers first-line therapy. Opiate analgesia should be prescribed to attenuate the sympathetic release of catecholamines to pain, with resultant tachycardia and hypertension. High-risk but asymptomatic patients with AAS, with the exception of Type A AD, can probably be followed up without urgent intervention if they do not have any early complications. All symptomatic patients will need surgical or interventional treatment, since AAS evolution is unpredictable with a high risk of severe complications. However, given the reasonable results with medical management of uncomplicated Type B AD, medical therapy is considered the best option that is difficult to surpass with surgery. However, some patients with Type B AD are initially managed medically, but then require intervention (TEVAR) at a later subacute or chronic stage (Table 9.2).

9.2.1 Pain control

First-line therapy is pain relief by morphine sulphate and intravenous beta-blockers. Opiate analgesia should be prescribed to attenuate the sympathetic release of catecholamines to pain with resultant tachycardia and hypertension [6]. Further management is dictated by the site of the lesion and evidence of complications (persistent pain, organ malperfusion) as well as evidence of disease progression on serial imaging [7].

9.2.2 Blood pressure control

The goals of treatment are to prevent the propagation of the dissection and aortic rupture [7], decrease left ventricular afterload and myocardial oxygen consumption. Few comparative randomised, controlled trials exist that provide definitive conclusions and/or recommendations regarding the efficacy and safety of comparative agents. Hypertensive crisis with AD and symptomatic aortic aneurysm is associated with major morbidity and mortality. Poorly-controlled hypertension may cause aortic disruption with potentially fatal bleeding as well as progression of the intimal flap in cases of AD [8]. A combination of a vasodilator and beta-blocker is preferred. A short-acting dihydropyridine calcium channel blocker may be used together with esmolol, labetalol or metoprolol. If further reduction in blood pressure (BP) is required, sodium nitroprusside, glyceryl trinitrate, or hydralazine are appropriate. Beta-blockers should be given first before vasodilators, as the reflex catecholamine release due to vasodilatation may increase left ventricular contractions. Once oral intake is established, parenteral antihypertensives are slowly switched to oral to maintain blood pressure and heart rate stable at all times [9].

9.3 Specific drugs

9.3.1 Beta-blockers

Intravenous β-blockers are the treatment of choice for patients with suspected AAD. β-blockers has a negative inotropic and chronotropic effect, which prolongs diastolic filling time and results in an increased left ventricle end-diastolic volume, thereby lowering blood pressure and heart rate [10]. Dosage is titrated for symptom control and to establish a target heart rate of 50-60 beats/minute and systolic blood pressure of 100-120 mmHg. The β-blocker of choice in this situation is usually esmolol and, alternatively, labetalol or metoprolol [11]. Esmolol is a β1 antagonist while labetalol is a combined α1, β1 and β2 antagonist with an alpha-to-beta blocking ratio of 1:7. Both slow down the heart rate and reduce myocardial oxygen demand. Esmolol lowers blood pressure by reducing cardiac output and inhibiting renin release, while labetalol reduces afterload directly and inhibits renin release. Their disadvantage is in the form of their negative inotropic effect, and possible reaction in patients with reactive airway disease. Half life of esmolol is around nine minutes, while that of labetalol is 5.5 hours [12]. The hypotensive effect of labetalol begins within 2-5 minutes after its intravenous administration, reaching a peak at 5-15 minutes following administration and lasting for 2-4 hours [13].

Labetalol may be administered as a loading dose of 20 mg, followed by repeated incremental doses of 20-80 mg at 10-minute intervals until the desired BP is achieved. Alternatively, after the initial loading dose, an infusion commencing at 1-2 mg/min and titrated up to until the desired hypotensive effect is achieved is particularly effective. Bolus injections of 1-2 mg/kg have been reported to produce precipitous falls in BP and should therefore be avoided.

9.3.2 Sodium nitroprusside

Nitroprusside is administered in patients with refractory hypertension after initiation of β-blocker therapy. It induces venous and arterial vasodilation, thereby increasing cardiac output [14]. Vasodilator therapy may be associated with reflex tachycardia that increases aortic wall stress, which can potentially cause expansion and propagation of thoracic AD. For this reason, vasodilator therapy should only be administered after heart rate is controlled. It has rapid onset of action, with a half-life of 3-4 minutes and thus is given in the form of continuous infusion. Dose is 0.3 μg/kg/min IV infusion; with titration q2 min until the desired response with a maximum dose 10 μg/kg/min is achieved. The hypotensive effects of nitroprusside can be unpredictable because it simultaneously causes potent venodilatation and peripheral arterial vasodilatation [8]. The most serious adverse effect is in the form of cyanide toxicity, which occurs due to accumulation of its metabolites thiocyanate/cyanide. Thus, it is recommended that this drug be used only when other intravenous antihypertensive agents are not available. Sodium nitroprusside in combination with an intravenous β-blocker effectively controls blood pressure in the majority of patients.

9.3.3 Non-dihydropyridine calcium channel blockers

In patients who do not respond, or poorly tolerate β-blockers, calcium channel blockers (Ca-blockers) can be used as an alternative. In addition, the use of Ca-blockers in Type B AD might reduce aortic expansion over time [10]. Standard dosage: Titrate dosage for symptom control, establish a target heart rate of 50-60 beats/minute and systolic blood pressure down to 100-120 mmHg.

9.3.4 Angiotensin converting enzyme inhibitors

In absence of adequate blood pressure control, angiotensin converting enzyme inhibitors (ACE-inhibitors) should be administered to reduce the blood pressure and to maintain adequate end-organ perfusion. Intravenous administration of an ACE-inhibitor is rarely needed for the treatment of AAD, due its effects including for hypotension, angioedema, dry cough. ACE-inhibitors can be useful in case of unirenal malperfusion with concomitant increasing renin levels [7].

9.3.5 Angiotensin receptor blockers

Angiotensin receptor blockers (ARBs) can be used as an alternative for ACE-inhibitors, when patients have persistent cough after administration of ACE-inhibitors. In addition, there is increasing controversy whether patients with Marfan syndrome may benefit from ARBs instead of ACE-inhibitors, as losartan seems to be associated with a reduced ascending aortic growth rate [9]. Standard dosage: Titrate dosage to establish a target systolic blood pressure down to 100 mmHg.

9.3.6 Alpha adrenergic blocking agents (α-blockers)

If the blood pressure is still uncontrolled despite using a combination of the earlier mentioned antihypertensive agents, addition of α-blockers can be a valuable option. It lowers the peripheral vascular resistance by dilation of the arterioles and venules.

9.3.7 Hydralazine

Hydralazine lowers blood pressure by exerting a peripheral vasodilating effect through direct relaxation of vascular smooth muscle. However, it is associated with reflex tachycardia and increases in left ventricular contractility, plasma renin levels and norepinephrine releases. For these reasons, this arteriolar dilator is considered to be relatively contraindicated for patients with suspected AAS, except when the heart rate is well controlled and hypertension persists [14].

9.4 Management of complications and specific conditions

9.4.1 Shock

Shock with diagnostic confirmation of a Type A AD (or any aortic disease involving the ascending aorta) should prompt undelayed surgery and open repair. Cardiogenic shock is caused either by pericardial tamponade (frequent with proximal dissection), acute aortic valve regurgitation or coronary compromise from the dissection lamella either progressing into the left coronary mainstem or just obstructing any coronary ostium, or from other rare conditions [15]. Interventions such as pericardiocentesis or coronary percutaneous procedures are not advised because they can worsen the acute problem and cost precious time until life-saving surgery. Shock from acute blood loss indicates rupture or contained rupture of the aorta and the need for immediate surgery; however, it often proves fatal.

In a Type B setting, haemodynamically unstable patients are either in haemorrhagic shock or septic/metabolic shock from visceral or limb malperfusion. They should be endotracheally intubated and fluid resuscitated with crystalloid, or other colloid. Shock call for immediate volume expansion (including blood transfusion) and swift endovascular management of such a life-threatening complication in an attempt to seal major communications to the false lumen and thereby stop further blood loss via the ruptured outer media layer of the false lumen.

9.4.2 Kidney failure

Acute kidney failure can result from kidney malperfusion from obstructed renal arteries. The obstruction often results from true lumen collapse or from static obstruction of renal arteries by either thrombus or invagination of dissected aortic wall components. In most cases, local interventions are not helpful and would delay urgent proximal repair in Type A AD; in Type B AD, malperfusion of renal arteries is best managed by endovascular scaffolding of the descending thoracic aorta with stent-graft in the true lumen, an intervention that depressurises the false lumen, redirects blood to the true lumen alone, and opens the true lumen by virtue of systolic pressure increase even at the level of abdominal side branches and iliac arteries. After such a procedure, stents in the ostia of renal arteries are rarely needed and fenestration procedures are obsolete. Kidney function usually recovers even after days of malperfusion.

9.4.3 Anticoagulation

Once a proximal or distal AD has been diagnosed, therapeutic management is focused on surgical repair in cases of Type A involvement and on proper triaging for complications, and thus endovascular treatment, of Type B AD. There is no place for anticoagulation strategies besides the use of prophylactic heparin to avoid deep venous thrombosis during immobilisation and bed rest. Similarly, no antiaggregation is required except for unrelated independent indications such as coronary or peripheral artery disease. Even after TEVAR, specific antithrombotic medication is not indicated. On the other hand, chronic dissection without signs of acute complications is not a contraindication for antithrombotic or anticoagulant medication if they are needed for another prognostically-relevant reason [16]. Surprisingly, evidence-based recommendations about heparinization and/or anticoagulation in acute Type B AD are so far completely missing.

9.4.4 Intramural haematoma and penetrating aortic ulcer

Medical management of intramural haematoma and penetrating aortic ulcer follows the same indications as AD. In Type A involvement, surgery should be considered in all cases except in the presence of comorbidities. Before surgery, or in cases where surgery is not indicated, medical treatment including control of symptoms and haemodynamic alterations is indicated (Table 9.3).

In Type B involvement, management is based on complications. In cases without complications, control of pain and blood pressure is paramount. Imaging controls during acute

Table 9.3 Initial medical treatment in patients with acute aortic dissection and hypertension

Name	Mechanism	Dose	Cautions/contraindications
Esmolol	Cardioselective β -1 blocker	Load: 500 μg/kg IV Drip: 50 μg kg^{-1} min^{-1} IV Increase by increments of 50 μg/min	– Asthma or bronchospasm – Bradycardia – 2nd- or 3rd-degree AV block – Cocaine or methamphetamine abuse
Labetalol	Nonselective β 1,2 blocker Selective α -1 blocker	Load: 20 mg IV Drip: 2 mg/min IV	– Asthma or bronchospasm – Bradycardia – 2nd or 3rd degree AV block – Cocaine or methamphetamine abuse
Enalaprilat	ACE inhibitor	0.625-1.25 mg IV q 6 hours Max dose: 5 mg q 6 hours	– Angioedema – Pregnancy – Renal artery stenosis – Severe renal insufficiency
Nitroprusside	Direct arterial vasodilator	Begin at 0.3 μg kg^{-1} min^{-1} IV Max dose 10 μg kg^{-1} min^{-1}	– May cause reflex tachycardia – Cyanide/thiocyanate toxicity – especially in renal or hepatic insufficiency
Nitroglycerin	Vascular smooth muscle relaxation	5-200 μg/min IV	– Decreases preload – contraindicated in tamponade or other preload-dependent states – Concomitant use of sildenafil or similar agents

phase are necessary to monitor the evolution of intramural or periaortic haemorrhage, progression of aorta size and disease extension. Treatment of an IMH in patients requiring anticoagulation therapy remains problematic, and no definitive data exist regarding the use of anticoagulants in these patients. Discontinuation of anticoagulants is common practice. In one report, by Cañadas et al. [17], the continued use of anticoagulants was not associated with progression of IMH. However, only three patients were included, and one of them had been treated with stenting for the newly-developed AD. In our opinion, anticoagulant therapy in patients with an acute IMH may facilitate re-bleeding of the aorta wall. We believe that when the thromboembolic risk is intermediate or low, interruption of anticoagulant treatment is advisable until the haematoma regresses significantly. If the thromboembolic risk is very high, as in patients with valvular prostheses, close monitoring with imaging techniques should be performed, and if evolution is not satisfactory, endovascular or surgical treatment should be considered. Individualisation of the risk/benefit of anticoagulation and monitoring of haematoma thickness by imaging techniques may facilitate the choice of the most appropriate therapeutic management [18].

9.4.5 Chronic phase

The 10-year actuarial survival rate of patients with AAS who are discharged ranges from 30 to 60% in different studies [19]. Several studies have suggested that 40-70% of late deaths in patients with Type A AD are due to comorbid diseases; mainly heart disease and stroke, emphasizing that cardiovascular risk factors should be thoroughly assessed and treated in this group. Interestingly, cigarette smoking does not seem to affect aortic expansion and rupture rates, although its detrimental role on cardiovascular risk is well established.

Dissection of the aorta represents a systemic problem with the entire aorta and its branches predisposed to dissection, aneurysm formation, and/or aortic rupture in the future. Systemic hypertension, advanced age, aortic size and the presence of a patent false lumen are all predictors of late complications [20]. Therefore, medical therapy including beta-blockers is needed to minimise aortic wall stress, and serial imaging to detect signs of progression, redissection or aneurysm formation. Regular assessment of the aorta should be made after discharge and annually thereafter. Significant imaging findings are progressive diameter, signs of aneurysm formation and haemorrhage at surgical anastomoses, or stent-grafted sites. The observation that both hypertension and aortic expansion/dissection are common and not difficult to predict early after discharge seems to justify such an aggressive follow-up strategy. There are no randomized, controlled trials of the different medications used to control the blood pressure in Type B AD. In a large retrospective series from Switzerland, the authors found that the use of beta-blockers significantly decreased ($p = 0.006$) the incidence of subsequent hospital admission and late dissection-related aortic complications. Cost of treatment and progression of aortic dilation were also reduced compared to other drugs [21]. This study demonstrates how beta-blockers not only reduce the blood pressure but also the pulsatile force or dP/dt, which can prevent the AD propagation. In the most recent publication from data of the International Registry of Acute Aortic Dissection (IRAD), data regarding medication prescription to patients with Type B AD at discharge was analysed to investigate the association of medications and mortality. Initial univariate analysis showed that use of beta-blockers was associated with improved survival in all patients ($p = 0.03$), and that use of calcium channel blockers was associated with improved survival in Type B patients receiving medical management ($p = 0.03$). Multivariate models further showed that use of calcium channel blockers was associated with improved survival in Type B medically-treated patients (OR 0.55; 95% CI, 0.35-0.88, $p = 0.01$) [22]. The findings of the IRAD analysis collectively demonstrated that while use of beta-blockers was associated with improved outcome in all patients with dissection, the use of calcium channel blockers was associated with improved survival selectively in

Type B AD. Use of ACE inhibitors did not improve survival. Consequently, the IRAD analysis suggests the possibility of type-selective benefits of medications in acute AD.

9.4.6 Specific aspects in the management of genetic aortic diseases

In patients with Marfan syndrome, the prophylactic use of β-blockers, angiotensin-converting enzyme (ACE) inhibitors, and angiotensin II receptor blockers seems to be able to reduce either the progression of the aortic dilation or the occurrence of complications [23]. However, there is no evidence for the efficacy of these treatments in aortic disease of other aetiologies. Medical management involves beta-blockers, sartans and statins to control blood pressure and inflammation. Losartan is an angiotensin II Type1 (AT1) receptor antagonist which attenuates canonical and non-canonical transforming growth factor-β (TGF-β) signalling in the aorta and inhibits TGF-β-mediated activation of extracellular signal-regulated kinase [24]. This drug significantly reduced the aortic dilation rate, first in a Marfan mouse model and later in a small observational study in children with MFS [25]. The COMPARE study revealed a significantly lower aortic dilation rate in patients treated with losartan-β-blocker therapy compared to β-blockers alone [23]. However, these results were not confirmed in the recent Marfan Sartan trial in which 86% of patients received β-blocker therapy [26]. Furthermore, a large clinical trial including children and young adults showed no benefit in aortic root dilation assessed by echocardiography when losartan was compared with atenolol over a 3-year period [27]. In our trial comparing atenolol vs. losartan in monotherapy, the changes in aortic root and ascending aorta indexed maximum diameters over three years of treatment did not differ significantly between treatment groups [28]. The results did not demonstrate differences between treatments in their efficacy to prevent aortic dilation in MFS.

Discrepancies in the results of these trials may be due to treatment study designs (additional beneficial effect of losartan vs. superiority over β-blockers), differences in drug doses, study population or imaging modality used to measure aorta dilation. Until future therapy directed at the fibrillin-1 gene or the TGF-β axis ultimately proves most effective at preventing the aortic complications of MFS, β-blocker therapy remains the "standard of care". Losartan as monotherapy is justified in patients with severe bradycardia, asthma or other beta-blocker contraindications. Effects of pharmacological therapy should be monitored closely during the initiation phase to ensure that heart rate goals and blood pressure management are optimal. Therefore, all patients who have had an AD and have been treated, either medically or surgically, should maintain a normal blood pressure and should be kept under surveillance by re-imaging for asymptomatic changes in the distal aorta that might require intervention.

9.5 Conclusions

While management of Type A AD is straightforward with the need for timely surgical repair after initial pain control and blood pressure control by intravenous drugs, sub-classification of Type B AD is more complex. Currently used recommendations suggest initial medical management (anti-impulse beta-blocker, sartans and/or Ca^{++}-channel blockers) with close surveillance for so-called uncomplicated Type B AD; emergent TEVAR is accepted and advised in all complicated scenarios of Type B AD. With better understanding of adverse predictors, the concept of pre-emptive repair of any Type B AD by TEVAR should be considered for Type B AD regardless of presenting symptoms and in addition to life-long pharmaceutical blood pressure control as long as they are anatomically suitable. All patients should be followed and offered sustained surveillance with focus on blood pressure control and progressive expansion. With this management, chances are that aneurysmatic expansion of dissected aortas could be prevented.

REFERENCES

1) Erbel R, Aboyans V, Boileau C, et al. 2014 ESC Guidelines on the diagnosis and treatment of aortic diseases: Document covering acute and chronic aortic diseases of the thoracic and abdominal aorta of the adult. The Task Force for the Diagnosis and Treatment of Aortic Diseases of the European Society of Cardiology (ESC). Eur Heart J 2014; 35(41): 2873-926.
2) Spencer KT, Kimura BJ, Korcarz CE, et al. Focused cardiac ultrasound: recommendations from the American Society of Echocardiography. J Am Soc Echocardiogr 2013; 26(6): 567-81.
3) Evangelista A, Flachskampf FA, Erbel R, et al. Echocardiography in aortic diseases: EAE recommendations for clinical practice. Eur J Echocardiogr 2010; 11(8): 645-58.
4) Goldstein SA, Evangelista A, Abbara S, et al. Multimodality imaging of diseases of the thoracic aorta in adults: from the American Society of Echocardiography and the European Association of Cardiovascular Imaging: endorsed by the Society of Cardiovascular Computed Tomography and Society for Cardiovascular Magnetic Resonance. J Am Soc Echocardiogr 2015; 28(2): 119-82.
5) Hiratzka LF, Bakris GL, Beckman JA, et al. 2010 ACCF/AHA/AATS/ACR/ASA/SCA/SCAI/SIR/STS/SVM guidelines for the diagnosis and management of patients with thoracic aortic disease: executive summary. A report of the American College of Cardiology Foundation/American Heart Association Task Force on Practice Guidelines, American Association for Thoracic Surgery, American College of Radiology, American Stroke Association, Society of Cardiovascular Anesthesiologists, Society for Cardiovascular Angiography and Interventions, Society of Interventional Radiology, Society of Thoracic Surgeons, and Society for Vascular Medicine. Catheter Cardiovasc Interv 2010; 76(2): E43-86.
6) Trimarchi S, Eagle KA, Nienaber CA, et al. Importance of refractory pain and hypertension in acute type B aortic dissection: insights from the International Registry of Acute Aortic Dissection (IRAD). Circulation 2010; 122(13): 1283-9.
7) Tolenaar JL, van Bogerijen GH, Eagle KA, Trimarchi S. Update in the management of aortic dissection. Curr Treat Options Cardiovasc Med 2013; 15(2): 200-13.
8) Khoynezhad A, Plestis KA. Managing emergency hypertension in aortic dissection and aortic aneurysm surgery. J Card Surg 2006; 21 Suppl 1: S3-7.
9) Khoynezhad A. Antihypertensive therapy in a patient with type B and de novo type A aortic dissection: case study. Crit Care Clin 2007; 23 Suppl1: 29-38.
10) Tran TP, Khoynezhad A. Current management of type B aortic dissection. Vasc Health Risk Manag 2009; 5(1): 53-63.
11) Varon J, Marik PE. The diagnosis and management of hypertensive crises. Chest 2000; 118(1): 214-27.
12) Gray RJ. Managing critically ill patients with esmolol. An ultra short-acting beta-adrenergic blocker. Chest 1988; 93(2): 398-403.
13) Varon J. Treatment of acute severe hypertension: current and newer agents. Drugs 2008; 68(3): 283-97.
14) Gupta PK, Gupta H, Khoynezhad A. Hypertensive emergency in aortic dissection and thoracic aortic aneurysm - a review of management. Pharmaceuticals 2009; 2: 66–76.
15) Tsai TT, Trimarchi S, Nienaber CA. Acute aortic dissection: perspectives from the International Registry of Acute Aortic Dissection (IRAD). Eur J Vasc Endovasc Surg 2009; 37(2): 149-59.
16) Nienaber CA, Eagle KA. Aortic dissection: new frontiers in diagnosis and management: Part I: from etiology to diagnostic strategies. Circulation 2003; 108(5): 628-35.
17) Cañadas MV, Vilacosta I, Ferreirós J, et al. [Intramural aortic hematoma and anticoagulation]. Rev Esp Cardiol 2007; 60(2): 201-4.
18) Ruggiero A, González-Alujas T, Rodríguez J, Bossone E, Evangelista A. Aortic intramural haematoma and chronic anticoagulation: role of transoesophageal echocardiography. Eur J Echocardiogr 2008; 9(1): 56-7.
19) Howard DP, Banerjee A, Fairhead JF, et al. Population-based study of incidence and outcome of acute aortic dissection and premorbid risk factor control: 10-year results from the Oxford Vascular Study. Circulation 2013; 127(20): 2031-7.
20) Evangelista A, Salas A, Ribera A, et al. Long-term outcome of aortic dissection with patent false lumen: predictive role of entry tear size and location. Circulation 2012; 125(25): 3133-41.
21) Genoni M, Paul M, Jenni R, et al. Chronic beta-blocker therapy improves outcome and reduces treatment costs in chronic type B aortic dissection. Eur J Cardiothorac Surg 2001; 19(5): 606-10.
22) Suzuki T, Isselbacher EM, Nienaber CA, et al. Type-selective benefits of medications in treatment of acute aortic dissection (from the International Registry of Acute Aortic Dissection [IRAD]). Am J Cardiol 2012; 109(1): 122-7.
23) Groenink M, den Hartog AW, Franken R, et al. Losartan reduces aortic dilatation rate in adults with Marfan syndrome: a randomized controlled trial. Eur Heart J 2013; 34(45): 3491-500.
24) Habashi JP, Judge DP, Holm TM, et al. Losartan, an AT1 antagonist, prevents aortic aneurysm in a mouse model of Marfan syndrome. Science 2006; 312(5770): 117-21.

25) Brooke BS, Habashi JP, Judge DP, et al. Angiotensin II blockade and aortic-root dilation in Marfan's syndrome. N Engl J Med 2008; 358(26): 2787-95.
26) Milleron O, Arnoult F2, Ropers J, et al. Marfan Sartan: a randomized, double-blind, placebo-controlled trial. Eur Heart J 2015; 36(32): 2160-6.
27) Lacro RV, Dietz HC, Sleeper LA, et al. Atenolol versus losartan in children and young adults with Marfan's syndrome. N Engl J Med 2014; 371(22): 2061-71.
28) Forteza A, Evangelista A, Sánchez V, et al. Efficacy of losartan vs. atenolol for the prevention of aortic dilation in Marfan syndrome: a randomized clinical trial. Eur Heart J 2016; 37(12): 978-85.

10

Aortic dissection in pregnancy

James H. Black, III and Bryan A. Ehlert

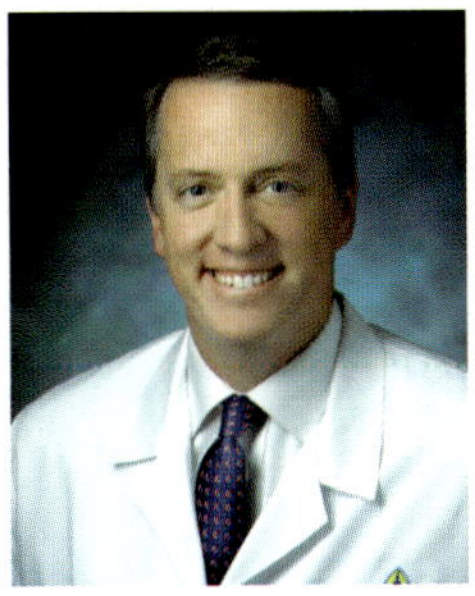

"I was at ease discussing the possibility of TEVAR for an acute dissection, even for a young expecting mother. But in the middle of this conversation, the fetal monitor decelerated and the labor and delivery nurse took on a very worried look. In that moment, I realized I was now treating two patients."

James Black, MD

10.1 Case presentation

10.1.1 Patient presentation

A 39 year old Asian female, who is 32 weeks pregnant (gravida 2, para 1), presents to an outside facility following acute onset tearing chest pain and shortness of breath. Her previous pregnancy was uncomplicated and she has no pertinent previous medical or surgical history. She has no family history of connective tissue disorders, aneurysms or dissections. A computed tomography angiogram (CTA) is obtained to rule out a pulmonary embolism and fetal monitoring confirms a viable fetus. Her CTA reveals an acute Type B aortic dissection (TBAD) with an entry tear distal to the left subclavian artery and extending into her visceral aorta (Fig. 10.1). Her physical exam reveals no evidence of malperfusion with a non-tender abdomen and palpable distal pulses. She presented with a systolic blood pressure of 158 mmHg and her baseline creatinine is 0.5 mg/dL. The maximum diameter of her aorta is 35 mm and she is initiated on β-blockade for heart rate and blood pressure control. She is transferred to our tertiary care center with stable hemodynamics.

10.1.2 Hospital course

Upon arrival, she is admitted to a cardiac surgery intensive care unit and continued on optimized medical therapy (OMT) with continuous infusion of an intravenous (IV) β-blocker, pain control and serial neurovascular exams. A maternal-fetal medicine consult is also obtained and continuous fetal monitoring is initiated. She initially responds well to OMT with cessation of symptoms; however, over the next 36 hours, fetal decelerations occurred with systolic blood pressures <120 mmHg. Her blood pressure goals were liberalized, resulting in improved fetal perfusion. After 72 hours, she developed recurrence of her chest pain and tighter hemodynamic management was once again instituted. Urgent repeat imaging is obtained, demonstrating growth of her descending thoracic aorta to 39 mm with expansion of the false lumen (Fig. 10.2). Despite appropriate anti-impulse therapy, she had persistent symptoms

James H. Black, III (jhblack@jhmi.edu)
The Johns Hopkins Hospital,
Baltimore, MD, USA

G. Melissano - R. Chiesa (eds), Aortic Dissection patients true stories and the innovations that saved their lives

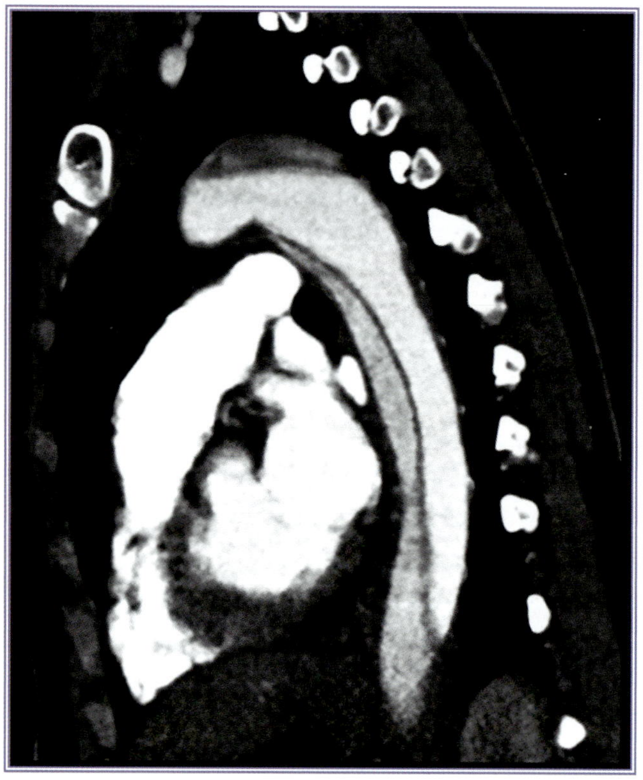

Fig. 10.1 Sagittal view of computed tomography arteriogram at presentation demonstrated acute Type B AD.

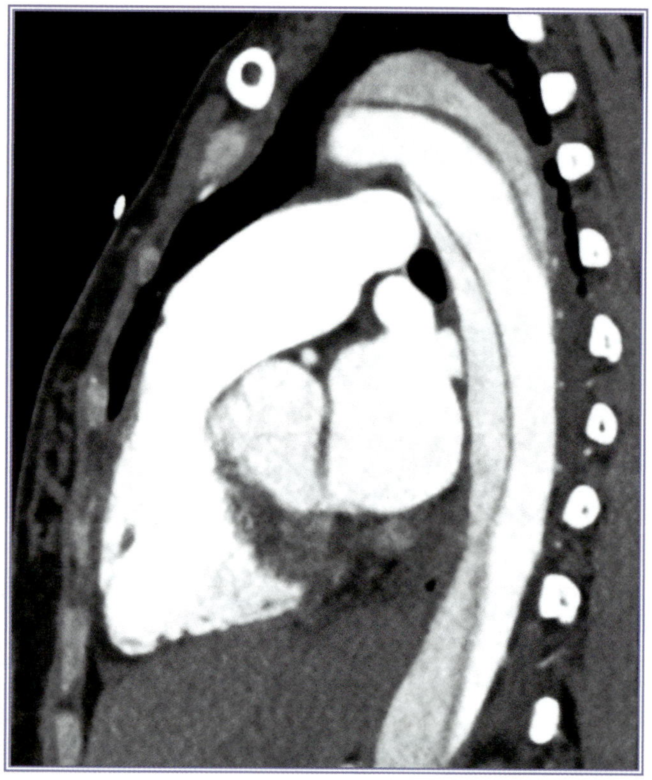

Fig. 10.2 Repeat computed tomography arteriogram at five days with increased aortic diameter and expansion of the false lumen.

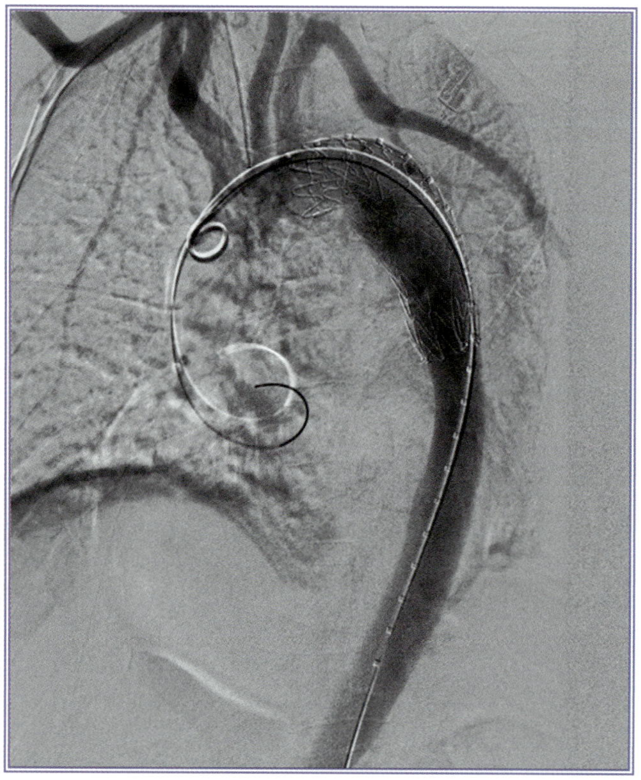

Fig. 10.3 Intraoperative aortogram following successful aortic stent graft deployment. The entry tear is covered with no flow into the false lumen and preservation of the left subclavian artery.

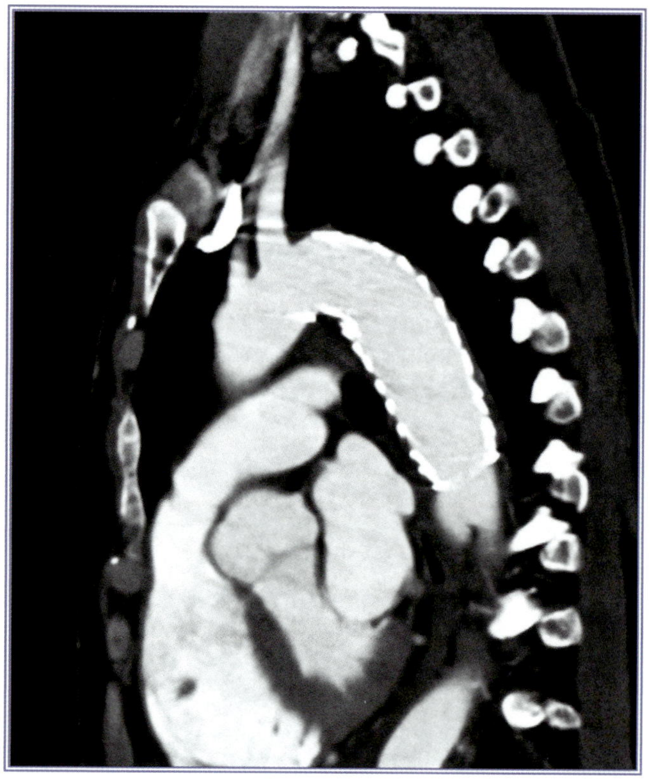

Fig. 10.4 Follow-up computed tomography arteriogram with thrombosis of the false lumen.

along with significant fetal decelerations returning to the fetus. Following multi-disciplinary discussion with the maternal-fetal medicine and obstetrics teams, the decision was made to proceed with emergent caesarian section to be followed by thoracic endovascular aortic repair (TEVAR) to cover the entry tear of the aortic dissection (AD). A healthy newborn was delivered and an aortic stent-graft was deployed following an aortogram via left femoral artery access with a seal obtained proximal to the entry tear (Fig. 10.3). The left subclavian artery was preserved and intravascular ultrasound (IVUS) was utilized to confirm there were no additional entry tears present.

10.1.3 Postoperative course

"The decision to go to surgery was an easy one... I knew I was going to have a baby and I wanted to be there for her after. Whatever it took, I would do". – The patient

The patient had an uneventful hospital recovery with resolution of her chest and back pain. She and her baby were discharged to home from the hospital. She was evaluated in our outpatient clinic at six weeks and she remained asymptomatic with continued β-blockade. She had a repeat CTA revealing an intact repair with thrombosis of the false lumen (Fig. 10.4).

10.2 Background and epidemiology

Despite advances in medical and surgical therapy, AD remains a morbid condition commonly associated with uncontrolled hypertension and connective tissue disorders. However, pregnancy is a unique predisposing risk factor and the leading cause of AD in females under the age of forty [1]. In the general population, the incidence of AD is 6/100,000 individuals per year [2]. In a review of the Nationwide Inpatient Sample (NIS) over a 10-year period, the incidence of AD in pregnancy was 3.9/10,000 individuals per year, an almost seven-fold increase in yearly incidence when compared to the general population [3]. A sub-analysis using the International Registry of Acute Aortic Dissection (IRAD) database identified a 0.6% incidence of AD during pregnancy [4]. Other reports have associated pregnancy with a 25% increased risk for acute AD with an incidence rate ratio of 4.0 (95% CI 2.0-8.2) [1, 5]. Stanford Type A AD are more prevalent than Type B AD (77.3% vs. 22.9%, $p < 0.01$) [6, 7]. Although AD during pregnancy remains a rare occurrence, it is significantly more common than in the general population and a predisposing risk factor amongst younger females.

Several physiologic and mechanical factors of pregnancy have been identified as precursors to AD. Maternal hemodynamics is altered during the course of a pregnancy. Physiologic changes of pregnancy include increases in blood volume, stroke volume, cardiac output, heart rate, and left ventricular mass; and, together, these alterations significantly increase the hemodynamic stress on the aortic wall [8-10]. The aortic diameter also increases with pregnancy, most pronounced during the third trimester and post-partum period, and may not revert back to baseline measurements [11, 12]. These findings may explain the relationship with multiparous patients having an increased risk for developing an AD [8]. Along with these hemodynamic influences, hormonal changes further impact the integrity of the aortic wall. The aortic wall possesses estrogen receptors, and as estrogen concentrations increase with pregnancy progression there is increased fragmentation of reticulin fibers [13]. Furthermore, a decrease in acid mucopolysacchrides results in a loss of normal corrugation of elastic fibers. Gestational hypertension accentuates these physiologic and hormonal changes and further increases the risk for AD [14]. Females diagnosed with hypertension and preeclampsia had more dramatic increases in aortic diameter [12]. Mechanical factors contribute to gestational hypertension as there is increased aortoiliac compression by the enlarging gravid uterus, resulting in increased outflow resistance [15, 16]. The interplay between all of these factors unique to pregnancy account for the increased incidence and risk for AD in this population.

Aortic dissection in the pregnant female, similar to the general population, is not a benign process. Aortic complications are responsible for 4% of all direct and indirect causes of maternal death [1]. Furthermore, in a case report from the Netherlands, aortopathies were found to be a major cause of maternal mortality; and, in over half of cases, there was a delay in diagnosis and appropriate therapy [17]. In another series from the Netherlands investigating the incidence and predictors of maternal cardiovascular mortality, AD had a mortality rate of 83% and accounted for nearly half of all cardiac deaths [18]. It has been established that patients are at highest risk for AD during the third trimester and immediate post-partum period, when the various physiologic and mechanical factors described above are at their peak [6, 15, 19]. A recent literature review identified the median gestational age for AD to be 32 weeks [6]. As expected, patients with known aortopathies, such as connective tissue disorders, have a higher incidence of AD during pregnancy. Multiple series report approximately half of ADs in pregnancy have a predisposing aortopathy, with most of these patients having Marfan syndrome [6, 7]. A recent report from the GenTAC investigators identified that 10.6% of all Marfan patients developed a pregnancy-related aortic complication [20]. They also found that the incidence of AD was markedly increased during pregnancy compared to non-pregnancy (incidence rate ration 8.4 [95% CI = 3.9-18.4]; $p < 0.0001$). Furthermore, patients with Marfan syndrome present earlier in the course of pregnancy than the general population (30.7 ± 8.6 weeks vs. 34.4 ± 4.4 weeks, $p = 0.03$) [19]. The relationship of AD in pregnancy with aortopathies may be underestimated, as a majority of studies were reported prior to the widespread recognition of more contemporary connective tissue disorders and aortopathies, such as Loeys-Dietz syndrome (LDS) and Familial Thoracic Aortic Aneurysm and Dissection (FTAAD) disorder.

10.3 Treatment

10.3.1 Prophylactic medical management

Patients known to have increased risk for AD, primarily those with diagnosed aortopathies, should be on β-blockade therapy for anti-impulse therapy [21]. Notably, β-blockers can cross the placental border, and this may contribute to reducing fetal heart rate. The effect of β-blockers to promote fetal decelerations is not clear, as such fetal decelerations should still be considered indicative of fetal distress. Patients who have been previously treated with angiotensin inhibitors or receptor blockers should be transitioned to β-blockade to avoid the teratogenic effects of this class of anti-hypertensives [22]. High-risk patients should also undergo routine screening and evaluations. Marfan syndrome patients with aortic root diameters <4 cm had only a 1% incidence of aortic complication; whereas, those with aortic root diameters >4 cm had an incidence of 10% [23, 24]. As such, for pregnant females with known aortopathy, current recommendations include monthly or bimonthly echocardiograms until delivery [25]. Although recently called into question, pregnancy in patients with diagnosed vascular Ehlers-Danlos syndrome remains contraindicated [26, 27].

10.3.2 Type A aortic dissection

Due to high morbidity and mortality rates associated with Type A AD during pregnancy, guidelines have been established for prophylactic surgical repair of the ascending aorta for females prior to conception [21, 28-30] (Table 10.1). Female patients with Marfan syndrome or FTAAD should undergo aortic surgery if ascending aorta diameter is ≥45 mm. In cases of LDS, prophylactic repair should be performed in cases where the diameter is 40-45 mm or

Table 10.1 Threshold diameters of the ascending aorta to undergo prophylactic operative repair prior to pregnancy in patients with known aortopathies

Aortopathy	Baseline ascending aorta diameter
Marfan syndrome	45 mm
FTAAD	45 mm
LDS	40-45 mm
Bicuspid aortic valve	50 mm
Aortic coarctation	All

FTAAD, Familial thoracic aortic aneurysm and dissection disorder; LDS, Loeys-Dietz syndrome

greater. Patients with bicuspid aortic valves and an aortic diameter of ≥50 mm should also be repaired. All patients with previously diagnosed aortic coarctation should undergo elective repair prior to pregnancy. It should be noted that all patients with pre-existing aortopathies that do not meet these criteria be evaluated in a multi-disciplinary approach involving genetics, obstetrics and surgical teams, as family history and history of aortic growth rate should be considered when discussing need for prophylactic surgical repair versus regular screening and medical management.

Open surgical repair remains the gold standard for patients presenting with acute Type A AD. A majority of the research involving the management of Type A AD has revolved around timing of repair, management of the fetus and cardiopulmonary bypass (CPB) adjuncts and strategies. The second trimester is the ideal time to perform semi-elective surgery in pregnant patients [31, 32]. This trimester avoids the increased risk of fetal developmental anomalies present with surgery during the first trimester. Furthermore, the maternal hemodynamic and hormonal changes that occur during the third trimester are not yet fully established. Others have reported that the presence of AD during the first two trimesters is an indication for immediate repair because of higher morbidity and mortality rates for surgical repairs performed during the third trimester [33]. Regarding management of the fetus, those with a gestational age of <28 should undergo repairs with the fetus in utero; while those with gestational age >32 week should have Caesarian section performed followed by aortic repair [34]. In cases between 28 and 32 weeks of gestation, the decision on fetal management should be made based on the fetal condition and following discussion with obstetrics and neonatal specialists. Given recent advancements in neonatal care, delivery of the fetus followed by aortic repair may be able to be performed at earlier gestational ages and should be evaluated on a case by case basis depending on available resources. Repair of Type A AD requires the utilization of CPB, and various adjuncts have been suggested to improve maternal and fetal morbidity and mortality. A literature review investigating outcomes of pregnant females placed on CPB found maternal mortality rates ranged from 3 to 13% with fetal mortality being 16-38% [35]. Factors that have been shown to improve outcomes in ascending aorta and arch repairs with fetus in utero include: normothermic CPB, increased pump flows (>2.5 L/min/m^2), shorter aortic cross clamp and CPB times, maintaining a hematocrit >28% and perfusion pressures >70 mmHg [36]. Increased fetal survival has been demonstrated with decreased CBP time. Hypothermia should be avoided as it may induce placental vasoconstriction and hypothermic CPB has been associated with fetal bradycardia [36]. Furthermore, deep hypothermic circulatory arrest mortality rates have been reported to be as high as 20% and 40% for the patient and fetus, respectively [6]. A recent report has emphasized avoiding hemodilution during CBP [37]. In the setting of hemodilution, progesterone levels are thought to decrease, inducing contractions. The initiation of contractions results in decreased uterine and placental blood flow and increases risk for fetal mortality. Although still experimental, it has been suggested that the utilization of pulsatile perfusion promotes placental vasodilation mediated by nitrous oxide pathways [38].

10.3.3 Type B aortic dissection

Similar to Type B AD in the general population, the gold standard remains OMT unless complicated by rupture, malperfusion or persistent symptoms despite OMT [25, 37]. As mentioned earlier, Type B AD are significantly less frequent than Type A AD and, as a result, the literature consists mainly of case reports for operative management. Both open and endovascular techniques have been described in patients that either failed OMT or were felt to be high-risk for rupture necessitating an elective repair [39-42]. More recently, aortic stent grafts have been used as a bridge to a more definitive open repair following delivery of the fetus [43]. This technique may be most beneficial in the setting of a connective tissue disorder, where open surgical repair remains the gold standard of care. As illustrated in our case and recent case reports, minimally invasive approaches have shown encouraging results with acceptable outcomes for both patient and fetus [41, 42]. Intravascular ultrasound and transesophageal echocardiogram have been efficacious in order to minimize radiation and intravenous contrast exposure [42]. However, in the absence of more robust case series, operative planning should be determined at the discretion of the operating surgeon.

10.4 Outcomes

Aortic dissection in pregnancy is associated with high maternal and fetal mortality rates. In patients with Type A AD, maternal and fetal mortality rates have been reported as high as 30% and 50%, respectively, in a series of 57 patients with AD [7]. However, a literature review of 56 case reports and three case series including 75 patients identified improved outcomes [6]. Their review showed equivalent maternal mortality rates between Type A and B AD (21% vs. 23%, $p = 1$). However, Type B AD were associated with significantly worse fetal outcomes compared to Type A AD (35 vs. 13%, $p < 0.05$). The improvement in fetal outcomes between these two studies may be the result of the CPB adjuncts described above, as these were published ten years apart. The increased fetal mortality in Type B AD is hypothesized to be the result of placental malperfusion secondary to intimal flap progression to the hypogastric arteries causing uterine artery insufficiency [39].

REFERENCES

1) Nasiell J, Lindqvist PG. Aortic dissection in pregnancy: the incidence of a life-threatening disease. Eur J Obstet Gynecol Reprod Biol 2010; 149(1): 120-1.
2) Howard DPJ, Banerjee A, Fairhead JF, et al. Population-based study of incidence and outcome of acute aortic dissection and premorbid risk factor control: 10-year results from the Oxford Vascular Study. Circulation 2013; 127(20): 2031-7.
3) Sawlani N, Shroff A, Vidovich MI. Aortic Dissection and mortality associated with pregnancy in the United States. J Am Coll Cardiol 2015; 65(15): 1600-1.
4) Nienaber CA, Fattori R, Mehta RH, et al. Gender-related differences in acute aortic dissection. Circulation 2004; 109(24): 3014-21.
5) Kamel H, Roman MJ, Pitcher A, Devereux RB. Pregnancy and the risk of aortic dissection or rupture: a cohort-crossover analysis. Circulation 2016; 134(7): 527-33.
6) Rajagopalan S, Nwazota N, Chandrasekhar S. Outcomes in pregnant women with acute aortic dissections: a review of the literature from 2003 to 2013. Int J Obstet Anesth 2014; 23(4): 348-56.
7) Immer FF, Bansi AG, Immer-Bansi AS, et al. Aortic dissection in pregnancy: analysis of risk factors and outcome. Ann Thorac Surg 2003; 76(1): 309-14.

11

Surgical treatment of acute Type A aortic dissection: Houston experience

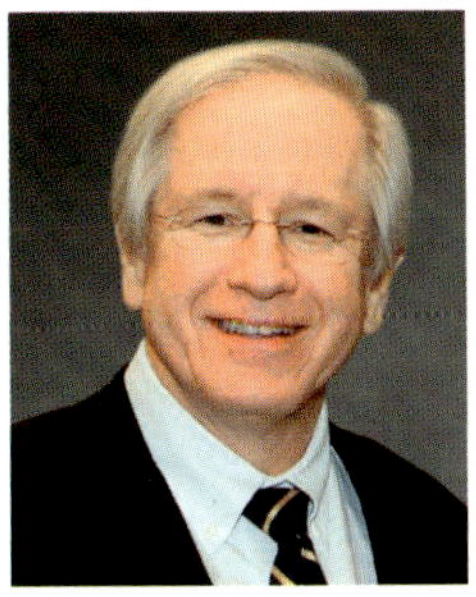

Joseph S. Coselli, Ourania Preventza, Alfred S. Song and Kim I. de la Cruz

11.1 Introduction

Aortic aneurysm and dissection are closely associated clinical entities and often exist together in the same patient at the time of presentation; however, the mechanism of aortic dissection (AD) is distinct. The aorta is composed of three layers: the intima (innermost layer), the media (middle layer), and the adventitia (outer layer). Aortic dissection involves the formation of an intimal tear that results in hydrodynamic delamination of the media, whereby blood under pulsatile arterial pressure flows through the media, creates a false lumen, and results in two competing channels of blood flow (Fig. 11.1) [1]. Often, as the false lumen expands, it compresses the true lumen; occasionally, malperfusion of branching arteries or downstream aorta may result from this compression or from the dynamic movement of the septum separating the two channels. Variants of classic AD include intramural hematoma and penetrating aortic ulcers; repair of these variants follows that of classic dissection.

Although the pathogenesis of AD involves degeneration of the aortic media, this is a complex process that is imperfectly understood – chronic inflammation, aortic injury, hemodynamic stress, cardiovascular risk factors, and genetic predisposition are all thought to play a role in its development [2]. Hypertension is the single greatest environmental risk factor for AD – 70 to 85% of patients with a thoracic AD have hypertension. Although atherosclerosis is fairly common in patients with AD, its role in the development and progression of AD is poorly understood. In classic cases of proximal AD, the originating tear tends to occur in a section of the aorta with minimal atherosclerosis [1]. After the establishment of an intimal tear, high blood pressure and heart rate can increase the rate of dissection through the media. Other risk factors for dissection include hypertension caused by drugs of abuse, such as cocaine and tobacco, and pregnancy, which has a poorly understood association with AD.

Aortic dissection tends to be common in patients with a connective tissue disorder in which connective tissue constituents are inherently weak, or with an inflammatory condition (e.g., atherosclerosis, vasculitis) in which there is degradation of structural components

---

Joseph S. Coselli (jcoselli@bcm.edu)
Baylor College of Medicine,
Houston, TX, USA

G. Melissano - R. Chiesa (eds), Aortic Dissection patients true stories and the innovations that saved their lives

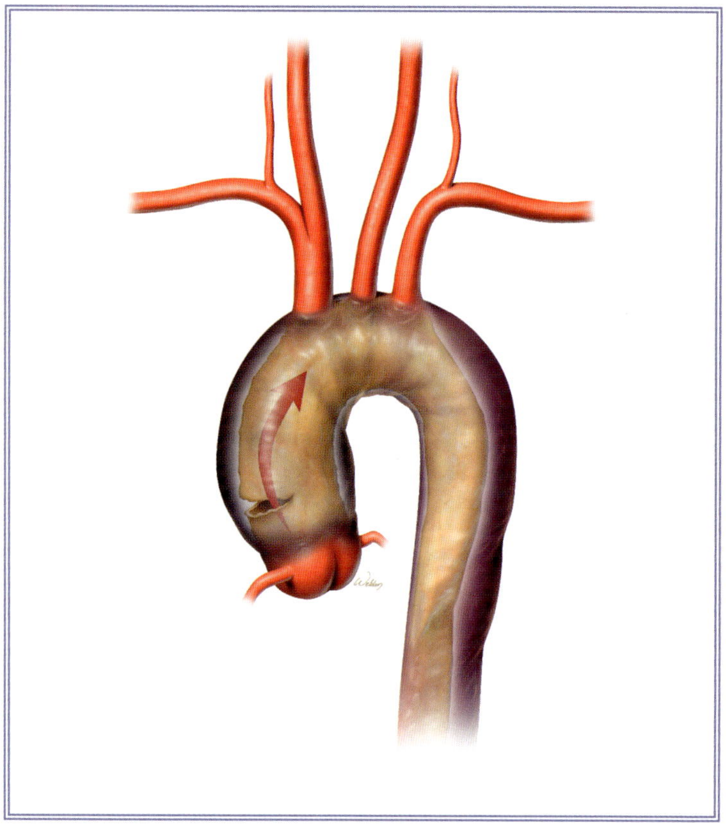

Fig. 11.1 Illustration of acute proximal AD with retrograde extension into the aortic root. The originating tear is shown above the sinutubular junction, and pulsatile blood is directed into the media, and thereby propagating a false channel into the distal aorta. Reproduced with permission of Baylor College of Medicine.

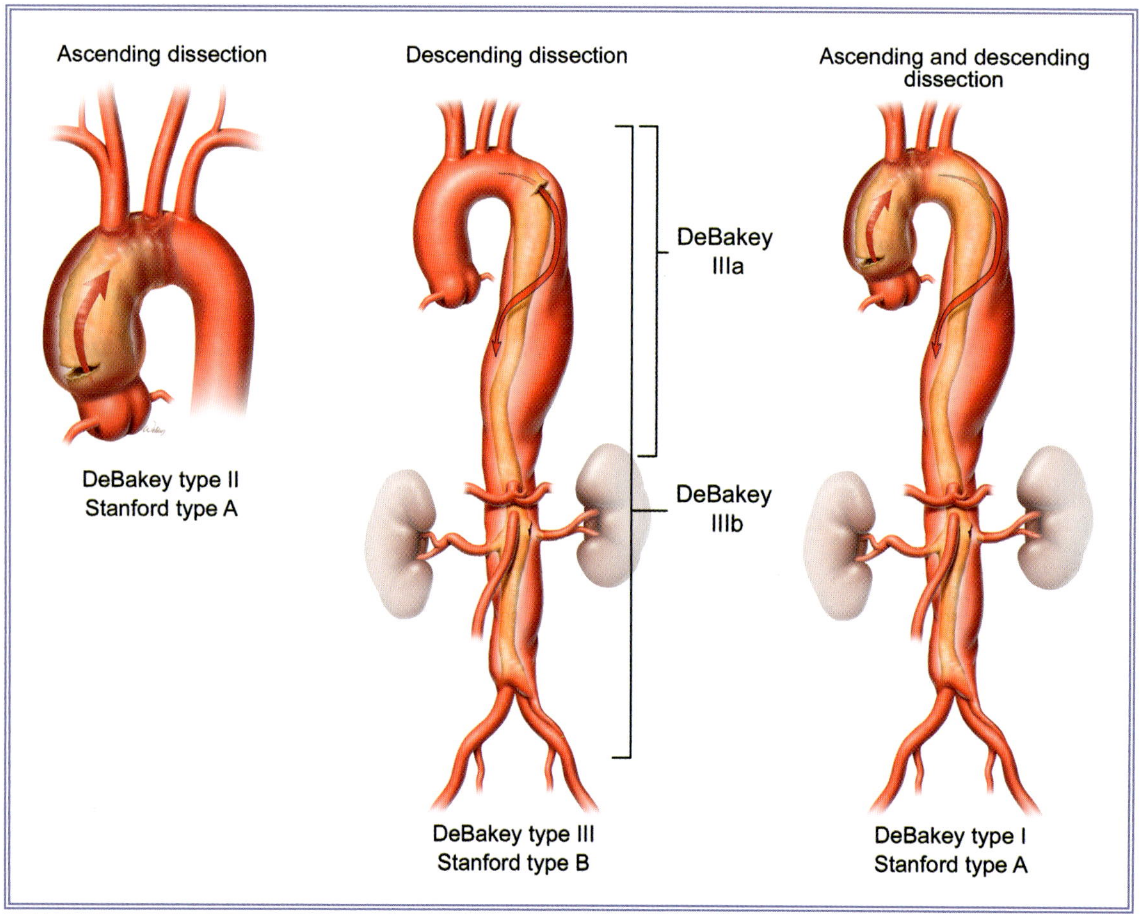

Fig. 11.2 Illustration of the DeBakey and Stanford classification schemas for acute AD. Dissection of the proximal aorta may be limited to the ascending aorta or it may extend distally to the aortic bifurcation. Reproduced with permission of Baylor College of Medicine.

of the connective tissue matrix. Marfan syndrome is the most well-studied connective tissue disorder associated with a weakened extracellular matrix, but others include Ehlers-Danlos syndrome and Loeys-Dietz syndrome. Patients with bicuspid aortic valves also have an increased risk of AD [1].

11.2 Categorization

Aortic dissection can be systematically categorized by either anatomic or temporal features. The two most common anatomic systems of categorization include the DeBakey and Stanford classifications, which describe how the proximal (i.e., ascending aorta and aortic arch) and distal aorta (i.e., the descending thoracic, thoracoabdominal, and abdominal aorta) are affected by AD (Fig. 11.2). Thc DeBakey system classifies dissections into one of three types: Type I, Type II, and Type III [3]. Type I dissections involve the ascending aorta, the transverse arch, and varying portions of the distal aorta, up to the aortic bifurcation. Type II dissections involve the ascending aorta up to but not including the transverse arch. Type III dissections are limited to the distal aorta. An alternative classification scheme called the Stanford system, described by Daily et al. in 1970 [4], delineates AD into two types, Type A or Type B, regardless of where the intimal tear began. Type A AD include all dissections involving the ascending aorta, whereas Type B AD are all other dissections not involving the ascending aorta. Dissections solely involving the transverse arch do not belong to any of the above classifications and are usually classified depending on the adjacent region of the aorta involved.

Historically, AD have been temporally categorized as acute or chronic. The starting time point is at the onset of the initial symptoms, which represents an intimal tear. The duration of time that distinguishes acute dissection is commonly defined as 2 weeks. This is based on early outcomes data showing that the risk of morbidity and mortality is highest in the first 2 weeks after dissection, after which a patient's prognosis begins to improve [5, 6]. Although attempts have been made to define a subacute phase that aligns with the physiology of remodeling, a complete consensus has not been reached. However, the subacute phase is usually defined as the interval between 15 and 90 days after dissection.

The physiologic significance of acute versus chronic dissection involves the strengthening of aortic tissue over time and the remodeling of the false lumen. In the acute phase, the aortic tissue is weakened, fragile, and difficult to suture. Over time, the tissue stabilizes and becomes less difficult to suture. Commonly, after the successful repair of an acute proximal AD, blood flow through the false lumen should be greatly reduced with subsequent aortic remodeling.

The application of these classification schemes is useful in discussions about management and repair approaches for proximal AD requiring timely, if not emergent, repair because of the potential for catastrophic outcomes and death. Acute proximal AD can result in cardiac tamponade, myocardial infarction, wide-open aortic insufficiency, stroke, and rupture, all of which increase the risk of death before and during operative repair.

11.3 Historical discussion of repair

King George II's personal physician, Frank Nicholls, provided one of the first written accounts of acute dissection in 1760. He described his patient as follows [6]:

> "...the pericardium was found distended with a quantity of coagulated blood, nearly a pint...; the whole heart was so compressed so as to prevent any blood contained in the veins from being forced into the auricles; therefore, the ventricles were found absolutely void of blood...; and in the trunk of the aorta we found a transverse fissure on its inner side, about

an inch and a half long, through which some blood had recently passed under its external coat and formed an elevated ecchymosis".

King George II died of a sustained cardiac tamponade caused by an acute Type A AD.

Up to the mid-20th century, many clinicians thought the surgical repair of AD was improbable. In 1955, Houston's DeBakey, Cooley, and Creech reported their emerging experience with such repair and described a series of 6 patients, including one with acute proximal AD that did not survive. All of those repairs involved the descending thoracic aorta, which was either transected to obliterate the dissection or replaced with a homograft [7]. The first successful repair of an acute proximal AD was performed by Houston's George Morris in 1962. In this case, the ascending aorta was transected to re-approximate the dissected aorta, and the aortic valve was resuspended [8]. In 1982, DeBakey et al. reported their 20-year results from the repair of 527 acute dissection cases, including 195 cases of acute proximal AD. From those cases, they found that operative mortality was more than doubled in DeBakey Type I repairs (30%) versus Type II repairs (14%) [9]. Using the results obtained from this group of acute dissection patients, they set precedents in the treatment and operative adjuncts used during the repair of AD, such as establishing that the method of surgical treatment should be dependent on the type of dissection. Cardiopulmonary bypass (CPB), resection of the ascending aorta, and aortic valvular replacement in patients with aortic valve insufficiency with proximal AD are all used today as the standard of care by cardiac surgery centers around the world.

11.4 Preoperative evaluation

In stable patients, computed tomography angiography (CTA) is useful for confirming a diagnosis of acute proximal AD by identifying the classic "curtain-like" flap traversing the ascending aortic lumen (Fig. 11.3A) and for evaluating the extent of dissection with or without involvement of the thoracoabdominal aorta. When CTA cannot be used because of concerns about contrast-induced nephropathy or allergy, an alternative is magnetic resonance angiography (MRA) (Fig. 11.3B). However, because the gadolinium contrast used in MRA has been implicated in fibrotic renal diseases such as nephrogenic fibrosing dermatopathy and systemic fibrosis, it should also be avoided in patients with prior kidney disease with concerns of worsening kidney function [10]. In the setting of absolute contraindication to both iodine- and gadolinium-based contrast agents, transesophageal echocardiography (TEE) can be also used.

Additionally, TEE can be used to evaluate the patient both preoperatively and intraoperatively to confirm the diagnosis, as well as to assess the extent of dissection and detect aortic root involvement or aortic insufficiency. If no other imaging modality is available, TEE should be performed when acute dissection is suspected.

11.5 Current surgical techniques

Most of the aortic cardiac surgery centers in the United States favor ascending and hemiarch replacement (Fig. 11.4) and limit total arch replacement to cases in which the originating tear involves the transverse arch or the arch measures more than 4.5-5 cm in diameter [11-16]. Others have advocated more aggressive repair as a standard approach [17-20]. Approaches to total arch repair include the island graft, branched graft, or Y-graft (single or double), with or without an elephant trunk for descending aortic involvement. Several options stemming from Borst's elephant trunk technique are available that address the distal arch and descending thoracic aorta at the time of emergent repair of the ascending aorta [21]. Borst's elephant

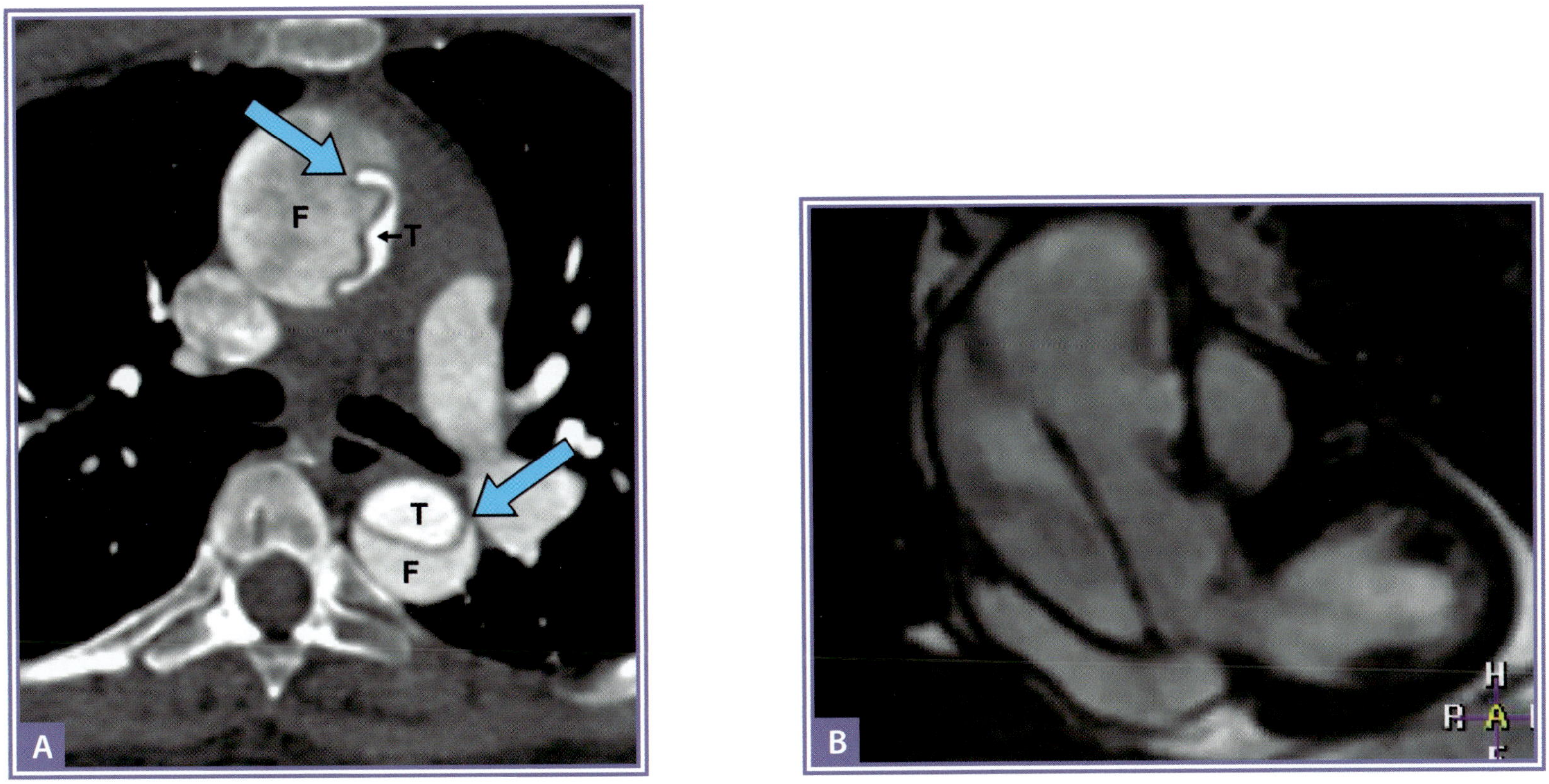

Fig. 11.3 Computed tomographic imaging scan (**A**) of acute DeBakey Type I AD. In this patient, the true lumen (T) has been nearly completely compressed by the false lumen (F) in the proximal aorta, although in the distal aorta, the lumens are approximately equal in size. Magnetic resonance imaging scan (**B**) of acute dissection in the proximal aorta. The dividing septum and entry tear are shown. Reproduced with permission of Baylor College of Medicine.

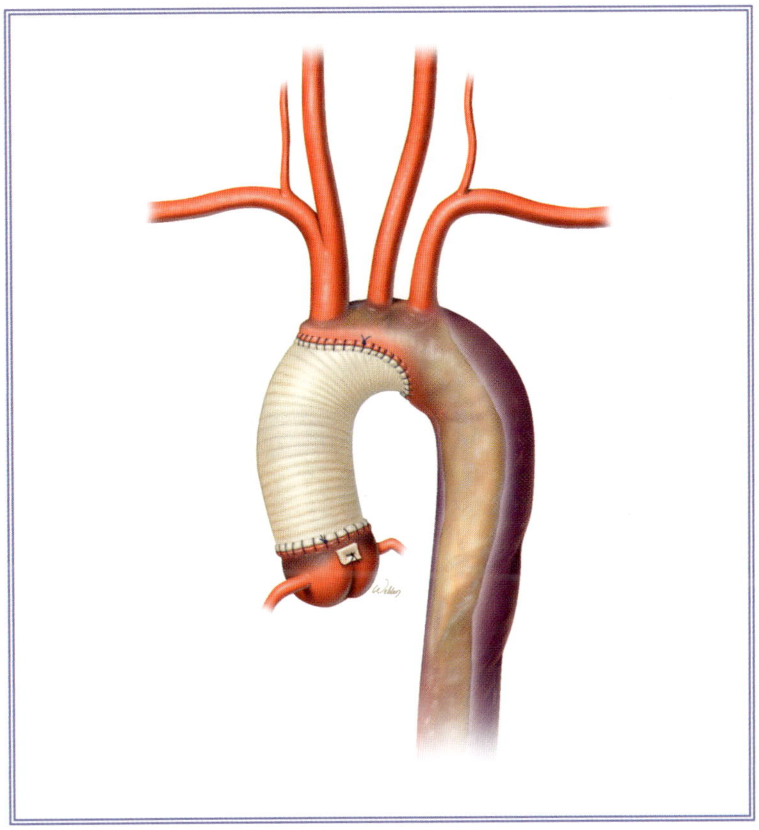

Fig. 11.4 Illustration of a hemiarch repair with resuspension of the aortic valve in a case involving acute DeBakey Type I AD. Reproduced with permission of Baylor College of Medicine.

trunk procedure is a two-stage repair that includes total arch replacement with an elephant trunk graft in the first stage. During the second stage, when the thoracoabdominal aorta is repaired, the elephant trunk provides a cross-clamp site and creates a secure endograft landing zone for potential endovascular repair in the future [22].

A variation of the total arch replacement with the elephant trunk is total arch replacement with the frozen elephant trunk (FET), in which a stent-graft device is used instead of a Dacron graft to "freeze" the elephant trunk into place. This technique has been used for aneurysmal disease and for Type A acute dissections [23-26].

It has been extensively debated in the literature what the appropriate extent of repair is (i.e., how much of the arch should be replaced, and should repair go beyond the arch?) Often, evidence has been conflicting. Balance is sought between limiting the initial repair (i.e., using a hemiarch approach) in hopes of reducing operative risk and extending initial repair (i.e., using a total arch with and without an elephant trunk extension) in hopes of reducing the late risk of distal aortic repair or of reduced survival. Traditionally, data from Crawford's classic paper from 1992 entitled "Surgery for acute dissection of the ascending aorta: Should the arch be included?" is used to support the argument for a limited initial repair [11]. However, there is considerable interest in developing extended repair approaches that do not increase early risk. Most approaches to extended repair aim to improve remodeling of the descending thoracic and thoracoabdominal aorta by limiting blood flow into the false lumen by redirecting blood into the true lumen, thereby reducing the rate of aortic dilatation in the chronic phase [27-29].

11.5.1 Evolution of hemiarch repair with antegrade or retrograde thoracic endovascular aortic repair

Emerging strategies include performing a hemiarch replacement with simultaneous antegrade, or less commonly, retrograde endovascular aortic repair of the proximal portion of the descending thoracic aorta (TEVAR) [22, 30-32]. Even though this technique is occasionally categorized as a frozen elephant trunk procedure, such categorization is misleading because this procedure does not entail total arch replacement with an elephant trunk as is done in the FET procedure. In the hemiarch replacement with TEVAR (Fig. 11.5), the arch branch vessels are preserved, and endograft material is used to repair a short portion of the descending aorta, thereby "sealing" the distal aortic portion of the AD [22]. In our experience, which has been previously described [32], we tend to use this approach in patients with malperfusion or in patients with severe compression of the true lumen by the false lumen. As a precaution against migration, we now secure the endograft circumferentially with 3-0 pledgeted sutures in the proximal descending thoracic aorta distal to the left subclavian artery, leaving only a small portion of native aortic arch.

Most commonly, operative repair of acute proximal AD necessitates a variable period of hypothermic circulatory arrest (HCA). Extending repair typically increases the duration of HCA. During HCA, cerebral protection strategies are commonly added and include antegrade cerebral perfusion, retrograde cerebral perfusion, or both. Different levels of hypothermia are in use today and include the categories listed in Table 11.1, which were established in 2013 in a consensus statement [33]. Temperatures in the deep range are the most commonly reported in the literature [12, 34], but with developments such as antegrade cerebral perfusion, the trend has been to use moderate rather than deep HCA [14, 16, 35]. Several different cannulation sites have been used during repair; these include the femoral, right axillary, and innominate arteries, as well as direct aortic cannulation [36-38].

In our contemporary approach, once the aorta has been opened, the left common carotid artery is cannulated to provide bilateral antegrade cerebral perfusion. Theoretically, the use of unilateral ACP is sufficient, which we have previously shown when the circulatory arrest time is less than 30 minutes [15]. However, other studies have shown that some patients have ana-

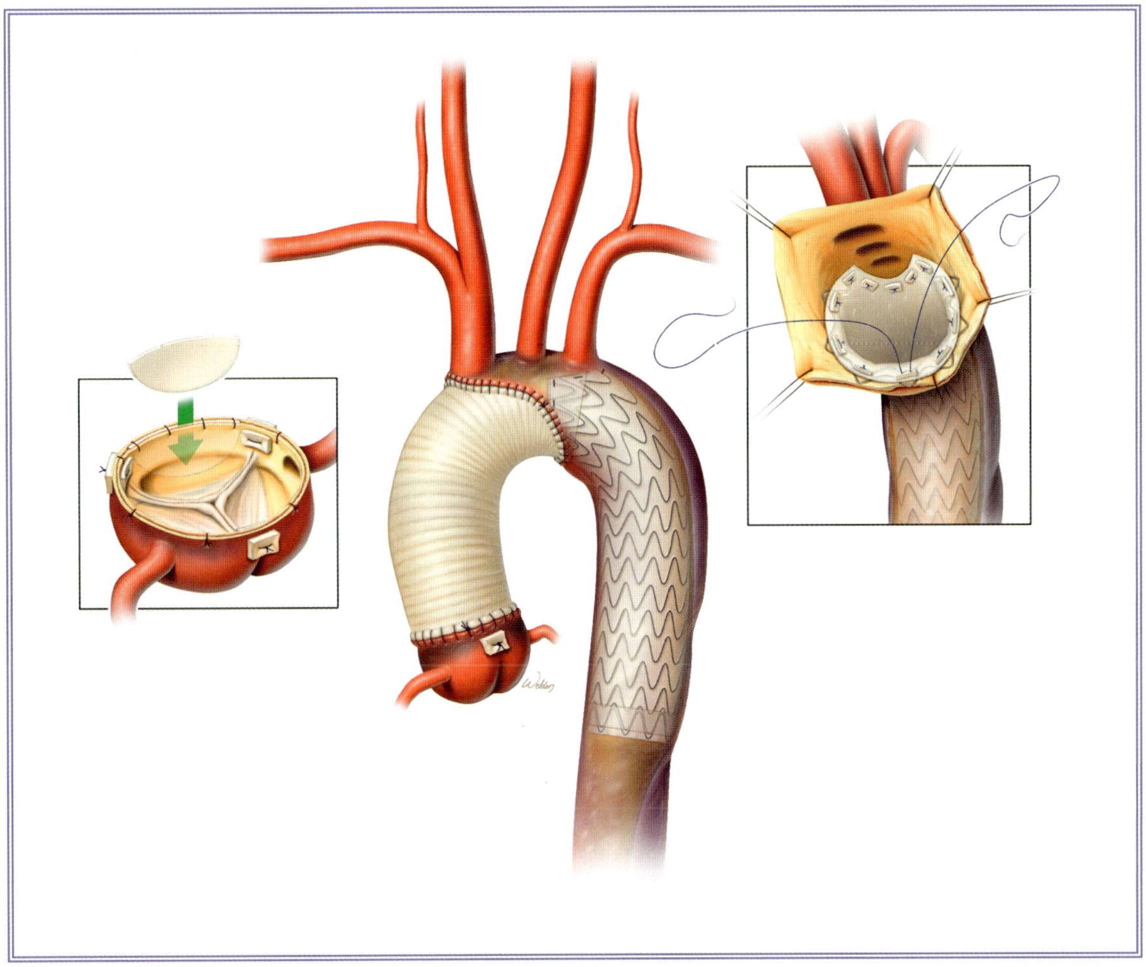

Fig. 11.5 Illustration of a hemiarch repair with antegrade endovascular repair in a case involving acute DeBakey Type I AD and distal malperfusion. During resuspension of the aortic valve, a tongue of Teflon has been added to support the noncoronary sinus. A small notch is cut into the endograft to permit blood flow into the left subclavian artery. To reduce the risk of distal endograft migration, the endograft is reinforced with pledgeted sutures circumferentially. Reproduced with permission of Baylor College of Medicine.

tomic variation in the circle of Willis and that the use of unilateral ACP in these individuals may result in inadequate perfusion to the brain [39, 40]. Recently, we have used bilateral ACP as a standard approach because it is easy to use and adds no time to the repair. Additionally, we monitor cerebral perfusion with near infrared spectroscopy oximetry as a surrogate measure of cerebral oxygenation.

Our contemporary approach to repairing acute proximal AD is as follows. To begin, we cool the patient down to 24 degrees. After the aorta is opened and transected at the proximal arch, the true and false lumens of the dissection are identified, as well as the origin of the intimal tear. If the arch itself and its branch vessels are uninvolved, hemiarch repair can be undertaken; otherwise, more comprehensive arch repair is typically performed. The

Table 11.1 Categories of hypothermia established by expert consensus

Category of hypothermia	Nasopharyngeal temperature
Profound	<14 °C
Deep	14.1-20 °C
Moderate	20.1-28 °C
Mild	28.1-34 °C

Adapted from [33]

distal anastomosis is formed by transecting the lesser curvature of the transverse arch in an oblique or beveled fashion to preserve the origins of the arch branches and should extend to just opposite of the left subclavian artery. The false lumen is obliterated by using BioGlue Surgical Adhesive (CryoLife, Inc., Kennesaw, GA) and a Foley catheter, which is inserted into the true lumen and inflated to provide pressure against the glued surfaces. Subsequently, pledgeted Prolene sutures may be used to reinforce the repair circumferentially. Then, in selected cases, we use antegrade endograft delivery in the descending thoracic aorta under direct vision.

The TEVAR system most commonly used by our group is an Imager II 5F Bern catheter (Boston Scientific Corp., Marlborough, MA) on an Amplatz stiff wire (Boston Scientific) that delivers the Conformable GORE TAG endovascular stent graft (W. L. Gore & Associates, Newark, DE) in the descending thoracic aorta. The nitinol mesh is expanded with the aid of warm irrigation solution. We typically deploy a single endograft that is oversized 10% to 15% of the long axis of the true lumen within the proximal descending thoracic aorta. The length of the endograft is based on the patient's body habitus and height. We typically use an endograft that is 10 or 15 cm in length.

The Dacron graft used for the repair of the ascending aorta and hemiarch should be sized to match the diameter of the transected arch. When the distal anastomosis is completed, the cross clamp is applied, and rewarming is initiated. With regards to the aortic valve, our preference is aortic resuspension with commissural plication, if needed. However, additional intervention may be needed to address the pathology of the aortic root or aortic valve. In patients with genetic tissue disorders, we generally prefer aortic root replacement; however, we are less likely to use valve-sparing approaches to root replacement in the setting of acute dissection. Concomitant procedures may include addressing coronary artery disease with bypass grafting.

With the antegrade delivery of the endograft into the descending thoracic aorta, there is heightened concern of spinal cord ischemia. Unlike traditional hemiarch repair, hybrid hemiarch repair with simultaneous antegrade TEVAR of the proximal portion of the descending thoracic aorta obstructs a few pairs of intercostal arteries and creates a potential risk of postoperative paraplegia.

11.6 Controversial delays in the surgical repair of aortic dissection

Although it is widely accepted that Type I or II dissections should be repaired emergently and without delay, surgical treatment of some patients may be delayed to permit stabilization of the aortic tissue. These include patients who have had prior cardiac surgery and/or prior aortic valve replacement. In patients who have previously had AVR, the valve replacement prevents wide-open aortic insufficiency. In the case of prior cardiac surgery, including valve replacements, postoperative adhesions and scarring may prevent or mitigate aortic rupture and tamponade, but patient results after delay have been contradictory [41-44].

11.7 Early postoperative care

In patients undergoing hemiarch repair with simultaneous placement of an endograft in the descending thoracic aorta, if a spinal cord injury is noticed when the sedation is discontinued, then a cerebrospinal fluid (CSF) drain is placed. In addition, we keep the mean arterial blood pressure between 80-90 mmHg. The drainage of CSF fluid reduces the intracranial pressure, which, in conjunction with an elevated mean arterial pressure, increases cerebral perfusion pressure.

Once recovered enough to be discharged either home or to a rehabilitation center, the patient should receive a CTA of the chest before discharge. Follow-up CTA and appointments are scheduled for approximately 3, 6, and 12 months after surgery and yearly thereafter to check for stability of the repair and the progression of remodeling. Other options for those intolerant to CTA have been discussed above in the section on preoperative evaluation.

11.8 Long-term management

Long-term patient education and surveillance protocols are initiated when patients prepare for discharge. Patients should be made aware that they should seek urgent treatment if concerning symptoms develop (e.g., the sudden onset of pain, any ischemic complications, persistent and unexplained low-grade fever, or unexplained weight loss). Additionally, patients should be counseled that they are at risk for subsequent aneurysm formation in any remaining native aortic segments, even if the patient has no connective tissue disorder or other major risk factors for aneurysm development. This is especially important in patients with extensive residual DeBakey Type I dissection. In patients with chronic dissection, the distal aorta (i.e., the descending thoracic, thoracoabdominal, or abdominal aorta) has been shown to dilate at a faster rate than in patients without AD, which may lead to late aneurysm formation [45]. Moreover, it is not yet clear what proportion of surviving patients will require further repair of the distal aorta or aortic arch. Some patients may not require any further repair. However, patients should be counseled that when further elective repair is needed, operative results tend to be good. We and others have reported our experience in survivors of acute Type I AD that have undergone further repair of the aortic arch or distal aorta [32, 46]. We recommend that the majority of patients in their 60s and 70s undergo at least yearly imaging of the chest and abdomen; in younger patients with connective tissue disorders, we recommend the use of MRA instead of CTA to reduce cumulative radiation exposure and adhere to the radiation safety principle of "as low as reasonably achievable" (ALARA).

Additional education regarding lifestyle modifications may be warranted. Maintaining a healthy blood pressure, heart rate, and weight is ideal. As needed, patients should be counseled on the importance of tobacco, cocaine, and methamphetamine cessation, especially if drug use has precipitated AD. Whereas light aerobic exercise remains beneficial to overall health, extreme isometric exercise (such as weightlifting) should be strictly limited. And although many patients can expect a full return to employment, strenuous manual labor should be avoided.

11.9 Outcomes

The International Registry of Acute Aortic Dissection (IRAD) represents the most comprehensive account of the European experience in treating Type A AD [47]. IRAD, which encompasses data collected from 18 referral centers across the world, provided data regarding surgical outcomes in 526 patients with acute AD in 2005 [47]. Investigators determined that, in patients with acute Type A AD, independent predictors of operative mortality were history of aortic valve replacement, migrating chest pain, hypotension as a sign of acute Type A AD, shock or tamponade, preoperative cardiac tamponade, and preoperative limb ischemia.

In a meta-analysis that compared hemiarch repair with total aortic replacement in patients with acute Type A AD, no significant difference was observed between the two groups in in-hospital mortality, whereas time on CPB, aortic cross-clamp time, and circulatory arrest times were significantly longer in the total arch replacement cases than in the hemiarch repair cases [48].

A few retrospective studies of hemiarch repair with TEVAR have been reported [22, 32, 49], each of which has concluded that hemiarch repair with TEVAR is technically safe and

Table 11.2 Preoperative characteristics, operative details, and early outcomes for 185 hemiarch repairs (2005-2016) in patients with acute DeBakey Type I AD

Variable	All (n = 185) n (%)	Hemiarch (n = 137) n (%)	Hemiarch + TEVAR (n = 48) n (%)
Preoperative characteristics			
Age (y)	61 [49-60.5]	57 [48.5-70]	66 [52.5-72.8]
Male	127 (68.6)	91 (66.4)	36 (75.0)
DeBakey Type I dissection	147 (79.5)	100 (73.0)	47 (97.9)
DeBakey Type II dissection	38 (20.5)	37 (27.0)	1 (2.1)
Hypertension	158 (85.4)	113 (82.5)	45 (93.8)
Genetic disorder	16 (8.6)	14 (10.2)	2 (4.2)
Operative details			
Elective repair	7 (3.8)	7 (5.1)	0 (0)
Urgent or emergent repair	178 (96.2)	130 (94.9)	48 (100)
Aortic root replacement	32 (17.3)	27 (19.7)	5 (10.4)
Aortic valve replacement (without root)	15 (8.1)	15 (10.9)	0
Aortic valve suspension or annuloplasty (without root or AVR)	119 (64.3)	81 (59.1)	38 (58.3)
Coronary artery bypass graft	17 (9.1)	15 (10.9)	2 (4.2)
Early outcomes			
Adverse event	38 (20.5)	30 (21.9)	8 (16.7)
Operative death	26 (14.1)	20 (14.6)	6 (12.5)
30-day death	21 (11.4)	16 (11.7)	5 (10.4)
Persistent* stroke	10 (5.4)	7 (5.1)	3 (6.3)
Persistent* paraplegia	1 (0.5)	1 (0.7)	0
Persistent* paraparesis	2 (1.1)	1 (0.7)	1 (2.1)
Persistent* renal failure necessitating dialysis	18 (9.7)	14 (10.2)	4 (8.3)

Data shown as median [interquartile range] or n (percentage).
* Persisting at time of final hospital discharge or early death.

effective. Regarding patients who underwent hemiarch repair with antegrade TEVAR as compared to those with traditional hemiarch repair, the patients with antegrade endograft delivery had improved resolution of preoperative malperfusion [32]. Our contemporary results are shown in Table 11.2.

11.10 Conclusions

Our approach for the emergent repair of acute proximal AD is performing the minimal amount of surgery needed to prevent death and morbidity and to reduce rates of complication associated with the surgery itself. Most commonly, we perform hemiarch replacement with resuspension of the aortic valve; however, the degree of aortic valve involvement and the presence of aortic root disease dictate our approach to the aortic valve and root. Recently, our contemporary approach to the repair of acute proximal AD has evolved to selectively include hemiarch replacement with additional anterograde stent delivery in patients with malperfusion and in whom the true lumen is severely compressed.

Acknowledgments

The authors express gratitude to Susan Y. Green, MPH, Hiruni S. Amarasekara, MS, and Nicole Stancel, PhD, ELS, for editorial assistance, and Scott A. Weldon, MA, CMI, for creating the illustrations and assisting with image selection. Images are used with permission from Baylor College of Medicine.

REFERENCES

1) LeMaire SA, Russell L. Epidemiology of thoracic aortic dissection. Nat Rev Cardiol 2011; 8: 103-13.
2) Wu D, Shen YH, Russell L, Coselli JS, LeMaire SA. Molecular mechanisms of thoracic aortic dissection. J Surg Res 2013; 184: 907-24.
3) DeBakey ME, Henly WS, Cooley DA, Morris GC, Jr., Crawford ES, Beall AC, Jr. Surgical management of dissecting aneurysms of the aorta. J Thorac Cardiovasc Surg 1965; 49: 130-49.
4) Daily PO, Trueblood HW, Stinson EB, Wuerflein RD, Shumway NE. Management of acute aortic dissections. Ann Thorac Surg 1970; 10: 237-47.
5) Crawford ES. The diagnosis and management of aortic dissection. JAMA 1990; 264: 2537-41.
6) Hirst AE, Jr., Johns VJ, Jr., Kime SW, Jr. Dissecting aneurysm of the aorta: a review of 505 cases. Medicine (Baltimore) 1958; 37: 217-79.
7) DeBakey ME, Cooley DA, Creech O, Jr. Surgical considerations of dissecting aneurysm of the aorta. Ann Surg 1955; 142: 586-610.
8) Morris GC, Jr, Henly WS, DeBakey ME. Correction of acute dissecting aneurysm of aorta with valvular insufficiency. Jama 1963; 184: 63-4.
9) DeBakey ME, McCollum CH, Crawford ES, et al. Dissection and dissecting aneurysms of the aorta: twenty-year follow-up of five hundred twenty-seven patients treated surgically. Surgery 1982; 92: 1118-34.
10) Grobner T. Gadolinium--a specific trigger for the development of nephrogenic fibrosing dermopathy and nephrogenic systemic fibrosis? Nephrol Dial Transplant 2006; 21: 1104-8.
11) Crawford ES, Kirklin JW, Naftel DC, Svensson LG, Coselli JS, Safi HJ. Surgery for acute dissection of ascending aorta. Should the arch be included? J Thorac Cardiovasc Surg 1992; 104: 46-59.
12) Crawford ES, Svensson LG, Coselli JS, Safi HJ, Hess KR. Surgical treatment of aneurysm and/or dissection of the ascending aorta, transverse aortic arch, and ascending aorta and transverse aortic arch. Factors influencing survival in 717 patients. J Thorac Cardiovasc Surg 1989; 98: 659-73.
13) Ehrlich MP, Ergin MA, McCullough JN, et al. Results of immediate surgical treatment of all acute type A dissections. Circulation 2000; 102: Iii248-52.
14) Leshnower BG, Thourani VH, Halkos ME, et al. Moderate versus deep hypothermia with unilateral selective antegrade cerebral perfusion for acute Type A dissection. Ann Thorac Surg 2015; 100: 1563-8; discussion 1568-9.
15) Preventza O, Simpson KH, Cooley DA, et al. Unilateral versus bilateral cerebral perfusion for acute type A aortic dissection. Ann Thorac Surg 2015; 99: 80-7.
16) Rylski B, Milewski RK, Bavaria JE, et al. Long-term results of aggressive hemiarch replacement in 534 patients with type A aortic dissection. J Thorac Cardiovasc Surg 2014; 148: 2981-5.
17) Kazui T, Washiyama N, Muhammad BA, et al. Extended total arch replacement for acute type a aortic dissection: experience with seventy patients. J Thorac Cardiovasc Surg 2000; 119: 558-65.
18) Kazui T, Yamashita K, Washiyama N, et al. Impact of an aggressive surgical approach on surgical outcome in type A aortic dissection. Ann Thorac Surg 2002; 74: S1844-7.
19) Trivedi D, Navid F, Balzer JR, et al. Aggressive aortic arch and carotid replacement strategy for Type A aortic dissection improves neurologic outcomes. Ann Thorac Surg 2016; 101(3): 896-903.
20) Urbanski PP, Lenos A, Schmitt R, Diegeler A. Extended arch resection in acute type A aortic dissection: PRO. Cardiol Clin 2010; 28: 335-42.
21) Borst HG, Walterbusch G, Schaps D. Extensive aortic replacement using "elephant trunk" prosthesis. Thorac Cardiovasc Surg 1983; 31: 37-40.
22) Roselli EE, Rafael A, Soltesz EG, Canale L, Lytle BW. Simplified frozen elephant trunk repair for acute DeBakey type I dissection. J Thorac Cardiovasc Surg 2013; 145: S197-201.
23) Ius F, Fleissner F, Pichlmaier M, et al. Total aortic arch replacement with the frozen elephant trunk technique: 10-year follow-up single-centre experience. Eur J Cardiothorac Surg 2013; 44: 949-57.

24) Ma WG, Zhu JM, Zheng J, et al. Sun's procedure for complex aortic arch repair: total arch replacement using a tetrafurcate graft with stented elephant trunk implantation. Ann Cardiothorac Surg 2013; 2: 642-8.
25) Preventza O, Al-Najjar R, LeMaire SA, Weldon SA, Coselli JS. Total arch replacement with frozen elephant trunk technique. Ann Cardiothorac Surg 2013; 2: 649-52.
26) Shrestha M, Kaufeld T, Beckmann E, et al. Total aortic arch replacement with a novel 4-branched frozen elephant trunk prosthesis: Single-center results of the first 100 patients. J Thorac Cardiovasc Surg 2016; 152: 148-159 e1.
27) Fattouch K, Sampognaro R, Navarra E, et al. Long-term results after repair of type a acute aortic dissection according to false lumen patency. Ann Thorac Surg 2009; 88: 1244-50.
28) Park KH, Lim C, Choi JH, et al. Midterm change of descending aortic false lumen after repair of acute type I dissection. Ann Thorac Surg 2009; 87: 103-8.
29) Rice RD, Sandhu HK, Leake SS, et al. Is Total arch replacement associated with worse outcomes during repair of acute Type a aortic dissection? Ann Thorac Surg 2015; 100: 2159-66.
30) Hofferberth SC, Newcomb AE, Yii MY, et al. Hybrid proximal surgery plus adjunctive retrograde endovascular repair in acute DeBakey type I dissection: superior outcomes to conventional surgical repair. J Thorac Cardiovasc Surg 2013; 145: 349-54.
31) Pochettino A, Brinkman WT, Moeller P, et al. Antegrade thoracic stent grafting during repair of acute DeBakey I dissection prevents development of thoracoabdominal aortic aneurysms. Ann Thorac Surg 2009; 88: 482-9.
32) Preventza O, Cervera R, Cooley DA, et al. Acute type I aortic dissection: traditional versus hybrid repair with antegrade stent delivery to the descending thoracic aorta. J Thorac Cardiovasc Surg 2014; 148: 119-25.
33) Yan TD, Bannon PG, Bavaria J, et al. Consensus on hypothermia in aortic arch surgery. Ann Cardiothorac Surg 2013; 2: 163-8.
34) Elefteriades JA. What is the best method for brain protection in surgery of the aortic arch? Straight DHCA. Cardiol Clin 2010; 28: 381-7.
35) Zierer A, Moon MR, Melby SJ, et al. Impact of perfusion strategy on neurologic recovery in acute type A aortic dissection. Ann Thorac Surg 2007; 83: 2122-8.
36) De Paulis R, Czerny M, Weltert L, et al. Current trends in cannulation and neuroprotection during surgery of the aortic arch in Europe. Eur J Cardiothorac Surg 2014; 47: 917-23.
37) Preventza O, Garcia A, Tuluca A, et al. Innominate artery cannulation for proximal aortic surgery: outcomes and neurological events in 263 patientsdagger. Eur J Cardiothorac Surg 2015; 48: 937-42.
38) Wong DR, Coselli JS, Palmero L, et al. Axillary artery cannulation in surgery for acute or subacute ascending aortic dissections. Ann Thorac Surg 2010; 90: 731-7.
39) Merkkola P, Tulla H, Ronkainen A, et al. Incomplete circle of Willis and right axillary artery perfusion. Ann Thorac Surg 2006; 82: 74-9.
40) Kapoor K, Singh B, Dewan LI. Variations in the configuration of the circle of Willis. Anat Sci Int 2008; 83: 96-106.
41) Hassan M, Carvalho EM, Macedo FI, Gologorsky E, Salerno TA. Paradigm change in the management of patients with acute type A aortic dissection who had prior cardiac surgery. J Card Surg 2010; 25: 387-9.
42) Estrera AL, Miller CC, Kaneko T, et al. Outcomes of acute type a aortic dissection after previous cardiac surgery. Ann Thorac Surg 2010; 89: 1467-74.
43) Teman NR, Peterson MD, Russo MJ, et al. Outcomes of patients presenting with acute type A aortic dissection in the setting of prior cardiac surgery: an analysis from the International Registry of Acute Aortic Dissection. Circulation 2013; 128: S180-5.
44) Collins JS, Evangelista A, Nienaber CA, et al. Differences in clinical presentation, management, and outcomes of acute type a aortic dissection in patients with and without previous cardiac surgery. Circulation 2004; 110: II237-42.
45) Coady MA, Rizzo JA, Hammond GL, Kopf GS, Elefteriades JA. Surgical intervention criteria for thoracic aortic aneurysms: a study of growth rates and complications. Ann Thorac Surg 1999; 67: 1922-6.
46) Coselli JS, Green SY, Zarda S, et al. Outcomes of open distal aortic aneurysm repair in patients with chronic DeBakey type I dissection. J Thorac Cardiovasc Surg 2014; 148: 2986-93 e1-2.
47) Trimarchi S, Nienaber CA, Rampoldi V, et al. Contemporary results of surgery in acute type A aortic dissection: The International Registry of Acute Aortic Dissection experience. J Thorac Cardiovasc Surg 2005; 129: 112-22.
48) Poon SS, Theologou T, Harrington D, Kuduvalli M, Oo A, Field M. Hemiarch versus total aortic arch replacement in acute type A dissection: a systematic review and meta-analysis. Ann Cardiothorac Surg 2016; 5: 156-73.
49) Vallabhajosyula P, Gottret JP, Robb JD, et al. Hemiarch replacement with concomitant antegrade stent grafting of the descending thoracic aorta versus total arch replacement for treatment of acute DeBakey I aortic dissection with arch. Eur J Cardiothorac Surg 2016; 49: 1256-61.

12

Open surgical management of patients undergoing operation for Type A aortic dissection: Moscow experience

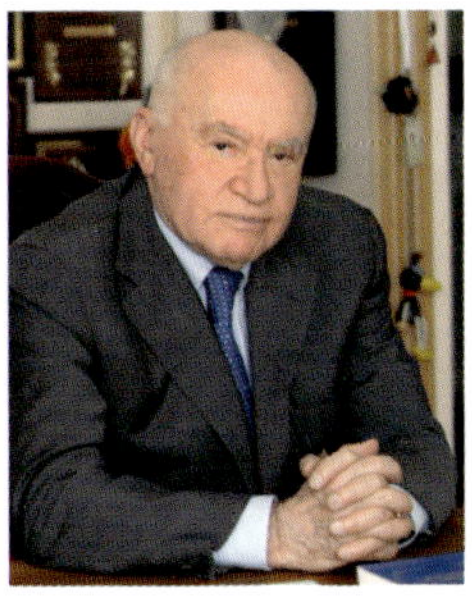

Leo A. Bockeria, Vladimir A. Mironenko and Sergey V. Rychin

12.1 Introduction

Cardiac surgery, open-heart surgery and surgery of the aortic aneurysms are the sites of the medicine by development of which can be represented the healthcare status in the whole country. Russia is no exception. The aortic surgery and the surgery of aortic dissection (AD) passed difficult way intimately associated with the foundation and the development of the cardiovascular surgery.

It is interesting that the group of British surgeons William Cleland, Hugh Bentall and Dennis Melrose performed first cases of operations with the use of cardiopulmonary bypass at A. N. Bakulev Scientific Center of Cardiovascular Surgery in 1959. A series of four successful operations for tetralogy of Fallot were performed with the assistance of the staff members S.A. Kolesnikov and V. A. Bukharin at the Institute of Thoracic Surgery of the Academy of Medical Sciences of the USSR (since 1961 – the Institute of Cardiovascular Surgery, and since 1993 – A.N. Bakulev Scientific Center for Cardiovascular Surgery) (Fig. 12.1).

Hugh Bentall was thus directly involved in the first procedures with cardiopulmonary bypass in our country. Subsequently he made a great contribution to cardiac surgery and especially to the surgery of aortic aneurysms.

Currently, over 5000 cases with cardiopulmonary bypass for all kind of cardiovascular pathology are performed at the Center. They include congenital and acquired heart diseases, coronary bypass, aortic aneurysms and AD, arrhythmia surgery, interactive pathology.

12.1.1 The background

Dissection is the most common catastrophic event affecting the aorta. The true frequency is not known due to improper and delayed diagnosis in many cases [1]. Mortality from acute AD is 1% per hour [2].

Leo A. Bockeria (leoan@bakulev.ru)
Bakulev Scientific Center for Cardiovascular Surgery,
Ministry of Health of Russian Federation, Moscow, Russia

G. Melissano - R. Chiesa (eds), Aortic Dissection patients true stories and the innovations that saved their lives

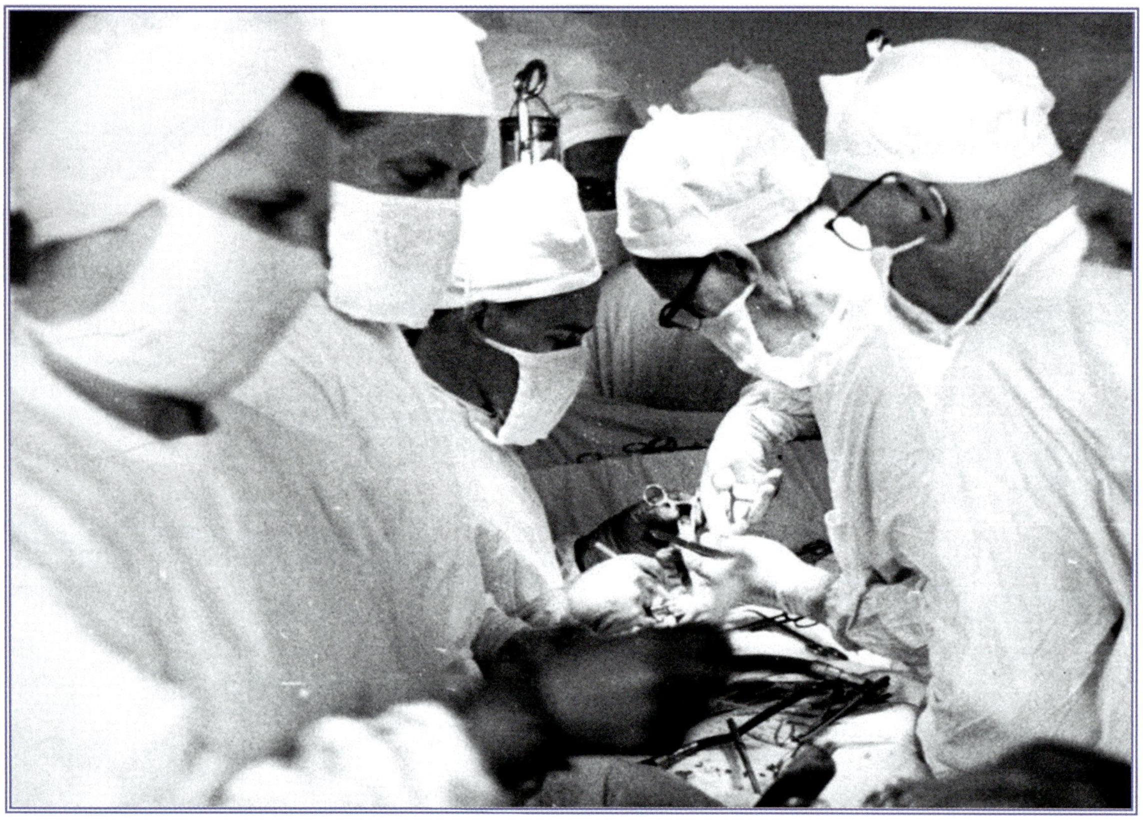

Fig. 12.1 The group of British and Soviet surgeons during the first procedures with cardiopulmonary bypass at the Institute of Thoracic Surgery of the Academy of Medical Sciences of the USSR (1959). From the left to the right: scrub nurse F. Bautly; surgeons: William Cleland, V. Bukharin; anesthesiologist G. Ryabov; surgeons: Hugh Bentall, S. Kolesnikov; scrub nurse D. Mikheeva.

12.1.2 The history

The term "dissecting aortic aneurysm" refers to a sudden formation of the inner aortic wall defect due to various reasons with subsequent penetration of blood flow and degenerative changes of the middle layer [3]. The first descriptions of the AD belong to Sennertus (1650) [4], Maunoir (1802) [5] and Scarpa (1804) [6]. They described the spontaneous "healing" of the dissecting aneurysms. Laennec [7] coined the term "dissection" in 1826.

Surgical treatment of the dissecting aortic aneurysms is a challenging problem of the modern cardiac surgery.

The first attempts of surgical treatment without cardiopulmonary bypass were palliative and were accompanied with unfavorable outcomes.

M. DeBakey [8] performed the first successful case using cardiopulmonary bypass in patient with chronic dissecting aortic aneurysm and aortic valve replacement in 1962. The next year, Morris reported the successful case of surgical correction of acute dissecting aortic aneurysm.

The critical stage in the surgical treatment of AD was the surgical technique, proposed by H. Bentall and A. De Bono [9] in 1968. Their technique made it possible to significantly reduce the rate of hemorrhagic complications and to improve immediate results. It has been recognized and has been widely used in clinical practice in Russia (G.I. Tsukerman [10], A.I. Malashenkov [11], M.L. Semenovsky [12], L.A. Bockeria [13], Y.V. Belov [14], A.M. Karaskov [15], and B.A. Konstantinov [16]).

B.V. Petrovsky [17] performed the first successful operation in the USSR for AD Type II in 1964. The operation consisted in the intersection of the aortic wall and suture of its walls with direct anastomosis.

The first successful surgical correction of chronic AD with the Bentall-De Bono technique at A.N. Bakulev CCVS was performed by G.I. Tsukerman in 1983. Professor A.I. Malashenkov was the first who performed this type of operation in acute Type A AD at the same institution, in 1985.

Since 1983 more than 1500 procedures for aneurysms and dissections of the ascending aorta were performed at our clinic. Of those, 646 were operations for Type A AD aneurysm.

In 2002, L.A. Bockeria, A.I. Malashenkov and G.I. Tsukerman, as part of the group of surgeons from the other centers, were awarded the State prize of the Russian Federation for their contribution to the practical success of surgical treatment of aneurysm of the ascending aorta.

12.2 Etiology

The causes of dissecting aortic aneurysm may be of congenital or acquired origin and are associated with the changes in the histological structure of the aortic wall. Congenital diseases include Marfan's syndrome, Ehlers-Danlos syndrome, Turner syndrome, familial AD, Loeys-Dietz syndrome, bicuspid aortic valve, coarctation of the aorta.

Acquired diseases such as long-persistent hypertension, dyslipidemia, atherosclerosis, cocaine abuse, chronic systemic inflammatory disease of blood vessels (syphilis, Takayasu's arteritis, giant cell arteritis, Behcet's disease, Ormond's disease) are associated with aortic aneurysms.

In addition to the above processes, an external mechanical impact, as well as iatrogenic effects, can be the cause of the dissection. Remote dissections after aortic valve replacement occur in 0.6% of cases.

Furthermore, the geometry of the ascending aorta and the degree of axial displacement of the aortic root have a direct influence on the mechanical stress acting on the wall of the aorta. This explains the cases of AD when its size is normal.

12.3 Diagnostics

Surgical approach for AD treatment depends on the extent of the pathological process. Therefore, the total diagnosis is extremely important. However, in case of acute AD a large amount of diagnostic examination may lead to higher mortality because of increased time prior surgery.

Diagnosis should be based on the use of imaging techniques to ensure a quick and correct diagnosis and determining the tactics and extent of surgical intervention.

In case of emergency admission to hospital, transthoracic echocardiography should be performed as well as blood analyses. It allows to identify or exclude immediately the dissection of the aortic root or cardiac tamponade and also to determine the heart contractility, the state of the aortic valve and also the presence or absence of concomitant valve pathology.

In case of relatively stable condition of the patient, the next step is computed tomography (CT) with contrast panaortography.

The patient at the critical state is transferred to the operating room immediately after the completion of CT. The time from admission to the beginning of the operation may not exceed 30-40 minutes.

The optimal procedure is to perform the complete diagnostics if the patient's condition allows. Echocardiography is supplemented by Doppler ultrasound. In some cases, when it is absolutely necessary, it is possible to perform transesophageal echocardiography (TEE) in the operating room. Computed tomography of the aorta may be supplemented by the imaging of the coronary arteries and brain vessels.

We do not use MRI in the acute stage of AD as well as an invasive coronary angiography and aortography, even in elderly patients.

Table 12.1 Diagnostic methods of examination depending on the stage of the dissection

Methods of examination	Acute dissection	Chronic dissection
EKG	+++	+++
X-Ray	+++	+++
TTE	+++	+++
TEE	++	+
Doppler sonography	+++	+++
CT	+++	+++
MRI	+	++
Aortography	–	+
Coronarography	–	+++

Note: +++, obligatory study; ++, commonly used study; +, rarely used study; –, not applicable study

It is extremely important to keep the balance of the information and the patient's condition.

In case of chronic dissection the list of diagnostic procedures is wider, not limited by time and may include MRI and angiography.

The diagnostic methods of examination are presented in Table 12.1.

12.4 The choice of cardiopulmonary bypass technique

12.4.1 General perfusion

Along with the diagnostics and the features of the AD, the determination of the surgical approach is carried out. An important element is the strategy of extracorporeal circulation: the arterial cannulation points, the level of hypothermia, the need for circulatory arrest, brain protection, the need for special perfusion techniques.

12.4.2 Arterial perfusion

Due to a variety of dissection types, ensuring of adequate perfusion can be a challenge. The rate of central nervous system and visceral organ complications varies widely: from 1% to 55% [18-23]. Some of the complications are directly related to the choice of the method of arterial perfusion. In most cases perfusion via femoral artery is used. In case of AD this technique has a high risk of emergence or amplification of the phenomena of malperfusion.

We believe that perfusion in case of Type A AD should be antegrade. We consider that the right subclavian artery is optimal to use [24-29].

We use the subclavian artery as the basic and optimal access to the surgical treatment of Type A AD from 2004. This has significantly reduced hospital mortality and number of post-operative complications caused by malperfusion syndrome (8.6% under subclavian vs. 28.7% under femoral perfusion).

The use of perfusion through the femoral artery is currently possible only as a forced procedure, in a very limited number of cases.

12.4.3 Brain protection

Protection of the brain in surgery of the ascending aorta and the aortic arch largely determines the success of the operation. The three methods are the most often used. They are: circulatory arrest under deep hypothermia, retrograde cerebral perfusion, selective antegrade brain perfusion.

We used deep hypothermic circulatory arrest until 1994, but a large number of neurological complications accompanied it. In the subsequent cases, circulatory arrest was used only for the revision of the aortic arch.

The results significantly improved when the use of a combination of hypothermia and selective antegrade perfusion began.

The unilateral antegrade perfusion of the brain is technically convenient to carry out – fewer cannulation points, easier blood circuit diagram. In case of its use the pre-operative evaluation of the circle of Willis (anatomical and functional) and intraoperative monitoring (transcranial doppler and cerebral oximetry) are extremely necessary. Intraoperative monitoring is particularly important in case of acute dissection when the preoperative evaluation is generally impossible due to lack of time. In any case of surgical treatment of aortic arch, we provide the possibility of quick modification of the arterial line with the ability to provide bihemispheric perfusion.

The technique of retrograde blood supply of the brain could be an alternative to the antegrade perfusion. The question of the effectiveness of retrograde perfusion remains debatable today. Retrograde perfusion in conjunction with hypothermia was applied in 21 patients. Despite the minor changes of parameters of cerebral perfusion and metabolism, we observed postoperative transient neurological disorders in 4 (19%) patients.

Thus, we believe that antegrade uni- or bihemispheric perfusion of the brain, which was used in most of our patients, is the most versatile and safe.

12.4.4 Special methods of cardiopulmonary bypass – Adaptive perfusion

In terms of patients with AD, we are faced with the fact that the standard methods of extracorporeal circulation do not always ensure adequate perfusion.

In standard cases, adequate perfusion during surgical interventions on the ascending aorta and the aortic arch is provided by connecting one of the lines through the subclavian or femoral artery. The length of the dissection, spreading it out on the main artery, the discharge of the arteries from the false lumen and fenestration at different levels define the peculiarity of the dissection. This dictates the choice of the connection point of the heart-lung machine.

For the complex types of AD with symptoms of malperfusion, combined lesions of the aorta and major arteries, the risk of perfusion via a single arterial trunk increases. In addition, circulatory arrest during intervention on the aortic arch represents the risk of occurrence or worsening of ischemia of the visceral organs.

Attempts to provide extracorporeal circulation through several blood lines were performed earlier, but at the present level the use of multiple arterial lines could solve the issue of malperfusion even in cases of emergency interventions.

On the basis of our own experience of the surgical treatment of non-standard forms of bundles, accompanied by malperfusion, we have formulated the concept of adaptive perfusion. It is the combination of methods of artificial circulation, aimed at ensuring of the adequate perfusion and protection of the brain, internal organs and extremities during the correction of complicated forms of aortic aneurysms.

The two groups were allocated by the type of adaptive perfusion:

- the group of variant connections of the extracorporeal circuit with the cannulation of one or more of the great arteries;

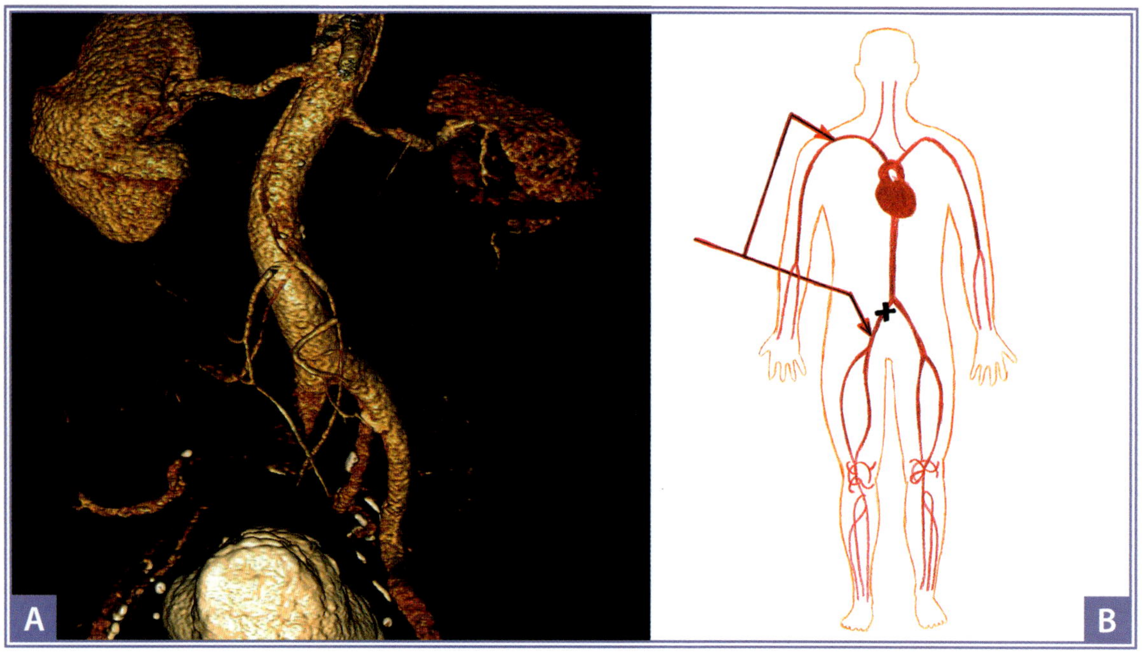

Fig. 12.2 The application of the regional perfusion. CT data of a patient with acute Type A AD complicated by ischemia of the right lower extremity (**A**). Diagram of the extracorporeal circuit connection (**B**).

- the group of combination of techniques of cardiopulmonary bypass: variable cerebral perfusion, perfusion of the visceral organs during the intervention on the aortic arch, regional perfusion of the separate areas of circulation.

The dual cannulation was used to ensure adequate volume perfusion rate in patients with a large body weight or in cases of high resistance in a standard connection of the arterial line in cases of anatomically narrow main arteries. But mostly we use a double cannulation to reduce the time of circulatory arrest and to perform complex surgical interventions on the aortic arch under moderate hypothermia within adaptive perfusion. One line is used for the unilateral antegrade cerebral perfusion, the second for the visceral perfusion.

We have used regional perfusion in patients with acute aortic Type A dissection complicated by ischemia of the lower limb due to the compression of the true lumen by the false, repeatedly (Fig. 12.2). This will be discussed below in more details.

Thus, the use of adaptive perfusion in complex forms of aneurysms of the ascending aorta enables an intervention in adverse clinical variant lesions of the aorta and its branches. It allows minimizing the time of circulatory arrest. It increases the time of safe operation on the aortic arch and the brachiocephalic vessels. Adaptive perfusion allows operating under moderate hypothermia and adjusting the perfusion protocol in cases of operation plan changing.

12.5 Current surgical techniques

Surgical management of AD can be divided into stages of proximal and distal aortic repair. The combination of these two interventions determines the final type of surgery, which depends on the type of dissection, density of tissues, involvement of the main trunk vessels and comorbidities.

Commonly we start the management of AD from the proximal (cardiac) side of the aorta. This allows efficient use of the cooling time of the patient.

12.5.1 Proximal anastomosis – Repair of cardiac side of the aorta

Supracoronary aortic replacement with prosthesis (prosthetic repair of the aorta) with root reconstruction

The intervention is performed in case the sinuses of Valsalva are not expanded, their wall thickness is normal and there are no aortic root fenestrations. When aortic regurgitation is caused by the expansion of sinotubular junction, the valve competence is being achieved by the right choice of the vascular prosthesis. In case the dissection extends into the aortic root with the rupture of the commissures, restoring the normal valve function is achieved by commissure fixation in physiological position followed by supracoronary prosthetic repair.

David procedure

The intervention is most applicable to the chronic AD with the expansion of the fibrous ring, sinuses of Valsalva. In case of acute dissection the condition of aortic root tissues should be evaluated as their imbibition with blood may complicate the intervention in this area and lead to bleeding from the area of fibrous ring sutures or appearance (persistence) of aortic insufficiency.

Bentall-De Bono procedure

The most radical intervention is performed in case of aortic root dilation, rough deformation of fibrous ring and aortic valve leaflets, as well as the presence of aortic root fenestrations or coronary ostia rupture.

In acute dissection we consider reliable to perform the conduit implantation as described by H. Bentall and A. De Bono [9], without complete excision of the aortic wall. This allows to perform the conduit wrapping with forming anastomosis between periconduit space and right atrium at the final stage of intervention [30]. This Cabrol maneuver is particularly useful in cases of thinned aortic tissue and annulus fibrosus, as well as during anticoagulation, such as after thrombolytic therapy applications.

Historical features of performing the Bentall procedure in the USSR and Russia

One of the main issues of prosthetic ascending aortic replacement is the problem of choosing the conduit. Despite a number of obvious advantages, synthetic conduits have disadvantages as well, such as a relatively thick wall, insufficient hemostatic properties of anastomosis, especially of the coronary ones, during procedures on acute dissection of the aorta and coronary ostia. Furthermore, tubular vascular prosthesis significantly limits the geometric options for correction and can lead to excessive tension on the sutures. This results in bleeding, suture incompetence, formation of hematoma and fistulae.

Early in 1987, a group of Brazilian cardiac surgeons from São Paulo published the first use of bovine pericardium for the ascending aortic replacement with success [31]. The experience of Brazilian doctors in implantation of xenopericardial conduits has been followed at our Institution.

Bioconduits in the ascending aortic surgery have been used at our Center since 1989. The first successful case using xenopericardial conduit of Brazilian production was performed by Professor A.I. Malashenkov. In the same year, the Laboratory of Biotissues at our Center created our own bioconduits (B.A. Fursov) (Fig. 12.3). Its first implantation was performed in 1990.

Conduit proved to be convenient during implantation, demonstrated high flexibility and hemostatic properties, which was particularly important for acute AD repair. Conduit was im-

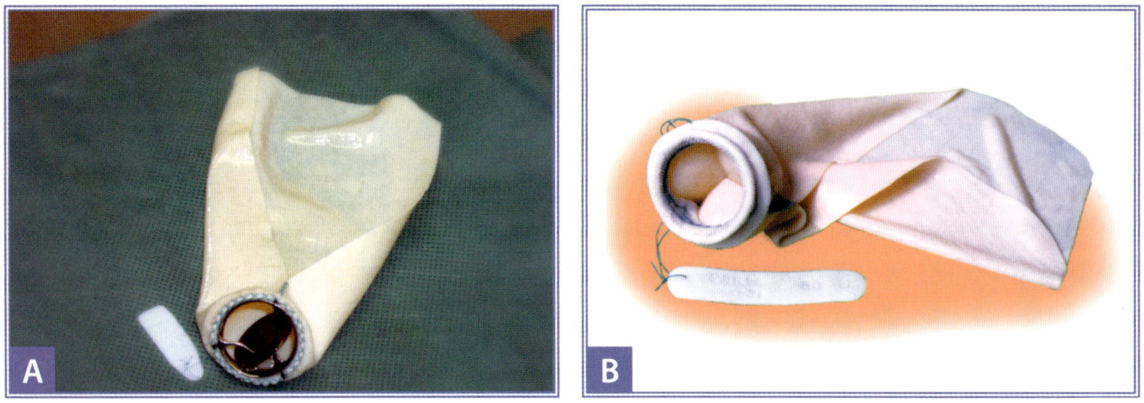

Fig. 12.3 Xenopericardial conduit: with a mechanical heart valve EMIKS (**A**); with the skeleton bioprosthetic valve (**B**).

planted accordingly to the Bentall-De Bono procedure with wrapping and forming an anastomosis between periconduit space and right atrium in Cabrol technique.

The total number of cases with xenopericardial conduits for the ascending aorta replacement is close to 500 implantations. In 216 cases the conduit was used for Type A AD.

The average hospital mortality was 11.1%: 17.2% in patients with acute dissection and 8.5% in elective surgery for chronic dissection. Hemorrhagic complications of anastomosis conduit were the cause of mortality in 1% of cases.

The problem of bioprosthesis is its limited viability. It is known that the age of patients at the time of surgery plays the key role in the duration of conduit functioning.

In our group the mean age of patients at the time of surgery was 38.9 ± 6 years. The highest percentage of biodegeneration happened in a limited group of patients with bioconduit containing frame valve bioprosthesis. At the same time, the biodegeneration process in the bioconduit wall was not so expressed and due to functional indifference had no practical value for maintaining physical integrity (Fig. 12.4).

The highest degree of biodegeneration was noted in young patients during the period of more than 10 years after implantation (Fig. 12.5).

In aged patients there were no significant signs of biodegeneration in conduit wall revealed, even against the expressed calcification of the native aortic wall. This is why in some cases we still use from time to time a valve containing xenopericardial conduits in old patients.

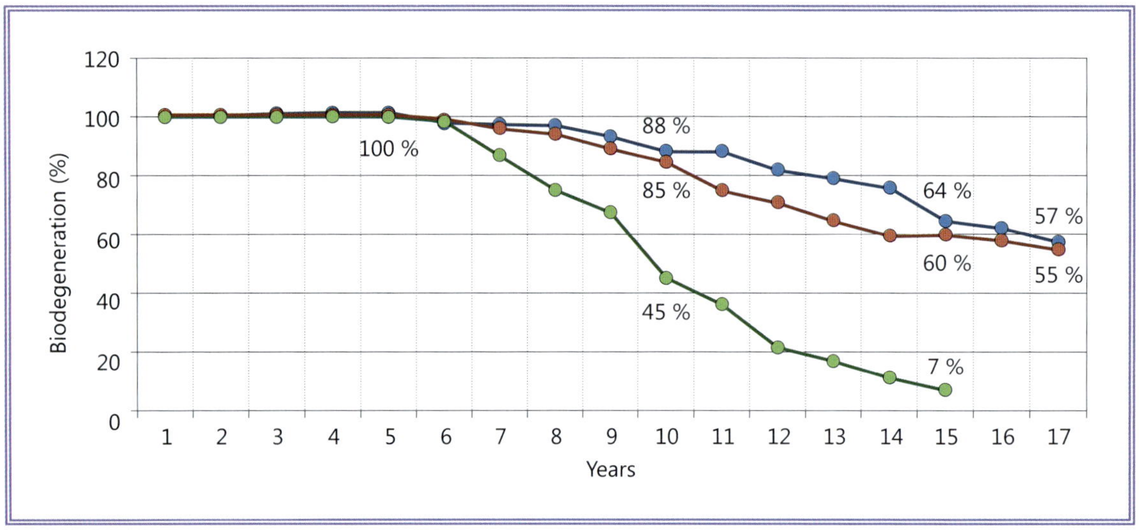

Fig. 12.4 Actuarial freedom from biodegeneration of bioconduit wall and leaflets of bioprosthesis.

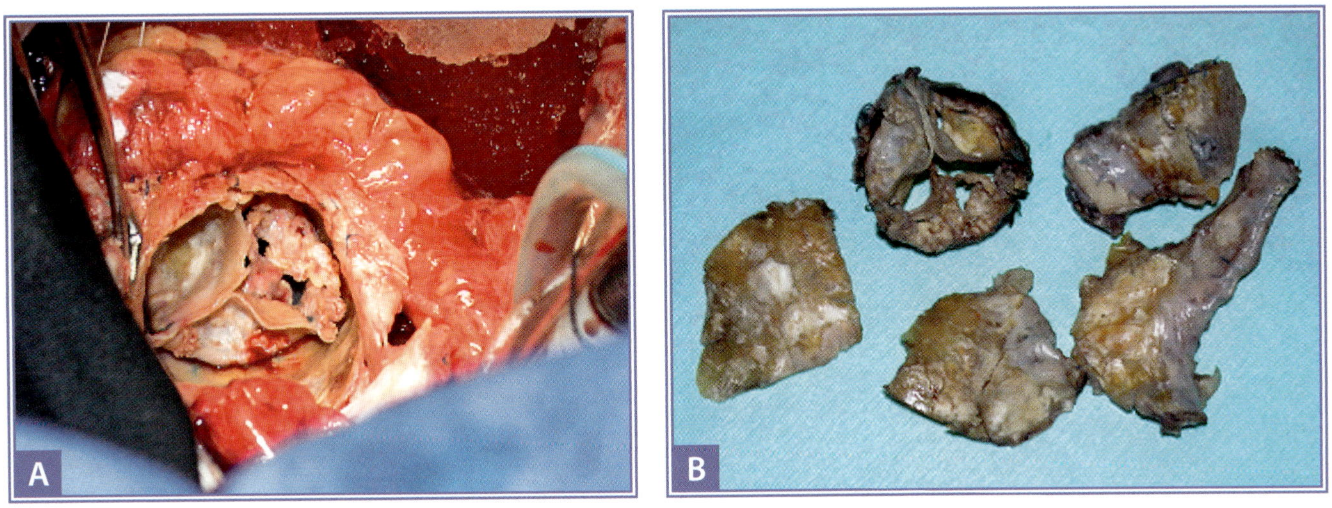

Fig. 12.5 Reoperation in patient H. (44 years), 13 years after xenopericardial conduit and bioprosthesis implantation. Intraoperative photo (**A**); removed materials: biologic prostheses and the wall of xenopericardial conduit (**B**).

12.5.2 Distal anastomosis

Depending on the level of distal anastomosis applications, the following options can be considered:

- anastomosis proximal to brachiocephalic trunk without aortic arch involvement;
- anastomosis proximal to brachiocephalic trunk with partial prosthesis along the "lesser curvature" of aortic arch ("hemiarch");
- prosthetic aortic arch replacement, the so called "elephant trunk" according to Borst [32];
- total prosthetic aortic arch replacement with anastomosis to brachiocephalic arteries on a common platform;
- total or partial prosthetic aortic arch replacement with linear prostheses in brachiocephalic arteries.

Regardless of the proximal anastomosis type, the location and type of the distal anastomosis is determined by the location of fenestration, its extension to the arch and brachiocephalic vessels, quality of ascending aorta and arch walls.

Anastomosis has to be applied to the true lumen with removal of proximal fenestration. We prefer to buttress the anastomosis with felt pads. Hemostasis is particularly important in acute dissection as in such case the adventitia is commonly thinned.

Anastomoses to brachiocephalic arteries

There are several options for restoring normal blood flow through brachiocephalic arteries. Commonly, the whole group of brachiocephalic arteries is implanted into the aortic arch prosthesis on a common platform. In case of thinned aortic wall, felt pads should be used in order to buttress the suture in the area of coronary ostia. If the proximal parts of brachiocephalic vessels are involved, the multi-branch prosthesis can be used for aortic replacement.

In this case "end-to-end" anastomosis between arterial ostia and branches of the prosthesis are applied with consistent blood flow restoration.

In case the dissection extends into the distal parts of the arteries (up to common carotid artery bifurcation or extension of the dissection into the internal carotid artery), we perform concomitant single-stage or staged brachiocephalic arteries and aortic arch repair.

12.6 Malperfusion

Malperfusion syndrome is a severe complication in patients with acute Type A AD that significantly worsens the prognosis of treatment and life expectance. In up to 33% of patients this syndrome manifests in the preoperative period. Of them, in 44% cases the clinical manifestations are due to coronary arteries, in 42% to brachiocephalic trunk involved in the process, in 34% to limb ischemia, in 11% to kidney vessels, and in 9% to mesenteric vessels. The malperfusion syndrome increases hospital mortality from 13.6% to 29% [33].

Special surgical techniques and the use of adaptive perfusion reduce the risks and improve immediate results.

12.6.1 Coronary ostia

The incidence of coronary arteries involvement in acute Type A AD varies widely from 11 to 70% [34-37]. Myocardial infarction can be a result of such involvement. Mortality in the group of patients with dissection of coronary arteries was four times (33.3%) higher than in patients without dissection (8.2%) [38].

In case of partial or complete coronary artery rupture from the true aortic root, every effort to apply direct anastomosis to graft should be made (Fig. 12.6).

In cases with a danger of eruption of coronary anastomosis sutures due to a sharp thinning of the aortic wall, we buttressed the coronary suture line with Teflon pads or autopericardial strips (Fig. 12.7). We used this technique in 27.5% of patients. In such cases xenopericardial conduit has the best hemostatic properties, providing almost 100% free from bleeding in this area.

In case the reconstruction of the artery is impossible, its ostium is sutured and Coronary Artery Bypass Graft (CABG) is subsequently performed. In our group such cases made up 5.3% of patients.

Having the installation for intraoperative coronary angiography, we are able to perform on-table stenting after restoration of the ascending aorta integrity. This expands our options in acute dissection treatment.

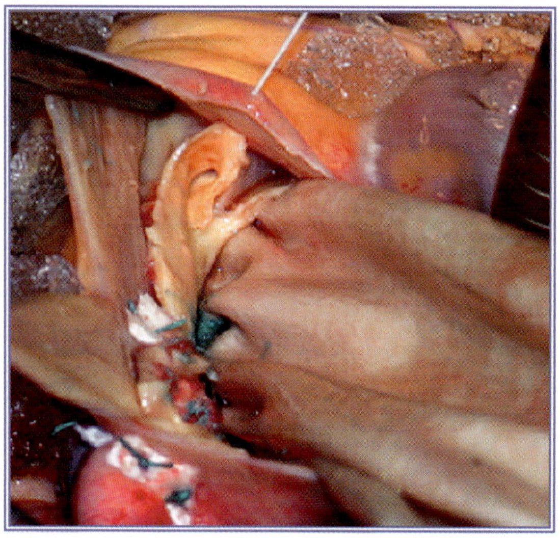

Fig. 12.6 The partial shearing of right coronary artery ostium, followed by implantation into the conduit.

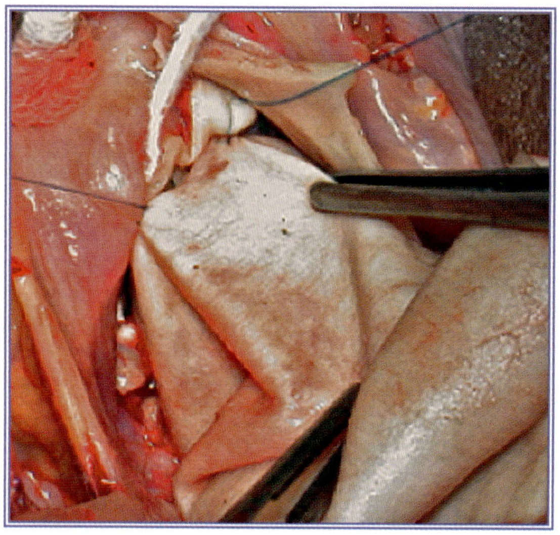

Fig. 12.7 Strengthening the mouth of the dissected right coronary artery by Teflon strip while implanting it into the xenopericardial conduit.

12.6.2 Brachiocephalic vessels

In case the dissection extends into the aortic arch and involves the brachiocephalic arteries, the risk of neurological deficit before surgery is of 14-20% [33, 39]. Manifestation of cerebral malperfusion increases mortality rate up to 43.7-50% [40, 41]. These patients pose a number of challenges for cardiac surgeon, such as the choice of surgical technique and location of arterial cannulation, ensuring adequate cerebral perfusion.

For concomitant brachiocephalic arteries and aortic arch repair a staged or single-stage intervention may be carried out. In the first case, the duration of each procedure shortens, and it is possible to assess the hemodynamic and neurologic status, including functional tests performance, between procedures. The most complex stage of repair takes place in more predictable conditions.

There are cases when the procedure cannot be divided into stages and a combined intervention is performed. Usually sternotomy incision is extended up to the neck and carotid artery or brachiocephalic trunk repair is performed. That became necessary for maintaining sufficient cerebral perfusion during ascending aorta or aortic arch repair. After restoration of cardiac activity and blood flow through the left main carotid artery, the brachiocephalic prosthesis is implanted in the prosthesis of ascending aorta.

Our experience consists of 16 combined (5 with an acute dissection) and 3 staged interventions, in which concomitant prosthetic brachiocephalic arteries repair in addition to ascending aorta and arch repair was performed (Fig. 12.8). There was no hospital mortality in this group. In one patient with acute dissection an ischemic stroke on the side of the affected brachiocephalic artery occurred.

It has to be noted that, unless concomitantly, it would be impossible to perform the aortic repair due to absence of cerebral perfusion supply.

All patients in this group underwent adaptive perfusion, including intermittent cerebral and visceral ones. All patients were operated on under moderate hypothermia.

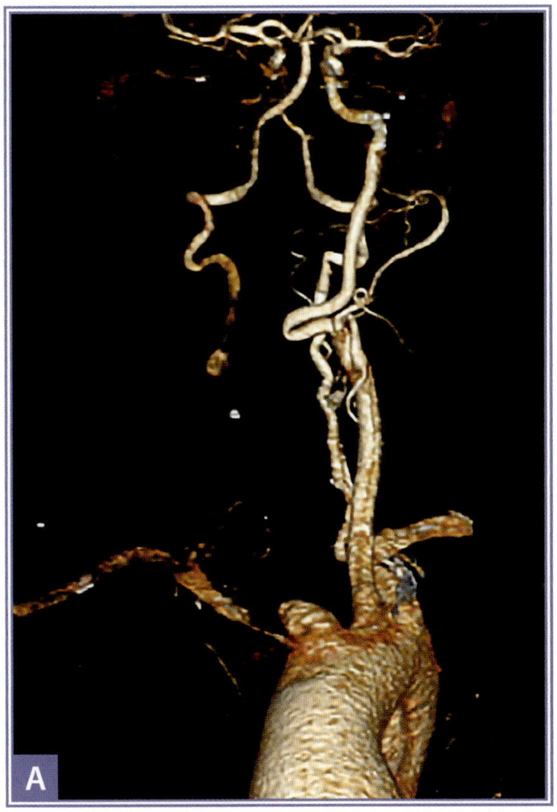

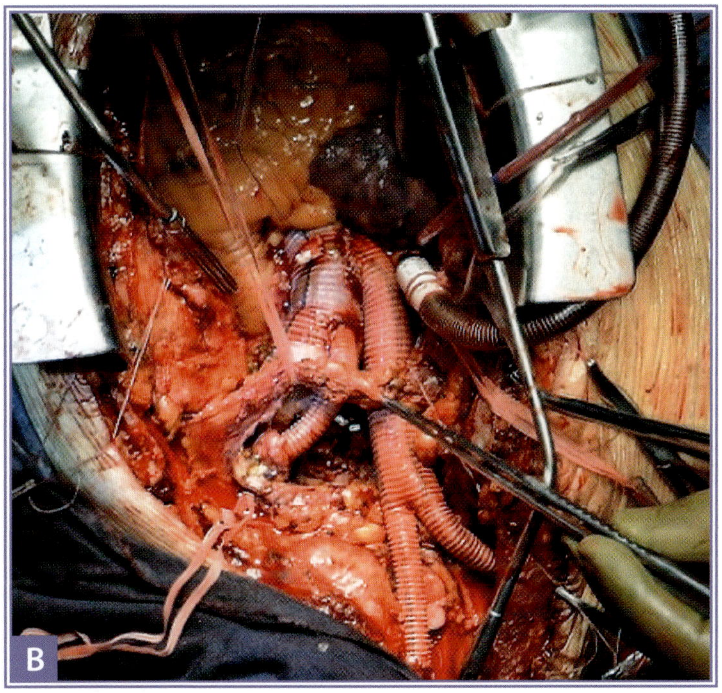

Fig. 12.8 Example of cerebral malperfusion in Type A AD (**A**). Prosthetic repair of left common carotid, right internal carotid and right subclavian artery in AD and cerebral malperfusion (**B**).

12.6.3 Malperfusion of the lower extremities

Limb ischemia in acute AD occurs in 12-30% of cases [33, 42]. Critical stenosis of the main artery is an absolute contraindication for elective Cardiopulmonary ByPass (CBP) cardiac surgery. However, in acute Type A AD, especially if there is a tamponade or pulmonary edema, emergency surgery is the only way to save the patient's life. Blood flow absence in the main artery may be either reversible or irreversible, even in case of a successful redirection of blood flow in the true lumen. In case of emergency intervention, it is extremely difficult to determine the prognosis of ischemia during the procedure. Long existing limb ischemia, especially during the cardiopulmonary bypass, may lead to fatal complications.

The sequence of those procedures may be different. Some authors recommend performing revascularization before the surgery on ascending aorta in order to avoid serious complications, while others carry it out after the main stage [43, 44].

One of the options for relatively fast treatment of the lower limb ischemia in acute AD is creating an artificial fenestration and stenting of the affected artery [45]. In some cases, you can make a subclavian-femoral or femoral-femoral bypass and perform the perfusion through it. This prevents the development of lower limb ischemia and renal failure [46, 47]. However, these techniques require performance of the first vascular stage of surgery, which in an emergency is not always possible or is not justified.

In such cases, we act differently. We established temporary perfusion of lower limb during the main phase of repair (Fig. 12.9) [48]. This option allows you to start the basic intervention as quickly as possible while guaranteeing the preservation of blood flow in the affected limb. The final decision on the restoration of blood flow in the ischemic limb is transferred to the final stage of the main procedure. It becomes possible to estimate the proximal blood flow in the artery after the dissection repair.

In our view, regional perfusion during AD complicated with lower limb ischemia is technically simple to be performed and effective in an emergency. We have the experience of three such cases. Only in one patient after the main stage of the intervention the femo-femoral bypass was required. In two other cases, after the dissection repair in the proximal aorta and the direction of blood flow into the true lumen, the blood flow in ischemic limb was restored (Fig. 12.10).

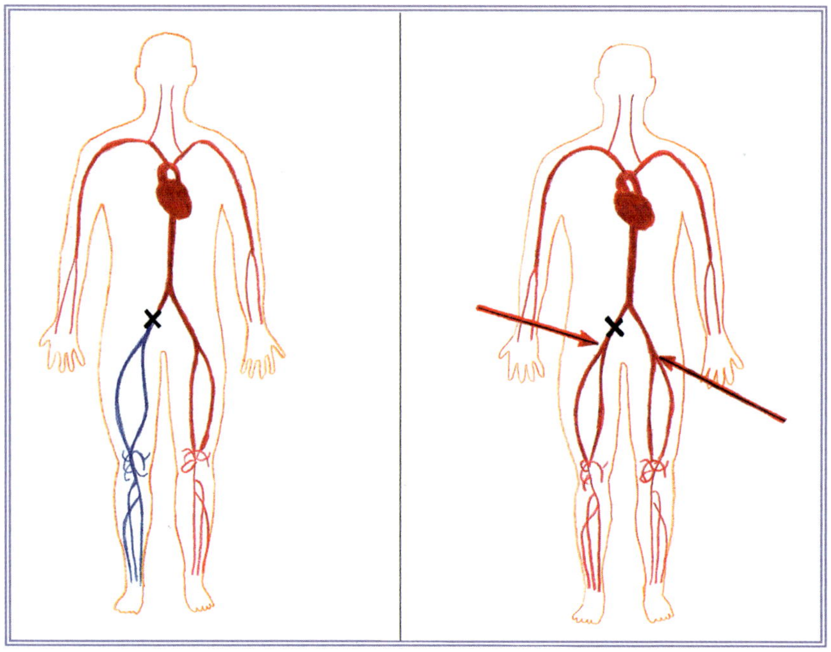

Fig. 12.9 Regional perfusion of the ischemic lower limb during acute Type A AD repair.

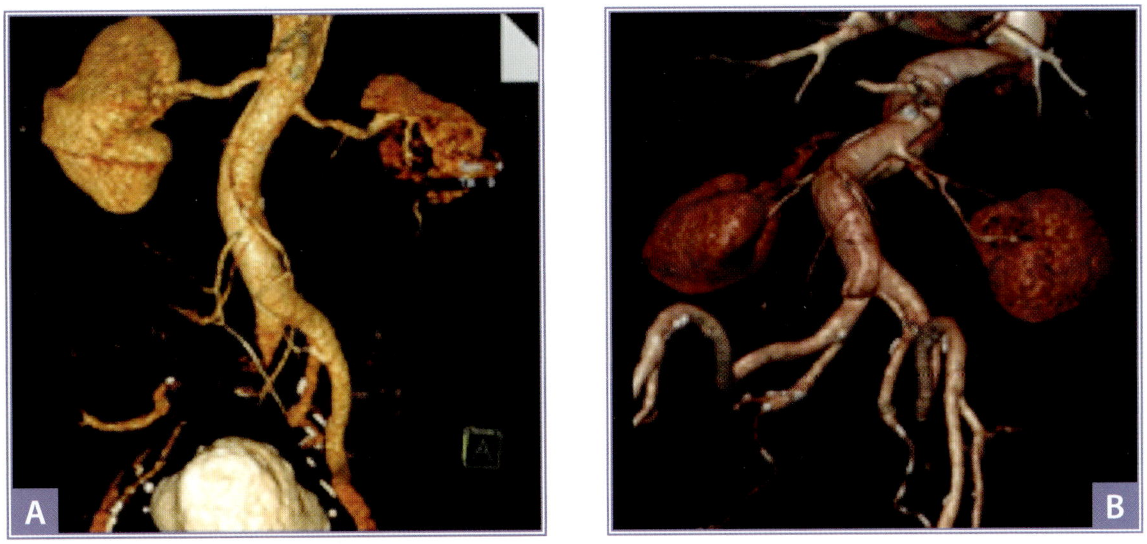

Fig. 12.10 Multiple detector computer aortography with contrast and 3D reconstruction; **A**, before surgery, occlusion of common iliac artery; **B**, after the surgery, no signs of occlusion.

12.7 Results

12.7.1 Immediate results

From 1983 to 2015, 646 patients with Type A AD underwent surgical treatment at our hospital. This group comprised 432 men (66.8%) and 214 women (33.2%). The average age was 48 ± 12.2 years (12 to 77). In 189 cases an emergent acute (up to 14 days) dissection repair was carried out. In the last 5 years the majority of cases are being performed in the first 24 hours after the dissection, due to improved diagnostic facilities of primary health care.

Over the years, the number of patients has increased (Fig. 12.11). At the same time, there has been a significant decrease in mortality rate.

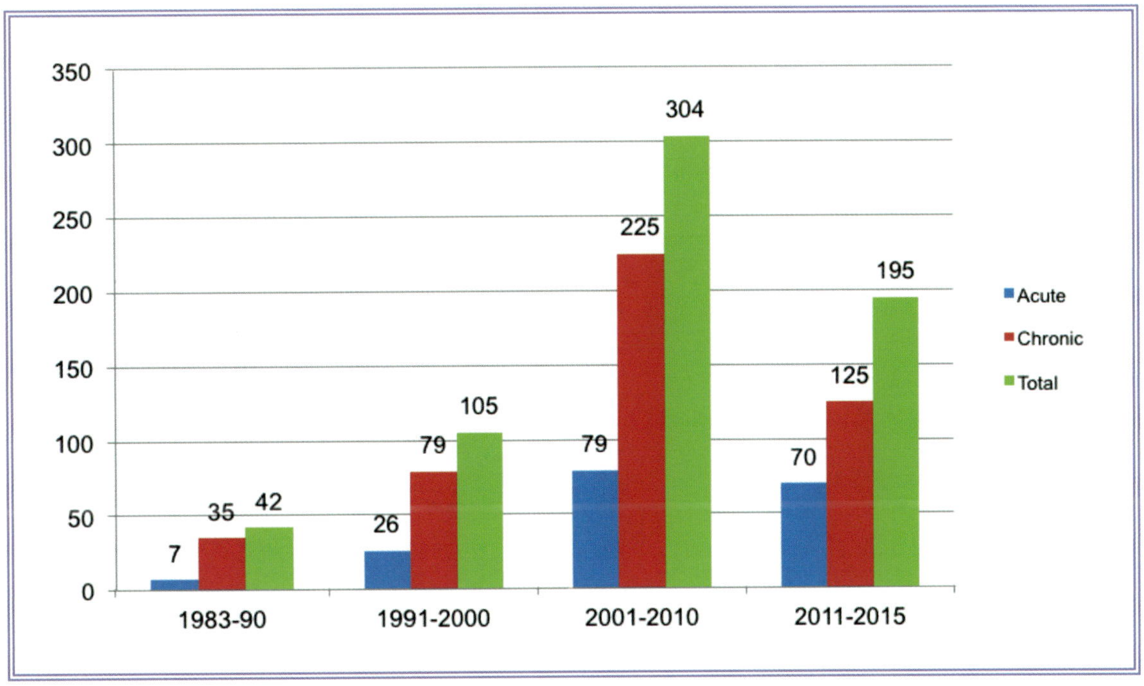

Fig. 12.11 Dynamics of the number of surgeries by year.

Table 12.2 The types of performed surgeries

	Acute aortic dissection	Chronic aortic dissection	Total
Number of patients/mortality rate	189/34(17.9%)	455/44(9.7%)	644/78 (12.1%)
Bentall-De Bono procedure	117	334	451
Xenoconduitis/Bioprosthesis	64/6	152/9	216/15
Cabrol procedure	2	17	19
Valve sparing procedure	70	104	174

Table 12.3 Concomitant procedures

	Acute aortic dissection	Chronic aortic dissection	Total
Concomitant arch interventions	28	100	128
Concomitant BCV interventions	3	10	13
Concomitant CABG	11	26	37
Concomitant AV valve interventions	4	41	45

AV, atrioventricular; BCV, brachiocephalic vessel; CABG, coronary artery bypass graft

The most common ascending aorta repair is Bentall-De Bono procedure. In 216 cases the xenopericardial conduit of our own production was used. The types of performed surgeries are presented in table 12.2.

In distal repair the intervention most often involved the aortic arch (128 patients). In 13 cases prosthetic BCV repair was carried out, right or left common carotid arteries due to their dissection and blood flow disorder (Table 12.3).

There were six cases of intraoperative deaths and four of them were due to uncontrolled bleeding in patients with acute dissection. All those patients were surgically treated before 1992. Once we started to use xenopericardial conduits, the bleeding problem has been solved in many ways.

In 2 cases, death was caused by coronary insufficiency due to the extension of the dissection into the left main coronary artery.

In-hospital deaths included 72 more patients. Overall hospital mortality was 12.1%. In case of emergency surgeries, the mortality rate made up 17.9%. In elective cases in patients with chronic dissection it was 9.7%.

12.7.2 Long-term results

Among the most demonstrative rates of successful treatment are mortality and survival of patients in long-term follow-up.

According to various data the rate of 10-year survival after surgery ranges from 53% to 88% [14; 49-52]. The results are influenced by many factors and include the initial patient's state, the urgency of surgery, comorbidities, the extent of surgery.

However, according to a number of authors, the main causes of mortality in the long-term period are a variety of cardiovascular complications and reoperations [53-56]. The aneurysm formation, ruptures and dissection of distal aorta take the first place in the structure of long-term mortality [57].

According to our data the actuarial survival rate at 5 and 10 years after surgery, excluding in-hospital mortality, made up 85% and 74% of cases, respectively. The main causes of long-term mortality were the complications of residual aorta and reoperations, as well as cardiovascular complications such as stroke, myocardial infarction and heart failure.

The analysis showed that the major risk factors for reoperation are functioning false lumen (OR = 1.26; 95% CI 1.06-1.50, $p < 0.05$), and age less than 45 years at the time of the initial intervention (OR = 1.29; 95% CI 1.08-1.53, $p < 0.05$).

In addition, the functioning false lumen (OR = 1.39; 95% CI 1.17-1.65; $p < 0.05$) and aggravated family history in patients with no outward signs of connective tissue disease (OR = 1.22; 95% CI 1.03-1.45; $p < 0.05$) increased the risk of an aneurysm in the long term period and, as a consequence, the need for re-operation.

Thus, redo operations on the aorta, young age, aggravated family history, functioning false lumen are the factors that have an adverse effect on the long-term surgical results. Therefore, ideally, the primary surgery has to ensure the elimination of the false lumen in distal aorta. In the late postoperative period these groups of patients should be carefully monitored.

12.8 Conclusion

We hope that our experience can be useful and will become part of the knowledge that allows to solve complex issues of AD surgical treatment.

REFERENCES

1) Cohn LH, Edmunds LH. Cardiac surgery in the adult. 2nd ed. New York: McGraw-Hill; 2003.
2) Hagan PG, Nienaber CA, Isselbacher EM, et al. The international registry of acute aortic dissection (IRAD): new insights into an old disease. JAMA 2000; 283: 897-903.
3) Burakovsky VI, Bockeria LA. Cardiovascular surgery. M. Medicine ; 1996: 608-646. [In Russian].
4) Sennertus D. Cap 42. Op Omn Lib; 1650; 5: 306.
5) Maunoir JP. Memoires physiologiques et pratiques sur l'aneurisme et la ligature des arteres. Geneva: JJ Paschoud; 1802 .
6) Scarpa A. Sull'aneurisma: riflessioni ed osservazioni anatomico-chirurgiche. Pavia; 1804.
7) Laennec RT. Traite de l'auscultation mediate et des maladies des poumons et du coeur. Paris: J.-S. Chaude; 1826.
8) DeBakey ME, Henly WS, Cooley DA, et al. Surgical management of dissecting aneurysms of the aorta. J Thorac Cardiovasc Surg 1965; 49: 130.
9) Bentall H, De Bono A. A technique for complete replacement of the ascending aorta. Thorax 1968; 23(4): 338-9.
10) Tsukerman GI, Malashenkov AI, et al. The surgery of ascending aorta aneurysms: retrospective view. J Thorac Cardiovasc Surg 1996; 3: 61-4. [In Russian].
11) Malashenkov AI, Rusanov NI, Padjaev MA, et al. Diagnosis and surgical treatment of acute dissecting aneurysm of ascending aorta. J Medical Practice 2004; 4: 16. [In Russian].
12) Semenovsky ML, Myakishev VB, Sokolov VV, et al. Immediate and long-term results of Bental de Bono operation. Angiology and Vascular Surgery 1997; 4: 12-6. [In Russian].
13) Bockeria LA, Malashenkov AI, Rusanov NI, et al. Surgical treatment of ascending aorta and arch aneurysm. J Thorac Cardiovasc Surg 2001; 3: 36-43. [In Russian].
14) Belov YV. Long-term results of surgical treatment of ascending aorta aneurysm. Angiology and Vascular Surgery 2005; 11(2): 105-11. [In Russian].
15) Karaskov AM, Chernyavsky AM, Porhanov VA, et al. Reconstructive Surgery of Aorta. Novosibirsk: Academician Publishing house «Geo»; 2006: 255. [In Russian].
16) Konstantinov BA, Belov YV, Kuznechevsky FV. Surgical treatment of ascending aorta and arch aneurysm. M. Medicine ; 2006: 335. [In Russian].

17) Petrovsky BV. Surgical treatment of ascending aorta aneurysm. J Surgery 1965; 7: 94-100.
18) Ricotta JJ, Faggioli GL, Castilone A, Hassett JM. Risk factors for stroke after cardiac surgery: Buffalo Cardiac-Cerebral Study Group. J Vasc Surg 1995; 21(2): 359-63.
19) Kincaid EH, Jones TJ, Stump DA, et al. Processing scavenged blood with a sell saver reduce cerebral lipid microembolization. Ann Thorac Surg 2000; 70: 1296-300.
20) Stamp DA, Newman SP, Hammon JW. Cerebral emboli and cognitive outcome after cardiac surgery. J Thorac Cardiovasc Surg 1996; 10(1): 113-8.
21) Stoica SC, Sharples LD, Ahmed I. Preoperative risk prediction and intraoperative events in cardiac surgery. Eur J Cardiothorac Surg 2002; 21(1): 41-6.
22) Nashef SA, Roques F, Hammill BG, et al. Validation of European System for Cardiac Operative Risk Evaluation (Euro SCORE) in North American cardiac surgery. Eur J Cardiothorac Surg 2002; 22(1): 101-5.
23) Geissler HJ, Fischer UM, Grunert S, et al. Incidence and outcome of gastrointestinal complications after cardiopulmonary bypass. Interact Cardiovasc Thorac Surg 2006; 5: 239-42.
24) Malashenkov AI, Rusanov NI, Arakelyan VS, et al. Surgical treatment of complicated forms of ascending aorta aneurysms under alternative methods of extracorporeal circulation. J Bulletin of A.N. Bakulev Center for CVS 2009; 10(3): 23. [In Russian].
25) Sukhanov SG, Katkov AI, et al. The choice of aortic cannulation as a method of brain protection in surgical treatment of ascending aorta dissecting aneurysm. J Bulletin of A.N. Bakulev Center for CVS 2006; 6(5): 61. [In Russian].
26) Watanabe K, Fukuda I, Osaka M, et al. Axillary artery and transapical aortic cannulation as an alternative to femoral artery cannulation. Eur J Cardiothorac Surg 2003; 23: 842-3.
27) Sinclair MC, Singer RL, Manley NJ, et al. Cannulation of the axillary artery for cardiopulmonary bypass: safeguards and pitfalls. Ann Thorac Surg 2003; 75: 931-4.
28) Neri E, Massetti M, Capannini G, et al. Axillary artery cannulation in type A aortic dissection operations. J Thorac Cardiovasc Surg 1999; 118: 324-9.
29) Hedayati N, Sherwood JT, Schomisch SJ. Axillary artery cannulation for cardiopulmonary bypass reduces cerebral microemboli. J Thorac Cardiovasc Surg 2004; 128: 386-90.
30) Cabrol C, Pavie A, Gandjbakhch I, et al. Complete replacement of the ascending aorta with reimplantation of the coronary arteries: new surgical approach. J Thorac Cardiovasc Surg 1981; 81: 309-14.
31) Ardito RV, Santos JL, Mayorquim RC, et al. Substituicao completa da aorta ascendente e da valva aortica com tubo valvulado de pericardio bovino. Rev Bras Cir Cardiovasc 1987; 2(2): 129-38.
32) Borst YG, Walterbusch G, Schaps D. Extensive aortic replacement using "elephant trunk" prosthesis. J Thorac Cardiovasc Surg 1983; 31: 37-42
33) Girdauskas E, Kuntze T, Borger MA, et al. Surgical risk of preoperative malperfusion in acute type A aortic dissection. J Thorac Cardiovasc Surg 2009; 138: 1363-9.
34) Kern MJ, Serota H, Callicoat P, et al. Use of coronary arteriography in the preoperative management of patients undergoing urgent repair of the thoracic aorta. Amer Heart J 1990; 119: 143-8.
35) DeBakey ME, McCollum CH, Crawford ES, et al. Dissection and dissecting aneurysms of the aorta: twenty-year follow-up of five hundred twenty-seven patients treated surgically. Surgery 1982; 92: 1118-34.
36) Rizzo RJ, Aranki SF, Aklog L, et al. Rapid noninvasive diagnosis and surgical repair of acute ascending aortic dissection. Improved survival with less angiography. J Thorac Cardiovasc Surg 1994; 108: 567-75.
37) Neri E, Toscano T, Papalia U, et al. Proximal aortic dissection with coronary malperfusion: presentation, management, and outcome. J Thorac Cardiovasc Surg 2001; 121: 552-60.
38) Kawahito K, Adachi H, Murata S, Yamaguchi A, Ino T. Ñoronary malperfusion due to type A aortic dissection: mechanism and surgical management. Ann Thorac Surg 2003; 76: 1471-6.
39) Krüger T, Weigang E, Hoffmann I, et al. Cerebral protection during surgery for acute aortic dissection type A: results of the German Registry for Acute Aortic Dissection Type A (GERAADA). Circulation 2011; 124: 434-43.
40) Tanaka H, Okada K, Yamashita T, Morimoto Y, Kawanishi Y, Okita Y. Surgical results of acute aortic dissection complicated with cerebral malperfusion. Ann Thorac Surg 2005; 80: 72-6.
41) Geirsson A, Szeto WY, Pochettino A, et al. Significance of malperfusion syndromes prior to contemporary surgical repair for acute type A dissection: outcomes and need for additional revascularizations. Eur J Cardiothorac Surg 2007; 32: 255-62.
42) Fann JI, Sarris GE, Mitchell RS, et al. Treatment of patients with aortic dissection and presenting with peripheral vascular compromise. Ann Surg 1990; 212: 705-13.
43) Charlton-Ouw KM, Sritharan K, Leake SS, et al. Management of limb ischemia in acute proximal aortic dissection. J Vasc Surg 2013; 57(4): 1023-9.
44) Girardi LN, Krieger KH, Lee LY, Mack CA, Tortolani AJ, Isom OW. Management strategies for type A dissection complicated by peripheral vascular malperfusion. Ann Thorac Surg 2004; 77: 1309-14.
45) Yamaguchi M, Sugimoto K, Tsuji Y, et al. Percutaneous balloon fenestration and stent placement for lower limb ischemia complicated with type B aortic dissection. Radiat Med 2006; 24: 233-37.

46) Long SM, Nair D, Halandras PM, Kasirajan K, Milner R, Chen EP. Ileofemoral malperfusion complicating type a dissection: revascularization prevents renal failure. Ann Thorac Surg 2007; 84(6): 2099-101.
47) Schönholz C, Ikonomidis JS, Hannegan C, Mendaro E. Bailout percutaneous external shunt to restore carotid flow in a patient with acute type A aortic dissection and carotid occlusion. J Endovasc Ther 2008; 15(6): 639-42.
48) Mironenko VA, Ruchin SV, Garmanov SV. The types of extracorporeal circulation in case of acute aortic dissection type 1, complicated with critical lower limb ischemia. J Thorac Cardiovasc Surg 2013; 6: 58-60. [In Russian].
49) Chiappini B, Schepens M, Tan E, et al. Early and late outcomes of acute type A aortic dissection: analysis of risk factors in 487 consecutive patients. Eur Heart J 2005; 26: 180-6.
50) Gariboldi V, Grisoli D, Kerbaul F, et al. Long-term outcomes after repaired acute type A aortic dissection. Interact Cardiovasc Thorac Surg 2007; 6: 47-51.
51) Geirsson A, Bavaria JE, Swarr D, et al. Fate of the residual distal and proximal aorta after acute type A dissection repair using a contemporary surgical reconstruction algorithm. Ann Thorac Surg 2007; 84: 1955-64.
52) Zierer A, Melby SJ, Lubahn JG, et al. Elective surgery for thoracic aortic aneurysms: late functional status and quality of life. Ann Thorac Surg 2006; 82: 573-8.
53) Yeh CH, Chen MC, Wu YC, Wang YC, Chu JJ, Lin PJ. Risk factors for descending aortic aneurysm formation in medium-term follow-up of patients with type A aortic dissection. Chest 2003; 124: 989-95.
54) Girdauskas E, Kuntze T, Borger MA, et. al. Long-term prognosis of type A aortic dissection in non-Marfan patients with histologic pattern of cystic medial necrosis. Ann Thorac Surg 2008; 85: 972-7.
55) Halstead JC, Meier M, Etz C, et al. The fate of the distal aorta after repair of acute type A aortic dissection. J Thorac Cardiovasc Surg 2007; 133: 127-35.
56) Olsson C, Ericsson N, Ståhle E, et al. Surgical and long-term mortality in 2634 consecutive patients operated on the proximal thoracic aorta. Eur J Cardiothorac Surg 2007; 31: 963-9.
57) Yu HY, Chen YS, Huang SC, Wang SS, Lin FY. Late outcome of patients with aortic dissection: study of a national database. Eur J Cardiothorac Surg 2004; 25: 683-90.

13

Acute aortic dissection in patients with bicuspid aortic valve

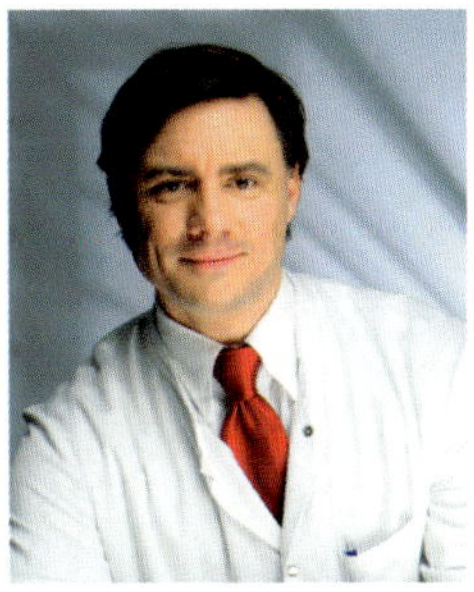

Christian D. Etz and Josephina Haunschild

13.1 The bicuspid aortic valve

The bicuspid aortic valve (BAV) is the most common congenital cardiac abnormality affecting up to 2% of the general population (Fig. 13.1) [1, 2]. According to contemporary expert consensus, BAV accounts for more morbidity and mortality than all other congenital heart malformation combined [1] and BAV-associated pathologies are considered so virulent that every BAV patient will – given enough time – develop valvular lesions or severe aortic complications such as aneurysm or acute dissection [3]. Interestingly, Leonardo da Vinci was the first scientist to describe the condition of a bicuspid aortic valve – considered an harmless anomaly for centuries to come [4]. Meanwhile, various morphologies have been recognized and there are several classification systems [5-7] to anatomically describe the valve's precise configuration, of which the Sievers classification [8] is probably the most established due to its clear and systematic approach.

Over the past decades, a lively discussion among experts was concerned with one of the major impacts of BAV: the associated proximal aortic pathology. Two major – most likely interacting – hypothesis have been identified:
1) genetic alterations [9-15]
2) altered blood flow architecture through the bicuspid valve [16-18].

Vast, yet unspecific evidence emerged supporting each hypothesis drawing the picture of BAV as a complex syndrome with wide and heterogeneous pattern.

Durable surgical solutions for patients with bicuspid aortic valve and proximal aortic disease are available achieving excellent long-term outcome [19, 20].

13.1.1 Genetics of bicuspid aortic valve

Echocardiographic screening of BAV families revealed that at least one out of ten siblings also carried a bicuspid aortic valve [10]. In 2004, a study collecting the family history over three

---

Christian D. Etz (Christian.Etz@medizin.uni-leipzig.de)
Herzzentrum Leipzig-Universitätsklinik,
Leipzig, Germany

G. Melissano - R. Chiesa (eds), Aortic Dissection patients true stories and the innovations that saved their lives

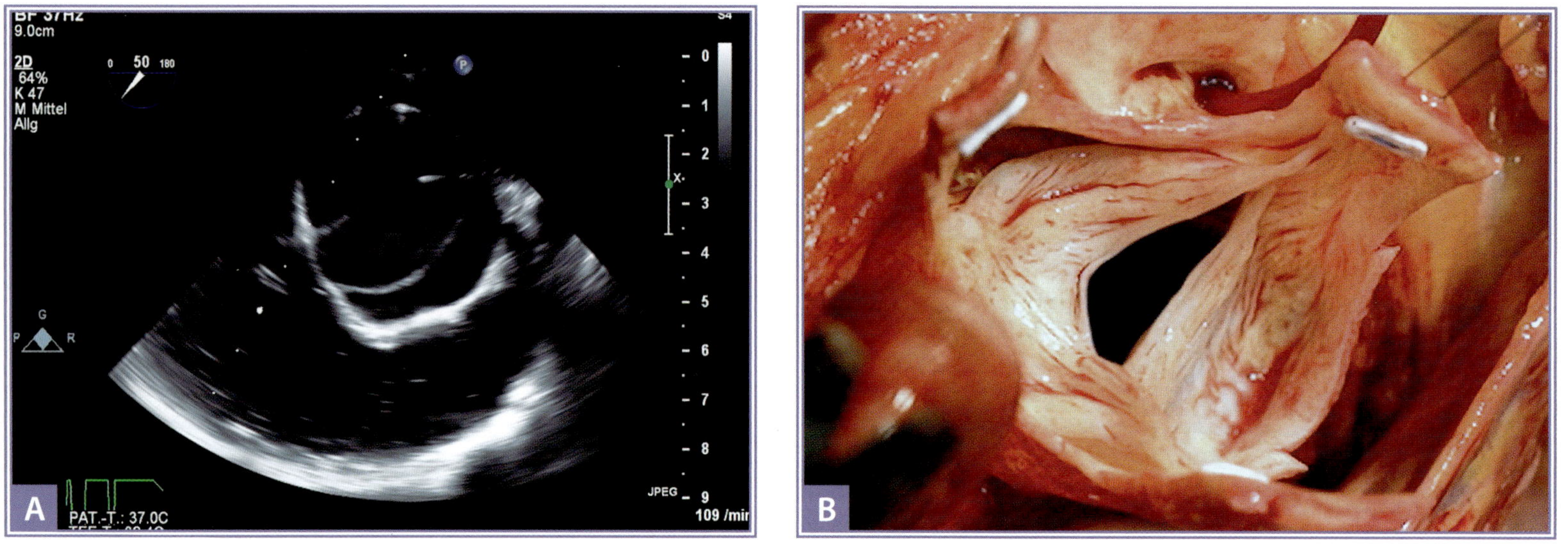

Fig. 13.1 Transesophageal echocardiographic imaging (**A**) and intraoperative situs (**B**). Bicuspid aortic valve (Sievers type I LR).

generations of fifty patients with BAV revealed that first-degree relatives had an increased risk of inheriting a BAV themselves (9%) – or various other congenital cardiac pathologies, such as aortic coarctation, ventricular or atrial septal defect, an abnormal mitral valve, aortic root dilation, or even hypoplastic left heart syndrome (31%) [15]. Biner et al. described that 32% of first-degree relatives of BAV patients (of whom 53% had a dilated aorta) also had dilated proximal aortas although they had a tricuspid aortic valve (TAV) [14] strongly supporting a genetic etiology. However, Dayan and colleagues examined first-degree relatives of BAV and TAV patients with no aortic dilation and could not detect any difference in aortic dimensions [21]. Meanwhile, several genes – *Fibrillin 1*, *NOTCH*, *GATA*, *eNOS* [22-25] – have been investigated but yet no culprit gene responsible for development of a BAV was identified (see also Chapter 6).

13.1.2 Alterations in flow architecture through the bicuspid aortic valve

More recently, evidence emerged that abnormal flow alterations through the functionally normal bi-leaflet BAV increase local wall stress, constituting not only flow alteration as a possible underlying factor for aneurysm formation but also as a major risk factor for acute Type A aortic dissection (AD) [26]. Since new technologies such as 4D-flow MRI analysis have recently become widely accessible, numerous studies have been published focussing on the blood flow architecture within the proximal aorta (Fig. 13.2) [16, 27-31]. A recent study revealed more intense helical flow ($p = 0.0098$) and suggested pronounced vortex formation in BAV patients.

Moreover, higher flow displacement possibly resulting in an increased peak systolic wall shear stress associated with BAV has been suggested [32]. Even in the absence of any valvular dysfunction the flow pattern in BAV patients is different compared to normal TAV patients and each BAV type may generate a distinctive flow architecture [17, 33, 34]. A research group at Stanford investigated the proximal blood flow after valve-sparing aortic root replacement in BAV patients with Sievers type 1 LR (fusion of left and right coronary cusp) and 0 lateral (true bicuspid) showing an elevated wall shear stress among 1 LR patients in the aortic root and proximal ascending aorta. Interestingly, type 0 patients revealed wall stress not significantly different from normal tricuspid patients [18]. These results should be kept in mind when isolated valve reconstruction is considered as opposed to full root reconstructions (e.g. David procedure) as wall shear stress alterations may trigger vascular remodeling processes [35, 36],

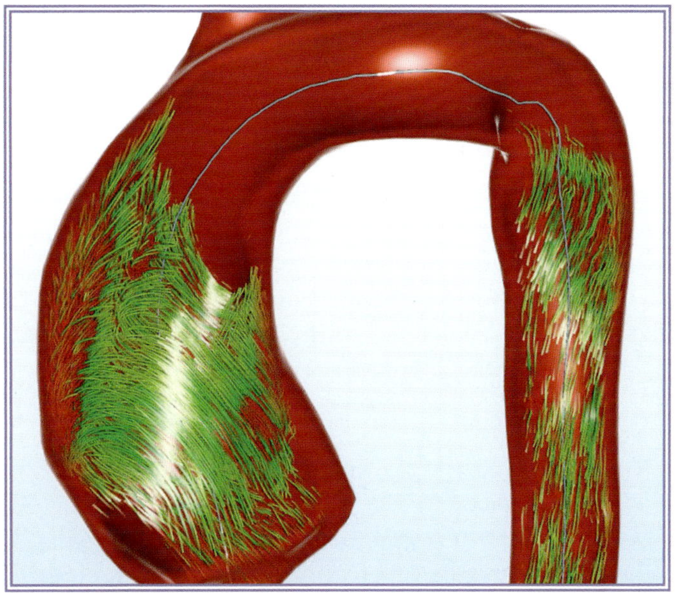

Fig. 13.2 4D MRI flow analysis in a BAV patient with Sievers type I LR morphology.

which could predispose these patients to further postoperative aortic dilation or, even worse, acute Type A AD. However, clinical evidence connecting various Sievers type with the actual risk for acute AD is scarce.

13.1.3 Molecular changes in the aortic wall

When analyzing regions of elevated wall shear stress, less elastin, thinner fibers and more space between the fibers have been detected [37]. Furthermore, enzymes of extracellular matrix degradation have increased activity suggesting abnormal blood flow as trigger for aortic wall remodeling possibly causing a thinning of the proximal aortic wall [37]. Not only areas of increased wall stress undergo alteration: several studies have demonstrated a decreased Fibrillin-1 content, increase in vascular smooth muscle cell apoptosis, a lower aortic distensibility and greater stiffness possibly exposing BAV patients more prone to acute Type A AD [38-41]. As potential underlying pathomechanism for acute Type A dissections among BAV patients, thinning of elastic lamellae and increased distance to one-another was assumed [42].

Due to the above described lack of profound understanding in the underlying pathomechanisms, individual risk stratification becomes virtually impossible and international guidelines are fluctuating, predominately based on expert opinion, rather than level one evidence.

13.2 Current guidelines

It is believed that carriers of a BAV have a lifetime risk for aortic valve and/or proximal aortic complications requiring surgery of up to 25% [43]. Current AHA/ACC guidelines are proposing an aggressive approach for replacement of proximal aorta in BAV patients with valvular dysfunction at 45 mm (vs. TAV patients at 50 mm). Without functional valvular lesion but in the presence of risk factors such as positive family history, the cut-off for elective, isolated ascending replacement in BAV is 50 mm (55 mm for TAV) [44, 45]. Just recently – in April 2016 – guidelines for aortic replacement in BAV patients with aortic dilatation were reviewed again by an expert consortium: for functionally normal, non-symptomatic BAV, ascending/root replacement is now recommended at 55 mm as a strong class I recommendation suggesting that the long-term benefits outweigh the operative risk. While a rather weak IIb recommendation is now implemented based on level B-NR evidence (non-randomized) setting the cut-off to 50 mm for BAV with no valvular lesion and no risk factor when an experienced aortic surgical team is performing the surgery [45].

The Olmsted County cohort study revealed – in the subset of BAV patients – that in patients with no aneurysm at time of BAV diagnosis the 25-year risk of aneurysm formation is 26% with an incidence of about 85 per 10,000 patient-years. Therefore, the age adjusted relative risk of developing an aortic aneurysm is 86.2 compared to the general population ($p < 0.001$) with 46% requiring aortic surgery within 15 years [46]. Consequently, Michelena et al. claim that the risk for AD in these patients is 8.4 times higher compared to general population ($p = 0.003$) with the 15-year risk for AD being 7% [46].

13.3 Bicuspid aortic valve and aortic dissection

Acute Type A AD is the most devastating, immediately life-threatening complication (with a significant mortality of 8 to 13% despite of immediate emergency treatment) [47-49] affecting up to 5% of BAV patients in a lifetime [50, 51]. In 1984, Larson and Edwards were the first to postulate that the incidence of Type A AD in BAV patients may be up to 11 times higher than in the normal tricuspid population (5.8 vs. 0.5%, $p > 0.001$) based on autopsy studies [51]. In 2007, analyses based on the International Registry of Acute Aortic Dissection (IRAD) data showed that, out of 591 patients with acute Type A AD, 349 (59%) had aortic diameters <55 mm while 229 (40%) even had a diameters below 50 mm [52]. A retrospective analysis from our Leipzig data revealed that there was no significant difference in the mean ascending aortic diameter between BAV and TAV patients at the time of acute Type A AD (61.59 vs. 53.2±13 mm, $p = 0.582$) [53], but a clear trend towards larger diameters at the time of acute Type A AD among BAVs. Based on these observations it currently becomes clear that 'maximum ascending/root diameter' may not be an ideal predictor for aortic catastrophes, particularly in BAV. New evidence to the question whether dissection among BAV patients occur at smaller or larger diameter was added by Eleid et al. demonstrating that Type A AD occurred over a wide range, however at larger diameters in most BAV patients [54]. They investigated 47 BAV patients, 31 with acute Type A AD, and revealed that in these patients aortic medial degeneration affected up to 75% of the aortic specimen. Though only 41% of the TAV specimen were affected ($p = 0.01$), the TAV patients had a higher incidence of arteriosclerosis (56 vs. 26%, $p = 0.02$). Also at the time of acute Type A AD patients with BAV were younger (58±14 vs. 66±13, $p = 0.0007$), had less hypertension (68 vs. 87%, $p = 0.03$) and higher maximum diameter (66±15 vs. 56±11 mm, $p = 0.0004$). The study also revealed that 50% of BAV patients with acute Type A AD had prior aortic dilatation (vs. only 20% of TAV) [54].

13.3.1 Functional bicuspid aortic valve status: stenosis vs. insufficiency

Eleid and colleagues also found the prevalence of severe aortic stenosis to be significantly higher at time of acute Type A AD (19 vs. 0%, $p = 0.002$) [54] reaching independence as a predictor of acute Type A AD and death among BAV patients (odds ratio 10.475) [55].

13.3.2 Dissection tear location and its implications: bicuspid aortic valve vs. tricuspid aortic valve

The Leipzig experience, summarized recently in a single center retrospective analysis of 460 patients with acute Type A AD of whom 8.4% had a BAV, suggested two major findings:

1) BAVs are significantly younger at the time acute dissection occurs (47±13 vs. 62±12, p <0.001);
2) BAV patients suffer the entry tear five times more often located in their aortic root compared to their tricuspid peers (31.3 vs. 6.3%, p <0.001).

Consequently, aortic root replacement was significantly more frequent (93.8 vs. 28.8%, p <0.001) among BAV dissection patients [53]. In contrast to Eleid and colleagues' data, however, our BAV population presented more frequently with severe aortic regurgitation (90.6 vs. 67.1%, p = 0.005) at time of acute Type A AD – possibly as a result of root tearing. These findings are in accordance with data from Rylski et al. published in 2014 – BAV patients were younger (55 vs. 61 years; p <0.001) and presented more frequently with moderate/severe aortic regurgitation (51 vs 34%; p = 0.039) [56]. Januzzi et al. analyzed acute Type A AD data from the IRAD focussing on young patients: among all patients under the age of 40 years 9% were carriers of a BAV, these patients had significantly larger aortic root diameter (49±1.7 mm vs. 41±1 mm, p = 0.01) and the dissection entry was more proximally located, adjacent or within the sinuses of Valsalva or sinotubular junction [57]. Of note, the diameter data in all studies need to be interpreted carefully as at time of dissection the diameter and geometry of the ascending aorta may change significantly [58].

Interestingly, BAV patients with previous, isolated aortic valve replacement (AVR due to valvular dysfunction) seem to remain at risk of dissection of the proximal aorta (estimated to about 0.6%) [59].

A recent meta-analysis by Girdauskas et al. in 2015 suggests that the risk for dissection after AVR in BAV patients is about 10 times higher in those with previous regurgitation than in those treated for stenosis (2.8 vs. 0.2%, p <0.01) [60]. In accordance, Benedik et al. developed a shear stress testing of aortic wall tissue and concluded that patients with aortic regurgitation have a worse wall cohesion than those with aortic stenosis [61].

Overall several studies revealed that patients with a BAV are younger at the time of dissection, and – although dissection may occur at any diameter – most BAVs dissect at an even larger diameter than their tricuspid peers, even though arterial hypertension is less frequent among them and the dissection entry located more proximally [53, 54, 56, 57]. Furthermore, downstream aortic aneurysm disease seems less frequent among BAV in general [19] as compared to TAV, and the dissection process seems more often restricted to the proximal aortic arch [53], hence BAV patients less frequently require treatment of downstream aortic pathologies following acute Type A AD.

13.4 Operative strategy

Emergency cardiac surgery is mandatory and an appropriate operative strategy is paramount. Perioperative mortality is high, ranging from 8 to 24% [48, 49, 53, 62] particularly in the presence of myocardial, cerebral and visceral ischemia.

13.4.1 Cannulation site for extracorporeal circulation and cerebral protection

In the majority of patients arterial access for cardiopulmonary bypass (CPB) is established at our center through the right axillary artery (>75% of cases) via a short subclavicular incision. In most cases direct cannulation is chosen, less frequently a short 6-8 mm dacron graft is sutured to the axillary artery to place the arterial cannula (e.g. if the diameter of the axillary is too small for direct cannulation). This technique allows for safe and rapid switch to unilateral antegrade/selective cerebral perfusion (aSCP) via the truncus during the procedure. Alternatively, also the femoral artery can be used for arterial cannulation (20% of cases at our center, valuable option as a last resort, i.e. used if the patient enters the operating room under cardiopulmonary resuscitation); rarely direct aortic cannulation (<5%) is the only option. Venous drainage is usually established via a wire-directed catheter through a femoral vein or through a double-stage cannula in the right atrium. Cooling begins immediately after extracorporeal circulation is started often times prior to median sternotomy.

At our institution in more than 50% of cases antegrade selective cerebral perfusion is conducted as an adjunct to mild to moderate hypothermic circulatory arrest either unilaterally via the axillary cannula in place. Balloon-occlusion perfusion catheters for direct cannulation of the head vessels may be utilized in selected cases – only if the dissection process does not involve the supraaortic arteries and this mode of cannulation is safe. In rare cases direct carotid artery cannulation via a side graft is the only option to secure cerebral perfusion in complex dissections involving the arch/head vessels. During cerebral perfusion efficacy of aSCP is monitored bilaterally via Near-infrared spectroscopy (NIRS monitoring) with optical sensors positioned over the forehead to monitor frontal lobe perfusion. In cases with severe destruction of the supraaortic vessels, deep hypothermic circulatory arrest without cerebral perfusion at mean temperatures of 20-24 °C (by perfusion cooling during the initial period of CPB) is utilized. The strategy for cerebral protection gradually changed during the past decade towards a more frequent utilization of antegrade bilateral cerebral perfusion in Leipzig.

After initiation of distal circulatory arrest (with or without aSCP) the dissected aorta is opened and myocardial protection initiated either antegrade (coronary ostia) or retrograde using Brettschneider (or cold blood) cardioplegia. Thereafter, all aortic tissue weakened by the dissection process including the entry tear is resected and the remaining aortic wall inspected for possible re-entry tears. In general principle, an open distal anastomosis is performed and the down-stream aorta (arch, proximal descending) thoroughly inspected.

13.5 Aortic root replacement for acute Type A aortic dissection in bicuspid aortic valve patients

Standard procedure in BAV patients at our center in acute Type A AD with root involvement is root replacement as a modified button Bentall procedure [7], utilizing either a biological or mechanical conduit (Fig. 13.3).

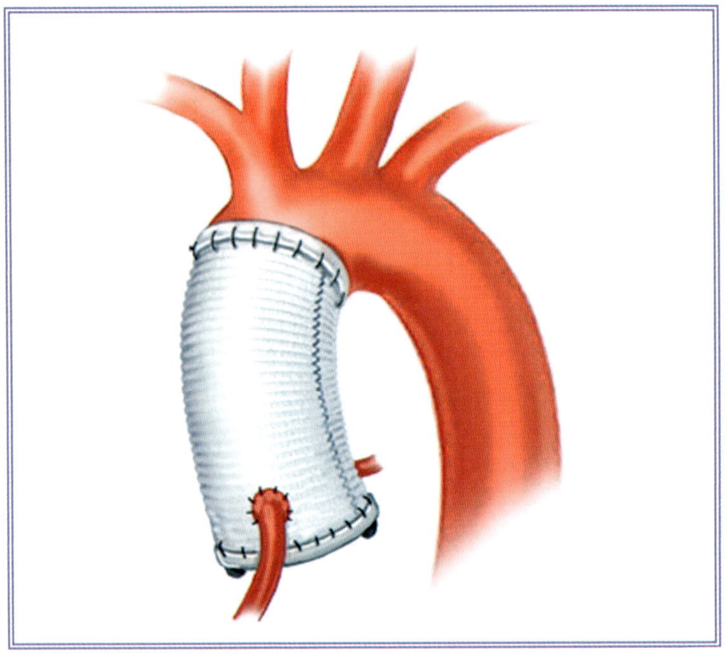

Fig. 13.3 Modified Bentall procedure with a biologically valved conduit for acute Type A AD in BAV (courtesy of Mount Sinai Hospital, New York).

Isolated root reconstruction is only appropriate if the integrity of the sinuses is not severely affected by the dissection process and is performed either by suture restoring sinus integrity with or without glue application or via valve-sparing repair techniques according to David or Yacoub [8]. Discussion remains, however, if this approach leaves 'genetically diseased' tissue behind, therefore almost 95% of BAV patients at our institution receive a complete replacement of the proximal aorta (Bentall procedure). In TAV patients, dissections strictly limited to the tubular ascending aorta are treated by supracoronary ascending aortic replacement (and additional aortic valve procedures if concomitant valve pathologies, not related to the dissection itself, are present). The overall ratio of mechanical and biological valves at our institution is roughly 50:50 for either isolated or composite replacement.

All dissections extending into the aortic arch (more often TAV patients), i.e. beyond the brachiocephalic trunk, were treated by partial or complete arch replacement with open anastomosis and hypothermic distal circulatory arrest with or without selective antegrade cerebral perfusion. If the dissection proceeds throughout the arch into the descending and thoracoabdominal aorta and visceral perfusion is not acutely compromised (e.g. abdominal arteries originating from the perfused true lumen) an elephant trunk procedure and subsequent, staged distal repair may be opted for. Alternatively, rapid restoration of distal perfusion via the true lumen may be achieved by placement of a frozen elephant trunk prosthesis to restore visceral perfusion (e.g. if the true lumen is collapsed). This approach has been suggested to decrease the risk of disease progression towards chronic dissecting thoracoabdominal aortic aneurysm.

When looking at surgical strategy of acute Type A AD in general, not focusing on BAV patients, a recently published study by Peterss et al. did not show an advantage for root replacement [63]. In our experience, however particularly BAV patients benefit from excellent longevity (significantly better than for tricuspid patients) after root replacement (Fig. 13.4) [53]. Our approach is supported by IRAD data: a propensity-score analysis demonstrated freedom from

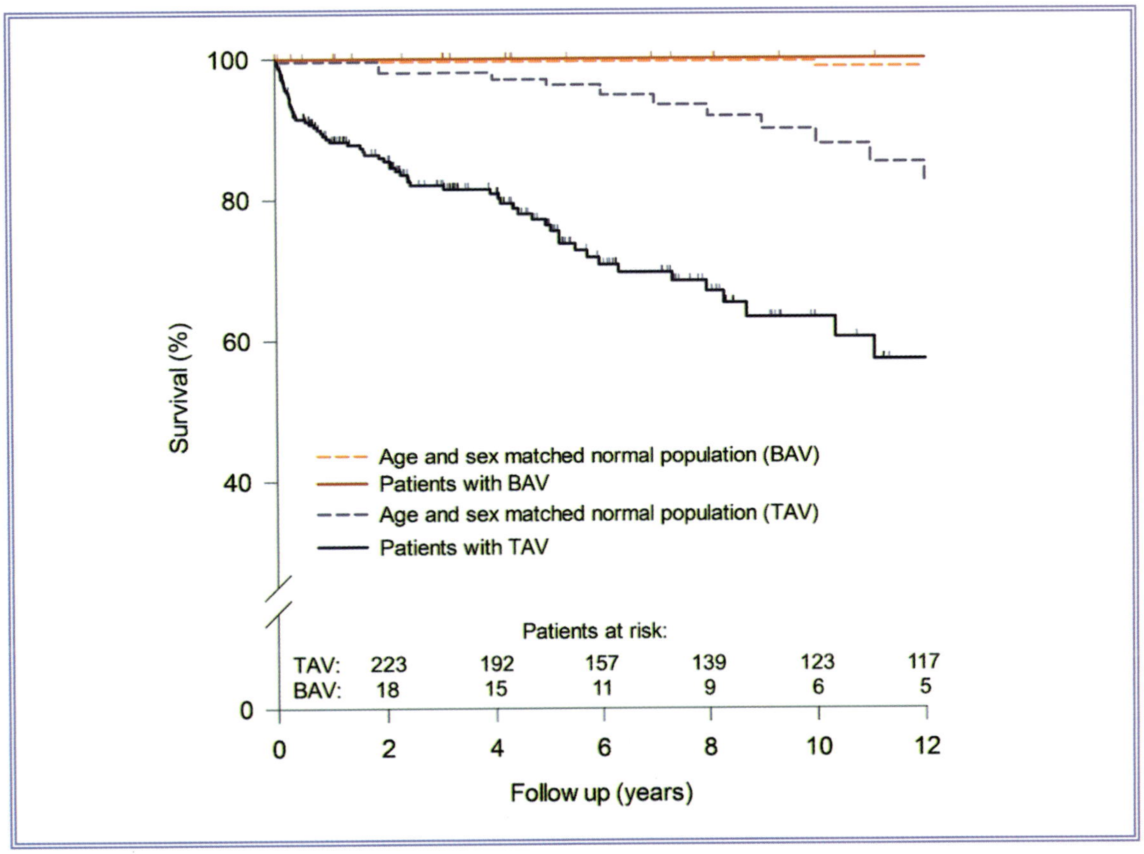

Fig. 13.4 Tricuspid versus bicuspid patients with age- and gender-matched normal population – survival after 30 days for patients with bicuspid aortic valves (BAVs) is equivalent to the norm, while the tricuspid (TAV) patient has worse survival than the corresponding matched normal population. Reprinted from [53], with permission.

aortic reintervention to be higher in patients with root replacement, reaching significance in the unmatched cohort (at 7 years: root replacement 96±3% vs. conservative root management 80±6%, p = 0.02) and slight superiority (98±2% vs. 86±6%, p = 0.06) after matching [64]. In line with our experience, Hysi et al. suggested a general advantage of root replacement over supracomissural ascending replacement, although cross-clamp times were longer in the root surgery group, the in-hospital mortality was lower (20 vs. 34%, p = 0.03), 10-year survival was higher (85.7 vs. 65.9%, p = 0.03) and significantly less aortic re-operations were needed in this group (freedom from re-operation: 93.4 vs. 82.9%, p = 0.02) [65]. As BAV patients are very young and have their dissection entry more often located in the aortic root [53, 54, 56, 57] the question of valve-sparing or composite conduit is of relevance and decision making has to take the individual experience of the surgeon and the patient clinical condition into account (i.e. suboptimal results with regard to valve repair may require additional cross clamping, e.g. after CPR possibly jeopardizing hospital survival). The risk of re-operation due to recurrent aortic valve regurgitation is another limiting factor that has to be taken into account [66]. In our center [53] almost 95% of BAV patients admitted for acute Type A AD receive a root replacement (vs. 29% of their tricuspid peers, p <0.001); during the past decades only 6% of BAV patients received an isolated supracommissural ascending replacement with concomitant aortic valve replacement. Overall operative mortality was not significantly different between BAV and TAV patients (BAV: 28.1 vs. TAV: 19.6%, p = 0.255 at 10-year follow up BAV patients had a significant better survival with 100% vs. 60.2% in TAV group, p = 0.011; however they were also significantly younger!). We identified age at surgery, preoperative CPR and acute myocardial infarction prior to surgery as independent factors influencing long-term outcome [53]. In this cohort none of the BAV patients received a valve-sparing root surgery.

Rylski et al. compared BAV patients receiving either valve replacement with or without root replacement (n = 53) or valve resuspension (n = 13). Additional aortic surgery included ascending replacement and hemiarch replacement with no difference within the groups. Groups did not differ significantly with regard to age (replacement 57±15 years vs. resuspension 62±13 years, p = 0.62). Patients in the replacement group had more sever regurgitation before surgery (45 vs. 15%, p = 0.06). Overall survival was not different between the groups [67].

13.6 Summary

- 1-2% of the general population carries a bicuspid aortic valve (BAV).
- BAV is associated with proximal aortic disease and up to 25% of carriers will need aortic valve or proximal aortic surgery during their life-time (it has been estimated that up to 5% of BAV may suffer acute Type A dissection).
- At time of acute dissection BAV patients are: younger, have in average a larger diameter of root and ascending aorta, have less hypertension and the entry is more often located in the aortic root.
- Long-term outcome after aortic root replacement for acute Type A AD in BAV patients is excellent.

REFERENCES

1) Ward C. Clinical significance of the bicuspid aortic valve. Heart 2000; 83(1): 81-5.
2) Hoffman J, Kaplan S. The incidence of congenital heart disease. J Am Coll Cardiol 2002; 39(12): 1890-900.
3) Friedman T, Mani A, Elefteriades JA. Bicuspid aortic valve: clinical approach and scientific review of a common clinical entity. Expert Rev Cardiovasc Ther 2008; 6(2): 235-48.
4) Mills P, Leech G, Davies M, Leathan A. The natural history of a non-stenotic bicuspid aortic valve. Br Heart J 1978; 40(9): 951-7.

5) Della Corte A, Bancone C, Dialetto G, et al. The ascending aorta with bicuspid aortic valve: a phenotypic classification with potential prognostic significance. Eur J Cardiothorac Surg 2014; 46(2): 240-7; discussion 247.
6) Rinnstrom D, Engstrom KG, Johansson B. Subtypes of bicuspid aortic valves in coarctation of the aorta. Heart Vessels 2014; 29(3): 354-63.
7) Waller BF, Carter JB, Williams HJ Jr, Wang K, Edwards JE. Bicuspid aortic valve. Comparison of congenital and acquired types. Circulation 1973; 48(5): 1140-50.
8) Sievers HH, Schmidtke C. A classification system for the bicuspid aortic valve from 304 surgical specimens. J Thorac Cardiovasc Surg 2007; 133(5): 1226-33.
9) Prakash SK, Bossé Y, Muehlschlegel JD. A roadmap to investigate the genetic basis of bicuspid aortic valve and its complications: insights from the International BAVCon (Bicuspid Aortic Valve Consortium). J Am Coll Cardiol 2014; 64(8): 832-9.
10) Hales AR, Mahle WT. Echocardiography screening of siblings of children with bicuspid aortic valve. Pediatrics 2014; 133(5): e1212-7.
11) Robledo-Carmona J, Rodríguez-Bailón I, Carrasco-Chinchilla F. Hereditary patterns of bicuspid aortic valve in a hundred families. Int J Cardiol 2013; 168(4): 3443-9.
12) Schnell S, Smith DA, Barker AJ, et al. Altered aortic shape in bicuspid aortic valve relatives influences blood flow patterns. Eur Heart J Cardiovasc Imaging 2016; pii: jew149 [Epub ahead of print].
13) Qu XK, Qiu XB, Yuan F, et al. A novel NKX2.5 loss-of-function mutation associated with congenital bicuspid aortic valve. Am J Cardiol 2014; 114(12): 1891-5.
14) Biner S, Rafique AM, Ray I, Cuk O, Siegel RJ, Tolstrup K. Aortopathy is prevalent in relatives of bicuspid aortic valve patients. J Am Coll Cardiol 2009; 53(24): 2288-95.
15) Cripe L, Andelfinger G, Martin LJ, Shooner K, Benson DW. Bicuspid aortic valve is heritable. J Am Coll Cardiol 2004; 44(1): 138-43.
16) Hope MD, Hope TA, Crook SE, et al. 4D flow CMR in assessment of valve-related ascending aortic disease. JACC Cardiovasc Imaging 2011; 4(7): 781-7.
17) Hope MD, Hope TA, Meadows AK. Bicuspid aortic valve: four-dimensional MR evaluation of ascending aortic systolic flow patterns. Radiology 2010; 255(1): 53-61.
18) Stephens EH, Hope TA, Kari FA. Greater asymmetric wall shear stress in Sievers' type 1/LR compared with 0/LAT bicuspid aortic valves after valve-sparing aortic root replacement. J Thorac Cardiovasc Surg 2015; 150(1): 59-68.
19) Etz CD, Homann TM, Silovitz D, et al. Long-term survival after the Bentall procedure in 206 patients with bicuspid aortic valve. Ann Thorac Surg 2007; 84(4): 1186-93; discussion 1193-4.
20) Etz CD, Zoli S, Brenner R, et al. When to operate on the bicuspid valve patient with a modestly dilated ascending aorta. Ann Thorac Surg 2010; 90(6): 1884-90; discussion 1891-2.
21) Dayan, Parma G, Drever M. First-degree relatives of bicuspid aortic valve patients with normal aortic dimensions do not carry an increased risk of aortic dilatation. Int J Cardiol 2014; 172(2): 518-9.
22) Lesauskaite V, Sepetiene R, Jariene G. FBN1 polymorphisms in patients with the dilatative pathology of the ascending thoracic aorta. Eur J Cardiothorac Surg 2015; 47(4): e124-30.
23) Laforest B, Andelfinger G, Nemer M. Loss of Gata5 in mice leads to bicuspid aortic valve. J Clin Invest 2011; 121(7): 2876-87.
24) Lee TC, Zhao YD, Courtman DW, Stewart DJ. Abnormal aortic valve development in mice lacking endothelial nitric oxide synthase. Circulation 2000; 101(20): 2345-8.
25) Niessen K, Karsan A. Notch signaling in cardiac development. Circ Res 2008; 102(10): 1169-81.
26) Robicsek F, Thubrikar MJ, Cook JW, Fowler B. The congenitally bicuspid aortic valve: how does it function? Why does it fail? Ann Thorac Surg 2004; 77(1): 177-85.
27) Hope MD, Dyverfeldt P, Acevedo-Bolton G, et al. Post-stenotic dilation: evaluation of ascending aortic dilation with 4D flow MR imaging. Int J Cardiol 2012; 156(2): e40-2.
28) Hope MD, Meadows AK, Hope TA, et al. Images in cardiovascular medicine. Evaluation of bicuspid aortic valve and aortic coarctation with 4D flow magnetic resonance imaging. Circulation 2008; 117(21): 2818-9.
29) Weigang E, Kari FA, Beyersdorf F, et al. Flow-sensitive four-dimensional magnetic resonance imaging: flow patterns in ascending aortic aneurysms. Eur J Cardiothorac Surg 2008; 34(1): 11-6.
30) Tsamis A, Phillippi JA, Koch RG, et al. Extracellular matrix fiber microarchitecture is region-specific in bicuspid aortic valve-associated ascending aortopathy. J Thorac Cardiovasc Surg 2016; 151(6): 1718-1728.
31) Allen BD, van Ooij P, Barker AJ, et al. Thoracic aorta 3D hemodynamics in pediatric and young adult patients with bicuspid aortic valve. J Magn Reson Imaging 2015; 42(4): 954-63.
32) von Knobelsdorff-Brenkenhoff F, Karunaharamoorthy A, Trauzeddel RF. Evaluation of aortic blood flow and wall shear stress in aortic stenosis and its association with left ventricular remodeling. Circ Cardiovasc Imaging 2016; 9(3): e004038.
33) Barker AJ, Lanning C, Shandas R. Quantification of hemodynamic wall shear stress in patients with bicuspid aortic valve using phase-contrast MRI. Ann Biomed Eng 2010; 38(3): 788-800.

34) Barker AJ, Markl M, Bürk J, et al. Bicuspid aortic valve is associated with altered wall shear stress in the ascending aorta. Circ Cardiovasc Imaging 2012; 5(4): 457-66.
35) Lehoux S, Tedgui A. Cellular mechanics and gene expression in blood vessels. J Biomech 2003; 36(5): 631-43.
36) Ando J, Yamamoto K. Effects of shear stress and stretch on endothelial function. Antioxid Redox Signal 2011; 15(5): 1389-403.
37) Guzzardi DG, Barker AJ, van Ooij P, et al. Valve-related hemodynamics mediate human bicuspid aortopathy: insights from wall shear stress mapping. J Am Coll Cardiol 2015; 66(8): 892-900.
38) Fedak PW, de Sa MP, Verma S, et al. Vascular matrix remodeling in patients with bicuspid aortic valve malformations: implications for aortic dilatation. J Thorac Cardiovasc Surg 2003; 126(3): 797-806.
39) Nataatmadja M, West M, West J, et al. Abnormal extracellular matrix protein transport associated with increased apoptosis of vascular smooth muscle cells in marfan syndrome and bicuspid aortic valve thoracic aortic aneurysm. Circulation 2003; 108 Suppl 1: II329-34.
40) Forsell C, Björck HM, Eriksson P, Franco-Cereceda A, Gasser TC. Biomechanical properties of the thoracic aneurysmal wall: differences between bicuspid aortic valve and tricuspid aortic valve patients. Ann Thorac Surg 2014; 98(1): 65-71.
41) Nistri S, Grande-Allen J, Noale M, et al. Aortic elasticity and size in bicuspid aortic valve syndrome. Eur Heart J 2008; 29(4): 472-9.
42) Bauer M, Pasic M, Meyer R, et al. Morphometric analysis of aortic media in patients with bicuspid and tricuspid aortic valve. Ann Thorac Surg 2002; 74(1): 58-62.
43) Tzemos N, Therrien J, Yip J, et al. Outcomes in adults with bicuspid aortic valves. Jama 2008; 300(11): 1317-25.
44) Nishimura RA, Otto CM, Bonow RO, et al. 2014 AHA/ACC guideline for the management of patients with valvular heart disease: a report of the American College of Cardiology/American Heart Association Task Force on Practice Guidelines. J Thorac Cardiovasc Surg 2014; 148(1): e1-e132.
45) 2010 ACCF/AHA/AATS/ACR/ASA/SCA/SCAI/SIR/STS/SVM Guidelines for the Diagnosis and Management of Patients With Thoracic Aortic Disease Representative Members, Hiratzka LF, Creager MA, et al. Surgery for aortic dilatation in patients with bicuspid aortic valves: A statement of clarification from the American College of Cardiology/American Heart Association Task Force on Clinical Practice Guidelines. J Thorac Cardiovasc Surg 2016; 151(4): 959-66.
46) Michelena HI, Khanna AD, Mahoney D, et al. Incidence of aortic complications in patients with bicuspid aortic valves. Jama 2011; 306(10): 1104-12.
47) Hagan PG, Nienaber CA, Isselbacher EM, et al. The International Registry of Acute Aortic Dissection (IRAD): new insights into an old disease. JAMA 2000; 283(7): 897-903.
48) Geirsson A, Bavaria JE, Swarr D, et al. Fate of the residual distal and proximal aorta after acute type a dissection repair using a contemporary surgical reconstruction algorithm. Ann Thorac Surg 2007; 84(6): 1955-64; discussion 1955-64.
49) Rylski B, Beyersdorf F, Blanke P, et al. Supracoronary ascending aortic replacement in patients with acute aortic dissection type A: what happens to the aortic root in the long run? J Thorac Cardiovasc Surg 2013; 146(2): 285-90.
50) Edwards WD, Leaf DS, Edwards JE. Dissecting aortic aneurysm associated with congenital bicuspid aortic valve. Circulation 1978; 57(5): 1022-5.
51) Larson EW, Edwards WD. Risk factors for aortic dissection: a necropsy study of 161 cases. Am J Cardiol 1984; 53(6): 849-55.
52) Pape LA, Tsai TT, Isselbacher EM, et al. Aortic diameter >or = 5.5 cm is not a good predictor of type A aortic dissection: observations from the International Registry of Acute Aortic Dissection (IRAD). Circulation 2007; 116(10): 1120-7.
53) Etz CD, von Aspern K, Hoyer A, et al. Acute type A aortic dissection: characteristics and outcomes comparing patients with bicuspid versus tricuspid aortic valve. Eur J Cardiothorac Surg 2015; 48(1): 142-50.
54) Eleid MF, Forde I, Edwards WD, et al. Type A aortic dissection in patients with bicuspid aortic valves: clinical and pathological comparison with tricuspid aortic valves. Heart 2013; 99(22): 1668-74.
55) Davies RR, Kaple RK, Mandapati D, et al. Natural history of ascending aortic aneurysms in the setting of an unreplaced bicuspid aortic valve. Ann Thorac Surg 2007; 83(4): 1338-44.
56) Rylski B, Desai ND, Bavaria JE, et al. Aortic valve morphology determines the presentation and surgical approach to acute type A aortic dissection. Ann Thorac Surg 2014; 97(6): 1991-6; discussion 1996-7.
57) Januzzi JL, Isselbacher EM, Fattori R, et al. Characterizing the young patient with aortic dissection: results from the International Registry of Aortic Dissection (IRAD). J Am Coll Cardiol 2004; 43(4): 665-9.
58) Rylski B, Blanke P, Beyersdorf F, et al. How does the ascending aorta geometry change when it dissects? J Am Coll Cardiol 2014; 63(13): 1311-9.
59) von Kodolitsch Y, Simic O, Schwartz A, et al. Predictors of proximal aortic dissection at the time of aortic valve replacement. Circulation 1999; 100(19 Suppl): II287-94.

60) Girdauskas E, Rouman M, Disha K, et al. Aortic dissection after previous aortic valve replacement for bicuspid aortic valve disease. J Am Coll Cardiol 2015; 66(12): 1409-11.
61) Benedik J, Dohle DS, Wendt D, et al. Comparison of ascending aortic cohesion between patients with bicuspid aortic valve stenosis and regurgitation. Eur J Cardiothorac Surg 2014; 46(6): e89-93.
62) Booher AM, Isselbacher EM, Nienaber CA, et al. The IRAD classification system for characterizing survival after aortic dissection. Am J Med 2013; 126(8): 730.e19-24.
63) Peterss S, Dumfarth J, Rizzo JA, et al. Sparing the aortic root in acute aortic dissection type A: risk reduction and restored integrity of the untouched root. Eur J Cardiothorac Surg 2016; 50(2): 232-9.
64) Castrovinci S, Pacini D, Di Marco L, et al. Surgical management of aortic root in type A acute aortic dissection: a propensity-score analysis. Eur J Cardiothorac Surg 2016; 50(2): 223-9.
65) Hysi I, Juthier F, Fabre O, et al. Aortic root surgery improves long-term survival after acute type A aortic dissection. Int J Cardiol 2015; 184: 285-90.
66) Zehr KJ, Orszulak TA, Mullany CJ, et al. Surgery for aneurysms of the aortic root: a 30-year experience. Circulation 2004; 110(11): 1364-71.
67) Rylski B, Siepe M, Beyersdorf F, et al. Bicuspid aortic valve resuspension in acute Type A aortic dissection patients. Ann Thorac Surg 2015; 100(3): 827-32.

14

When and how to replace the aortic arch for Type A dissection

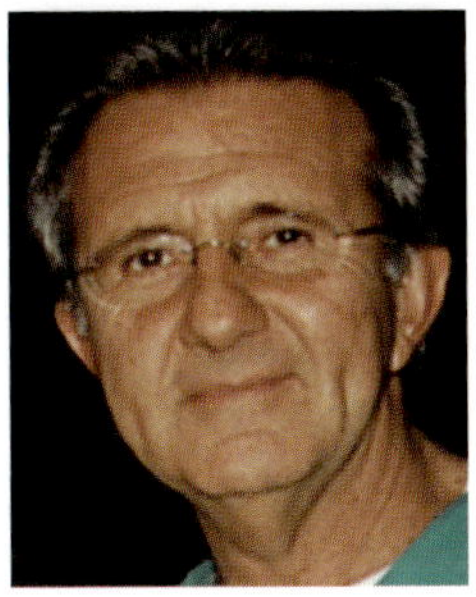

Roberto Di Bartolomeo, Alessandro Leone, Luca Di Marco and Davide Pacini

14.1 Introduction

Acute Type A aortic dissection (AD) remains one of the most challenging diseases in cardiothoracic surgery and, despite numerous innovations in medical and surgical management, early mortality still remains high. The preoperative status of the patient is an important risk factor for hospital mortality, however also the different techniques of aortic repair used are well-known influence factors of the postoperative course.

Important aspects of the management are still to be clarified, in order to refine the technique's selection criteria and the extension of replacement.

Among the various open issues in this field, the management of the dissected aortic arch is one of the most discussed topics.

There is still not a full consensus in the cardiothoracic surgery community about the best management of the aortic arch in acute Type A AD. Some surgeons advocate a more conservative tear oriented approach (hemiarch replacement) to reduce postoperative mortality and morbidity [1].

On the other hand, others authors support a more aggressive approach for acute Type A AD, mainly consisting in total arch replacement with or without the use of "frozen elephant trunk" (FET) or classic "elephant trunk" (ET) technique [2-5].

The rationale behind this more invasive operation is to contrast late aneurysm formation at the distal aorta and to avoid distal malperfusion due to the compression of the true lumen.

Our purpose is to delineate when and how to replace aortic arch in acute Type A AD, analyzing different solutions and approaches.

14.2 Indications to aortic arch replacement

The standard treatment of acute Type A AD is represented by emergency surgery of the proximal aorta, preventing rupture and consequent cardiac tamponade. Resection of the primary intimal tear and repair of the aortic root and aortic valve are well-established surgical principles.

Roberto Di Bartolomeo (roberto.dibartolomeo@unibo.it)
S. Orsola-Malpighi Hospital, University of Bologna,
Bologna, Italy

G. Melissano - R. Chiesa (eds), Aortic Dissection patients true stories and the innovations that saved their lives

Even though many surgeons advocate this kind of approach with the replacement of the proximal arch in addition to the repair of the aortic root, in such cases, the dissection in the aortic arch and descending untreated aorta remains, with the risk of subsequent false lumen dilatation and even rupture, true lumen compression and distal malperfusion.

Fattori and associates followed very closely a cohort of 70 patients after surgical intervention for acute Type A AD with serial magnetic resonance imaging. They reported a growth rate of the descending aorta of 3.7 mm/y in patients with patent false lumen, significantly higher than in patients without patent false lumen (only 1.1 mm/y) [6]. Zierer demonstrated that the expansion of the aorta was more common and more rapid at the level of the descending segment, and he identified three independent predictors for aortic dilatation: 1) aortic diameter, 2) elevated systolic blood pressure at late follow-up, and 3) patent false lumen [7]. Another study by Park et al. [8] evaluated the postoperative CT images of 122 patients who underwent aortic repair for acute Type A AD. All patients underwent open distal repair and in all of them the primary entry tear was always resected. The thoracic false lumen remained patent in 85 patients (69.7%) while a thrombosis occurred in the remaining 37 patients. The false lumen of the abdominal aorta was more frequently patent, namely, in 91% (111 of 122) of the patients. Enlargement of the descending aorta, during follow up, occurred in 58 patients (47.5%) and in 50 of those, the proximal thoracic aorta was involved. Dilatation of the aorta was significantly related with the false lumen characteristics. It occurred more frequently when the false lumen was patent or larger than the true lumen.

A direct association between patency of the false lumen and reoperation on the remaining distal aorta has been also demonstrated [9-11].

The presumed rate of distal reoperation is 15 to 30% at 10 years; however, this has probably been underestimated because most publications have not differentiated between extension of false lumen beyond the arch and extension solely in the proximal aorta [12].

Differences in late reoperation rate after total arch replacement, as reported by various authors, may also be due to the number and the dimensions of the intimal tears in the descending and abdominal aorta that represent important factors influencing the fate of the distal false lumen. In fact, complete resection of all entry sites is required for thrombosis of the residual false lumen but initial surgery for acute Type A AD fails to achieve this objective, particularly in patients with primary or secondary entry located in the descending thoracic or abdominal aorta.

Complete thrombosis of the false lumen is one of the main objectives. On the other hand, formation of a partial thrombosis in the distal aorta after surgery is not desirable because it may occlude the distal tears, impede outflow, and in the most extreme situation result in a blind sac. An increase in false lumen pressure will increase wall tension, which may elevate the risk of distal aortic aneurysmal change and eventually result in rupture [13].

This pathophysiologic effect has been clearly demonstrated by Tsai and colleagues for patients with Type B AD. They were also able to demonstrate that partial thrombosis of the false lumen represents a predictor of poor late events [14].

Recently, similar results have been also reported after acute Type A AD repair. Song et al. [13] evaluated a series of 118 patients operated on for acute AD and a total of 66 out of the 97 survived patients had sufficient imaging data to be analyzed. The incidence of residual patent false lumen was 77% (51/66): 24 (47%) had a completely patent false lumen and in the remaining 27 patients (53%) a partial thrombosis was observed. Moreover, partial thrombosis occurred more frequently after ascending or hemiarch replacement than total arch replacement (55% [47/86] vs. 34% [11/32], $p = 0.0001$). The median segmental aortic growth rate for the aortic arch, proximal descending thoracic aorta, and abdominal aorta was higher in the partially thrombosed group than in the completely patent or completely thrombosed group. Nine of the 13 patients who underwent late aortic reoperation had partial thrombosis of the false lumen. They were able to demonstrate that partial thrombosis of the false lumen was an independent risk factor for rapid aortic dilatation and aorta-related repeat procedures.

To reduce the risk of distal reoperation, surgeons have attempted to extend the replacement specially when, after carefully inspection, the primary entry tear is found directly on the aortic arch. Considering that the mainstay of therapy of AD is closing the entry site, this may be considered a rationale indication for a total arch replacement. In fact avoiding a proximal perfusion of the false lumen should, at least theoretically, reduce the pressurization and the following dilatation of the false lumen during time.

Evangelista was able to demonstrate that in 184 patients, 108 surgically treated Type A and 76 medically treated Type B, in addition to Marfan syndrome and aortic diameter, large and proximal entry tear were independent risk factors for dissection related adverse event [15].

Another consideration has to be made for patients with previous history of severe and untreated hypertension and chronic aneurysm of the ascending aorta and aortic arch that evolved in acute Type A AD eventually. Often in such cases a severe dilatation of the aortic arch can be found and has to be replaced, independently from the primary entry tear location.

In the last decades a step forward has been made with the introduction of the well-known endovascular techniques (Thoracic EndoVascular Aortic Repair, TEVAR) for treatment of aortic pathologies.

TEVAR is a less invasive treatment option for patients with thoracic aortic aneurysm and dissection. Moreover, growing technical experience and improving stent graft devices have resulted in better patient outcomes and expanded clinical indications. However, TEVAR bears the risk of unusual and severe complications. One of the most feared complication is Retrograde Ascending Aortic Dissection (RAAD), which has been highlighted as a potentially lethal complication, ranging from 1.3 to 3% [16-18]. This event cannot only occur during the procedure, but even after long time from the operation [19]. In those cases patients have to be immediately operated and replacement of the aortic arch is mandatory.

Aortic arch replacement represents a more complex and time demanding procedure, requiring expertise and experience. However, even if conflicting data are available in the literature [20], aortic arch replacement does not seem to be associated with higher early mortality and morbidity.

Kazui, in a series of 130 patients, reported an overall in-hospital mortality of 19.2% without significant difference in in-hospital mortality among the three groups having different extents of distal aortic replacement: 26% in ascending aorta replacement group, 14% in hemiarch replacement group, and 17% in the total arch replacement group [21]. Similar results are also reported by others well experienced "aortic" surgeons [22].

Even registry data demonstrated no differences in early mortality in patients who had more extensive aortic replacement [23, 24]. The German Registry for Acute Aortic Dissection Type A (GERAADA registry) [24], which represents the largest registry worldwide documenting patients undergoing surgery for acute Type A AD, showed a lower postoperative mortality in those receiving hemiarch replacement compared with total arch replacement (18.7% vs. 25.7%), but the difference was not statistically significant. Similar results have been also reported by the International Registry for Aortic Dissection (IRAD registry): early mortality rate was 22.9%, 20.9%, and 23.7% for patients who underwent ascending aorta replacement, hemiarch replacement, and total arch replacement, respectively [25]. Unfortunately, registry papers did not give any significant follow-up information about reoperation rate related to the extension of aortic replacement.

14.3 Techniques of aortic arch replacement

The classic aortic arch operation consists in the replacement of the arch with re-implantation of the supraaortic vessels. Effective methods of cerebral, myocardial as well as visceral protection are necessary to obtain acceptable results in terms of hospital mortality and morbidity. The best method to protect the brain has demonstrated to be the bilateral antegrade selective cerebral perfusion (ASCP) with moderate hypothermia according to Kazui's technique [26]. In fact, very favorable outcomes are reported in literature indicating ASCP as the best method to protect the brain, especially when time consuming and complex arch repairs are required [27].

Total arch replacement in acute Type A AD may be an effective strategy, especially when, in complex cases, the left subclavian artery re-implantation is not feasible or in case of excessive dilatation of the distal arch. In such cases the distal anastomosis can be performed after the left carotid artery, thus allowing a necessary landing zone for a further endovascular extension. However the left subclavian artery must be ligated, and a carotid-subclavian bypass performed.

The elephant trunk procedure (ET) [28] can be an alternative technique for total arch replacement. This technique, in which a segment of prosthetic graft beyond the distal arch anastomosis floats freely within the descending aorta, facilitates interval repair of distal aortic aneurysms.

The ET was initially studied to facilitate the second-stage operation where the descending aorta would be replaced through left thoracotomy access, allowing an easier end-to-end anastomosis during this phase. With the increasing of the experience with this technique the indication has been progressively expanded from the arch and descending aorta aneurysm, to chronic Type A, acute Type B and finally to acute Type A AD.

However in case of acute AD, ET can present some technical difficulties due to the small dimension of the true lumen and, if the false lumen is pressurized, the floating graft can result compressed. In that case, the dissected layers should be united during the anastomosis using Teflon felt strips in order to avoid tearing of the fragile tissue. Moreover, the graft should be slightly oversized so that the “ET” presses against the dissected aorta.

In case of cannulation of femoral artery for cardiopulmonary bypass, it is essential to switch perfusion from retrograde (femoral artery) to antegrade, preventing ET kinking.

During years, several graft modification occurred. Modern grafts with four side branches as well as sewing collars for the distal anastomosis simplified the ET implantation. These modern grafts incorporate radio-opaque markers at the distal end, which are helpful to identify the proximal landing zone in case of endovascular extension as second stage of the procedure. A recent modification of the ET is the frozen elephant trunk (FET) technique, initially developed by some Japanese authors [29-31], mainly consisting in treating complex lesions of the thoracic aorta in a single-stage procedure combining endovascular treatment with conventional surgery.

The graft is composed of a proximal part consisting of vascular prosthesis and a distal part of self-expandable nitinol stent graft (Fig. 14.1).

During the early experience with this technique, the prosthesis used where basically custom made; afterwards the first commercially available was the E-vita JOTEC hybrid graft (JOTEC GmbH, Hechingen, Germany) [32], and recently the Thoraflex™ Hybrid multi-branched graft and distal stent (Vascutek Terumo, Renfrewshire, Scotland, UK) [33].

The technique consists in the implantation of the stented distal segment of the hybrid-prosthesis into the descending aorta through the opened aortic arch, while the proximal non-stented segment is used for conventional replacement of the upstream aorta.

Indications for the use of the FET are chronic aneurysm of the ascending, arch and descending aorta, chronic dissection involving all the thoracic aorta, retrograde Type A AD after TEVAR procedure, rupture of the arch and also chronic aneurysm involving the distal part of the aortic arch and the upper part of the descending aorta. The FET technique facilitated single-stage arch and descending aorta replacement in complex lesion; afterwards the indication has been extended to selected patients with AD [34].

In some patients with acute Type A AD this technique can resolve the entire aortic pathology, especially in case of Type I or retrograde dissection limited to the descending thoracic aorta. Moreover patients with organ malperfusion and consequent visceral ischemia, such as for true lumen collapse in the thoraco-abdominal aorta or for branch vessel obstruction for extending dissection into visceral arteries with narrowed true lumen compressed by false lumen, may represent another viable indication for the use of FET. In such cases the stented part of the prosthesis can easily re-expand the compressed true lumen in the descending aorta.

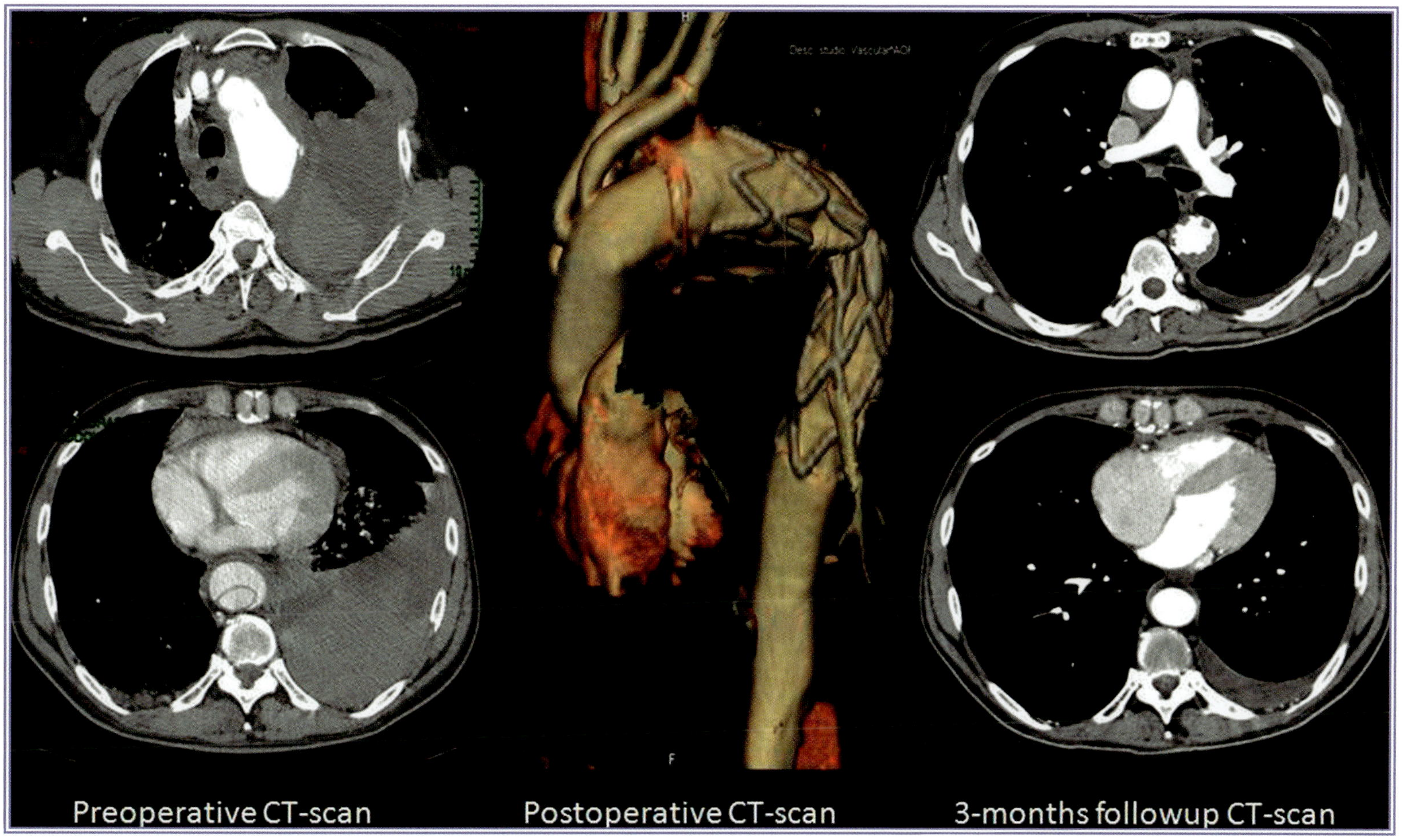

Fig. 14.1 Case of acute Type A AD treated with the frozen elephant trunk technique, with the complete resolution of the dissection three months after surgery.

FET is undoubtedly a major aortic procedure and requires very accurate pre-operative planning. For this reason, the assessment of the aortic anatomy is essential. In details, great care has to be taken when assessing the extent of the intimal flap, the relationship existing between the true and false lumen, the location of entry and re-entry tears and the origin of visceral vessels from the false lumen. In fact, in patients with visceral arteries rising from the false lumen not communicating with the true by the presence of near re-entry tears, organ malperfusion can be a lethal complication after FET [35]. Moreover, oversizing of the stent graft is not indicated in patients with AD, whereas a 10-20% oversizing should be performed in patients with degenerative aneurysms. Furthermore, if the patients are not selected carefully, or the disease progresses into the downstream aorta, a second-stage procedure may be necessary even with FET.

A recent new development for the treatment of acute Type A AD is the Lupiae technique. Originally studied for the treatment of complex pathologies of thoraco-abdominal aorta, afterwards it has been used also for the treatment of acute Type A AD.

The prosthesis used is the Vascutek Lupiae Graft (Vascutek Terumo, Renfrewshire, Scotland, UK), designed for this procedure. The main features of this graft are the presence of a bovine trunk at the proximal end dividing into three branches for the neck vessels and a fourth branch opposite to the bovine trunk used to resume the antegrade perfusion once the distal anastomosis is completed.

The technique consists of a first surgical step, in which the ascending aorta and the aortic arch are replaced while the rerouting of the supraaortic vessels on the proximal ascending aorta is performed. This creates a Dacron landing zone in Criado zone 0, which allows a TEVAR procedure as second step to exclude any residual intimal tear. Rerouting the origin of the epiaortic vessels closer to the sinotubular junction allows to have the necessary distance between the bovine-like trunk and the distal anastomosis, normally positioned for the Lupiae between the origin of left common carotid artery and the left subclavian artery, never shorter than 2.5 cm. The length and the position of the proximal landing zone, together with the systematic reimplant of the LSA and the choice to address the problem of the patent/partially thrombosed false lumen when the descending aorta is not already extremely dilated, could probably improve results in terms of endoleaks [36].

It is well know that acute Type A AD represents one of the most feared and catastrophic pathology in cardiothoracic surgery and that all the recent developments in this field stimulated the cardiothoracic surgeons to perform more complex and time demanding procedure, replacing the aortic arch with or without two-stage approach techniques.

However in some cases the aortic arch replacement has to be considered as part of a complex operation that may also include aortic root procedure as root replacement or valve sparing operation. This has to be taken into consideration, especially for the myocardial ischemia and cardiopulmonary bypass time, for the expertise and the experience required to the surgeon and for the patient's clinical condition at admission.

Patient's conditions represent one of the most important turning point in the decision-making. Sometimes even if the anatomy of the dissection is suitable for a multi-stage or a single-stage approach, total arch replacement may not be indicated, as in patients with advanced age or in extremely poor clinical condition.

On the other hand young patients, Marfan patients and patients in stable condition can benefit more from a radical treatment of the thoracic aorta even in terms of hospital mortality and above all at long term.

14.4 Conclusion

In the last decades, different techniques for total arch replacement have been developed, allowing more complex operation with satisfactory results.

Dilatation of the aortic arch as well as the presence of a tear and retrograde dissection can be all considered indication for a total arch replacement in acute Type A AD.

The ET and the Lupiae technique are viable two-stage strategies that can offer a solution for the problem of the fate of the false lumen in the descending thoracic aorta, reducing rate of future reoperation, dilatation and rupture.

Furthermore, FET is a single-stage approach that can be extremely useful in case of Type I dissection, retrograde dissection or in case of true lumen compression with consequent malperfusion syndrome.

However a correct assessment of the anatomy of the dissection in addition to the clinical condition of the patients remain the decision points for the best arch repair strategy to use in acute Type A AD.

REFERENCES

1) Westaby S, Saito S, Katsumata T. Acute type A dissection: conservative methods provide consistently low mortality. Ann Thorac Surg 2002; 73: 707-13.
2) Kazui T, Washiyama N, Muhammad BA, et al. Extended total arch replacement for acute type A aortic dissection: experience with seventy patients. J Thorac Cardiovasc Surg 2000; 119: 558-65.
3) Urbanski PP, Siebel A, Zacher M, Hacker RW. Is extended aortic replacement in acute type A dissection justifiable? Ann Thorac Surg 2003; 75: 525-9.
4) Shrestha M, Fleissner F, Ius F, et al. Total aortic arch replacement with frozen elephant trunk in acute type A aortic dissections: are we pushing the limits too far? Eur J Cardiothorac Surg 2015; 47: 361-6.
5) Di Eusanio M, Castrovinci S, Tian DH, et al. Antegrade stenting of the descending thoracic aorta during DeBakey type 1 acute aortic dissection repair. Eur J Cardiothorac Surg 2014; 45: 967-75.
6) Fattori R, Bacchi-Reggiani L, Bertaccini P, et al. Evolution of aortic dissection after surgical repair. Am J Cardiol 2000; 86(8): 868-72.
7) Zierer A, Voeller RK, Hill KE, Kouchoukos NT, Damiano RJ Jr, Moon MR. Aortic enlargement and late reoperation after repair of acute type A aortic dissection. Ann Thorac Surg 2007; 84(2): 479-86; discussion 486-77.
8) Park KH, Lim C, Choi JH, et al. Midterm change of descending aortic false lumen after repair of acute type I dissection. Ann Thorac Surg 2009; 87(1): 103-8.
9) Concistre G, Casali G, Santaniello E, et al. Reoperation after surgical correction of acute type A aortic dissection: risk factor analysis. Ann Thorac Surg 2012; 93(2): 450-5.
10) Fann JI, Smith JA, Miller DC, et al. Surgical management of aortic dissection during a 30-year period. Circulation 1995; 92(9 Suppl): II113-21.
11) Moore NR, Parry AJ, Trottman-Dickenson B, Pillai R, Westaby S. Fate of the native aorta after repair of acute type A dissection: a magnetic resonance imaging study. Heart 1996; 75(1): 62-6.
12) Uchida N, Shibamura H, Katayama A, Shimada N, Sutoh M. Total arch replacement with an open stent graft for acute type A aortic dissection: fate of the false lumen. Eur J Cardiothorac Surg 2009; 35(1): 83-8.
13) Song SW, Chang BC, Cho BK, et al. Effects of partial thrombosis on distal aorta after repair of acute DeBakey type I aortic dissection. J Thorac Cardiovasc Surg 2010; 139(4): 841-7 e841; discussion 847.
14) Tsai TT, Evangelista A, Nienaber CA. Partial thrombosis of the false lumen in patients with acute type B aortic dissection. N Engl J Med 2007; 357(4): 349-59.
15) Evangelista A, Galuppo V, Gruosso D, Cuéllar H, Teixidó G, Rodríguez-Palomares J. Role of entry tear size in type B aortic dissection. Ann Cardiothorac Surg 2014; 3(4): 403-5.
16) Kpodonu J, Preventza O, Ramaiah VG, et al. Retrograde type A dissection after endovascular stenting of the descending thoracic aorta. Is the risk real? Eur J Cardiothorac Surg 2008; 33: 1014-8.
17) Eggebrecht H, Thompson M, Rousseau H, et al. Retrograde ascending aortic dissection during or after thoracic aortic stent graft replacement: insight from the European Registry on Endovascular Aortic Repair Complications. Circulation 2009; 120: S276-81.
18) Czerny M, Bavaria JE, Weigang E, et al. Targeting landing zone 0 by total arch rerouting and TEVAR: midterm results of a transcontinental registry. Ann Thorac Surg 2012; 94: 84-9.
19) Eggebrecht H, Thompson M, Rousseau H, et al. Retrograde ascending aortic dissection during or after thoracic aortic stent graft placement. Circulation 2009; 120: S276-81.
20) Kim JB, Chung CH, Moon DH, et al. Total arch repair versus hemiarch repair in the management of acute DeBakey type I aortic dissection. Eur J Cardiothorac Surg 2011; 40(4): 881-7.
21) Kazui T, Washiyama N, Bashar AH, et al. Surgical outcome of acute type A aortic dissection: analysis of risk factors. Ann Thorac Surg 2002; 74(1): 75-81; discussion 81-2.
22) Ochiai Y, Imoto Y, Sakamoto M, et al. Long-term effectiveness of total arch replacement for type A aortic dissection. Ann Thorac Surg 2005; 80: 1297-1302.
23) Trimarchi S, Nienaber CA, Rampoldi V, et al. Contemporary results of surgery in acute type A aortic dissection: The International Registry of Acute Aortic Dissection experience. J Thorac Cardiovasc Surg 2005; 129(1): 112-22.
24) Easo J, Weigang E, Holzl PP, et al. Influence of operative strategy for the aortic arch in DeBakey type I aortic dissection: analysis of the German Registry for Acute Aortic Dissection Type A. J Thorac Cardiovasc Surg 2012; 144(3): 617-23.
25) Trimarchi S, Eagle KA, Nienaber CA, et al. Role of age in acute type A aortic dissection outcome: report from the International Registry of Acute Aortic Dissection (IRAD). J Thorac Cardiovasc Surg 2010; 140(4): 784-9.
26) Kazui T, Inoue N, Yamada O, Komatsu S. Selective cerebral perfusion during operation for aneurysms of the aortic arch: a reassessment. Ann Thorac Surg 1992; 53: 109-14.
27) Khaladj N, Shrestha M, Meck S, et al. Hypothermic circulatory arrest with selective antegrade cerebral

perfusion in ascending aortic and aortic arch surgery: a risk factor analysis for adverse outcome in 501 patients. J Thorac Cardiovasc Surg 2008; 135: 908-14.
28) Borst HG, Walterbusch G, Schaps D. Extensive aortic replacement using "elephant trunk" prosthesis. Thorac Cardiovasc Surg 1983; 31(1): 37-40.
29) Kato M, Ohnishi K, Kaneko M, et al. New graft-implanting method for thoracic aortic aneurysm or dissection with a stented graft. Circulation 1996; 94(9 Suppl): II188-93.
30) Suto Y, Yasuda K, Shiiya N, et al. Stented elephant trunk procedure for an extensive aneurysm involving distal aortic arch and descending aorta. J Thorac Cardiovasc Surg 1996; 112(5): 1389-90.
31) Usui A, Fujimoto K, Ishiguchi T, Yoshikawa M, Akita T, Ueda Y. Cerebrospinal dysfunction after endovascular stent-grafting via a median sternotomy: the frozen elephant trunk procedure. Ann Thorac Surg 2002; 74(5): S1821-4; discussion S1825-32.
32) Di Bartolomeo R, Di Marco L, Armaro A, et al. Treatment of complex disease of the thoracic aorta: the frozen elephant trunk technique with the E-vita open prosthesis. Eur J Cardiothorac Surg 2009; 35(4): 671-5.
33) Shrestha M, Pichlmaier M, Martens A, Hagl C, Khaladj N, Haverich A. Total aortic arch replacement with a novel four-branched frozen elephant trunk graft: first-in-man results. Eur J Cardiothorac Surg 2013; 43(2): 406-10.
34) Di Bartolomeo R, Pantaleo A, Berretta P, et al. Frozen elephant trunk surgery in acute aortic dissection. J Thorac Cardiovasc Surg 2015; 149(2 Suppl): S105-9.
35) Tsagakis K, Pacini D, Di Bartolomeo R, et al. Arch replacement and downstream stent grafting in complex aortic dissection: first results of an international registry. Eur J Cardiothorac Surg 2011; 39: 87-93; discussion 93-4.
36) Esposito G, Cappabianca G, Bichi S, Cricco A, Albano G, Anzuini A. Hybrid repair of type A acute aortic dissections with the Lupiae technique: ten-year results. J Thorac Cardiovasc Surg 2015; 149(2 Suppl): S99-104.

15

Treatment options for aortic arch dissecting aneurysm in patients with previous surgery for acute Type A aortic dissection

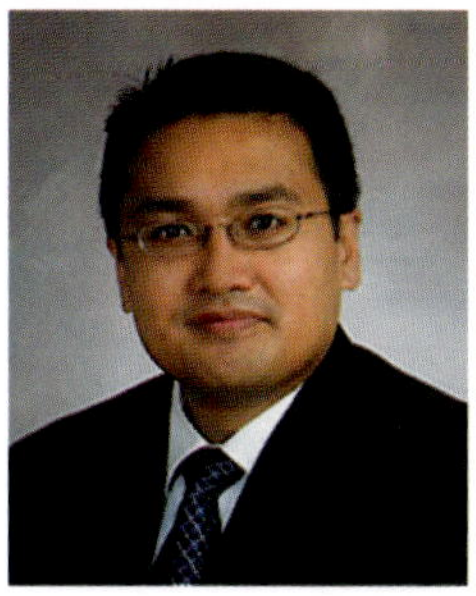

Anthony L. Estrera and Akiko Tanaka

15.1 Introduction

The survival after acute Type A aortic dissection (AD) has improved over the past two decades [1] with advancements in both surgical techniques and perioperative care. The incidence of distal reoperation after limited aortic repair for acute Type A AD, such as graft replacement of the ascending and proximal arch, is reported as high as 8 to 16% in contemporary series [2-6]. In this chapter, we will describe the current challenge of how to approach and treat an aortic arch aneurysm after repaired Type A AD.

15.2 Preoperative assessment

As the index Type A AD repair is almost always performed emergently, a new full preoperative evaluation is required. History taking and physical exam are the first steps in making a surgical plan. The underlying comorbidities and presence of connective tissue disorders are important in the decision making of the extent of aortic repair. A careful review of computed tomography (CT) or magnetic resonance imaging (MRI) is mandatory to make a surgical plan. CT and MRI with or without contrast will give us the following information: the extent of an aortic aneurysm; the distance between the sternum and underlying structures (i.e., the right ventricle/atrium, aorta, graft, bypass graft, innominate vein, and pericardium); and depth of the surgical field. If the patient's condition permits, we perform a contrast CT of the chest, abdomen, and pelvis as it provides better images to observe the extent of AD and the presence of thrombus. It also helps with decision making, such as which artery to access when peripheral cannulation is required. Transthoracic echocardiogram is obtained to evaluate the

---

Anthony L. Estrera (Anthony.L.Estrera@uth.tmc.edu)
McGovern Medical School at The University of Texas Health Science Center (UTHealth), Houston, TX, USA

G. Melissano - R. Chiesa (eds), Aortic Dissection patients true stories and the innovations that saved their lives

cardiac function, aortic root diameter, and valve disease, especially the aortic valve. Other routine preoperative workup includes carotid Doppler study, electrocardiogram, and pulmonary function test. Cardiac catheterization is performed in patients with high risk or history of coronary artery disease.

15.3 Surgical approach

The open surgical approach is either redo median sternotomy or left thoracotomy. The decision depends on the extent of an aneurysm and residual diseased aorta, as well as the patient's comorbidities, such as chronic lung disease, cerebrovascular disease, or valve/coronary artery disease. Nonetheless, since 1991, our preferred approach for aortic arch aneurysm has been aortic arch replacement with elephant trunk technique via median sternotomy [7]. Also, our standard approach has been a two-stage repair for extensive aortic aneurysm [7].
We avoid left thoracotomy, especially in cases in which proximal control is expected to be difficult and requires circulatory arrest, because the procedure is associated with high incidence of cerebral complications [8]. Left thoracotomy approach is only selected when a patient has symptomatic descending or thoracoabdominal aortic aneurysm (i.e., rapidly growing aneurysm, aortic diameter exceeding 60 mm, or abdominal/back pain).

Redo aortic arch surgery with AD is challenging [9]. However, with meticulous planning and operative procedures, postoperative mortality may be comparable to primary aortic arch repair [10, 11]. The key to successful treatment is: 1) safe re-entry of the chest; 2) appropriate perfusion strategy; and 3) staging of the procedures in extensive aortic aneurysm.

15.4 Redo median sternotomy approach

15.4.1 Monitoring and considerations

External defibrillating paddles are placed on the patient. In addition to the routine cardiac monitoring, regional cerebral oxygen saturation with near infrared spectroscopy is monitored for cerebral perfusion. Nasopharyngeal/tympanic and rectal/bladder temperatures are measured for cerebral and core temperatures. Cardiopulmonary bypass circuit needs to be ready and primed before starting the sternotomy. The groin areas are also prepared but not opened.

Some authors recommend elective femoro-femoral (or jugular) bypass cannulation to avoid and minimize catastrophic events during reentering the chest [6]. However, we do not routinely use this technique because: 1) femoro-femoral bypass before sternotomy increases prolonged pump time and bleeding; 2) flow patterns from femoral arterial return in chronic dissection is unpredictable and may cause organ ischemia (on the other hand, once arterial cannulation is established from the previous ascending graft, theoretically, the blood should flow with similar flow pattern, which currently the patient has); 3) thrombus in the false lumen or atheromatous plaque in the aorta may cause embolus; and 4) we prefer to spare femoral access for future reoperations (i.e., descending/thoracoabdominal aortic aneurysm repair).

15.4.2 Sternal re-entry

The sternum can be reopened with either an ordinary sternal saw or an oscillator saw. The oscillator saw may be more commonly used but it carries higher risk of injury to the underlying structures. The sternal reentry with the ordinary sternal saw can be performed quickly and safely, as previously described [11].

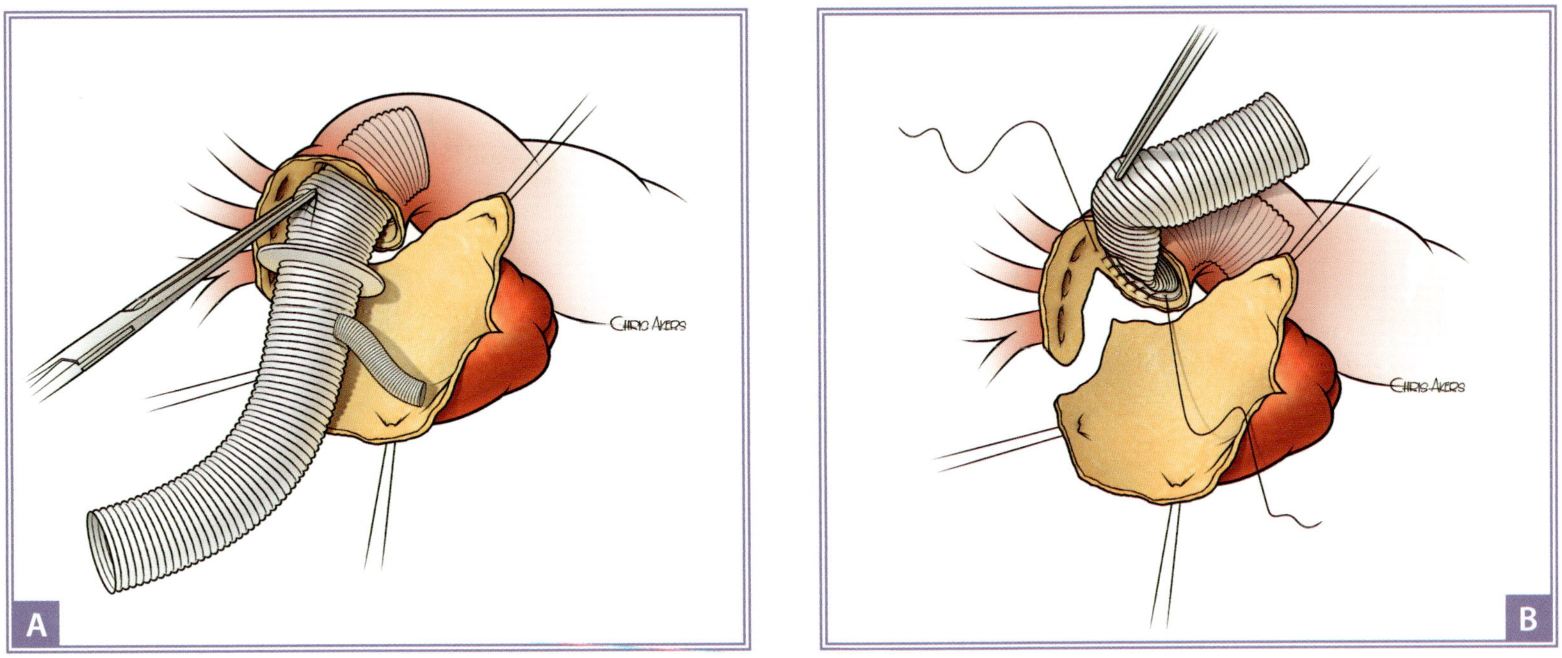

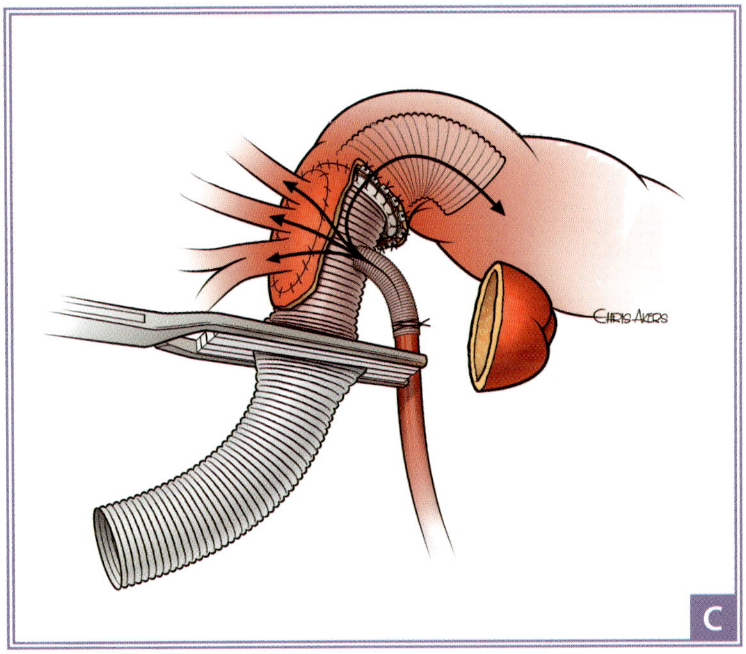

Fig. 15.2 Elephant trunk procedure with collared graft. **A**, Insertion of the collared graft to the descending aorta. **B**, Anastomosis to the proximal descending aorta. **C**, Reinstitution of the cerebral and lower body circulation (copyright Chris Akers®, reproduced with permission).

coronary buttons. In such circumstances, we use modified Cabrol graft technique with a 10 or 12-mm Dacron graft (Vascutek® Terumo, Gelweave™) to reconstruct the coronary arteries (Fig. 15.3) [14]. After completion of the proximal anastomosis, the patient's heart is rewarmed to a myocardial septal temperature of 30 °C, and then we release the ascending aortic clamp and restore the flow to the coronary circulation. Once the patient's core body temperature is 35-36 °C and can maintain systemic blood pressure and sinus rhythm, they are weaned from cardiopulmonary bypass. Ventricular fibrillation after the release of the aortic clamp may be encountered, and if the lateral wall of the heart is difficult to dissect, left pleural space is opened, and defibrillation is performed by placing the pads on the inferior wall and lateral wall via the left pleural space.

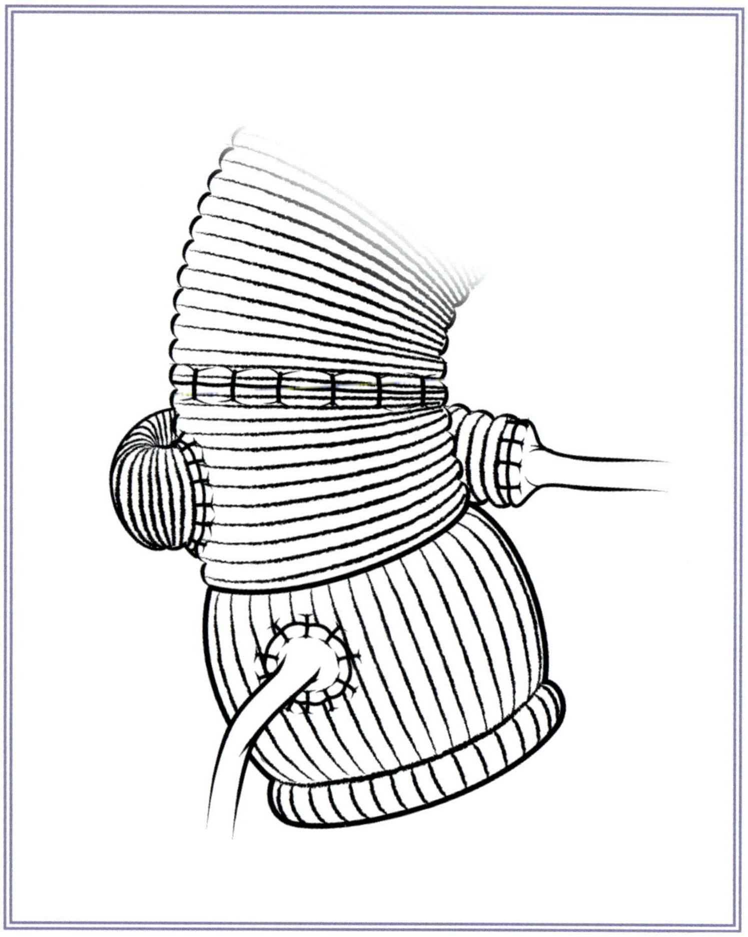

Fig. 15.3 Modified Cabrol technique (copyright Chris Akers®, reproduced with permission).

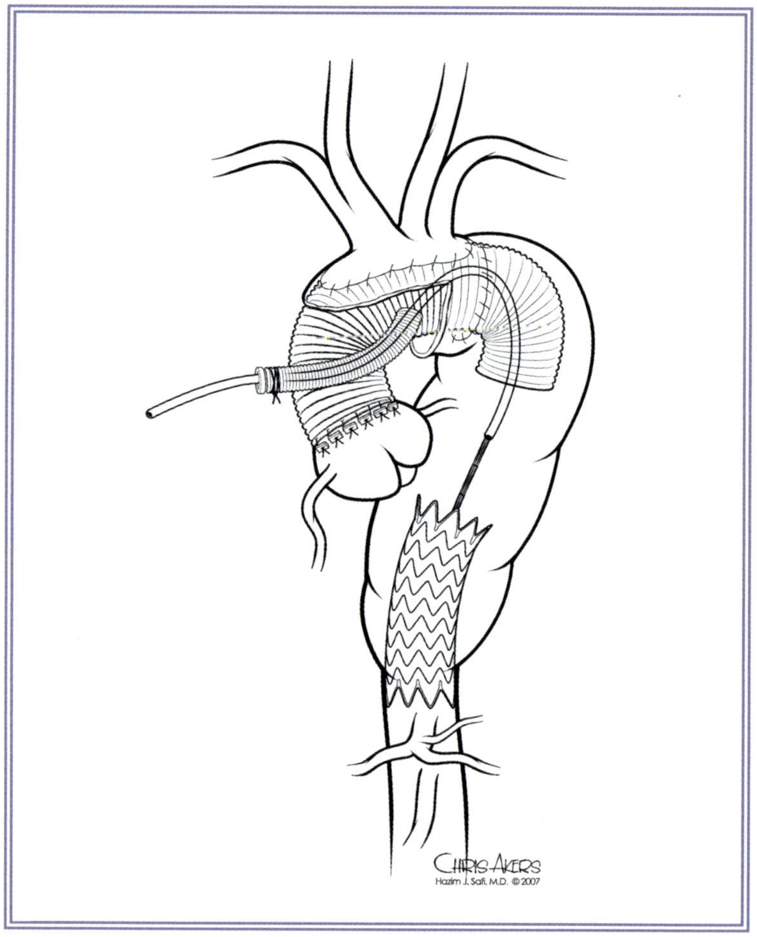

Fig. 15.4 Concomitant thoracic endovascular aortic repair via median sternotomy (copyright Chris Akers®, reproduced with permission).

15.4.6 Concomitant thoracic endovascular aortic repair

Due to the concern of spinal cord injury, we prefer staged thoracic endovascular aortic repair (TEVAR). However, symptomatic descending aorta with proximal and/or transverse arch aneurysm can be treated with concomitant TEVAR through median sternotomy. After finishing the proximal anastomosis, the side arm can now be utilized as an access route for TEVAR. Under fluoroscopy guidance, the stent graft is advanced toward the descending aorta and released (Fig. 15.4).

15.5 Left thoracotomy approach

15.5.1 Monitoring and considerations

A left thoracotomy is chosen when the aneurysm is located at the distal arch or proximal descending aorta without involvement of the transverse aortic arch. In case of a symptomatic large descending thoracic/thoracoabdominal aortic aneurysm with transverse arch involvement, we usually stage the procedures: repair descending/thoracoabdominal aortic aneurysm with reversed elephant trunk and perform total arch replacement as a second stage procedure.

After general anesthesia, the patient is placed in the right lateral decubitus position, and a cerebrospinal fluid (CSF) drain catheter is placed to allow CSF drainage and monitoring of CSF pressure. Somatosensory and motor-evoked potentials are monitored [15]. The patient is placed on right decubitus position with hips rotated 45 degrees to the left. The left common femoral artery is exposed with an oblique incision in the left groin.

15.5.2 Thoracotomy and exposure of the aorta

The skin incision is tailored to complement the extent of the aneurysm and the left pleural space is entered through the 5th or 6th intercostal space (Fig. 15.5). The costal cartilage is excised, and the 4th or 5th rib may be cut at the back if the proximal surgical view is insufficient.

If the patient has an elephant trunk inserted in the descending aorta from the index surgery, periaortic ultrasound or transesophageal echocardiography is useful to reassure the presence and location of the elephant trunk. The proximal aorta does not need to be dissected with the presence of the elephant trunk because after opening the aorta, the elephant trunk can be easily secured manually and clamp under direct vision. We use rapid ventricular pacing to reduce cardiac output when we open the aorta and apply a clamp on the elephant trunk.

After exposure of the aorta, the patient is heparinized.

15.5.3 Establishing left heart bypass

The left heart bypass is established with the left atrium drainage through the left inferior pulmonary vein and the arterial return with direct cannulation through a purse-string suture or cannulation through an 8-mm Dacron graft sutured end-to-side to the left common femoral artery. If the left common femoral artery is difficult to access (e.g. previous aortofemoral artery bypass, or morbid obesity, etc.), distal-first approach is selected.

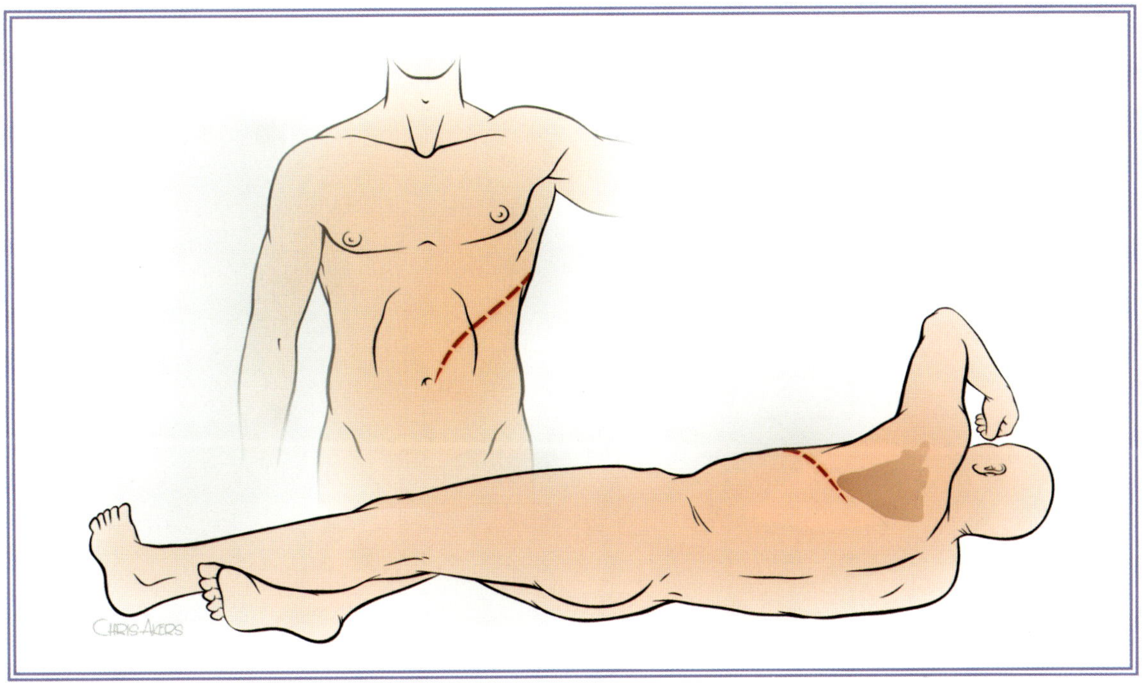

Fig. 15.5 Thoracoabdominal aortic repair skin incision (copyright Chris Akers®, reproduced with permission).

Distal aortic perfusion begins as the cross-clamp is applied, or after the distal anastomosis is completed in the case of the distal-first approach.

15.5.4 Descending thoracic aneurysm and thoracoabdominal aortic aneurysm repair

A side-branched thoracoabdominal graft (STAG; MAQUET Cardiovascular, Wayne, NJ) is selected to repair thoracoabdominal aortic aneurysm in patients with connective tissue disorder or aneurysmal visceral branches, and the visceral branches are reconstructed separately (Fig. 15.6). Otherwise, a single side-arm Dacron graft is selected and the visceral branches are reconstructed as an island patch in thoracoabdominal aortic aneurysm. Before clamping

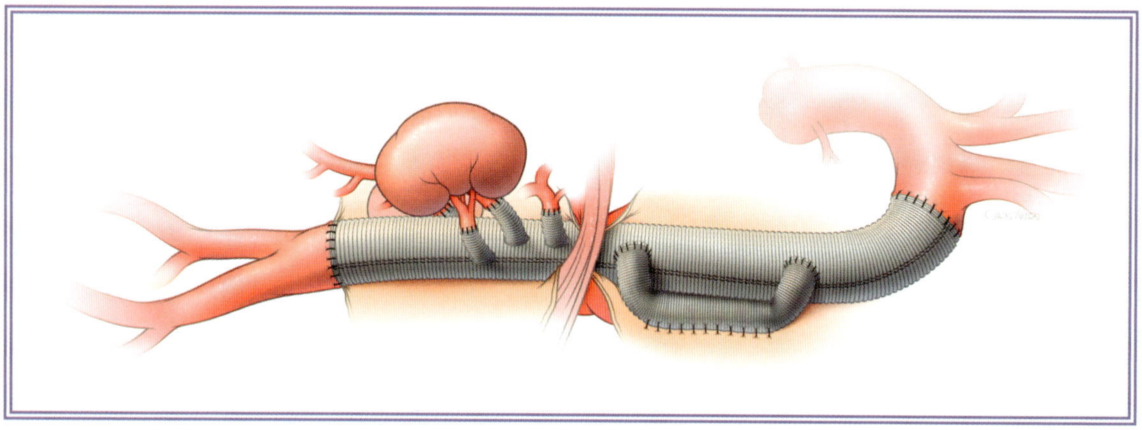

Fig. 15.6 Thoracoabdominal aortic aneurysm repair with side-branched thoracoabdominal graft with reconstruction of intercostal arteries (copyright Chris Akers®, reproduced with permission).

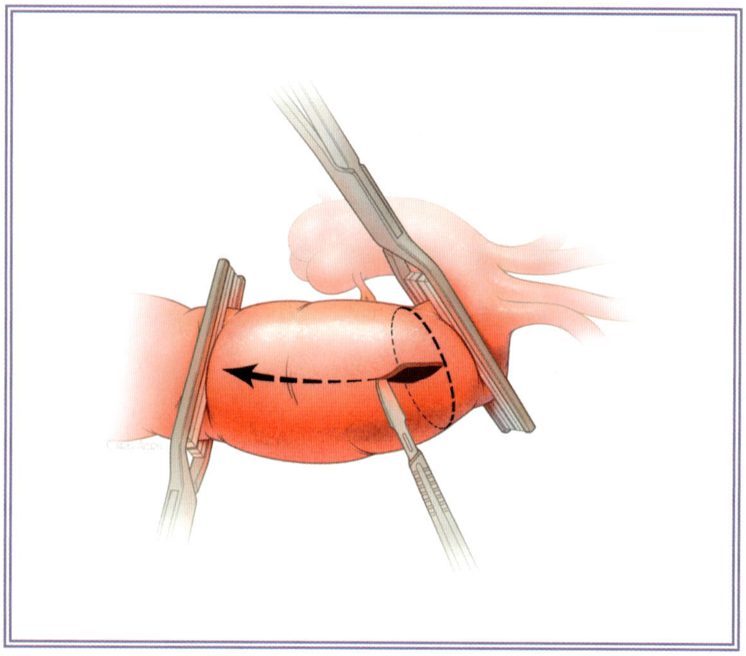

Fig. 15.7 Segmental clamping (copyright Chris Akers®, reproduced with permission).

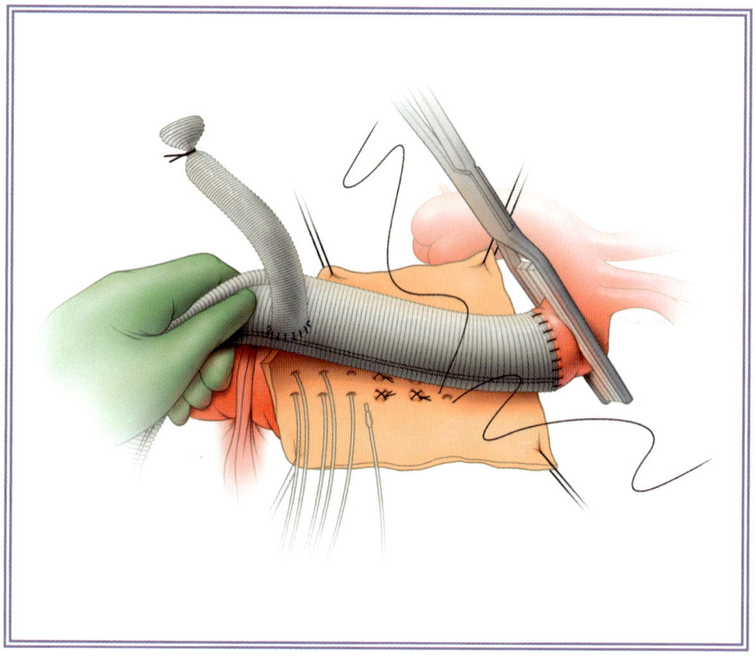

Fig. 15.8 Ligation and preservation of intercostal arteries (copyright Chris Akers®, reproduced with permission).

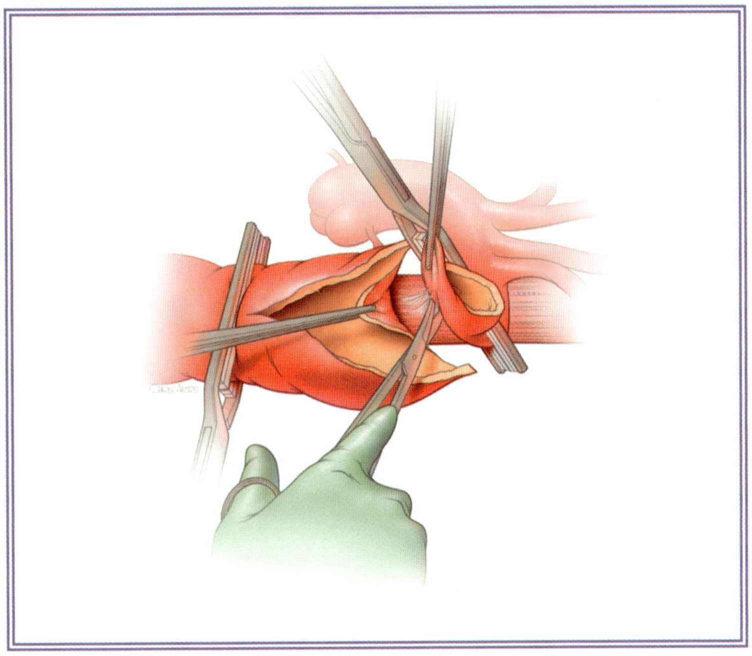

Fig. 15.9 Transection of the proximal descending aorta and dissection from the esophagus (copyright Chris Akers®, reproduced with permission).

and opening the aorta, the size and type of Dacron graft are selected and opened on the table. The reversed elephant trunk is prepared by invaginating the proximal end of the graft, 5 cm in length, if the aortic arch has not been replaced at the time of index surgery.

Sequential clamp is applied to minimize organ ischemic time, beginning proximal/distal to the left subclavian artery or the elephant trunk and mid-descending thoracic aorta (Fig. 15.7). The aorta is opened, and the intercostal arteries found within this segment are all ligated to prevent the steal phenomenon (Fig. 15.8). The aorta is transected and separated from the underlying esophagus for proximal anastomosis to avoid esophageal fistula (Fig. 15.9). The proximal anastomosis is performed with 2-0 Prolene® CT-1 or 3-0 Prolene® SH continuous suture, in a fashion to eliminate the proximal false lumen.

Following the completion of the proximal anastomosis, the upper clamp is moved to the graft and hemostasis is checked. Then the lower clamp is moved to the distal thoracic aorta at the diaphragm, and the distal descending aorta is opened. Patent intercostal arteries in this segment are preserved and 3-Fr Fogarty® occlusion catheters (Edwards Lifescience Co., Irvine, CA) are inserted (see Fig. 15.8).

For descending thoracic aortic aneurysm, the graft is cut and sewn to distal thoracic aorta. When the dissection extends beyond the distal anastomosis, the dissection flap needs to be fenestrated to maintain the flow to both the true and false lumens, which is done with a very short open distal procedure. The distal anastomosis can be performed with either inclusion or exclusion technique using 2-0 Prolene® CT-1 or 3-0 Prolene® SH.

For thoracoabdominal aortic aneurysm, we further move the distal clamp to the infrarenal abdominal aorta, and the longitudinal incision of the aorta is elongated caudad. The celiac axis, superior mesenteric, right renal and left renal arteries are identified, cannulated with balloon perfusion catheters (9 Fr: renal arteries, 12 Fr: celiac axis, superior mesenteric arteries; B-lumen irrigation arterial embolectomy catheter, Lucas Medical Inc., Anaheim, CA), perfused and cooled using Ringer's lactate solution for renal arteries and blood for celiac axis and superior mesenteric artery at a flow rate of 300-600 mL/min. Left renal temperature is monitored and maintained below 15 °C. However, we maintain the patient's body temperature at about 33-34 °C by warming the lower circulation to avoid ventricular fibrillation.

After the final anastomosis, all the clamps are removed and pulsatile flow is restored. The pump is weaned after warming the patient to 36 °C. The intercostal arteries are reattached selectively based on neuromonitoring [15]. We currently use loop technique with a 14-mm Dacron graft attached to the main graft and reconstruct the intercostal arteries with inclusion technique (side-to-side anastomosis) (see Fig. 15.6). If there is no change in the monitoring, intercostal arteries are ligated at the end of the procedure. The local analgesics are injected for paravertebral block before the closure.

15.6 Endovascular approach

If the aneurysm is limited to distal arch/proximal descending thoracic aorta and the patient is old (>65 years old) without connective tissue disorders, thoracic endovascular aortic repair (TEVAR) is a feasible treatment option. If zone 2 TEVAR is to be performed, left carotid artery to left subclavian artery bypass or transposition of left subclavian artery to left carotid artery is considered to reduce the risk of paraplegia.

There are reports of coiling the false lumen [16] or debranching TEVAR [17, 18] in high-risk patients. However, long-term results are not available.

15.7 Results

We performed a total of 489 acute Type A AD repairs between October 1999 and December 2014. Of those, 19 patients underwent distal reoperation (23 procedures) at our institution. Index procedure was ascending and proximal arch replacement in 17 patients (+ root replacement in one patient) and total arch replacement with elephant trunk technique in two patients. Five patients had total arch replacement with redo median sternotomy, nine patients had descending thoracic aortic aneurysm repair (two extent A, seven extent C), six patients had thoracoabdominal aortic aneurysm repair (one extent I, three extent II, one extent III, one extent IV), and three patients received TEVAR. All of the patients who underwent total arch replacement had uneventful re-entry of the sternum without requirement of femoro-femoral bypass, and no mortality was observed. There were two deaths after descending thoracic aortic aneurysm repairs (one ruptured extent A, one extent C; both died of coagulopathies). One patient died of intraoperative myocardial infarction after extent II thoracoabdominal aortic aneurysm repair. There was no adverse event after TEVAR.

15.8 Summary

Preoperative careful assessment of the imaging studies and meticulous surgical plan are required for optimal outcomes in patients undergoing aortic arch aneurysm after Type A AD repair. Our preferred approach is redo median sternotomy if the aneurysm involves transverse arch. Aortic aneurysm localized distal to the subclavian artery is treated with left thoracotomy approach, or TEVAR may be indicated in high-risk patients. However, it is important to emphasize that TEVAR complete false lumen thrombosis are infrequently obtained (only 20%) [19] and careful follow-up is required for the downstream aorta. Debranching TEVAR or other hybrid approaches have been reported and we await long-term results.

REFERENCES

1) Pape LA, Awais M, Woznicki EM, et al. Presentation, diagnosis, and outcomes of acute aortic dissection: 17-year trends from the International Registry of Acute Aortic Dissection. J Am Coll Cardiol 2015; 66(4): 350-8.
2) Geirsson A, Bavaria JE, Swarr D, et al. Fate of the residual distal and proximal aorta after acute type a dissection repair using a contemporary surgical reconstruction algorithm. Ann Thorac Surg 2007; 84: 1955-64.
3) Zierer A, Voeller RK, Hill KE, et al. Aortic enlargement and late reoperation after repair of acute type A aortic dissection. Ann Thorac Surg 2007; 84: 479-86.
4) Zhang H, Lang X, Lu F, et al. Acute type A dissection without intimal tear in arch: proximal or extensive repair? J Thorac Cardiovasc Surg 2014; 147: 1251-5.
5) Omura A, Miyahara S, Yamanaka K, et al. Early and late outcomes of repaired acute DeBakey type I aortic dissection after graft replacement. J Thorac Cardiovasc Surg 2016; 151: 341-8.
6) Luciani N, De Geest R, Lauria G, et al. Late reoperations after acute aortic dissection repair: single-center experience. Asian Cardiovasc Thorac Ann 2015; 23(7): 787-94.
7) Safi HJ, Miller CC 3rd, Estrera AL, et al. Staged repair of extensive aortic aneurysms: morbidity and mortality in the elephant trunk technique. Circulation 2001; 104(24): 2938-42.
8) Safi HJ, Miller CC 3rd, Subramaniam MH, et al. Thoracic and thoracoabdominal aortic aneurysm repair using cardiopulmonary bypass, profound hypothermia, and circulatory arrest via left side of the chest incision. J Vasc Surg 1998; 28(4): 591-8.
9) Moz M, Misfeld M, Leontyev S, Borger MA, Davierwala P, Mohr FW. Aortic arch reoperation in a single centre: early and late results in 57 consecutive patients. Eur J Cardiothorac Surg 2013; 44(1): e82-6.
10) Etz CD, Plestis KA, Homann TM, et al. Reoperative aortic root and transverse arch procedures: a comparison with contemporaneous primary operations. J Thorac Cardiovasc Surg 2008; 136: 860-7.
11) Estrera AL, Miller CC 3rd, Porat E, et al. Determinants of early and late outcome for reoperations of the proximal aorta. Ann Thorac Surg 2004; 78(3): 837-45.
12) Estrera AL, Miller CC 3rd, Lee TY, Shah P, Safi HJ. Ascending and transverse aortic arch repair: the impact of retrograde cerebral perfusion. Circulation 2008; 118(14 Suppl): S160-6.
13) Estrera AL, Sandhu HK, Miller CC, et al. Repair of extensive aortic aneurysms: a single-center experience using the elephant trunk technique over 20 years. Ann Surg 2014; 260(3): 510-6.
14) Svensson LG. Approach for insertion of aortic composite valve grafts. Ann Thorac Surg 1992; 54: 376-8.
15) Estrera AL, Sheinbaum R, Miller CC 3rd, Harrison R, Safi HJ. Neuromonitor-guided repair of thoracoabdominal aortic aneurysms. J Thorac Cardiovasc Surg 2010; 140(6 Suppl): S131-5; discussion S142-6.
16) Zink JN, Maness MR, Powell CS, et al. Coil embolization of persistent false lumen after type A dissection repair. Ann Thorac Surg 2014; 97(6): 2193-6.
17) Murphy EH, Dimaio JM, Jessen ME, Arko FR. Technique for branched thoracic stent-graft repair of a chronic type A aortic dissection in a patient with multiple prior sternotomies. J Endovasc Ther 2011; 18(3): 359-64.
18) Canaud L, Gandet T, Ozdemir BA, Albat B, Marty-Ané C, Alric P. Hybrid aortic repair of dissecting aortic arch aneurysm after surgical treatment of acute type A dissection. Ann Vasc Surg 2016; 30: 175-80.
19) Kimura N, Itoh S, Yuri K, et al. Reoperation for enlargement of the distal aorta after initial surgery for acute type A aortic dissection. J Thorac Cardiovasc Surg 2015; 149(2 Suppl): S91-8.

16

Endovascular treatment of residual arch dissection after open repair of Type A aortic dissections

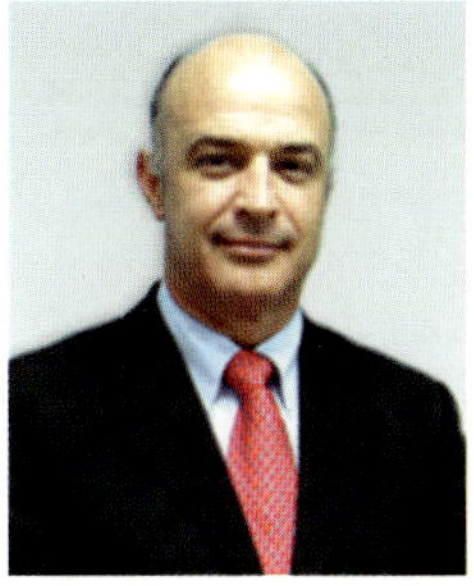

Marcelo Ferreira, Eduardo Rodrigues, Diego Ferreira,
Rodrigo Cunha and Guilherme Bicalho

16.1 Introduction

As previously described in other chapters of this book, the development of Type A aortic dissection (AD) is a life-threatening disease with a high mortality rate. A mortality of 1% per hour and an expected mortality of 70 to 90% during the first three months have been reported if left untreated [1].

In-hospital mortality ranges from 15 to 30% according to the International Registry of Acute Aortic Dissection (IRAD). Unfortunately, surviving the operation does not guarantee freedom from subsequent aortic events, because in many cases the distal intimal tear cannot be removed, and the false lumen frequently remains patent, leading to progressive descending aortic dilatation and rupture [2].

Despite initial treatment, progressive dilatation of the false lumen in the arch and descending aorta has been encountered in one-third of survivors as late sequelae, following repair of ascending AD [3].

Key factors may be attributed to explain residual arch dissection. Patients with descending aortas greater than 3.5 cm, and high blood pressure are prone to dissection. If the false lumen presents itself with sizes superior to 2 cm and the initial tear is greater than 10 cm, there are bigger chances of residual dissection [2].

The indications of surgical intervention rely upon accelerated growth rates and upon aortic dilatation that exceeds 5.5 cm [2].

The best treatment strategy for aortic arch pathologies is currently being studied and under big debate. There are four main surgical options: open repair, hybrid surgery with aortic debranching associated with thoracic endograft, parallel grafts (chimneys/ snorkels) and total endovascular repair (fenestrated or branched endografts).

Conventional treatment of this delayed complication involves open arch repair with elephant trunk. This procedure requires cardiopulmonary bypass and deep hypothermic circulatory arrest, with its inherent high morbidity and mortality [3].

Many different surgical techniques may be applied to treat residual arch dissections. Given the scope of this chapter, strictly endovascular techniques will be further elucidated.

Marcelo Ferreira (marceloferreira1959@gmail.com)
SITE – Serviço Integrado de Técnicas Endovasculares,
Rio de Janeiro, Brazil

G. Melissano - R. Chiesa (eds), Aortic Dissection patients true stories and the innovations that saved their lives

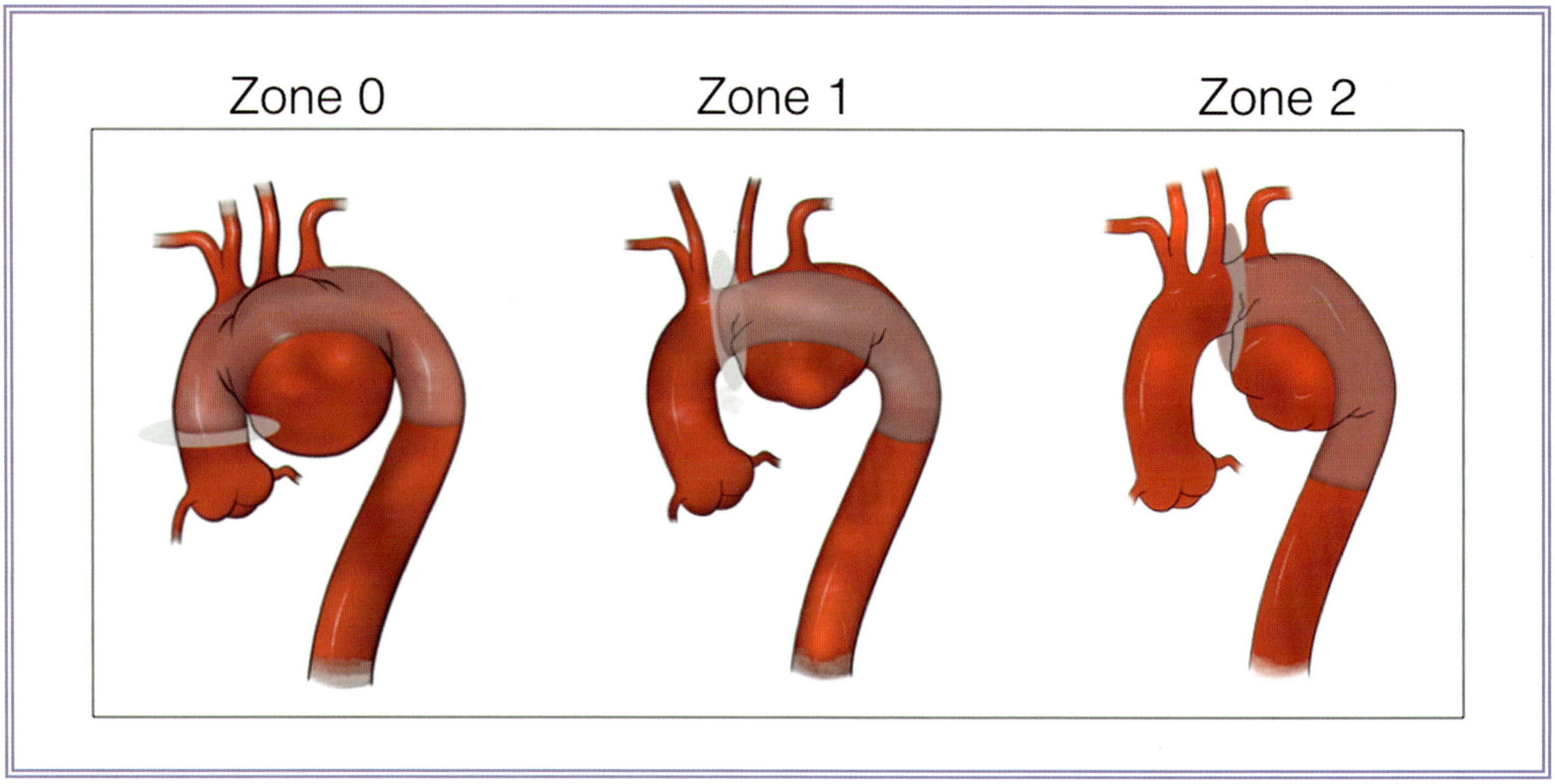

Fig. 16.1 Ishimaru's classification of arch aneurysms. Reproduced from [5], with permission.

16.1.1 Anatomical considerations

The aortic arch is marked by its distinct morphology, hemodynamic forces, and lack of proximal seal given its proximity to the coronary arteries. Ascending aortic pathology is often associated with concomitant aortic valve, coronary artery, and distal aortic disease. When treating the aortic arch it is of utmost importance to take in consideration the three-dimension angulation of the aorta, and the position and variation of each of the three arch vessels.

The anatomical features of the aortic arch impose different hemodynamic characteristics. Pulsatility in this region has been shown to be two-three times higher than the descending aorta. These characteristics may result in wrong graft positioning, with consequent graft, kinking and endoleaks.

Ishimaru proposed a novel classification for landing zones regarding the treatment of the diseases of the ascending aorta, suggesting that the fixation of the proximal endograft should be indicated by a line from the distal side of the branch artery orifice in the aortic arch. Landing zone 0 is the region between the coronary arteries and the innominate artery . Next, is landing zone 1 that extends itself from the innominate artery until the left carotid artery. Landing zone 2 comes next, and is the region that contains the left subclavian artery (Fig. 16.1). The following two regions marked as three and four lies beyond the subclavian artery and in the descending aorta.

In order to apply endovascular technique it is necessary to assure that the patient has no prior aortic valve replacement (biological or mechanical valves) and to achieve adequate sealing, the ascending aorta must have 20 mm in length, 38 mm in diameter. The innominate must measure at least 8 mm whereas the carotid should measure 6 mm in diameter to accommodate an endograft [4].

16.2 Type of treatments

16.2.1 Hybrid technique

The hybrid technique consists in minimizing surgical exposition time by mixing endovascular techniques and extra anatomical bypasses. Similar to other endovascular interventions, it is necessary to obtain a good landing zone for complete sealing.

Usually this type of approach is based on Ishimaru classification [5] and four different scenarios can be drawn.

Each scenario precludes a different technique. Most aortic arch grafts tend to revascularize both the innominate and the left carotid, thus only a left carotid-subclavian transposition is necessary.

Landing zone 0

It is necessary to revascularize all three supra aortic vessels. Once the debranching is done, a thoracic graft can be adequately implemented.

Landing zone 1

Landing zone 1 preserves the origin of the innominate artery. The landing zone is the origin of the left carotid artery thus a carotid-carotid bypass is deemed necessary (Fig. 16.2).

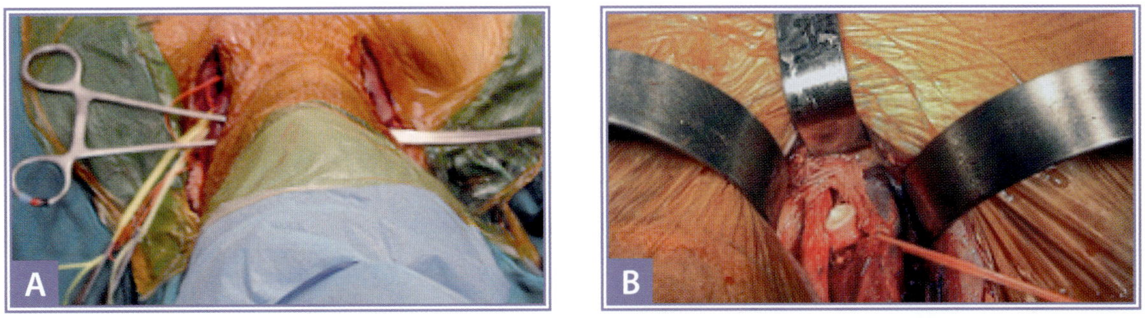

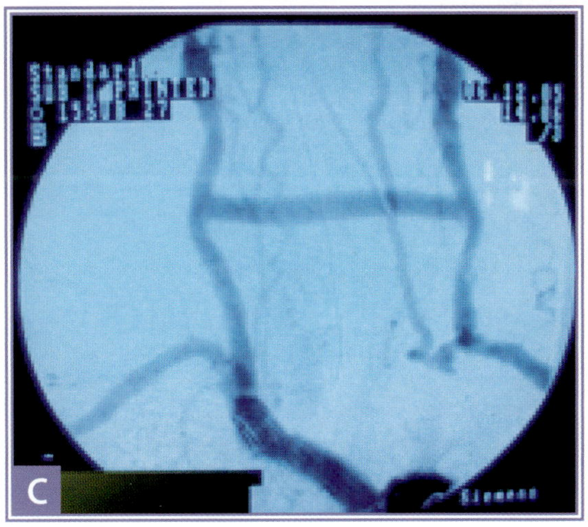

Fig. 16.2 Preparing the carotid for bypass (**A**, **B**); final angiogram (**C**).

Landing zone 2

Both the innominate and the left carotid arteries are left patent. Only the subclavian is occluded. In these cases a carotid-subclavian bypass or transposition may be performed.

Although literature denotes that the subclavian artery may be occluded without risk in specific populations our group tends to revascularize all patients in order to preserve adequate flow to the vertebral arteries and other important collaterals, minimizing risks of paraplegia.

Landing zone 3 and 4

Both landing zone 3 and 4 preclude traditional thoracic endograft techniques, without further adjuvance.

16.2.2 Endovascular solutions

Bare metal stents

In the beginning, in order to address tears in the residual dissected aorta and avoid complications, bare metal stents were used as first line treatments. The concept was to join the dissected layers without occluding important side branches.

The Zenith® (Cook Medical, Bloomington, IN), the E-xl (JOTEC GmbH, Hechingen, Germany) and the Djumbodis® dissection system (Saint Come Chirurgie, Marseille, France) are three examples of bare metal stents. Today these stents are only used in specific situations.

The E-xl stent is a self-expandable nitinol bare stent, which combines flexibility through the open cell structure in the middle section of the stent. The closed cell structure on both ends provides adequate fixation.

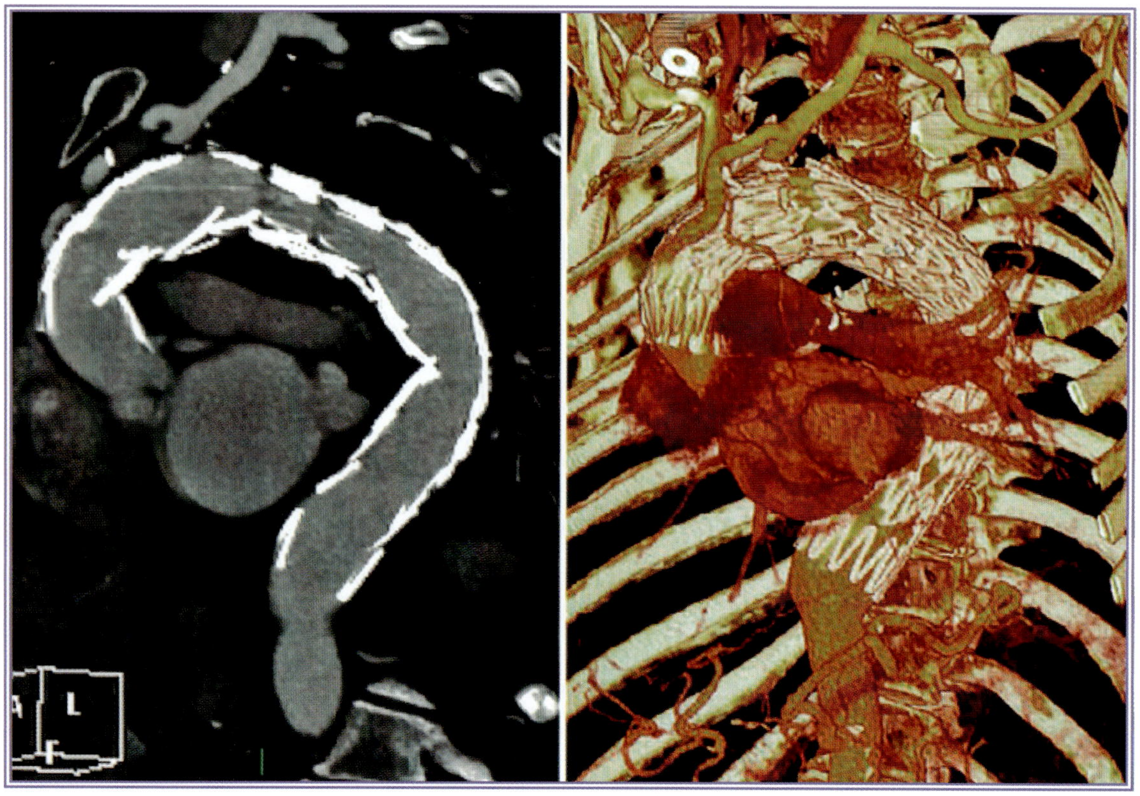

Fig. 16.3 CTA at 18 months after implantation of the bare stents, which are seen at the ascending aorta and along the stent-graft in the ascending aorta, arch, and descending aorta.

The Djumbodis® dissection system is a balloon expandable stent where the balloon allows adequate conformation to the anatomy of the aorta and the mesh is large enough to preserve flow to the collaterals.

Our group published in 2009 on the *Journal of Endovascular Therapy* [6] the employment of the Zenith® dissection bare metal stents in the aortic arch to correct a residual dissection [5] (Fig. 16.3).

Although feasible, the results of bare metal stents were not comparable to those obtained by regular cardiac techniques such as the frozen elephant. Today these devices are only used in selected cases.

Parallel grafts

The chimney technique first described by Greenberg, as a mean of rescuing a renal artery inadvertently covered by the stent graft, during endovascular aneurysm repair, has been applied to revascularize aortic arch branches [7].

It consists of placing a bare metal stent or a covered stent in a target vessel alongside the main aortic stent-graft.

Although this technique has been applied in patients with thoracic aortic pathology, reports regarding the application of chimneys grafts in the arch are limited to few case reports and small series.

The diameter of the innominate artery poses an issue with sealing, and the added distance of the second chimney resulted in a longer graft and a higher chance of compression and occlusion.

According to the paper published in 2014 by Stephen Cheng [8] on the journal *Endovascular Today*, chimneys require an average of 20 to 30% oversizing of the endograft. Because most patients with arch aneurysms are elderly and have degenerations in the ascending aorta, the applicability of chimneys in the context of a dilated ascending aorta is questionable.

Some reports indicate that gutter endoleaks increase with the size of the chimneys. Aggressive oversizing and ballooning in this area, as is recommended in most chimney procedures, may produce adverse results. The hemodynamic forces on the stent graft components in this area remain unknown, and there may be a theoretical higher chance of retrograde Type A AD [9].

These poor results, of both bare stents and chimney procedures, paved the way for the development of branched devices.

Branched devices

Inoue et al. reported the first use of a branched endovascular device for treatment of arch aneurysms [9]. From 1995 to 2002, 48 total patients were treated with this design.

Although the technical feasibility of the procedure has been demonstrated, the procedure related mortality was 23%. Additionally, severe complications including stroke, dissection, and persistent endoleak were reported in 17% of the patients.

The major challenges with the Inoue graft were that the branches protruded externally to the aortic component, thus complicating cannulation of the target vessels and proper placement of covered stents in each of the branches.

Chuter and coll. first reported the use of a modular branched stent graft for arch repair in 2003 [10]. Unlike the Inoue system, the custom-made endografts devised by Tim Chuter had a modular design, with a proximal bifurcated graft with one branch opening into the innominate artery and the distal end opened into another aortic endograft that extended into the descending thoracic aorta below the aneurysm.

The proximal graft was inserted through a conduit anastomosed to the common carotid or innominate artery, and the distal component was inserted through a standard femoral approach. In order to maintain the supra aortic vessels patent, it was necessary to perform a ca-

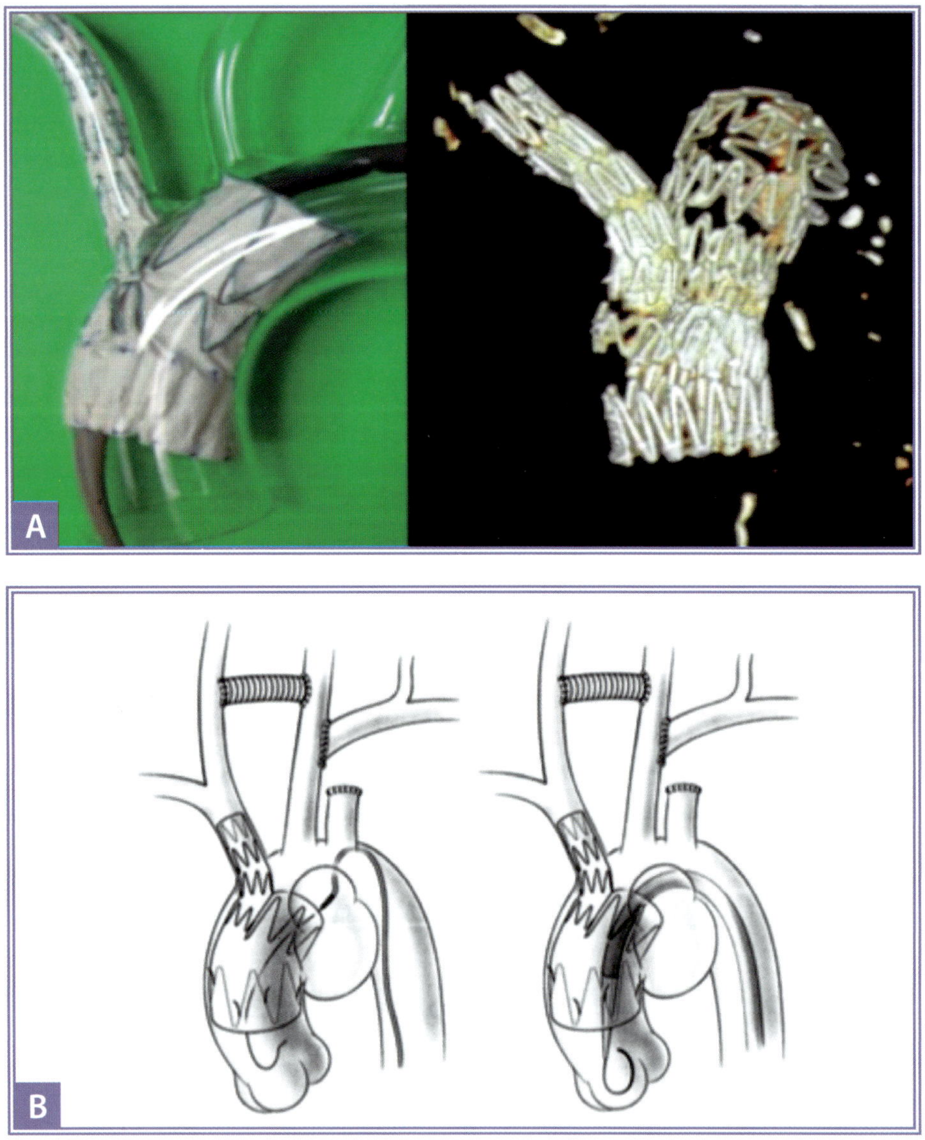

Fig. 16.4 **A**, Custom made Chuter endograft. **B**, Final configuration of graft and bypass. Reproduced from [10], with permission.

rotid-carotid retropharyngeal bypass and a left subclavian to carotid transposition (Fig. 16.4).

Since Chuter's pioneer endograft in 2003 many studies have taken place and many modifications have been done to the original graft.

In 2009, our group together with Tim Chuter published an initial experience in the Journal Vascular [11].

As seen in Figure 16.5, outer branch devices were used to attend the necessities of the aortic arch anatomy.

Nowadays, the most used graft is a double inner branch endograft manufactured by Cook Medical.

As seen in Figure 16.6, each endograft has two internal side branches with an enlarged external opening at their distal ends. Diamond-shaped radio opaque markers are placed on both ends of each inner side branch to facilitate positioning under fluoroscopy [12].

Both ends of the endograft are wide and flexible, whereas the middle, the side branch bearing portion, is narrow and straight. The design objective was to separate the orifices of the side

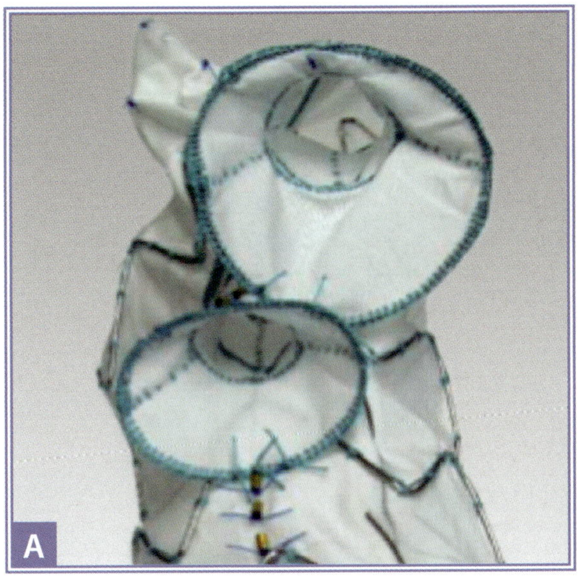

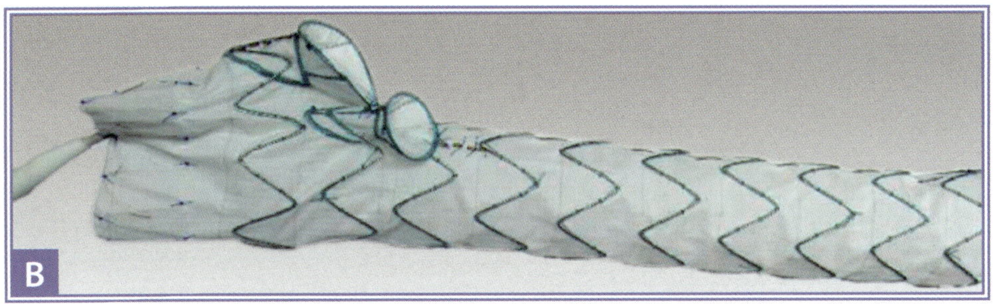

Fig. 16.5 **A**, **B**, Arch device with external branches. Courtesy of Cook Medical.

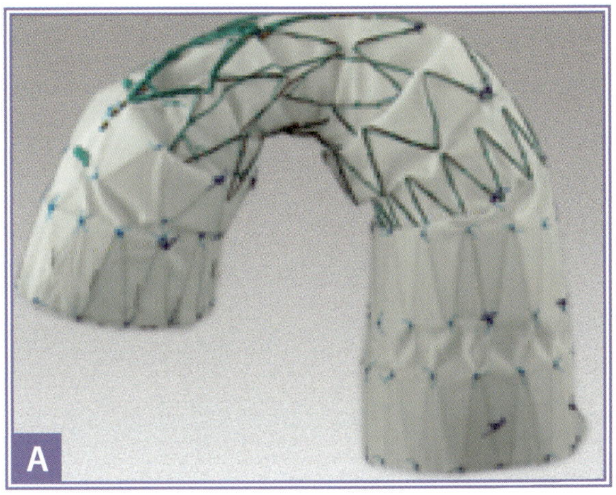

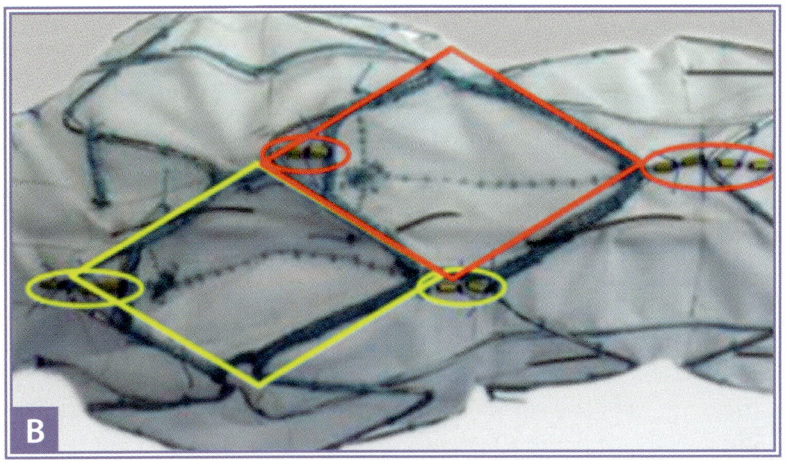

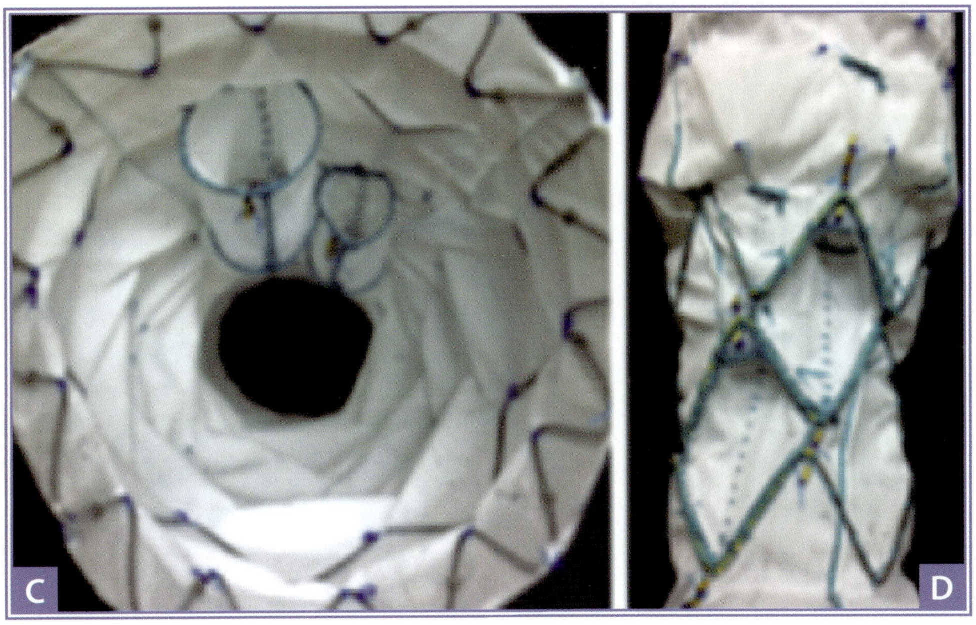

Fig. 16.6 **A**, Arch device with inner branches. **B**, Diamond disposition. **C**, Inner view of arch device. **D**, Detail. Courtesy of Cook Medical.

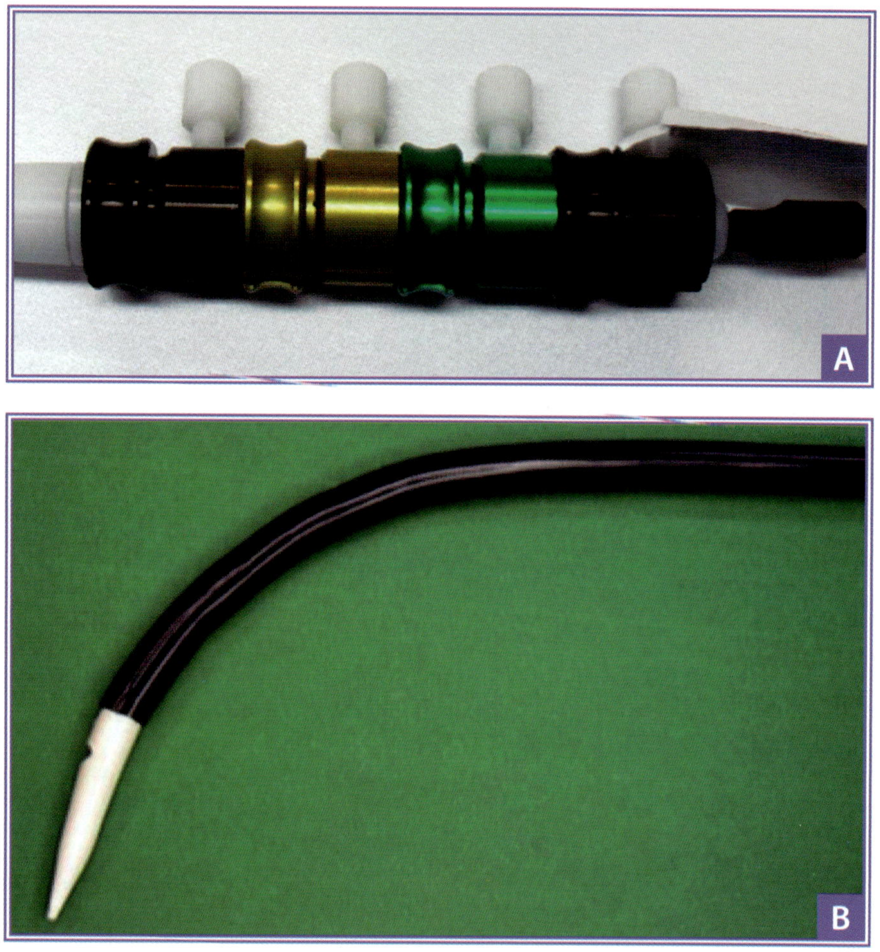

Fig. 16.7 **A**, Four trigger wires. **B**, Curved hydrophilic sheath. Courtesy of Cook Medical.

branches from the orifices of the supra-aortic trunks, preserving perigraft flow and facilitating branch cannulation [12].

As seen in Figure 16.7A, four trigger wires attach the proximal edge of the graft to the central shaft of the delivery system just behind the fusiform tip. The first is a spiral stabilizing wire, and the second is an inner curve proximal attachment, the release of which ensures medial wall attachment of the proximal stent. The third releases the diameter-reducing ties that give the "proform" effect for first stent deployment, which helps to prevent bird-beak configuration along the medial curve of the ascending aorta, and the fourth secures the distal end of the stent graft to the central shaft of the delivery system [12].

All four trigger wires are attached to a single ring on the outer end of the shaft. Placement of the bridging stents is from a retrograde approach via access to the supra-aortic vessels. The device seals distally in the descending thoracic aorta and may be used with additional thoracic grafts to achieve a seal in a healthy segment of the thoracic aorta [12].

The device is loaded into a curved introducer with a hydrophilic sheath (Fig. 16.7B). The curved system facilitates alignment of the branches with the greater curve of the aortic arch. The innominate artery distally is usually too large for a standard-size covered stent and requires a customized graft. The bridging component for the innominate artery is manufactured with low-profile graft fabric and loaded into a short 14 Fr Flexor delivery system. This is usually a modified iliac limb placed on a shorter delivery system [12]. A commercially available covered stent Fluency® (Bard, Murray Hill, NJ) or Viabahn® (W.L. Gore, Flagstaff, AZ) can be used as the bridging component for the left common carotid (LCC) artery.

16.3 Case planning

When considering the hemodynamics involved with aortic arch surgery, special care must be taken for correct deployment of the graft.

The first step in performing any endovascular surgery and specially when attending the arch is adequate planning. All patients should have CT scans with symmetrical and thin cuts to allow proper three-dimensional reconstruction. The supra aortic vessels should be visualised and the cerebral circulation should be studied. All our cases are planned in the office using Osirix Medical Version, all projects that are completed are revised with the team. The diameters, angulations and landing zones should be considered. It is important to anticipate any anatomical difficulty during planning so that adequate planning is done (Fig. 16.8).

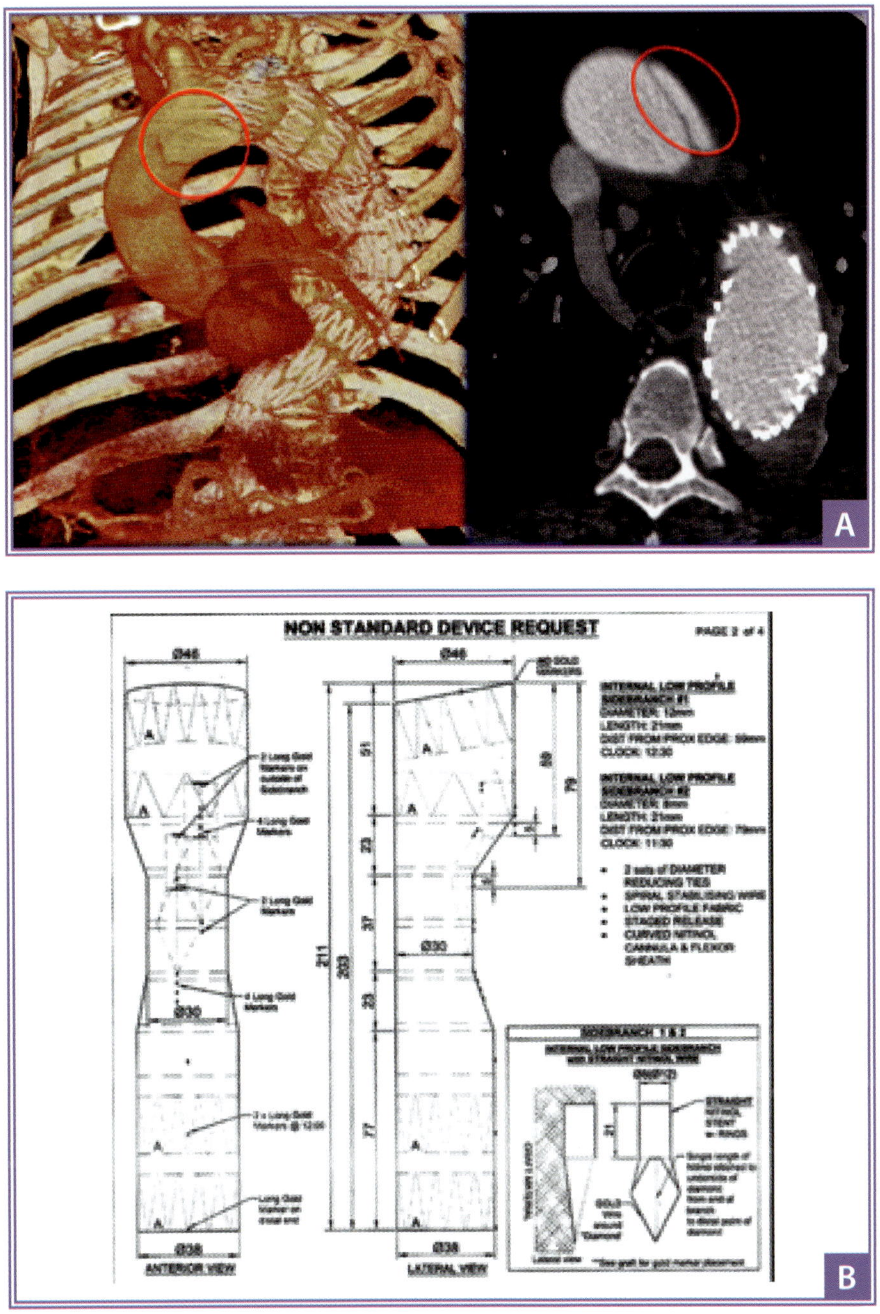

Fig. 16.8 **A**, CT scan demonstrating arch dissection. **B**, Custom made device, graft planning.

16.4 Technical aspects of branched devices

Accurate deployment depends on excellent imaging and stable hemodynamics. Traditionally, the blood pressure was lowered pharmacologically using various vasodilators in intravenous bolus. Because adenosine has a transient negative chronotropic effect it was used to create a temporary state of asystole to reduce the post load and facilitate navigation and deployment. However because of the uncertainty of duration, dose, and reproducibility of asystole, as well as the possibility of inadequate return of rhythm it is not used anymore in majority of places.

In order to correctly deploy the graft it is necessary to induce a temporary fibrillation of the heart. Such condition may be obtained through means of pacemaker. Nowadays, the use of rapid ventricular pacing is the gold standard.

This method temporarily abolishes ejection forces during graft deployment. It is done by accessing the femoral vein and positioning the pacemaker inside the heart. It is important to observe any instability while electrically stimulating the heart.

In order to perform arch endovascular surgery a minimum of three access sites are necessary. The most commonly used are the femoral artery, and both carotids. Depending on the anatomic situation axillary arteries and ventricular apex may also be considered.

The transapical approach can be used when the regular aortic route is calcified and tortuous, the pitfall is that only straight tubes may be employed. Crossing the aortic valve for a prolonged time with an 18 Fr sheath may produce a transient hypotension [13].

Considering the comorbidities presented by the patients, and the close relationship with the coronaries, most endovascular arch corrections are executed with transesophagic eco assistance.

It is important to consider neurological surveillance as well. During surgery transcranial doppler and continuous electroencephalogram are used.

Both carotids are exposed and used as surgical access. During surgery the key issue is to manipulate each carotid at a different moment, this way cerebral perfusion is maintained with the contralateral side. Such protocol minimizes the total clamping involved thus reducing the ischemia time and stroke rate.

Cherrie Abraham described that some aortic centers have been using neurological protection to prevent strokes [12].

The first step of the surgery consists in a left subclavian artery transposition. The transposition is useful to maintain cerebral flow while the carotid is clamped. It is routine to occlude the origin of the subclavian artery with the placement of a Amplatzer™ plug (St. Jude Medical, St. Paul, MN) after the transposition has been performed.

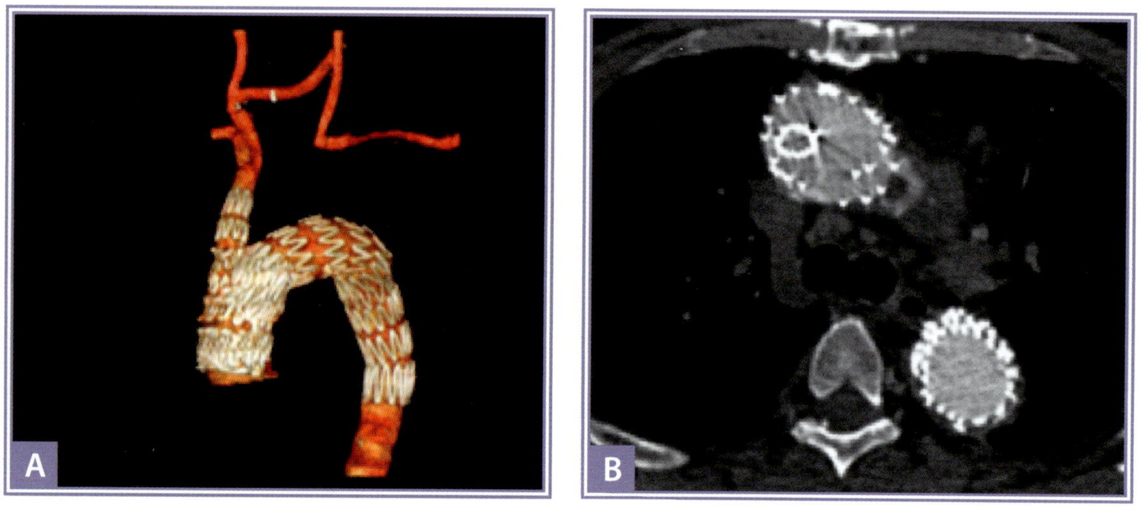

Fig. 16.9 **A**, Three-dimensional reconstruction. **B**, Control CT scan.

Once the surgical part has been completed, it is necessary to carry on the endovascular part. From the femoral access a hydrophilic wire is placed across the aortic valve and then exchanged for a stiff wire with the tip of the wire positioned inside the left ventricle.

The graft is loaded into a large Flexor sheath that has a pre-curved inner nitinol cannula to ensure orientation of the branches with the arch vessels.

The delivery system for the arch branch graft is advanced through the aortic valve. Once positioned the rapid pacing is initiated and the graft positioned. It is important to correctly align the diamonds and the gold markers with the branches of the arch.

After the graft is deployed, the inner branches are cannulated. The cannulation is done with a straight catheter and a hydrophilic wire. Once cannulated, the sheath is advanced through the inner marks and covered stent grafts are deployed to seal the branches.

Attention should be drawn towards the anatomical curve of the arch so that the graft is properly deployed (Fig. 16.9).

16.5 Possible complications

As with any surgery, access remains a potential complication site. Although feasible and elegant option, the trans-apical access site remains a concern. Apart from bleeding from the left ventricle (LV) apex (generally managed with extra sutures and blood transfusion and ECMO – extracorporeal membrane oxygenation support as required), more rare complications include the formation of an LV apex pseudoaneurysm and the presence of a late ventricular septal defect. Follow-up with echo is mandatory after surgical approach via the LV apex procedures [13].

Other possible complications that may occur include perforation of the heart, acute aortic valve insufficiency and retrograde dissection of the coronary arteries. When considering complete coverage of the aorta, paraplegia becomes a concern. Whenever possible, staged procedures should be performed.

In Haulon published series, the 30-day mortality rate was 13.2%, technical success rate 84%. Median intensive care unit stay was 2 days (range, 1.5-4 days) and median hospital stay was 10 days (range, 7.5-15.5 days) [4].

Initially, these arch branched procedures were hampered by a relatively high incidence of stroke. The initial experience hindered a stroke rate ranging from 0 to 11%. Early cerebrovascular complications were diagnosed in 6 patients (15.8% [95% CI, 4.0-27.6]), including 4 transient ischemic attacks, 1 stroke, and 1 subarachnoid hemorrhage [4].

In 2014, Haulon published in the *Journal of Thoracic and Cardiovascular Surgery* that after the "learning curve", which in the author's opinion is a difficult number to establish, the mortality was lowered to 7% in the latter part of his series.

Many factors are related to stroke; these include carotid thrombosis, emboli due to the graft manipulation in the arch. This specific mechanism can almost be recognized and prevented by looking carefully the preoperative CT scan. Air emboli released from the delivery system and low cerebral perfusion during cross clamping are also important mechanisms of strokes.

More significantly, an ascending aortic diameter bigger than 38 mm was found to be the main independent risk factor of mortality and neurologic complications, which would make this procedure contraindicated in patients with dilated ascending aortas [4].

Those patients with previous aortic interposition grafts that do present with significant angulation do impose an extra challenge. The stiffness of the graft may present some difficulty in conforming to the arch's angulation.

In our Brazilian experience, technical success was obtained in 75% of the cases. Only one surgery could not be completed given that the patient died. During graft deployment through the aortic valve, the patient presented with a hypotension non responsive to any medication and consequent death.

Late analysis attributes this unfavorable outcome to partially coverage of the right coronary artery thus resulting in heart ischemia and cardiac arrest.

None of the other cases presented with neurological sequelae or any other side effects. All patients are enrolled in our follow-up program and do return on a regular basis for consultations.

16.6 Discussion

Historically, these arch pathologies have been treated with conventional surgical techniques requiring cardiopulmonary bypass and deep hypothermic circulatory arrest (DHCA) with a mortality rate ranging from 2 to 16.5% and a stroke rate ranging from 2 to 18% [4].

The indication for redo surgery varies and was established in cases of progressive aortic enlargement, development of a false aneurysm/rupture, proven graft infection, or aortic valve incompetence. The isolated persistence of false lumen in the aortic arch is not an indication for intervention and can be observed carefully with sequential CT scans.

Until today, open surgery is the gold standard to treat residual dissections. In order to address this late aortic risk, the Mayo Clinic analyzed the performance of a total arch replacement at the time that acute dissection repair was done. The theory was that this additional aortic replacement would decrease the patency of the false lumen with its late aortic complications [14-16].

Despite the hope that such radical proximal dissection treatment would improve results, experience has shown that total arch replacement at the time of acute dissection increases operative time, morbidity (especially neurological give numbers), and mortality without significant improvement in long-term outcome [17, 18].

According to Cherrie Abraham in his paper published in the *Annals of Cardiothoracic Surgery* in 2013, only low risk patients with no history of cardiac procedures should be offered conventional open or hybrid surgery [12].

Chiesa [19] in 2010 published a series of 116 patients that underwent hybrid surgery. Although the hybrid surgery avoids crossclamping and circulatory bypass it does carry a certain risk.

The arch branch procedure should only be considered in patients deemed high risk for conventional treatment or in patients for whom difficult redo surgery is anticipated. The major advantage of this approach is the avoidance of DHCA and cardiopulmonary bypass.

Initial worldwide results concerning total endovascular arch repair are relatively sparse, but very promising. Stoke rates in the later part of Haulon's series are comparable to those of conventional surgical repair.

Continued development and evolution of endografts in the visceral segment have constructed expertise to allow for the application of total endovascular repair of complex aortic aneurysms and dissections involving the aortic arch segment.

For this purpose, highly specialized arch debranching grafts have been developed, with better trackability and conformation, so that the graft deployment can be done in a more precise manner.

A recent paper published by Tsilimparis et al. (2016) in the *Journal of Vascular Surgery* analysed 29 patients that underwent both fenestrated and branched endografts. They concluded that both methods are acceptable and play an important role in the treatment of arch pathologies. Although feasible, branched devices are surely more suitable for extended, complex arch diseases, especially in the presence of previous ascending aortic repair [20].

Until today, the main surgical indications are defined by the cardiac surgery team. Only exceptional cases are carried out in a total endovascular fashion. Maybe with growing experience and better results, specially concerning strokes rates, these limited indications might broaden up.

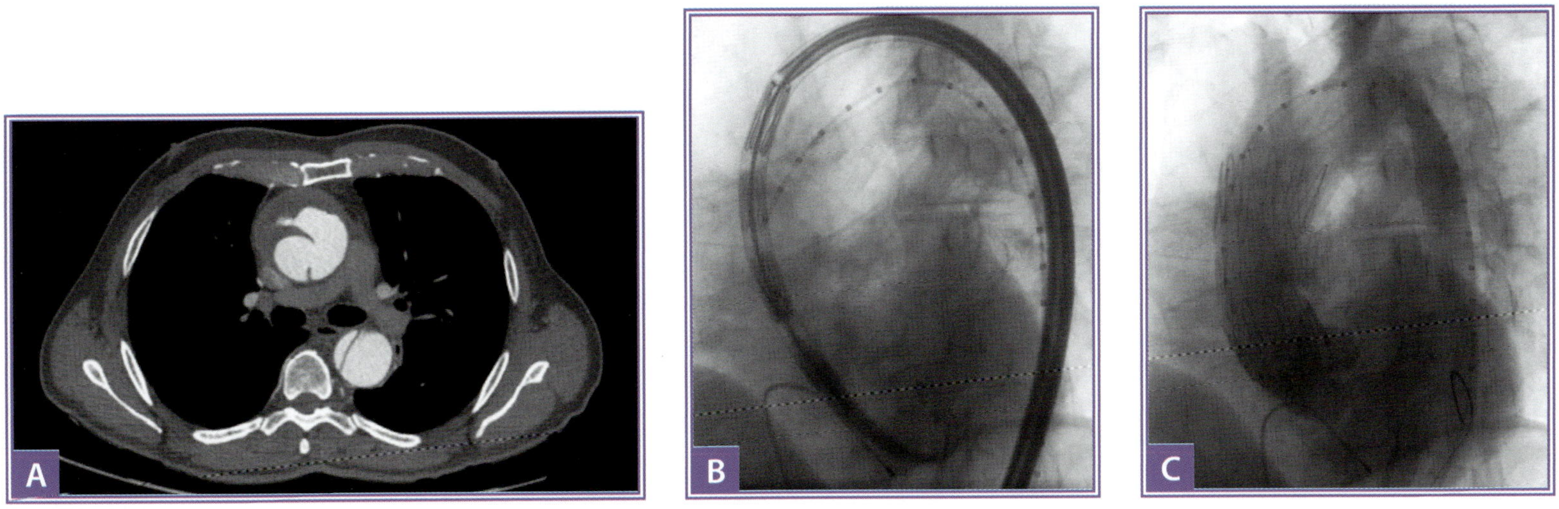

Fig. 16.10 **A**, CT scan demonstrating proximal tear. **B**, Adequate positioning of the graft. **C**, Final angiogram, demonstrating complete seal.

The international experience is still very limited given that only exceptional cases are treated in a total endovascular manner. There are many issues such as branch patency, presence of endoleaks, aortic conformation that are being put under evaluation. The follow-ups on patency of these total arch replacement are still very limited.

16.7 Perspectives

Many companies are developing newer grafts that are able to address physiological demands concerning arch pathologies. Today, in order to manufacture a proper arch graft it is necessary to wait 6 to 8 weeks. This condition imposes a limitation for emergency repairs.

Most companies today are developing branched device, pursuing the revascularization of the left subclavian artery. It has been proven that the vertebral artery is very important to the irrigation of the medulla specially when considering extensive coverage of the aorta.

Device alignment and capability of conforming to aortic structure is crucial to obtain good results. With experience better adapting devices, with auto aligning features, may be warranted.

To avoid lower limb ischemia as well as other complications, and considering the close proximity to the aortic valve, a non-traumatic delivery systems is very important.

Despite significant efforts to minimize the profile of the device by using low profile graft fabric and stents the sheath size is 24 Fr. These large profiles have been associated with increased access site complications. In the future smaller profiles certainly will be available.

With the advance of image fusion, precise identification of the tears and re-entries can be done, resulting in a more directed strategy with better results and less covering of the aorta.

Our group has recently done a case, where the patient presented with a Type A AD that extended throughout the aorta. With adequate imaging we were able to identify a tear in the ascending aorta. With the positioning of a proximal cuff we were able to seal the dissection and expand the true lumen (Fig. 16.10).

16.8 Conclusion

With growing endovascular demands, surgeons are gaining more experience and recent complication rates have been decreasing, thus demonstrating to be a viable option for patients specially those with prohibitive risk.

As with any new therapy, it takes time to establish itself as first line treatment. International experience lack long-term follow-up. Key issues such as patency of the branches, presence of endoleaks, are still being studied and analysed.

More multicentric studies are warranted to address these issues. Maybe in the future the indications for total arch repair might broaden more. Meanwhile we understand that, although feasible, it carries caveats that do need improvement.

REFERENCES

1) Myrme IT, Lai DT, Miller DC. Can the principles of evidence-based medicine be applied to the treatment of aortic dissections? Eur J Cardiothorac Surg 2004; 25: 236-45.
2) Fattouch K, Sampognaro R, Navarra E, et al. Long-term results after repair of type A acute aortic dissection according to false lumen patency. Ann Thorac Surg 2009; 88: 1244-50.
3) Viswanathan S, Agrawal V, Parameshwarappa SK, Savlania A, Kumar S, Madathipat U. Hybrid strategy for residual arch and thoracic aortic dissection following acute type A aortic dissection repair. Case Rep Vasc Med 2014; 2014: 165425.
4) Haulon S, Greenberg RK, Spear R, et al. Global experience with inner branched arched endograft. J Thorac Cardiovasc Surg 2014; 148(4): 1709-16.
5) Chiesa R, Melissano G, Tshomba Y, et al. Endovascular treatment of aortic arch aneurysms. J Vasc Bras 2008; 7(2): 90-8.
6) Ferreira M, Lanziotti L, Monteiro M, Abuhadba G. The arch and beyond: bare stents in the ascending aorta. J Endovasc Ther 2009; 16(3): 310-13.
7) Greenberg RK, Clair D, Srivastava S, et al. Should patients with challenging anatomy be offered endovascular aneurysm repair? J Vasc Surg 2003; 38: 990-6.
8) Cheng S. Arch debranching is best (Debate aortic arch aneurysms). Endovascular Today 2014; 13(11): 74-6.
9) Inoue K, Hosokawa H, Iwase T, et al. Aortic arch reconstruction by transluminally placed endovascular branched stent graft. Circulation 1999; 100(19 Suppl): II316-21.
10) Chuter TA, Schneider DB, Reilly LM, Lobo EP, Messina LM. Modular branched stent graft for endovascular repair of aortic arch aneurysm and dissection. J Vasc Surg 2003; 38(4): 859-63.
11) Ferreira M, Chuter T, Hartley D, et al. Hybrid repair of aortic arch aneurysms: a totally extrathoracic approach with branched endografts in two patients. Vascular 2007; 15: 79-83.
12) Neequaye S, Abraham CZ. Total endograft replacement of aortic arch. Ann Cardiothorac Surg 2013; 2(3): 362-6.
13) Ramponi F, Stephen MS, Wilson MK, Vallely MP. Think differently: trans-apical platform for TEVAR. Ann Cardiothorac Surg 2012; 1(3): 412-6.
14) Iturra A, Pochettino A. Should the dissected aortic arch be replaced in acute type A dissection? The Mayo Clinic perspective. Ann Cardiothorac Surg 2013; 2(2): 202-4.
15) Urbanski PP, Siebel A, Zacher M, Hacker RW. Is extended aortic replacement in acute type A dissection justifiable? Ann Thorac Surg 2003; 75: 525-9.
16) Hirotani T, Nakamichi T, Munakata M, et al. Routine extended graft replacement for an acute type A aortic dissection and the patency of the residual false channel. Ann Thorac Surg 2003; 76: 1957-61.
17) Watanuki H, Ogino H, Minatoya K, et al. Is emergency total arch replacement with a modified elephant trunk technique justified for acute type A aortic dissection? Ann Thorac Surg 2007; 84: 1585-91.
18) Kim JB, Chung CH, Moon DH, et al. Total arch repair versus hemiarch repair in the management of acute DeBakey type I aortic dissection. Eur J Cardiothorac Surg 2011; 40: 881-7.
19) Chiesa R, Melissano G, Tshomba Y, et al. Ten years of endovascular aortic arch repair. J Endovasc Ther 2010; 17(1): 1-11.
20) Tsilimparis N, Debus ES, von Kodolitsch Y, et al. Branched versus fenestrated endografts for endovascular repair of aortic arch lesions. J Vasc Surg 2016; 64(3): 592-9.

17

Aortic intramural hematoma and penetrating atherosclerotic ulcer

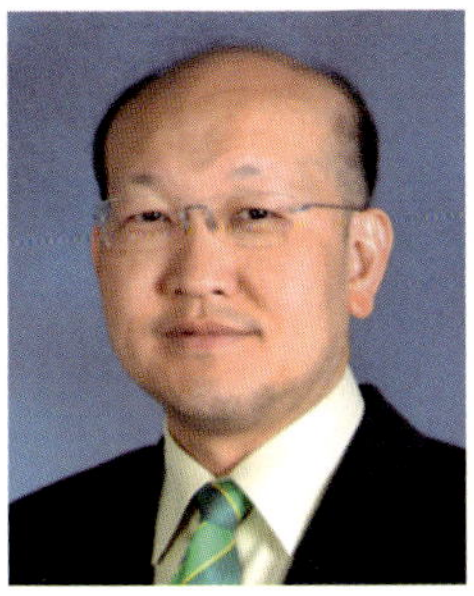

Worawong Slisatkorn, Wanchai Wongkornrat and Teerawoot Jantarawan

17.1 Aortic intramural hematoma

17.1.1 Definition

Aortic intramural hematoma (IMH) is defined as aortic wall dissection without detectible intimal tear and lack of blood flow in the false lumen.

17.1.2 Etiology

IMH is histologically believed to originate from ruptured vasa vasorum within the outer third of aortic media. Krukenberg reported the first case of aortic wall dissection without an intimal tear in 1920 [1]. However, there are increasing reports of intimomedial tears found at time of surgery that were not demonstrated at preoperative imaging and it is not clear whether it is the true pathogenesis rather than vasa vasorum rupture [2, 3]. Some consider IMH as a subtype of aortic dissection (AD) and propose the use of the term "thrombosed-type aortic dissection or aortic dissection with a closed and thrombosed false lumen" [4-6]. The location of the media dissection in IMH is closer to the adventitial side when compared to its location in acute AD. This may explain why IMH has no re-entry tear and is more likely to rupture and why AD has a re-entry tear [7]. IMH may occur spontaneously in elderly and hypertensive patients or as secondary phenomenon after the rupture of an atheromatous plaque through the internal elastic lamina and the formation of a penetrating atherosclerotic ulcer allowing extravasation of blood into the aortic wall [8].

17.1.3 Incidence

The incidence of IMH was reported to be 10-30% of all acute aortic syndromes [9-11]. It appears to be significant higher in Asian than in European and North American countries. IMH

Worawong Slisatkorn (wslisatkorn@gmail.com)
Faculty of Medicine Siriraj Hospital, Mahidol University,
Bangkok, Thailand

G. Melissano - R. Chiesa (eds), Aortic Dissection patients true stories and the innovations that saved their lives

occurs in older patients compared to acute AD (mean age 69-70 vs. 63 years) and more frequently in female patients (56% vs. 44%) [12, 13]. The majority of IMH lesions occurred in the descending aorta (67%) [12]. The incidence of Type A IMH (ascending aorta) relative to classic AD in Asian, Western countries and International Registry of Acute Aortic Dissection (IRAD) is 25.5%, 10.9% and 3.5%, respectively [14-17].

17.1.4 Natural history and prognostic factors

The natural history of IMH is variable and not clearly known. It may spontaneously regress (10%), remain stable, enlarge or progress to aneurysm or dissection and rupture. Conversion of the IMH to classic AD occurs in 3-14% of cases involving descending aorta and 11-88% in cases involving ascending aorta [18]. Risk of rupture is higher than in AD, but less frequent in organ malperfusion and aortic insufficiency, probably because false lumen in IMH is closer to adventitia than that in acute AD and false lumen pressure is lower than true lumen pressure.

In the IRAD series, the in-hospital mortality of Type A IMH was similar to acute Type A AD [14]. Acute Type B IMH has an in-hospital mortality less than 10%, similar to that observed with acute Type B AD [18]. Stanford Type A IMH has a high risk of adverse event if maximal diameter is more than 48-55 mm [18-21], while Type B IMH is at high risk if maximal diameter exceeds 40-41 mm [22, 23].

Intramural blood pool (IBP) is an intramural contrast medium-filled pool with tiny intimal orifice (<2 mm in diameter). It can be found at multidetector computed tomography (CT) in patients with descending intramural hematoma more than 10 mm in thickness and may connect to the intercostal or lumbar artery. IBP is associated with benign clinical course that shows complete resorption or stability in 86% of patients [24]. IBP with larger transmural diameter and connected with intercostal or lumbar artery is associated with incomplete resorption.

Ulcer-like projection (ULP) is a localized blood-filled pouch protruding into the IMH with communication with the true lumen and its opening usually wide (>3 mm). It is usually not observed at the initial CT and more common in the ascending aorta. The focal intima usually demonstrated no atherosclerotic plaque, which was different from penetrating atherosclerotic ulcer (PAU). ULP represents a new intimal disruption and shows a poor prognosis.

Predictors of IMH complications in the acute phase are [25]:

1) persistent and recurrent pain despite aggressive medical treatment
2) difficult blood pressure control
3) ascending aortic involvement
4) maximum aortic diameter >50 mm
5) progressive maximum aortic wall thickness (>11 mm)
6) enlarge aortic diameter
7) recurrent pleural effusion
8) penetrating ulcer or ulcer-like projection secondary to localized dissection in the involved segment
9) detection of organ ischemia (brain, myocardium, bowel, kidneys, etc.).

17.1.5 Clinical presentation

IMH is one of the entities of acute aortic syndrome. The common presentation is acute chest pain with history of chronic hypertension. Malperfusion manifestation is less frequent than in acute dissection. Similar to AD, IMH is divided according to Stanford classification system:

Stanford Type A IMH involves the ascending aorta, with or without involvement of the descending aorta; Stanford Type B IMH includes lesions in aortic arch or descending aorta but does not involve the ascending aorta.

17.1.6 Diagnosis

IMH is diagnosed in the presence of a circular or crescent shaped thickening of >5 mm of aortic wall in the absence of detectible blood flow [25]. CT and magnetic resonance imaging (MRI) are the leading techniques for diagnosis classification of acute aortic IMH.

CT is widely used as the first modality of choice to detect thoracic aortic pathology because it is easily accessible, noninvasive and has rapid scan time. Nonenhanced CT demonstrates hyperattenuation crescentic or circular thickening of aortic wall, in a longitudinal, non-spiral fashion and displacement of intimal calcification in a curvilinear distribution. This is the hallmark of IMH (Fig. 17.1). Aortic lumen is rarely compromised and no intimal flap or enhancement of the aortic wall after contrast administration is observed, in contrast to AD [25] (Fig. 17.2). Decreasing of aortic luminal diameter in enhanced CT is often better appreciated on oblique or sagittal reformatted images and can be useful in differentiating IMH from contained aortic rupture which revealed diffuse enhancement of hematoma [3].

Subacute IMH may be isoattenuating relative to the blood pool in nonenhanced CT.

MRI has been found to be superior to CT in differentiation of IMH from atherosclerotic aorta, thrombus and thrombosed dissection. It may provide a determination of the age of hematoma, based on the signal characteristics of different degradation products of hemoglobin. Acute hemorrhage displays isointense or more intense signal compared with the aortic wall on T1-weighted images and high signal intensity on T2-weight images [26, 27]. Subacute hemorrhage appears with high signal intensity on T1 images and less signal intensity on T2 images.

Transesophageal echocardiography (TEE) is an excellent method to demonstrate circumferential or crescentic aortic wall thickening without intimal tear [28, 29].

Transthoracic echocardiography (TTE) alone is inadequate for detection of an acute IMH because of its low sensitivity (<40%) [30].

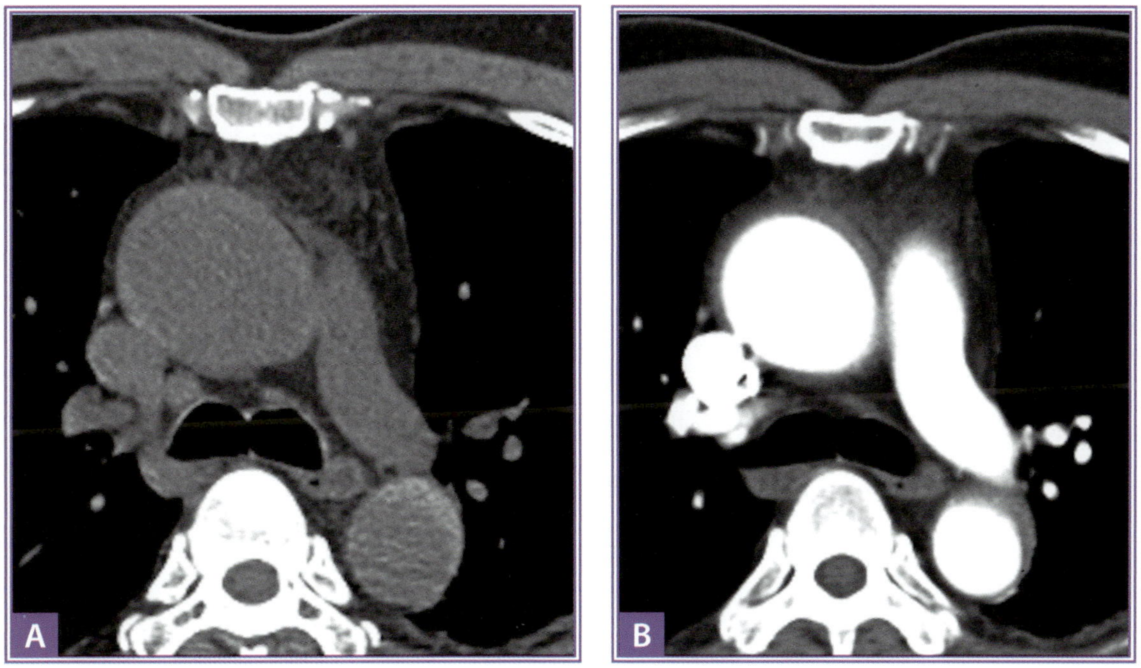

Fig. 17.1 Demonstrated acute aortic intramural hematoma Type A. **A**, Nonenhanced CT showed hyperattenuation crescentic thickening of aortic wall. **B**, Contrast enhanced CT showed no blood flow in aortic wall.

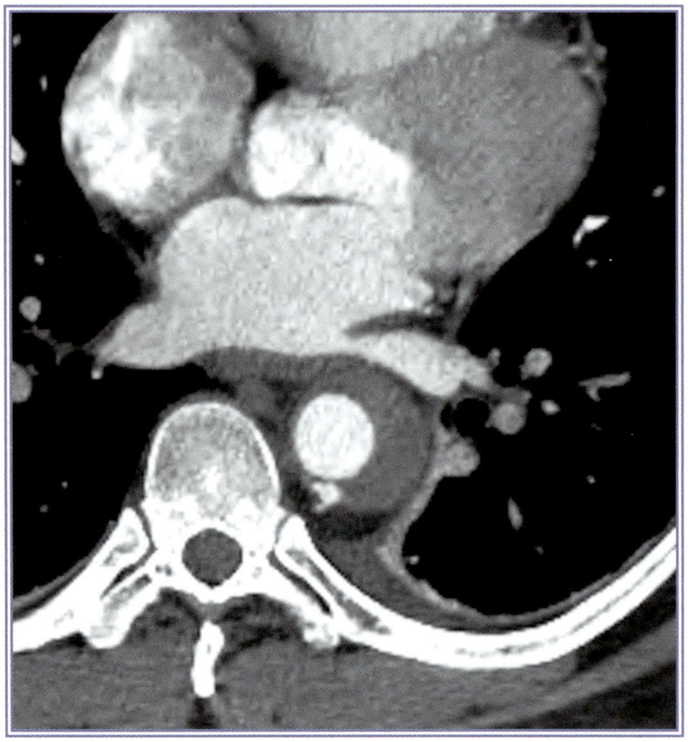

Fig. 17.2 Demonstrated acute aortic intramural hematoma Type B from contrast enhanced CT and intramural blood pool, which connects to intercostal artery.

17.1.7 Management

Initial management of IMH should be directed at decreasing aortic wall stress by controlling heart rate and blood pressure. Intravenous beta blockade should be initiated to target a heart rate of 60 beats per minutes or less. Non-dihydropyridine calcium channel blocking agents should be used as an alternative for rate control in patients with clear contraindications to beta blockade. Angiotensin-converting enzyme inhibitors and/or other vasodilators should be administered intravenously to reduce blood pressure if the systolic blood pressures remain greater than 120 mmHg [18].

Definite therapeutic management in acute IMH should be similar to that for acute AD [18, 25].

Type A intramural hematoma

Emergency surgery is indicated in complicated Type A IMH with pericardial effusion, periaortic hematoma or large aneurysm. Urgent surgery is required in most Type A IMH [12, 14, 25, 31]. Optimal medical therapy and repetitive imaging may be a reasonable option in elderly patients with significant comorbidities, particularly in the absence of aortic dilatation (<50 mm) and IMH thickness <11 mm [25]. Early medical treatment with alternative surgical conversion for selected, complicated cases is the management strategy in some Asian countries [16, 17, 20, 32].

Type B intramural hematoma

Initial medical therapy with blood pressure and pain control is the standard treatment for uncomplicated Type B IMH [14, 25, 33]. Thoracic endovascular repair is preferred rather than surgery in complicated Type B IMH with expansion despite optimal medical therapy and the disruption of intimal tear on contrast enhanced CT [25].

Patients with aortic dilatation or ulcer-like projection (ULP) should be followed closely and treated more aggressively if symptoms persist or reappear or progressive aortic dilatation is observed.

17.1.8 Outcomes

Type A intramural hematoma

From IRAD study, early medical treatment was 39.1%, overall hospital mortality was 20.7%, early medical and surgical hospital mortality were 33.3 and 42.9% [14].

In Eastern countries, early medical treatment was 80.8%, overall hospital mortality was 6.6%, early medical and surgical hospital mortality were 5.9 and 9.4% [6, 15, 16]. In less aggressive strategy centers, at 2-year follow-up, survival was 86.9%, progression to AD was 18%, need of surgical treatment 29.5% [32]. In more aggressive approach, no hospital mortality was observed and at 5-year, freedom from IMH related event was 92.6±4.1% [31].

Different clinical experience between Western and Eastern countries also affected the approach strategy and clinical outcomes in Type A IMH.

Type B intramural hematoma

In hospital mortality for Type B IMH was 0-7% [33, 34] and 5-year survival rate was 97% [34].

Overall long-term survivals for IMH were 75, 69, 64 and 39% at 1, 3, 5 and 10 years [12].

IMH patients had higher 5-year survival after surgery than AD patients (97.2% vs. 85.9%, $p = 0.006$) [13].

17.1.9 Long-term follow-up

Follow-up imaging by CT or MRI, chest plus abdomen and examination at 1, 3, 6, 9 and 12 months after discharge and annually thereafter was recommended similar to patients with classic AD to detect potential complications [14, 18].

Data from Siriraj Hospital, Mahidol University, between January 2007 and June 2016, shows that there were 9 IMH patients, 7 Type A IMH and 2 Type B IMH, who needed operation. Mean age was 63.5 years (range 44-79 years), 8 males and 1 female.

Our strategy is open repair in Type A IMH. There was no mortality, 1 patient developed ischemic stroke post ascending, arch and proximal descending replacement. One patient with thin Type A IMH and symptomatic descending AD had TEVAR performed at descending aorta. He developed classic Type A AD after 3 months and needed ascending and total arch replacement; no retrograde dissection was found intraoperatively. For 2 complicated Type B IMH, TEVAR was performed without mortality. Surgery in acute Type A IMH and TEVAR in indicated Type B IMH showed a good outcome in our experience.

17.1.10 Conclusion

IMH is an entity of acute aortic syndrome with higher incidence in old age and female and higher risk of rupture rate at presentation than in classic acute AD. CT, MRI and TEE can demonstrate crescentic or circular wall thickening without blood flow. Treatment strategies for IMH are similar to those for acute AD and depend on whether hematoma is Stanford Type A or Type B. Long-term follow-up with imaging was recommended to detect potential complication.

17.2 Penetrating atherosclerotic ulcer

Penetrating atherosclerotic ulcers (PAU) or penetrating aortic ulcer is an ulcerating atherosclerotic lesion that tunica intima and progresses into the tunica media [8]. In the early stages the lesions just invade the tunica intima and are asymptomatic. With further progression they invade the tunica media and lead to a hematoma of variable size within the tunica media. This is one of the causes of an acute aortic syndrome and related to AD and aortic intramural hematoma.

17.2.1 Epidemiology

PAU affects older patients with a history of hypertension, diabetes mellitus, smoking, coronary artery disease, chronic renal insufficiency and chronic obstructive pulmonary disease. PAU accounts for 7.5% of all cases of acute aortic syndrome. In about 50% of cases, there are concurrent aortic aneurysms [35].

17.2.2 Clinical presentation

Patients present with symptoms of an acute aortic syndrome, acute chest pain, described as tearing and migrating pain. Some of the patients with PAU are asymptomatic and the diagnosis is made incidentally. The PAU can resolve completely or stay stable, but they can also progress to the media forming AD, or progress to the adventitia becoming aortic saccular pseudoaneurysms and even spontaneous aortic rupture. The rate of rupture in PAU is 42.1%, higher than in IMH (35.3%) or in AD (3.6-7%) [35]. Usually the ulcer is found in the descending thoracic aorta in 61.2% of patients, 29.7% in the abdominal aorta, 6.8% in the aortic arch and 2.3% in the ascending aorta. PAU may present with multiple ulcers and several ranges of diameter and depth [36].

17.2.3 Investigation

Computed tomography angiography of the aorta

The typical finding is a contrast-filled, pouch-like protrusion of the aorta into the thickened aortic wall with absence of intimal flap and false lumen. Often there is extensive atherosclerosis apart from the ulceration [37] (Fig. 17.3).

Transesophageal echocardiography

Transesophageal echocardiography (TEE) demonstrates a localized, crater-like protrusion of the aortic lumen into the thickened aortic wall with absence of intimal flap and false lumen.

17.2.4 Treatment

Penetrating atherosclerotic ulcer at ascending aorta

Urgent or emergent open surgical repair is recommended for PAU at ascending aorta because of high risk of rupture.

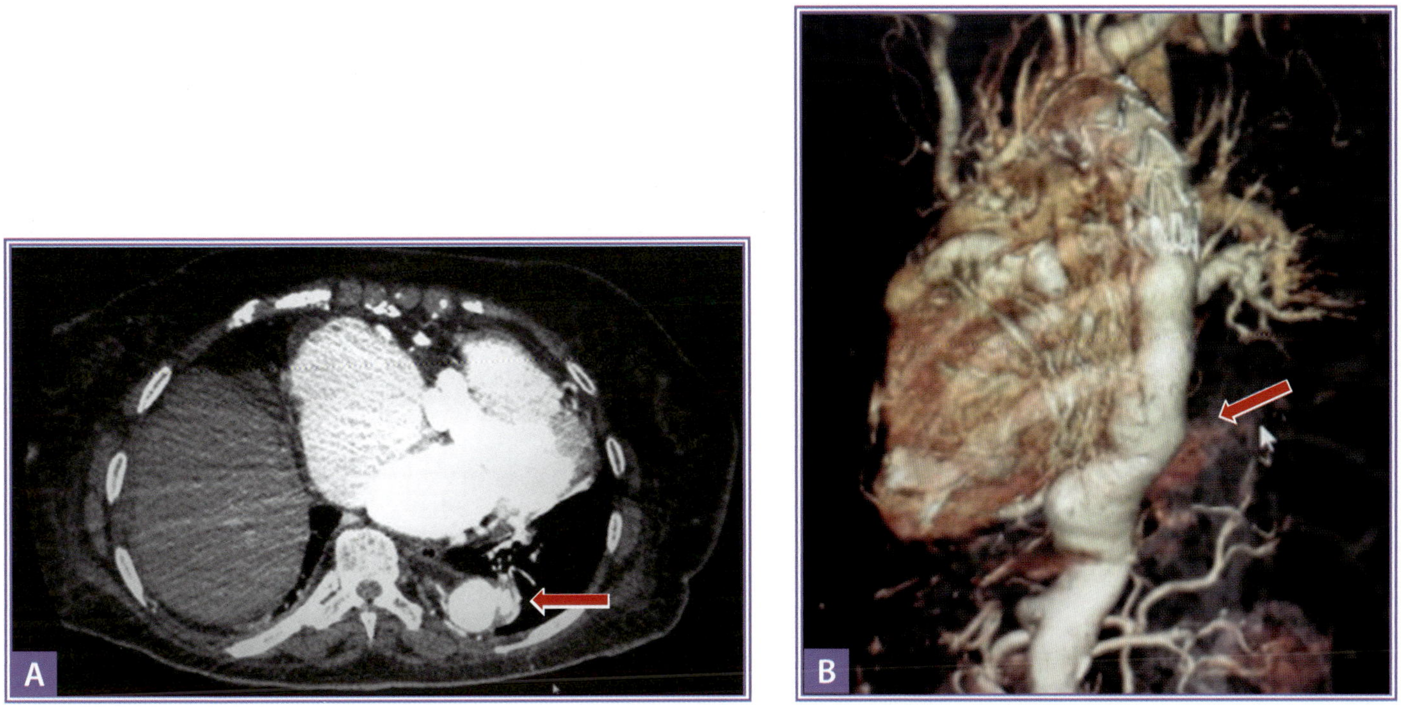

Fig. 17.3 A 77-year-old woman presenting with asymptomatic penetrating atherosclerotic ulcer of descending thoracic aorta after she underwent total aortic arch replacement and frozen elephant trunk 2 years before for treatment of Type A AD, DeBakey Type 2. CTA aorta shows PAU (arrow) filling with contrast media. **A**, Axial scan. **B**, 3D reconstruction.

Penetrating atherosclerotic ulcer at descending aorta

It is difficult to determine that PAU is the source of a patient's pain or it is just an incidental finding. However, associated pleural effusion correlates with complicated PAU. Asymptomatic PAU at descending aorta is initially treated with antihypertensive drug with closed CTA aorta follow-up, which is important to prevent aortic complications. Increasing diameter and depth of the ulcer is a sign of PAU progression. For patients with symptomatic PAU at descending aorta or with signs of progression, open surgical repair or thoracic endovascular aortic repair (TEVAR) become necessary (Fig. 17.4).

Many successful TEVAR have been reported [18, 25]. This method offers the possibility to treat patients who are not suitable for open surgical repair, especially older and high comorbidity patient. The endovascular device has developed over the years, including the smaller size of the delivery systems, the better quality and design of stent graft and the variety of size of stent graft. However, CTA aorta follow-up is important to detect complications after treatment with TEVAR (Fig. 17.5).

In 2010 ACCF/AHA/AATS/ACR/ASA/SCA/SCAI/SIR/STS/SVM Guidelines for the Diagnosis and Management of Patients with Thoracic Aortic Disease [18], localized lesions and lesions involving a limited segment of the aorta are mentioned. They included uncomplicated aortic ulcers and saccular aneurysms of the aorta. The guideline recommended treatment as saccular aneurysms based on their maximum diameter and clinical feature. These lesions can be treated with open surgical repair or TEVAR. According to the summary of the Society of Thoracic Surgeons, the classification of recommendation and level of evidence was IIa/C for TEVAR in symptomatic PAU (benefit >risk) and III/C for asymptomatic PAU (risk >benefit).

In the study by Jánosi RA et al. [38], they analyzed an 11-year single-center experience of complicated PAU treatment using TEVAR. This study included 63 patients with complicated PAU (42 symptomatic, 22 with rupture). The PAUs were located in the aortic arch (n = 11), the

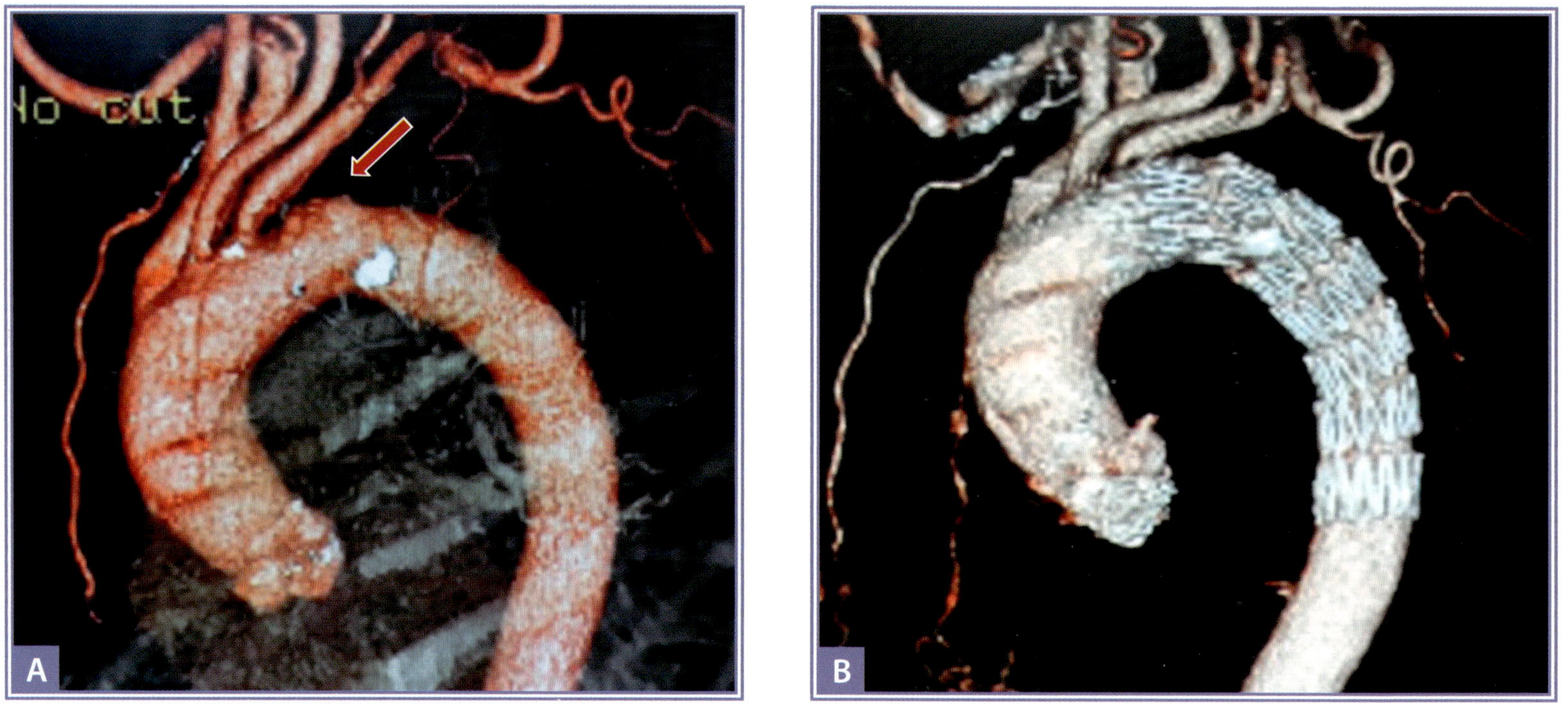

Fig. 17.4 **A**, A 73-year-old woman presenting with acute chest pain. CTA aorta shows ruptured aorta due to PAU at proximal descending thoracic aorta (arrow). **B**, Post TEVAR CTA aorta shows no endoleak complication.

descending thoracic aorta (n = 43), and the thoracoabdominal aorta (n = 9). Technical success was 98.4%. One patient had a type I endoleak in the aortic arch. No patient experienced spinal cord ischemia. Five (7.9%) patients died in-hospital; 3 had cardiac complications, 1 died from aortic rupture, and 1 died from septic shock. Mean follow-up was 45.6±47.2 months; during follow-up 19.0% of patients needed a secondary intervention because of late endoleaks (6.3%) or new complications due to disease progression (12.6%). Multivariate analysis indicated that a PAU depth >15 mm was an independent predictor of mortality (p = 0.03).

In the literature review by D'Annoville et al. [39], they studied the results of TEVAR for PAU patients. Thirty-one articles were included in this literature, and 310 PAU patients treated by TEVAR. 9% were asymptomatic PAU. 76% were a single PAU, located in the descending thoracic aorta (81%), with associated intramural hematoma in 45%. The technical success of TEVAR was 98.3%. Surgical conversion was required in 1 patient. The overall 30-day mortality was 4.8%. The endoleak was 8% and access problem was 16.1%. After a mean follow-up of 17.7

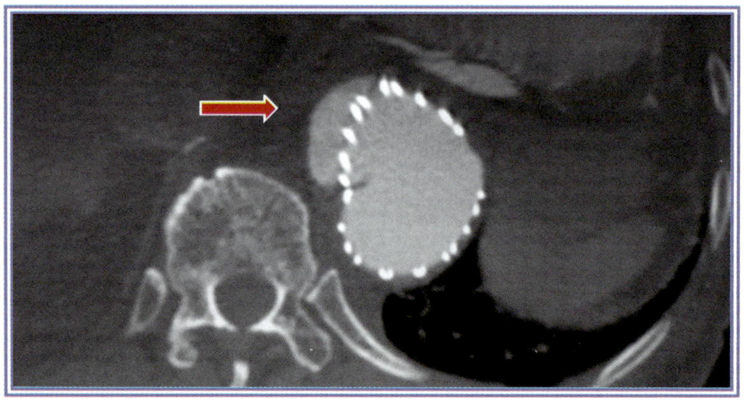

Fig. 17.5 CTA aorta shows endoleak at distal end of stent graft (arrow), which is a complication after TEVAR.

months (range, 1 to 52), the all-cause mortality was 22.9%, and the aortic-related mortality was 4.1%. During follow-up, new endoleak and ulcer recurrence were 5.4 and 4.5% respectively.

In the study by Clough RE et al. [40], TEVAR showed similar late results in the high-risk PAU patients when compared to open surgical repair. The 5-year freedom from cardiovascular events rate was 67.8%. However, TEVAR resulted in a higher rate of perioperative stroke (8.4% vs. 16.2%).

In 2014 ESC Guidelines on the diagnosis and treatment of aortic diseases [25], the indication for treatment is symptomatic PAU including recurrent and refractory pain, signs of contained rupture, rapidly growing aortic ulcer, periaortic hematoma, or pleural effusion. There is no randomized study to compare open surgical repair and TEVAR. The choice of treatment is based on anatomical features of the aorta, clinical presentation, and comorbidities. If the anatomical feature of the aorta is suitable for endovascular stenting and the patients are poor candidates for open surgical repair due to old age or severe comorbidities, TEVAR should be the treatment of choice. The classification of recommendation and level of evidence was IIa/C (benefit >risk) for TEVAR in symptomatic PAU, but there is no classification of recommendation and level of evidence for asymptomatic PAU.

However, asymptomatic PAU patients with an ulcer diameter >20 mm and/or an ulcer depth >20 mm are associated with high risk of disease progression and should be evaluated as possible candidate for early endovascular or surgical repair [41].

Data from Siriraj Hospital, between January 2007 and June 2016, shows that 26 patients, with mean age of 67.31 years (29-82 years), 18 males and 8 female, were diagnosed with penetrating atherosclerotic ulcer. PAU was the principle diagnosis for 14 cases, the left 12 cases were associated diagnosis. Eleven cases underwent emergency operation and 15 cases were in elective operation. The location of PAU was at descending aorta in 21 cases (80.7%), aortic arch in 4 cases (15.3%) and ascending aorta in 1 case (3.8%). The operation included 15 TEVAR, 5 open surgical repair and 7 hybrid surgery. There was 1 death (3.8%) from hybrid group and the cause of death was aspiration pneumonia and sepsis. One case of endoleak was observed (3.8%), requiring re-TEVAR. The mean ICU (intensive care unit) stay was 4.5 days, the mean hospital stay was 11.7 days.

17.2.5 Conclusion

Penetrating atherosclerotic ulcers is an ulcerating atherosclerotic lesion. The patients with PAU can be asymptomatic or symptomatic with chest pain related to AD, pseudoaneurysm or aortic rupture. CTA aorta is the gold standard for investigation. Penetrating atherosclerotic ulcers at ascending aorta should be treated with urgent or emergent open surgical repair because of high risk of rupture. Symptomatic PAU at descending aorta including recurrent and refractory pain, signs of contained rupture, rapidly growing aortic ulcer, periaortic hematoma, or pleural effusion should be treated with TEVAR or open surgical repair. Asymptomatic small PAU at descending aorta can initially be treated with antihypertensive drug with closed CTA aorta follow-up until an ulcer diameter >20 mm and/or an ulcer depth >20 mm, which are associated with risk of rupture, are observed, when early endovascular or surgical aortic repair should be considered.

REFERENCES

1) Krukenberg E. Beiträge zur Frage des Aneurysma dissecans. Beitr Pathol Anat Allg Pathol 1920; 67: 329-51.
2) Mukohara N. Intramural hematoma - contradiction to the theory of rupture of the vasa vasorum at onset. Ann Thorac Cardiovasc Surg 2014; 20: 949-50.
3) Gutschow SE, Walker CM, Martinez-Jimenez S, Rosado-de-Christensen ML, Stowell J, Kunin JR. Emerging concepts in intramural hematoma imaging. Radiographics 2016; 36: 660-74.

4) Kitai T, Kaji S, Yamamuro A, et al. Detection of intimal defect by 64-row multidetector computed tomography in patients with acute aortic intramural hematoma. Circulation 2011; 124(11 suppl): S174-8.
5) Uchida K, Imoto K, Karube N, et al. Intramural haematoma should be referred to as thrombosed-type aortic dissection. Eur J Cardiothorac Surg 2013; 44: 366-9.
6) Song JK. Update in acute aortic syndrome: intramural hematoma and incomplete dissection as new disease entities. J Cardiol 2014; 64: 153-161.
7) Kan CB, Chang RY, Chang JP. Optimal initial treatment and clinical outcome of Type A aortic intramural hematoma: a clinical review. Eur J Cardiothorac Surg 2008; 33(6): 1002-6.
8) Stanson AW, Kazmier FJ, Hollier LH, et al. Penetrating atherosclerotic ulcer of the thoracic aorta: natural history and clinicopathologic correlations. Ann Vasc Surg 1986; 15-23.
9) Yamada T, Tada S, Harada J. Acute aortic dissection without intimal rupture: diagnosis with MR imaging and CT. Radiology 1988; 168: 347-52.
10) Nienaber CA, von Kodolitsch Y, Peterson B, et al. Intramural hemorrhage of the thoracic aorta. Diagnostic and therapeutic implications. Circulation 1995; 92: 1465-72.
11) Harris KM, Braverman AC, Gutierrez FR, Barzilai B, Dávila-Román VG. Transesophageal echocardiographic and clinical features of aortic intramural hematoma. J Thorac Cardiovasc Surg 1997; 114: 619-26.
12) Chou AS, Ziganshin BA, Charilaou P, Tranquilli M, Rizzo JA, Elefteriades JA. Long-term behavior of aortic intramural hematomas and penetrating ulcers. J Thorac Cardiovasc Surg 2016; 151: 361-73.
13) Matsushita A, Fukui T, Tabata M, Sato Y, Takanashi S. Preoperative characteristics and surgical outcomes of acute intramural hematoma involving the ascending aorta: a propensity score-matched analysis. J Thorac Cardiovasc Surg 2016; 151: 351-8.
14) Evangelista A, Mukherjee D, Mehta RH, et al. Acute intramural hematoma of the aorta: a mystery in evolution. Circulation 2005; 111: 1063-70.
15) Pelzel JM, Braverman AC, Hirsch AT, Harris KM. International heterogeneity in diagnostic frequency and clinical outcomes of ascending aortic intramural hematoma. J Am Soc Echocardiogr 2007; 20: 1260-8.
16) Kitai T, Kaji S, Yamamuro A, et al. Clinical outcomes of medical therapy and timely operation in initially diagnosed type A aortic intramural hematoma: a 20-year experience. Circulation 2009; 120(suppl1): S292-8.
17) Song JK, Yim JH, Ahn JM, et al. Outcomes of patients with type A aortic intramural hematoma. Circulation 2009; 120: 2046-52.
18) Hiratzka LF, Bakris GL, Beckman JA, et al. 2010 ACCF/AHA/AATS/ACR/ASA/SCA/SCAI/SIR/STS/SVM guidelines for the diagnosis and management of patients with Thoracic Aortic Disease: a report of the American College of Cardiology Foundation/American Heart Association Task Force on Practice Guidelines, American Association for Thoracic Surgery, American College of Radiology, American Stroke Association, Society of Cardiovascular Anesthesiologists, Society for Cardiovascular Angiography and Interventions, Society of Intervention Radiology, Society of Thoracic Surgeons, and Society of Vascular Medicine. Circulation 2010; 121: 266-369.
19) von Kodolitsch Y, Csösz SK, Koschyk DH, et al. Intramural hematoma of the aorta: predictors of progression to dissection and rupture. Circulation 2003; 107: 1158-63.
20) Sawaki S, Hirate Y, Ashida S, Takanohashi A, Yagami K, Usui M. Clinical outcomes of medical treatment of acute type A intramural hematoma. Asian Cardiovasc Thorac Ann 2010; 18: 354-9.
21) Park KH, Lim C, Choi JH, et al. Prevalence of aortic intimal defect in surgically treated acute type A intramural hematoma. Ann Thorac Surg 2008; 86: 1494-500.
22) Sueyoshi E, Sakamoto I, Uetani M, Matsuoka Y. CT analysis of growth rate of aortic diameter affected by acute type B aortic intramural hematoma. AJR Am J Roentgenol 2006; 186(6 suppl 2): S414-S420.
23) Sueyoshi E, Imada T, Sakamoto I, Matsuoka Y, Hayashi K. Analysis of predictive factors for progression of type B aortic intramural hematoma with computed tomography. J Vasc Surg 2002; 35: 1179-83.
24) Wu MT, Wang YC, Huang YL, et al. Intramural blood pools accompanying aortic intramural hematoma: CT appearance and natural course. Radiology 2011; 258: 705-13.
25) Erbel R, Aboyans V, Boileau C, et al. 2014 ESC Guidelines on the diagnosis and treatment of aortic diseases. Document covering acute and chronic aortic diseases of the thoracic and abdominal aorta of the adult. The Task Force for the Diagnosis and Treatment of Aortic Diseases of the European Society of Cardiology (ESC). Eur Heart J 2014; 35: 2873-926.
26) Murray JG, Manisali M, Flamm SD, et al. Intramural hematoma of the thoracic aorta: MR image findings and their prognostic implications. Radiology 1997; 204: 349-55.
27) Litmanovich D, Bankier AA, Cantin L, Raptopoulos V, Boiselle PM. CT and MRI in the diseases of the aorta. AJR Am J Roentgenol 2009; 193: 928-40.
28) Mohr-Kahaly S, Erbel R, Kearny P, Puth M, Meyer J. Aortic intramural hemorrhage visualized by transesophageal echocardiography: findings and prognostic implications. J Am Coll Cardiol 1994; 23: 658-64.
29) Song JK. Diagnosis of aortic intramural hematoma. Heart 2004; 90: 368-71.
30) Cecconi M, Chirillo F, Costantini C, et al. The role of transthoracic echocardiography in the diagnosis and management of acute type A aortic syndrome. Am Heart J 2012; 163: 112-8.

31) Shimokawa T, Ozawa N, Takanashi S, Itoh T. Intermediate-term results of surgical treatment of acute intramural hematoma involving the ascending aorta. Ann Thorac Surg 2008; 83: 982-6.
32) Choi YJ, Son JW, Lee SH, et al. Treatment patterns and their outcomes of acute aortic intramural hematoma in real world: multicenter registry for aortic intramural hematoma. BMC Cardiovasc Disord 2014; 14: 103.
33) Tolenaar JL, Harris KM, Upchurch GR, et al. The differences and similarities between intramural hematoma of the descending aorta and acute type B dissection. J Vasc Surg 2013; 58: 1498-504.
34) Kaji S, Akasa T, Katayama M, et al. Long-term prognosis of patients with type B aortic intramural hematoma. Circulation 2003; 108(suppl1): II307-11.
35) Coady MA, Rizzo JA, Elefteriades JA. Pathologic variants of thoracic aortic dissections. Penetrating atherosclerotic ulcers and intramural hematomas. Cardiol Clin 1999; 17: 637-57.
36) Nauta F, Kamman A, Trimarchi S. Penetrating aortic ulcer and intramural hematoma, an update on how to differentiate and manage two potentially devastating diagnoses. Endovasc today 2014; 13: 11.
37) Coady MA, Rizzo JA, Hammond GL, Pierce JG, Kopf GS, Elefteriades JA. Penetrating ulcer of the thoracic aorta: what is it? How do we recognize it? How do we manage it? J Vasc Surg 1998; 27: 1006-15.
38) Jánosi RA, Gorla R, Tsagakis K, et al. Thoracic endovascular repair of complicated penetrating aortic ulcer: an 11-year single-center experience. J Endovasc Ther 2016; 23: 150-9.
39) D'Annoville T, Ozdemir BA, Alric P, Marty-Ané CH, Canaud L. Thoracic endovascular aortic repair for penetrating aortic ulcer: literature review. Ann Thorac Surg 2016; 101: 2272-8.
40) Clough RE, Mani K, Lyons OT, et al. Endovascular treatment of acute aortic syndrome. J Vasc Surg 2011; 54: 1580-87.
41) Nathan DP, Boonn W, Lai E, et al. Presentation, complications, and natural history of penetrating atherosclerotic ulcer disease. J Vasc Surg 2012; 55: 10-15.

18

Type B aortic dissection complicated by visceral ischemia

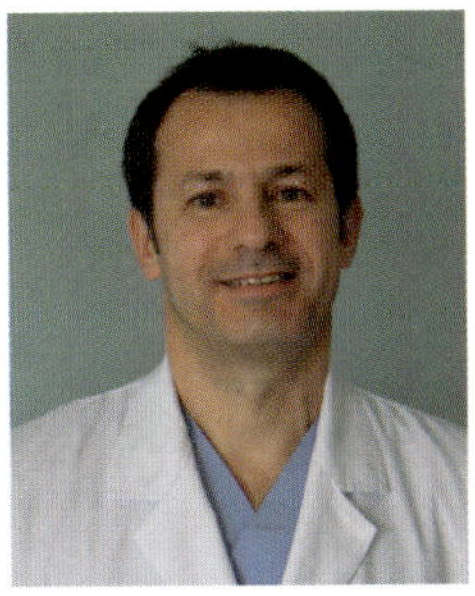

Santi Trimarchi, Hector W.L. de Beaufort and Arnoud V. Kamman

18.1 Introduction

Acute Type B aortic dissection (AD) can lead to obstruction of aortic branch vessels, causing ischemia of the spinal cord, lower extremities, or vital abdominal organs. Obstruction of the celiac and/or mesenteric arteries leads to visceral ischemia, which is present in 7-8% of all acute Type B AD patients [1, 2]. It is one of the most lethal complications of AD, and a timely diagnosis is crucial to increase the chances of survival. Endovascular methods are the most frequently adopted in order to restore blood flow to the intestines, while open surgical procedures may be used in those rare cases of endovascular management failure. The outcomes of this aortic catastrophe are humbling, with overall mortality rates of 30% [1]. Data from the International Registry of Acute Aortic Dissection (IRAD) suggest that visceral ischemia is responsible for 15% of the mortality observed with acute AD [3]. In this chapter, the presentation, management, and outcomes of this aortic catastrophe will be described.

18.2 Pathophysiology

Malperfusion syndromes can be due to dynamic or static branch vessel obstruction. In about 80% of cases, branch vessel obstruction is dynamic (Fig. 18.1). The pressure difference between false and true lumen causes movement of the intimal membrane over the origin of a branch vessel, compression of the true lumen, and vessel obstruction during part of the cardiac cycle (usually systole), while vessel perfusion is still present during diastole. Dynamic obstruction is affected by hemodynamic factors such as blood pressure, heart rate and peripheral resistance of the branch vessel. The percentage of aortic circumference that is dissected and distal communications between true and false lumen also impact dynamic obstruction. Regulation of these factors might reverse obstruction in some patients. However, in case of overt malperfusion syndrome, more invasive therapy aimed at re-establishing the aortic true lumen is necessary.

Santi Trimarchi (Santi.Trimarchi@grupposandonato.it)
Policlinico San Donato IRCCS, University of Milan,
Milan, Italy

G. Melissano - R. Chiesa (eds), Aortic Dissection patients true stories and the innovations that saved their lives

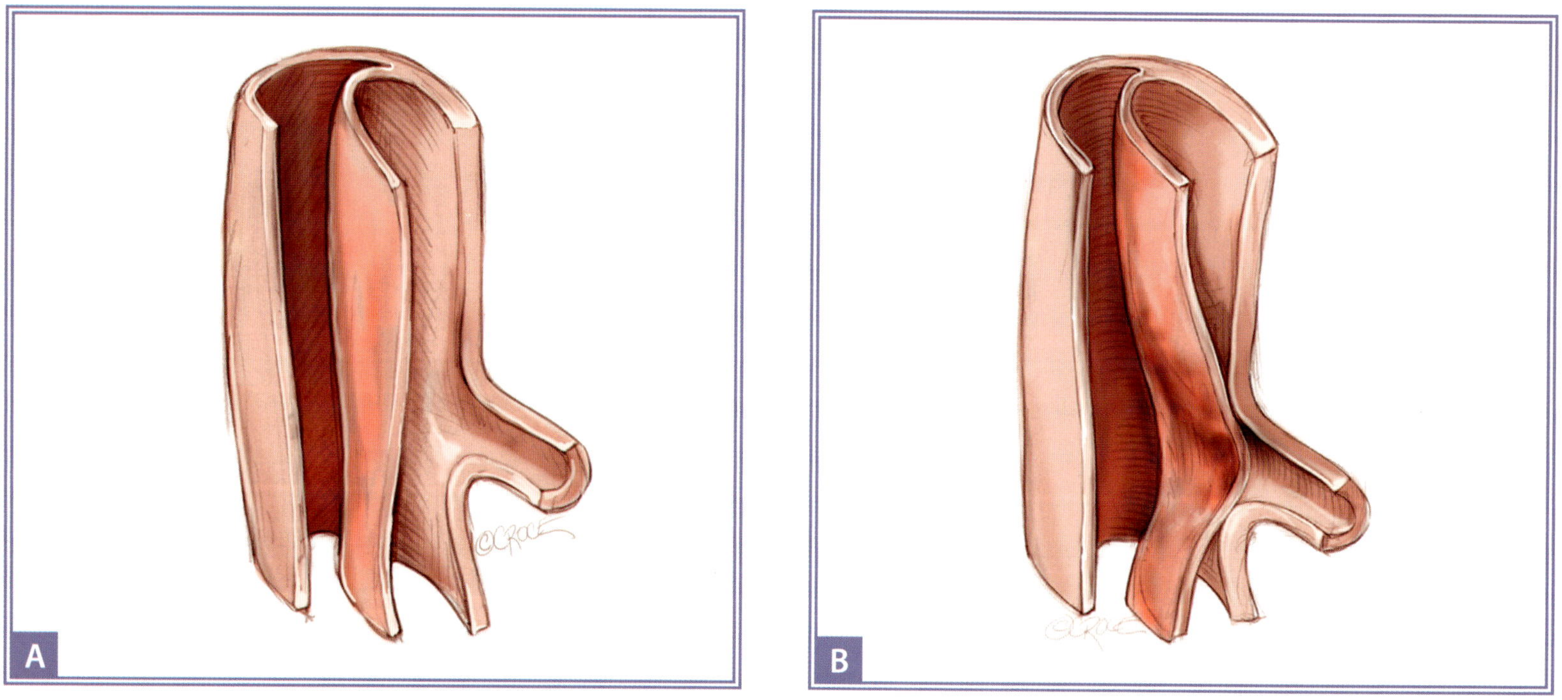

Fig. 18.1 In dynamic obstruction (**A**, **B**), the septum may prolapse into the vessel ostium during the cardiac cycle, and the compressed true lumen flow is inadequate to perfuse branch vessel ostia, which remain anatomically intact. Reproduced from [14], with permission.

Static obstructions are caused by extension of the intimal flap into the branch artery, which can be aggravated by distal arterial thrombosis due to stasis and false lumen hypercoagulability related to exposure of the adventitia and tunica media (Fig. 18.2). In these cases, revascularization of the branch vessel is necessary to restore end-organ perfusion.

Whether dynamic or static, the obstruction of the celiac and/or mesenteric arteries and consequent visceral ischemia leads to activation of an inflammatory cascade. These inflammatory molecules not only enhance local tissue damage, but cause negative systemic effects

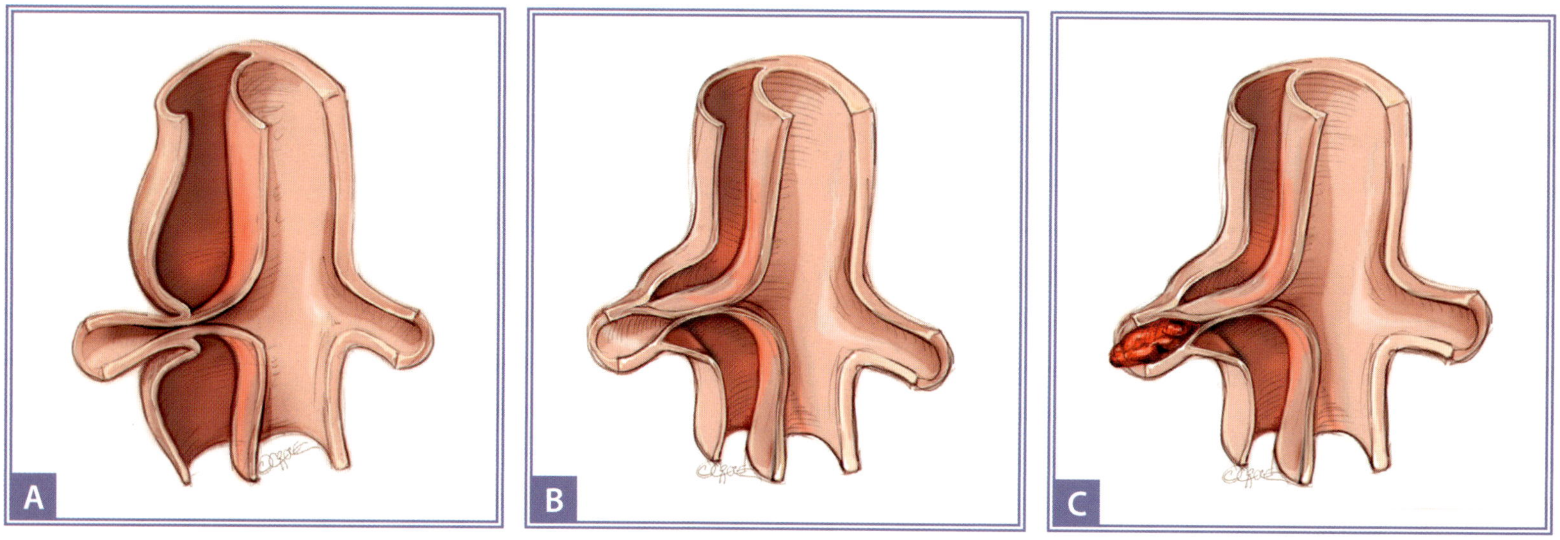

Fig. 18.2 Mechanism of static obstruction. **A**, Compression of the vessel by blind ends of the false lumen. **B**, Presence of true and false lumen in the vessel causing further compression. **C**, Thrombosis of the vessel distal to the compromised ostia. Reproduced from [14], with permission.

as well, particularly on the lungs. The intestinal ischemia-reperfusion injury that results from this inflammation depends on the duration of ischemia and may continue even after reversal of obstruction, thus negatively impacting operative success [4]. The risks related to prolonged visceral ischemia outweigh the risks of aortic rupture, possibly even in Type A AD. This has led to some controversy regarding the optimal treatment strategy in Type A AD [5] in terms of treating the patients initially with central open aortic repair or visceral aortic endovascular therapy.

18.3 Presentation

On average, Type B AD patients with visceral ischemia are younger than patients without visceral ischemia [1, 6]. Malperfusion due to AD can cause evident symptoms related to the affected end-organs. This might be more frequent in case of static malperfusion, while diagnosis can be delayed in cases of dynamic malperfusion, when signs and symptoms may be intermittent and of varying intensity, which may delay diagnosis, with all consequences that this entails. Abdominal pain is frequently the first manifestation of mesenteric malperfusion, which may also cause diarrhea or bloody defecation. Moreover, malperfusion syndromes of other organs are frequently present simultaneously to visceral ischemia. Limb ischemia has been reported in up to 28%, acute renal failure in 40%, and spinal cord ischemia in 5% of patients with visceral ischemia [1]. Symptoms related to those arterial beds can therefore be present; for example, femoral pulse deficits are seen in a third of patients with visceral ischemia, which is significantly more frequent than in Type B AD patients without visceral ischemia [1].

Subtle biochemical markers often precede symptoms. Raised serum levels of creatinine, amylase, bilirubin, liver enzymes, and lactates should increase suspicion of visceral ischemia. In many cases, biochemical changes may be absent in the early stage and develop when end-organ ischemia has led to irreversible damage and when intervention may come too late. Therefore, absence of such biochemical markers should not delay intervention if there is a strong suspicion of visceral malperfusion, for example in cases of peritonitis. Radiological evidence of visceral malperfusion syndrome includes true lumen compression, branch vessel dissection and thrombosis, and reduced late-phase visceral enhancement on computed tomography angiography (CTA) (Fig. 18.3).

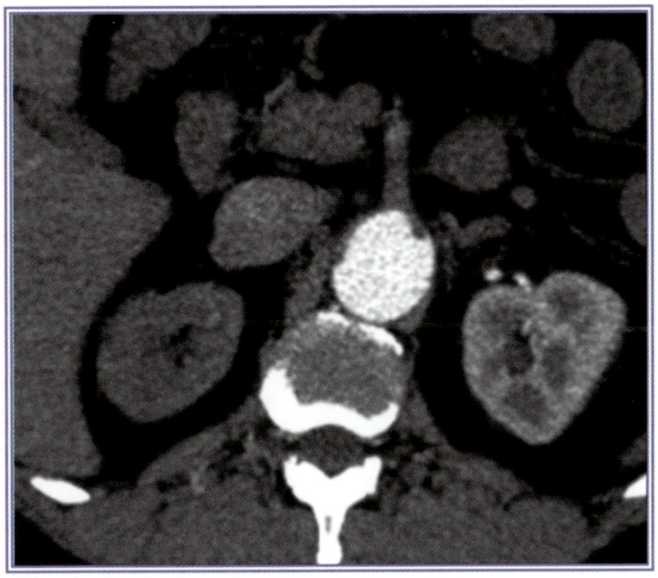

Fig. 18.3 Computed tomography angiography (CTA) image of visceral malperfusion syndrome.

18.4 Management options

There is overall consensus that thoracic endovascular aortic repair (TEVAR) is the first choice of treatment in acute complicated Type B AD patients [7]. By covering the proximal entry tear and expanding the true lumen, TEVAR can reverse celiac or mesenteric artery obstruction (Fig. 18.4). Additional branch vessel stenting may be necessary in 0-20% of these patients [8-10]. Thus, TEVAR effectively corrects mesenteric malperfusion in the setting of dynamic obstruction [8]. However, TEVAR can be associated with in-hospital mortality rates of 20-40% [9-11].

Furthermore, a number of TEVAR-specific complications may occur in a small percentage of AD patients, such as retrograde Type A AD and stent graft induced new entry tears. To decrease the risk of these complications, stent graft oversizing in Type B AD should not exceed 10%, and stent graft deployment should be avoided in the presence of an intramural hematoma in the proximal landing zone. There are still some concerns regarding late dilatation and reintervention rates. The use of a proximal stent graft in combination with a distal aortic bare metal stent (PETTICOAT – Provisional Extension To Induce Complete ATtachment – technique, Fig. 18.5) [12] and the use of dedicated stent grafts for dissection, some of these currently under development, may improve long-term outcomes of TEVAR in Type B AD.

Endovascular fenestration of the intimal flap is a valid alternative treatment option, if necessary accompanied by branch vessel stenting if static obstruction of a branch vessel is present.

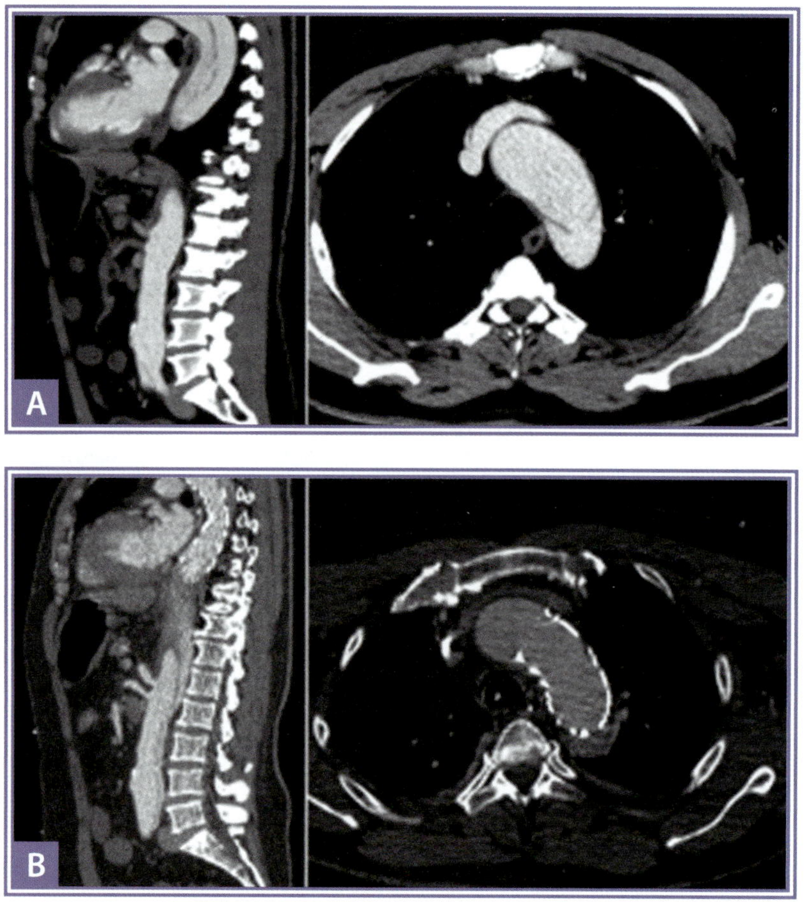

Fig. 18.4 Preoperative (**A**) and postoperative (**B**) computed tomography angiography images of a patient with visceral ischemia based on dynamic obstruction successfully treated by covering the proximal entry tear with a stent graft.

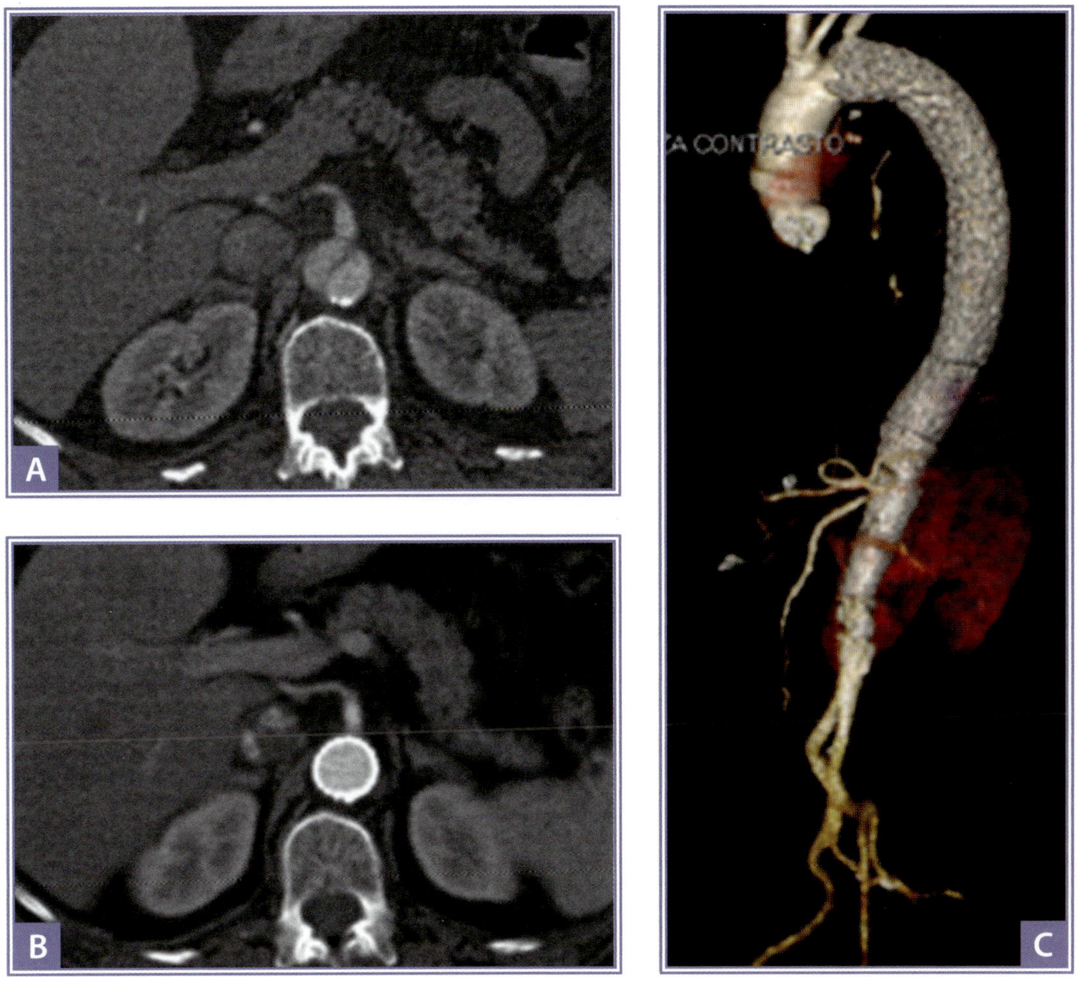

Fig. 18.5 **A**, Preoperative computed tomography angiography (CTA) image of a patient with mesenteric malperfusion syndrome. **B**, Postoperative CTA image after treatment with a proximal stent graft and distal bare metal stent (PETTICOAT technique) to reoppose the dissection flap. **C**, 3D reconstruction of the postoperative CTA scan.

In an experienced center, a 17% early mortality rate was noted after endovascular fenestration in a cohort of 69 Type B AD patients with malperfusion, of which 7% was due to aortic rupture and 10% due to malperfusion complications [13]. A downside of fenestration is the risk of late aortic dilatation. Long-term results show freedom from aortic rupture or aortic repair rates at 1, 5, and 8 years of 80.2, 67.7 and 54.2% [13].

In order to perform endovascular fenestration with or without branch vessel stenting, true and false lumen access must be obtained. Intravascular ultrasound is useful to distinguish the relationship of the intimal membrane with aortic branch vessels. Especially in cases of renal malperfusion, it is beneficial to decrease contrast burden by injecting iodated contrast only in selected branches to prove that the catheter is beyond the dissection [12]. Pressure measurements, comparing branch vessel pressure with aortic root pressure, provide further evidence of malperfusion if a pressure gradient is present between the two lumens. All aortic branches need to be visualized before intervention because relief of obstruction in one branch vessel may lead to changes in mobility of the intimal membrane and could thus lead to dynamic obstruction of other branch vessels. In case of static obstruction of a branch vessel, wire access into the distal true lumen of the vessel should be obtained. A self-expanding stent may then be deployed. This should be done before aortic fenestration, which leads to unpredictable changes of aortic flow and can make it difficult to regain access to branch vessels. After stenting of compromised branch vessels, fenestration of the aortic intimal membrane can be performed. This is usually done from the true lumen to the false lumen, the latter being larger. Re-entry tears, which are often present at the level of branch vessels, can be used as a starting point for further fenestration. If not, a first fenestration is made at the level of the obstructed artery using a stiff guidewire. A low profile catheter can then be advanced through the fenestration into the false lumen before an angioplasty balloon is used to enlarge the fenestration, eventually leading to the desired equalization of peak systolic pressures in true and false lumen. In some cases, an uncovered stent may be placed in the true lumen to preserve patency of the fenestration. Angioplasty balloons are superior to alternative fenestrating techniques such as the scissors technique or the use of a snare wire to pull the dissection flap down the aorta, because the latter carry a risk of circumferential separation of the dissection flap from the aortic wall causing aortic intussusception, and are no longer used [12].

In general, TEVAR is suitable for the majority of patients, and is especially valuable in patients with advanced age, aortic dilatation, and uncontrollable hypertension. Fenestration may be more appropriate than TEVAR in patients at an increased risk of spinal cord ischemia (i.e. previous abdominal aortic repair, left subclavian, vertebral, or iliac artery obliteration), in whom the false lumen feeds a large number of intercostal and lumbar vessels. Together, endovascular methods are chosen as treatment for almost 70% of patients with visceral ischemia enrolled in the IRAD in recent years [1].

The use of open surgery has been decreasing in favor of endovascular treatment options, and nowadays only a small percentage of patients is treated with open surgical methods [1]. Patients with peritonitis, refractory lactic acidosis, or hemodynamic instability due to ongoing intestinal malperfusion require immediate laparotomy for inspection of the intestines and, if needed, resection of necrotic tissue (Fig. 18.6). Delaying operative closure may be favorable to allow repeated bowel inspection at a later stage. Apart from this situation, open surgical methods should only be considered if endovascular options are contraindicated or have previously failed [7]. Contraindications to TEVAR, which have been reported to be infrequent, are mainly anatomical and include unsuitable access vessels or insufficient proximal landing zones. Furthermore, in patients suffering from connective tissue disease, open surgical repair is the treatment of choice, although TEVAR can be applied as a bridge to more definitive therapy. Open surgery might also be considered in younger patients, since long-term durability of TEVAR is not well defined.

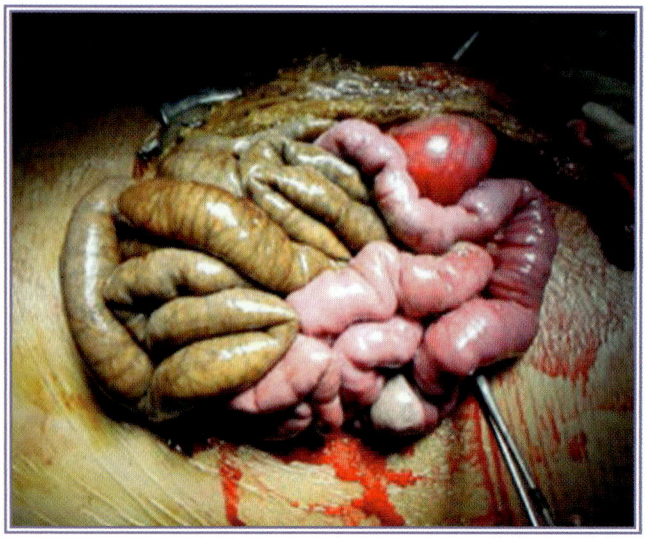

Fig. 18.6 Intraoperative appearance of a patient with Type B AD showing necrotic intestinal tissue.

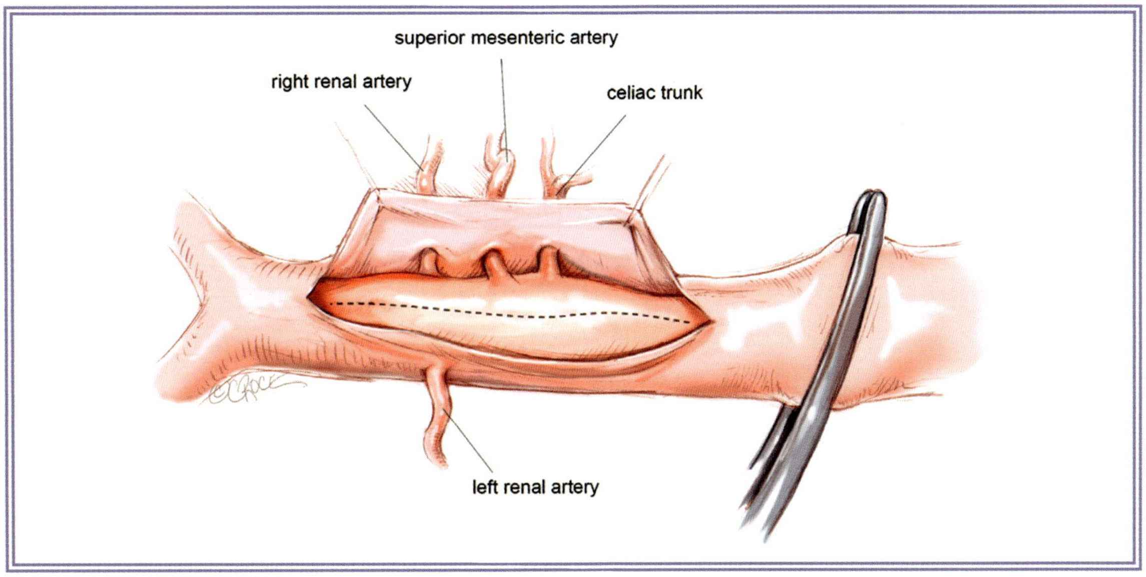

Fig. 18.7 Open fenestration technique. Supraceliac clamping allows inspection of the visceral segment of the aorta. A longitudinal aortotomy is made left anteriolaterally. The intimal septum is widely resected to maximize the size of the single aortic lumen. Reproduced from [14], with permission.

Open surgical options to treat visceral malperfusion include open fenestration and aortic graft replacement.

The technique of open fenestration relies on creating a single lumen by wide resection of the intimal flap, thereby restoring inflow to any compromised branch vessels (Fig. 18.7). There is little available evidence about the outcomes after open surgical fenestration, but it appears to be effective at relieving malperfusion [14]. Nevertheless, rates of in-hospital mortality after open fenestration of about 20% have been reported [14]. There are concerns about late aortic dilatation after surgical fenestration, however positive results have been reported about this issue when reduction of aortic diameter to close the aortotomy was adopted; based on Laplace's law, this decreases tension on the aortic wall [14].

Aortic graft replacement via a thoracotomy or thoracoabdominal incision is a potential/suitable treatment option [1]. However, when applied to acute AD patients, this type of surgery is associated with about 30% rate of mortality [15] and a substantial risk of spinal cord ischemia in case of extensive distal thoracoabdominal resection [1].

In about 20% of patients with visceral ischemia, only medical management is attempted [1]. These patients may have radiological or angiographic evidence of mesenteric ischemia without any related symptoms [2]. More frequently, they may be in such a poor clinical condition that either endovascular or surgical intervention is deemed futile. As a result, the mortality rate of patients treated medically is very high (50%); in fact, medical management was found to be the only independent predictor of in-hospital mortality in a multicenter study [1]. In contrast, mortality rates were similar after surgical and endovascular management of visceral ischemia (25.8% and 25.5%). General consensus, however, is that endovascular techniques are associated with reduced mortality [7].

18.5 Conclusion

Acute Type B AD complicated by visceral ischemia is a lethal condition that requires adequate management in order to restore flow to the affected branch vessels. TEVAR is the first choice of treatment. In selected patients, endovascular fenestration can also offer favorable outcomes. Open surgical techniques should be limited to patients in whom endovascular repair is contraindicated. Another primary issue is the timeliness of diagnosis and subsequent reversal of end-organ ischemia.

REFERENCES

1) Jonker FH, Patel HJ, Upchurch GR, et al. Acute type B aortic dissection complicated by visceral ischemia. J Thorac Cardiovasc Surg 2015; 149(4): 1081-6 e1.
2) Lauterbach SR, Cambria RP, Brewster DC, et al. Contemporary management of aortic branch compromise resulting from acute aortic dissection. J Vasc Surg 2001; 33(6): 1185-92.
3) Hagan PG, Nienaber CA, Isselbacher EM, et al. The International Registry of Acute Aortic Dissection (IRAD): new insights into an old disease. JAMA 2000; 283(7): 897-903.
4) Caty MG, Guice KS, Oldham KT, Remick DG, Kunkel SI. Evidence for tumor necrosis factor-induced pulmonary microvascular injury after intestinal ischemia-reperfusion injury. Ann Surg 1990; 212(6): 694-700.
5) Patel HJ, Williams DM, Dasika NL, Suzuki Y, Deeb GM. Operative delay for peripheral malperfusion syndrome in acute type A aortic dissection: a long-term analysis. J Thorac Cardiovasc Surg 2008; 135(6): 1288-95; discussion 95-6.
6) Jonker FH, Trimarchi S, Muhs BE, et al. The role of age in complicated acute type B aortic dissection. Ann Thorac Surg 2013; 96(6): 2129-34.
7) Fattori R, Cao P, De Rango P, et al. Interdisciplinary expert consensus document on management of type B aortic dissection. J Am Coll Cardiol 2013; 61(16): 1661-78.
8) Szeto WY, McGarvey M, Pochettino A, et al. Results of a new surgical paradigm: endovascular repair for acute complicated type B aortic dissection. Ann Thorac Surg 2008; 86(1): 87-93; discussion 93-4.
9) Sfyroeras GS, Rubio V, Pagan P, Diethrich EB, Rodriguez JA. Endovascular management of malperfusion in acute type B aortic dissections. J Endovasc Ther 2011; 18(1): 78-86.
10) Ryan C, Vargas L, Mastracci T, et al. Progress in management of malperfusion syndrome from type B dissections. J Vasc Surg 2013; 57(5): 1283-90; discussion 90.
11) Khoynezhad A, Donayre CE, Omari BO, Kopchok GE, Walot I, White RA. Midterm results of endovascular treatment of complicated acute type B aortic dissection. J Thorac Cardiovasc Surg 2009; 138(3): 625-31.
12) Canaud L, Faure EM, Ozdemir BA, Alric P, Thompson M. Systematic review of outcomes of combined proximal stent-grafting with distal bare stenting for management of aortic dissection. Ann Cardiothorac Surg 2014; 3(3): 223-33.
13) Patel HJ, Williams DM, Meerkov M, Dasika NL, Upchurch GR Jr, Deeb GM. Long-term results of percutaneous management of malperfusion in acute type B aortic dissection: implications for thoracic aortic endovascular repair. J Thorac Cardiovasc Surg 2009; 138(2): 300-8.
14) Trimarchi S, Segreti S, Grassi V, et al. Open fenestration for complicated acute aortic B dissection. Ann Cardiothorac Surg 2014; 3(4): 418-22.
15) Conrad M, Cambria R. Aortic dissection. In: Cronenwett J, Johnston KW (eds). Rutherford's vascular surgery, eighth edition. Philadelphia (PA): Elsevier Saunders, 2014; p. 2179-85.

19

Post-dissection and degenerative thoracoabdominal aortic aneurysms

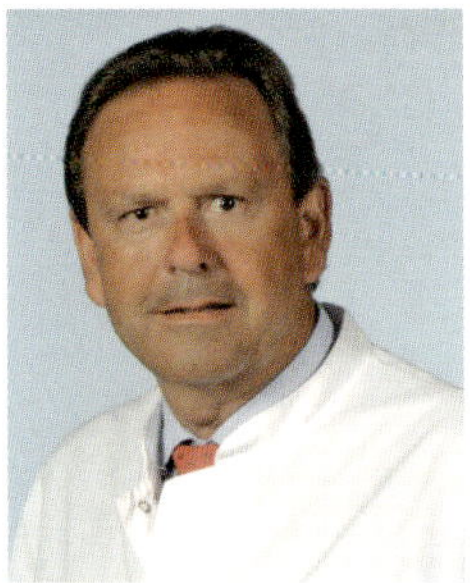

Michael J.H.M. Jacobs, Barend Mees, Noud Peppelenbosch and Geert Willem Schurink

Aneurysms involving the thoracic and abdominal aorta constitute an enormous challenge for the patient and the team managing this complex pathology. Especially in extensive thoracoabdominal aortic aneurysms (TAAA), the surgical trauma and associated potential adverse events are massive threats for our patients. Surgical results have significantly improved over time, especially in experienced and high-volume centers, however, mortality and morbidity rates remain high. Endovascular strategies are increasingly performed in TAAA patients, both in degenerative and post-dissection aneurysms, showing encouraging results. This chapter addresses some important differences between degenerative and post-dissection aneurysm.

19.1 Ascending versus descending thoracic aneurysms

Aneurysms can develop in any part of the aorta and it has long been assumed that etiologies were similar for thoracic and abdominal aortic aneurysms. Recent research has shown that aortic structure and function differ along the length of the entire aorta. Ito et al. [1] have shown that abdominal aortic aneurysms are mainly associated with risk factors like atherosclerosis, dyslipidemia and coronary artery disease in contrast to thoracic aneurysms in which these factors are less apparent. Differences between aneurysms in the chest have not really been assessed. Vapnik et al. [2] researched etiologic differences and clinical outcomes associated with repetitive anatomic distributions of thoracic aneurysms. They distinguished different groups: isolated ascending thoracic aortic aneurysms (ATA), isolated descending thoracic aneurysms (DTA) and combined ascending and descending thoracic aneurysms (CTA). Patients with DTA suffered more from hypertension and atherosclerosis than ATA. Patients with ATA were younger and genetically triggered thoracic aneurysms occured in almost all patients. Patients with isolated DTA were demographically similar to patients with CTA. Patients with DTA and CTA had more aortic events like dissection and rupture and

Michael J.H.M. Jacobs (m.jacobs@mumc.nl)
Maastricht University Medical Center,
Maastricht, The Netherlands

G. Melissano - R. Chiesa (eds), Aortic Dissection patients true stories and the innovations that saved their lives

increased mortality as compared to patients with ATA. Adverse aortic events were higher in patients with larger aneurysms and those with atherosclerosis. The authors concluded that patients with DTA with or without associated ATA predominantly suffer from hypertension, atherosclerosis and advanced age, whereas in isolated ATA genetic factors play a more important etiologic role.

19.2 Hereditary factors in thoracic aortic dissection and aneurysm

The understanding of the pathogenesis of thoracic aortic aneurysms has significantly improved over the last years, mainly due to the discovery of genetic predisposition. Isselbacher et al. [3] recently summarized the current knowledge of human genetic discoveries. Gene research in affected families with thoracic aneurysms has identified different groups of gene alterations. The first group shows mutations in genes encoding components of the transforming growth factor beta signaling cascade. The second group consists of genes which encode components of the smooth muscle contractile apparatus.

Marfan syndrome, Loeys-Dietz syndrome and vascular Ehlers-Danlos syndrome, clustered as connective tissue diseases, are typical "syndromic" aortic aneurysm conditions. Connective tissue diseased patient can suffer from aortic pathologies but also have non cardiovascular features. It should be emphasized that patients with connective tissue diseases not necessarily have cardiovascular risks. In nonsyndromic thoracic aortic aneurysms, however, pathologies are limited to the cardiovascular system. These patients most often have hereditary aneurysm conditions [3]. Gene defects causing familial thoracic aneurysms and dissections represent defects in proteins with functionality specific to the aorta, specifically to vascular smooth muscle cells. Another identified gene found in familial thoracic aneurysms and dissections is *ACTA2*. Patients with this mutation mainly suffer from ascending aortic aneurysm and dissection.

This very interesting research indicates that thoracic aneurysms have different etiologies than abdominal aortic aneurysms but also that the ascending aorta behaves different than the descending aorta.

19.3 Degenerative versus post-dissection aneurysms

Degenerative aneurysms are the most common type of descending and thoracoabdominal aortic aneurysms and occur as the result of breakdown of the connective tissue and muscular layer. The main causing factors are hypertension, cigarette smoking, genetic conditions, affecting patients at higher age. Post-dissection aneurysms develop after a Type A or Type B aortic dissection (AD) over time. These post-dissection aneurysms can also occur in elderly patients but the larger group of affected patients are those with severe hypertension or syndromic aortic conditions.

For therapeutic purposes it is relevant to understand the differences between degenerative and post-dissection aneurysms. In general, the indication for treatment depends on the maximal diameter of the aneurysm and no difference is made between degenerative and post-dissection aneurysm: larger than 6 cm is accepted as a threshold for intervention. In connective tissue disease patients this threshold is 5 cm.

The open surgical techniques do not differ in degenerative and post-dissection aneurysms.

Post-dissection thoracoabdominal aneurysms can develop following extensive Stanford Type A or Stanford Type B AD in which the longitudinal extension of the dissection involved the descending thoracic and abdominal aorta, most often including the iliac arteries as well. Such late aneurysmal degeneration of the outer wall of the false lumen occurs in 30-40% [4]. One of the main differences between degenerative and post-dissection aneurysms is patency of intercostal and lumbar arteries: in the latter group almost all segmental arteries are patent whereas in atherosclerotic aneurysms the majority of segmental vessels is occluded. In post-dissection aneurysms, the important segmental vessels most often originate from the true lumen, which is technically an advantage for revascularization since the quality of tissue is better than in the false lumen.

The surgical strategy is similar to the standard open surgical principles in degenerative aneurysms. However, some different approaches can be considered. First, sequential clamping, if feasible, allows stepwise aortic reconstruction and limits substantial blood loss caused by profound back bleeding from intercostal arteries due to the distal perfusion; blocking with balloon catheters or over sewing these arteries requires significant amount of time and therefore sequential steps are preferred. Second, reversing the direction of aortic reconstruction from distal to proximal in order to avoid insufficient perfusion of visceral, renal and segmental arteries due to changed flow patterns induced by retrograde perfusion: Type B AD cause a wide range of morphologic changes with different false and true lumens, entries and re-entries with subsequent visceral and renal circulation via separate pathways. Cross clamping the proximal descending aorta and starting retrograde aortic perfusion can change these alternative perfusion channels to the visceral organs, potentially causing malperfusion and subsequent organ ischemia. Therefore it can be considered to start the reconstruction at the distal part, by either implanting a bifurcated graft to the iliac arteries or a tube graft to the aortic bifurcation, clearly dependent on whether the anatomy would permit such a strategy. While performing these anastomoses, the aortic cross clamp is distal to the renal arteries and all organs are perfused in antegrade direction. Following, the arterial cannula is inserted and fixed in the polyester graft and the venous cannula in the right atrium via the femoral vein, allowing extra corporeal circulation and perfusion of the legs. Next, the left renal artery can be reconstructed with a separate graft and perfused via the prosthesis. Following, the visceral and right renal artery are reconstructed, either as an island reimplantation or with separate grafts if the dissection injured these arteries as well.

Treatment and handling of the dissected layers require utmost care because severe complications can develop if the true lumen is not correctly identified and controlled. The true lumen is often much smaller and can even be compressed in such a way that it can be disregarded. If the aorta is not entirely encircled and cross clamped, significant bleeding through the incomplete clamped true lumen occurs as soon as the aorta is opened. An important technical principle of dealing with the dissected aorta is to circumferentially divide the aorta at all suture lines to ensure adequate adventitial purchase of the suture bites; an exception is the posterior-inferior aspect of the visceral inclusion button. Another potential danger of overlooking the small true lumen is leaving intercostal arteries without reattachment. Therefore it is essential to open the septum between the true and false lumen over the entire length of the aortotomy. The septum is subsequently resected, leaving a small rim of 1-2 millimeters septum between both lumens. Revascularizing segmental arteries originating from the false lumen might be hazardous because the aortic tissue is thin and of inferior quality. Intercostal and lumbar arteries coming from the true lumen are reimplanted, limiting the amount of aortic tissue as much as possible by suturing on the edge of the vessels. In general, most surgeons reimplant segmental arteries between T8 and L1, depending on patency and quality of the aortic wall. Our strategy of revascularizing depends on monitoring motor evoked potentials [5].

At the site of the planned proximal anastomosis in post Type B AD, the origin of the initial intimal tear is often at the level of the left subclavian artery. Also, the aortic wall at the tear can be thickened and contain false lumen thrombosis, compromising an adequate proximal anastomosis. Therefore it is frequently necessary to cross clamp between the left carotid and left subclavian arteries, allowing resection of the diseased aortic tissue until adequate and relatively normal aortic material is reached. Finally, the end-to-end anastomosis to a circumferentially divided aorta is performed, either at the edge of the left subclavian artery or distal to the carotid artery with reimplantation or bypass of the left subclavian artery.

19.4 Relevant differences in spinal cord vasculature between degenerative and post-dissection aneurysms

Maintenance of spinal cord perfusion is one of the main targets during TAAA repair. Blood supply to the spinal cord must be guaranteed in order to limit ischemic damage during and after the procedure. Under normal conditions, the anterior spinal artery (ASA) is supplied by several anterior radiculomedullary arteries, the largest of which is the Adamkiewicz artery (AKA). The blood supply to the spinal cord is from the aorta through the segmental arteries

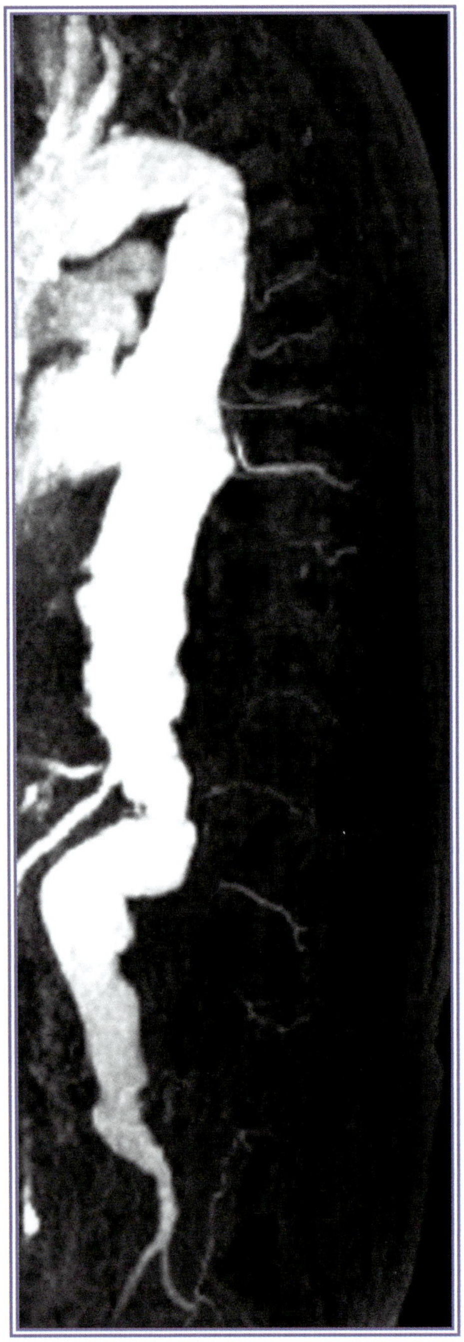

Fig. 19.1 MRA of degenerative thoracoabdominal aortic aneurysm. The majority of intercostal and lumbar arteries are occluded.

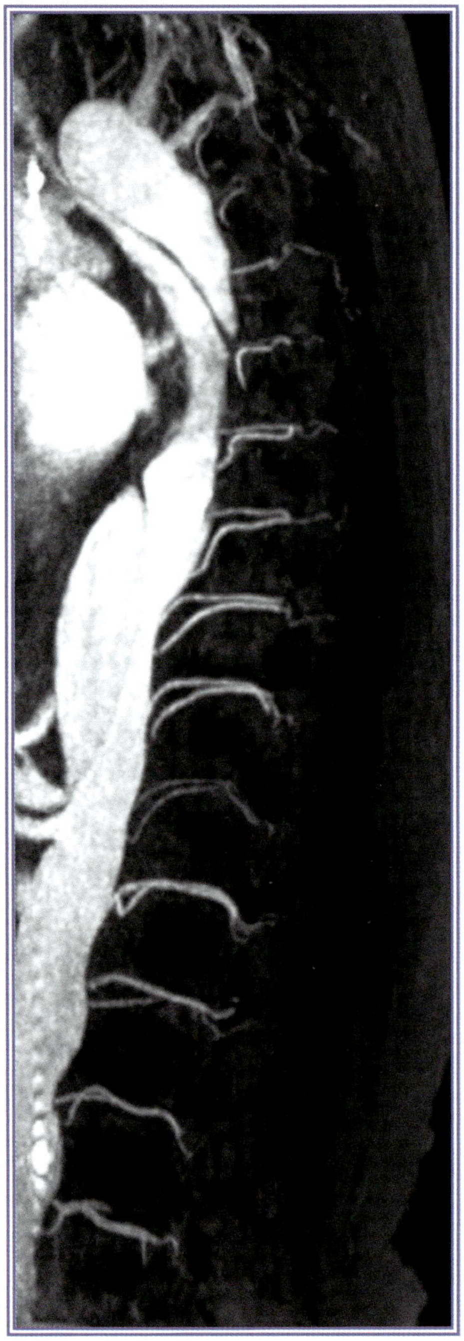

Fig. 19.2 MRA of post-dissection thoracoabdominal aortic aneurysm. All intercostal and lumbar arteries are patent.

(SA), the AKA and the ASA [6]. If the blood supply is via the SA and the AKA, it is referred as direct spinal cord blood supply. However, in patients with aneurysm, the segmental artery feeding the AKA might be occluded by thrombus or plaque formation. In these cases, spinal cord perfusion is provided by collateral vessels and referred as indirect spinal cord blood supply.

The main difference in blood supply to the spinal cord between patients with degenerative and post-dissection aneurysms is the number of patent intercostal and lumbar arteries. We have systematically assessed the feeding arteries to the spinal cord by means of magnetic resonance angiography (MRA) techniques [7, 8]. It appeared that in degenerative aneurysms the majority of intercostal and lumbar arteries were occluded (Fig. 19.1). Patients with post-dissection aneurysms had significantly more patent segmental arteries than patients with degenerative aneurysms (Fig. 19.2). In addition, in degenerative aneurysms, more than half of the patients had indirect intersegmental supply, indicating that spinal cord blood supply depends more strongly on collaterals. This was in contrast to patients with post-dissection aneurysms in whom only a minority had indirect perfusion to the cord.

19.5 Moving from open to endovascular thoracoabdominal aortic aneurysm repair?

Open surgical repair of degenerative and post-dissection TAAA is still the gold standard in patients "fit" for surgery. However, the majority of patients are not fit enough for this huge surgical trauma. The best results with open repair are obtained in patients with Marfan syndrome who most often have a TAAA following Type A or B AD [9]. These patients are significantly younger than patients with degenerative aneurysms, contributing to lower mortality rates. They frequently have undergone multiple aortic procedures of the ascending and/or aortic arch already.

The surgical trauma in isolated descending thoracic aortic aneurysm repair is significantly lower than in open thoracoabdominal aortic repair. In intact descending thoracic aneurysms, surgical mortality is approximately 7% and comparable to mortality rates after TEVAR. Von Allmen et al. [10] assessed 30-day mortality, long-term survival (5 years) and aortic-related interventions and found similar short-term mortality after open and endovascular repair in a large group with degenerative descending thoracic aortic aneurysms. However, 5-year survival was significantly worse after TEVAR.

Open TAAA repair in the elderly patient is associated with higher mortality and major adverse events, both for degenerative and post-dissection aneurysms . Therefore it is encouraging that endovascular solutions with branched and fenestrated grafts provide acceptable outcomes and that results are improving over time [11]. Even post-dissection thoracoabdominal aneurysms are currently treated by endovascular means, however, experience is still limited and results are reported by highly experienced and high-volume centers [12]. These complex procedures, either open surgical or endovascular, should therefore be centralized in centers of excellence with the full infrastructure and multidisciplinary teams to master the procedures and handle adverse events.

REFERENCES

1) Ito S, Akutsu K, Tamori Y, et al. Differences in atherosclerotic profiles between patients with thoracic and abdominal aortic aneurysms. Am J Cardiol 2008; 101(5): 696-9.
2) Vapnik JS, Kim JB, Isselbacher EM, et al. Characteristics and outcomes of ascending versus descending thoracic aortic aneurysms. Am J Cardiol 2016; 117(10): 1683-90.
3) Isselbacher EM, Lino Cardenas CL, Lindsay ME. Hereditary influence in thoracic aortic aneurysm and dissection. Circulation 2016; 133(24): 2516-28.
4) Song JM, Kim SD, Kim JH, et al. Long-term predictors of descending aorta aneurysmal change in patients with aortic dissection. J Am Coll Cardiol 2007; 50(8): 799-804.

5) Schurink GW, Peppelenbosch AG, Mees BM, De Haan MW, Jacobs MJ. Strategies to prevent spinal cord ischemia in thoracoabdominal aortic aneurysm repair. J Cardiovasc Surg (Torino) 2015; 56(2): 281-6.
6) Melissano G, Bertoglio L, Rinaldi E, Leopardi M, Chiesa R. An anatomical review of spinal cord blood supply. J Cardiovasc Surg (Torino) 2015; 56(5): 699-706.
7) Nijenhuis RJ, Jacobs MJ, Schurink GW, Kessels AG, van Engelshoven JM, Backes WH. Magnetic resonance angiography and neuromonitoring to assess spinal cord blood supply in thoracic and thoracoabdominal aortic aneurysm surgery. J Vasc Surg 2007; 45(1): 71-7; discussion 77-8.
8) Backes WH, Nijenhuis RJ, Mess WH, Wilmink FA, Schurink GW, Jacobs MJ. Magnetic resonance angiography of collateral blood supply to spinal cord in thoracic and thoracoabdominal aortic aneurysm patients. J Vasc Surg 2008; 48(2): 261-71.
9) Coselli JS, Green SY, Price MD, et al. Results of open surgical repair in patients with Marfan syndrome and distal aortic dissection. Ann Thorac Surg 2016; 101(6): 2193-201.
10) von Allmen RS, Anjum A, Powell JT. Outcomes after endovascular or open repair for degenerative descending thoracic aortic aneurysm using linked hospital data. Br J Surg 2014; 101(10): 1244-51.
11) Verhoeven EL, Katsargyris A, Bekkema F, et al. Ten-year experience with endovascular repair of thoracoabdominal aortic aneurysms: results from 166 consecutive patients. Eur J Vasc Endovasc Surg 2015; 49(5): 524-31.
12) Spear R, Sobocinski J, Settembre N, et al. Early experience of endovascular repair of post-dissection aneurysms involving the thoraco-abdominal aorta and the arch. Eur J Vasc Endovasc Surg 2016; 51(4): 488-97.

20

Dissection true stories; options for the management of non-A, non-B Type aortic dissection

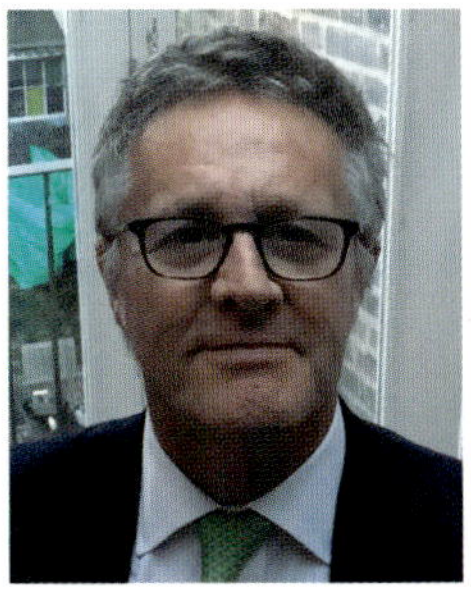

Nicholas J.W. Cheshire and Ulrich P. Rosendahl

20.1 Introduction

We are rapidly approaching consensus on the management of classical aortic dissections (AD). The results of recent trials, and evidence gained from large case series, mean that most major centres now have evidence-based policies for the management of Type A and Type B lesions, in both acute and chronic phases.

In this chapter we describe two recent, atypical cases – which do not fit standard definition or management protocols – which we managed using different approaches. We urge flexibility and a whole team approach to such cases.

20.2 Case 1

A previously fit 52-year-old man presented with classic chest and back pain suggestive of acute AD whilst on holiday. Initial computed tomography (CT) images showed a dissection with an entry point in the distal transverse aortic arch, around the medial border of origin of the left subclavian artery (Fig. 20.1). He was treated conservatively with anti-impulse, anti-hypertensive therapy and analgesia. After 2 days in hospital, he was discharged and returned to London. After a further episode of chest pain on day 5, he presented to his local hospital and was transferred to The Royal Brompton aortic centre.

On day 8 after initial presentation, with ongoing chest pain, he underwent hybrid surgery with a Thoraflex™ (Vascutek Terumo, Renfrewshire, UK) frozen elephant trunk through a median sternotomy; bypass was established with femoral, innominate and left common carotid arterial lines. The stent component was placed into the descending aorta during circulatory arrest in the lower body, the sewing ring was sutured into the distal arch and the supra-aortic vessels sutured onto the dacron component of the device on a Carrel patch.

Nicholas J.W. Cheshire (nick.cheshire@imperial.ac.uk)
Royal Brompton & Harefield Hospitals,
London, United Kingdom

G. Melissano - R. Chiesa (eds), Aortic Dissection patients true stories and the innovations that saved their lives

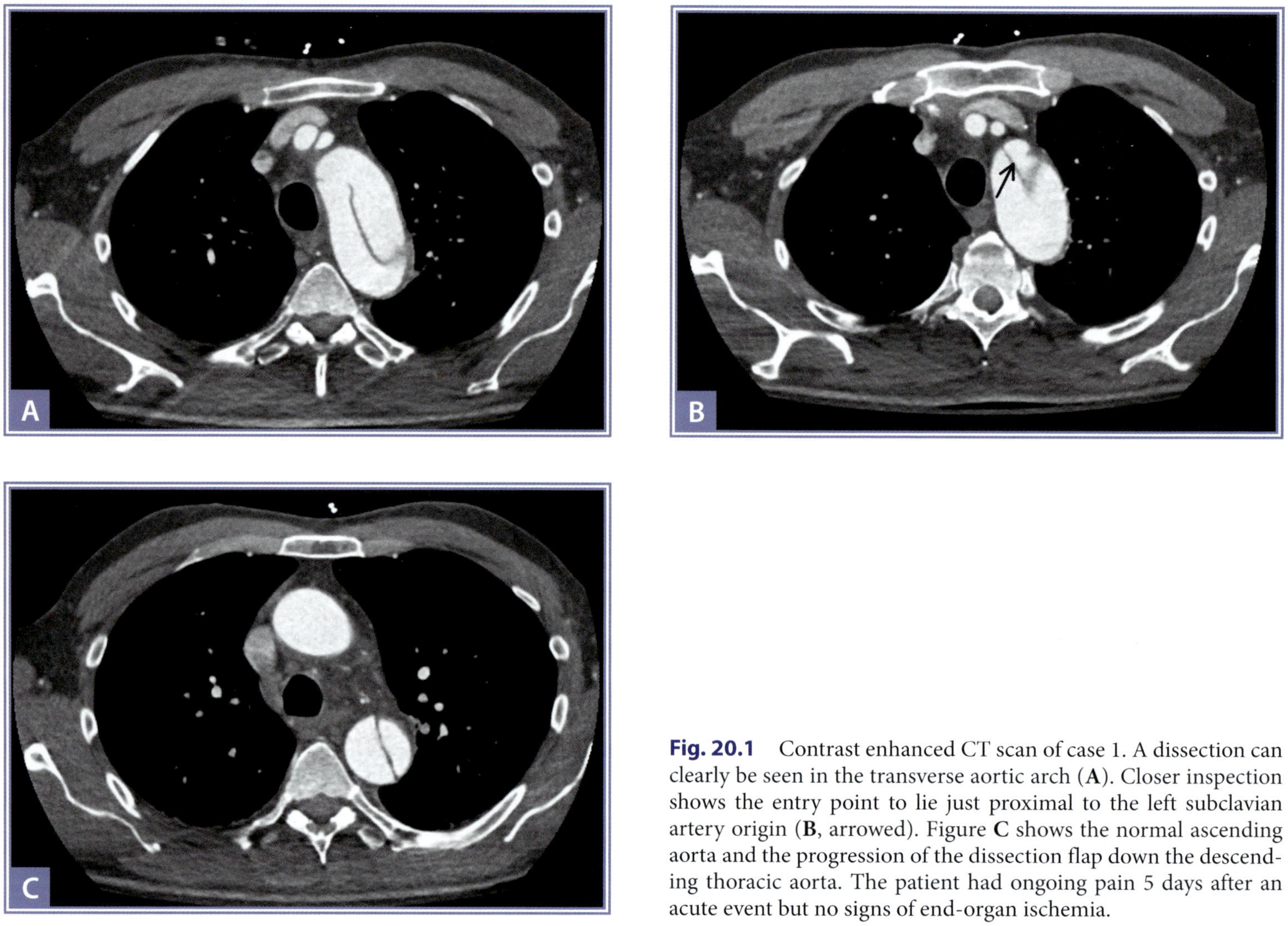

Fig. 20.1 Contrast enhanced CT scan of case 1. A dissection can clearly be seen in the transverse aortic arch (**A**). Closer inspection shows the entry point to lie just proximal to the left subclavian artery origin (**B**, arrowed). Figure **C** shows the normal ascending aorta and the progression of the dissection flap down the descending thoracic aorta. The patient had ongoing pain 5 days after an acute event but no signs of end-organ ischemia.

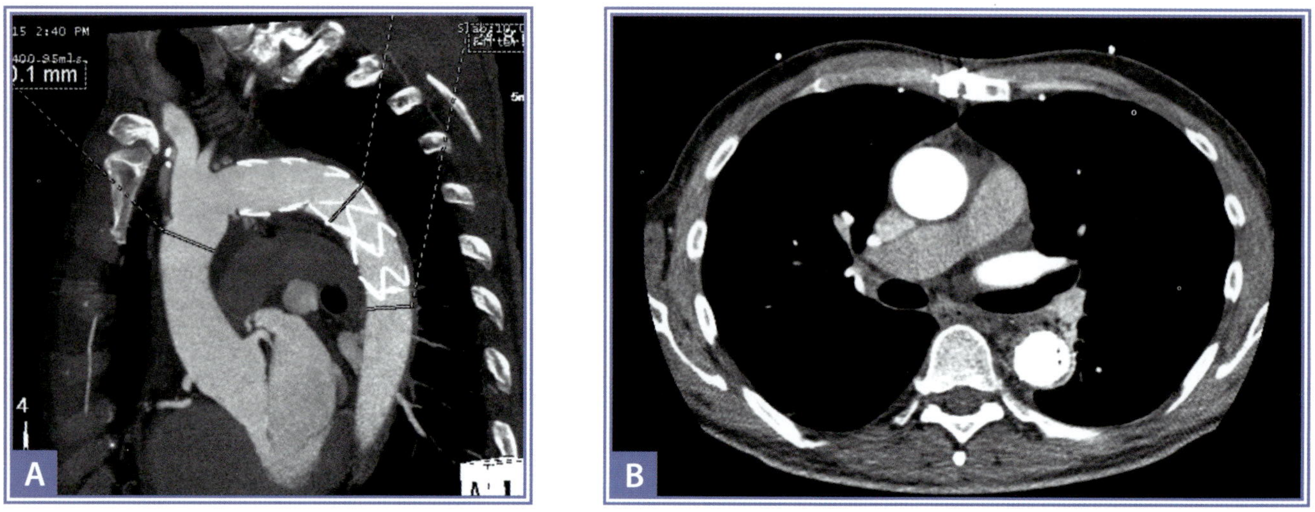

Fig. 20.2 Contrast enhanced CT scan of case 1 three months after frozen elephant trunk repair of acute non-A, non-B Type AD. The lateral view in figure **A** shows a good position of the Thoraflex™ stent graft with the supra-aortic vessels reconstructed on a Carrel patch. In figure **B** almost complete remodelling of the dissection in the descending aorta is seen even at this early stage. There has thus far not been any indication for further stenting to the descending aorta.

He made an uneventful recovery and was discharged from hospital on day 7 after surgery. Repeat CT scans 3 months after surgery showed normal circulation in the supra-aortic vessels with remodeling of the distal aorta (Fig. 20.2).

20.3 Case 2

A 69-year-old lawyer presented with an episode of acute chest pain, diagnosed as Type B AD and managed conservatively in his local hospital. At follow-up three months after the initial event, a CT scan showed early dilatation of the upper descending thoracic aorta to a maximum diameter of 5.9 cm, with a large distal entry point visible (Fig. 20.3A, B). There was also abnormality in the aortic arch, with a dissection/false aneurysm originating around the left subclavian artery – seemingly separate from the dissected descending thoracic aorta (Fig. 20.3C, D). The distal transverse arch of the aorta between the two dissections was also thickened and abnormal.

We elected to treat this complex lesion with open surgery and first approached the proximal arch through a median sternotomy. Under hypothermic circulatory arrest the distal ascending

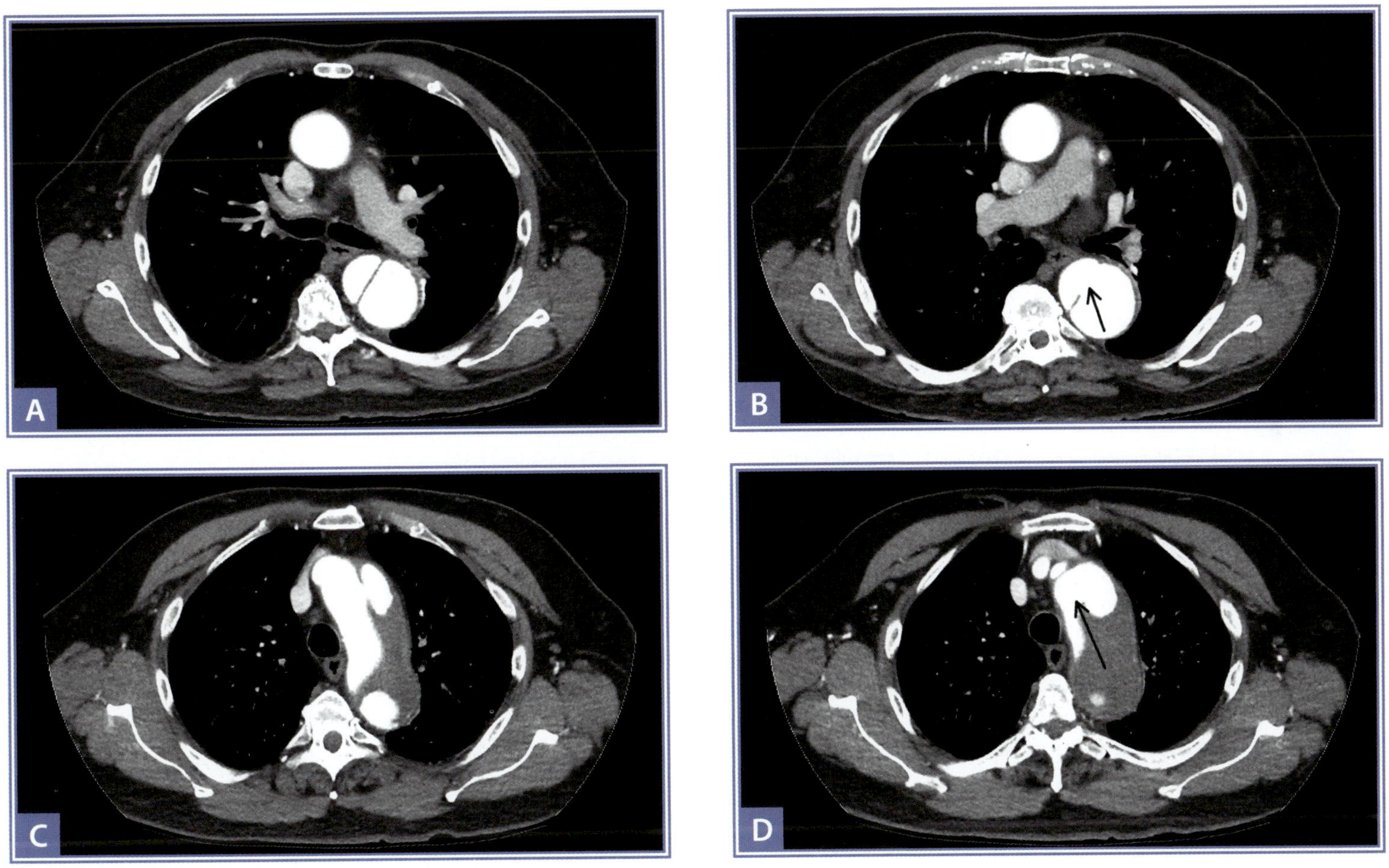

Fig. 20.3 Contrast enhanced CT scan of case 2, four months after conservative management of an acute dissection event; in figures **A** and **B** the normal ascending aorta and early dilatation of the dissected descending thoracic aorta can be seen. There appeared to be an entry point in the upper 1/3 descending aorta (**B**, arrowed). The maximum diameter was 5.9 cm. Scrutiny of the aortic arch (**C**) demonstrated a seemingly separate dissection – or even a false aneurysm – in the more proximal arch. This pathology had an entry point around the origin of the left subclavian artery (**D**, arrowed). The clue that the two areas of dissection were linked is provided by the abnormal area of thickened aortic wall lying distal to the left subclavian artery. At arch surgery through sternotomy, this proved to be a thrombosed false lumen in an area of classically dissected aorta.

aorta and the arch were replaced using an elephant trunk technique; at surgery the distal arch was classically dissected and the false lumen filled with thrombus. This was removed during the period of arrest and the inner and outer walls of the aorta repaired with Teflon. The distal anastomosis was performed distal to the left subclavian origin. All three supra-aortic vessels were sutured onto the dacron graft on a Carrel patch. Despite a relatively prolonged period of circulatory arrest (40 mins) the patient recovered well and was discharged from hospital on day 12 after surgery. Three months later he underwent Thoracic EndoVascular Aortic Repair (TEVAR) into the elephant trunk, covering the thoracic aorta to just above the diaphragm. He made an uneventful recovery.

20.4 Discussion

The Stanford classification of AD has become the predominant system used in western literature. Type A is a lesion with an endothelial entry point in the ascending aorta, going on to involve the arch and descending aorta. Type B is a distal lesion with an entry point distal to the left subclavian artery. Both are life threatening in the acute situation. Increasingly, consensus about the management of Type A (open surgery) and uncomplicated Type B (initial blood pressure and pain control, followed by TEVAR) is becoming clear, and is supported by trial data.

But what of dissection that does not meet either the classic Stanford Type A or Type B pattern, where the entry point is most likely in the arch? How to manage these lesions?

The DeBakey classification system includes a third type (the DeBakey Type II lesion) – an endothelial entry point in the ascending but dissection involving only the ascending aorta – but this is not informative when considering complex dissection, particularly in acute presentations, that do not fit common patterns.

The two cases presented above represent our recent experience with entry points around the level of the left subclavian artery. In keeping with many major centres we are now much more interventional in our management of dissection and prefer to offer TEVAR to Type B lesions in the early acute phase or when there is early dilatation of the upper thoracic segment. In the two cases presented here, however, we were presented with a dilemma.

Case 1 required early intervention because of ongoing symptoms; we could not wait for our ideal of 4-6 weeks after presentation to allow for stabilization. The entry point of the dissection around the medial border of the left subclavian artery mandated stent graft coverage of that artery to get a seal. The patient had around 14 mm of space between the left common carotid artery and the left subclavian artery – sufficient for a seal in our experience – but we were concerned about the risk of retrograde Type A dissection in such an acute lesion, with a stent graft landing in abnormal tissue within the aortic arch. The prospect of a right-to-left carotid-carotid cross over graft in the neck was considered to allow the TEVAR to be placed more proximally in the arch but was discounted because of the relatively young age of the patient. In these circumstances the frozen elephant trunk technique is a very controlled and elegant way of dealing with the aortic arch and descending aorta in one procedure with complete ability to prevent retrograde Type A AD. The patient was young and fit and made a complete recovery.

Case 2 presents related arguments. He was referred to us for open surgery to the early descending dilatation by an experienced team who was concerned that TEVAR posed a risk of retrograde Type A AD because of the abnormal arch. Understandably, the proximal lesion had been interpreted as a second problem, distinct from the descending dissection. We were concerned that an open surgical approach to the descending thoracic aorta through a left thoracotomy could be very challenging; we would be limited at the upper end of the approach and were concerned that we could find we were unable to completely exclude the disease. We therefore considered an anterior approach first would give us more control over the disease. We discussed a frozen elephant trunk for this patient but the position of the entry point in the descending aorta was just too distal to be covered by the stent component of the device – in which case TEVAR would be required anyway. We therefore elected to do classical surgery, which turned out to be challenging but undoubtedly the correct decision. Both primary TEVAR and open surgery from left thoracotomy would have put this patient at great risk.

Our two cases represent only a fraction of the spectrum of dissection presentations that do not fit the classic Stanford Type A or Type B definitions, but we believe they illustrate some common themes. In keeping with our practice for classic Type B AD, we believe that early intervention is preferable to conservative therapy, not least because of the significant challenge – and high mortality – of post-dissection aneurysm management. Retrograde Type A AD is the most feared complication of stent graft therapy for dissection and carries a high risk of death. What evidence there is suggests that the risk of retrograde Type A AD is highest when stents are placed within the first month after acute presentation (as with case 1) or are required to land within the aortic arch (both of our cases). Alternative strategies require an approach that secures the ascending aorta – usually therefore via sternotomy – and thus need multi-disciplinary team working both in planning the approach and performing the procedure. Both classical open surgery and the frozen elephant trunk techniques are suitable and both may require subsequent stent grafting to the descending aorta.

21

When TEVAR fails: secondary interventions and direct false lumen adjuncts

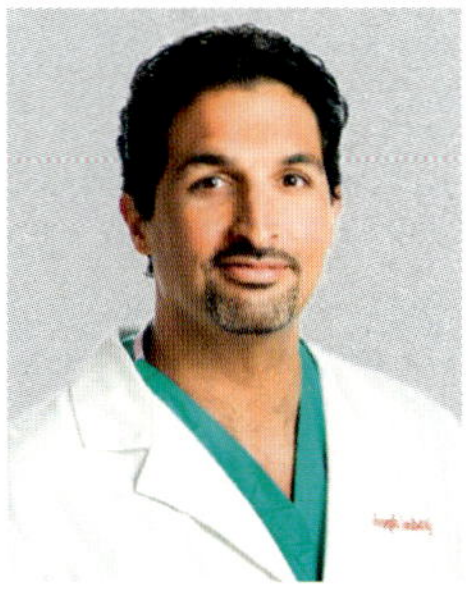

Joseph V. Lombardi and Marissa Famularo

21.1 Introduction

In endovascular repair of Type B aortic dissection (AD), the proximal entry tear is covered by a stent graft in an attempt to redirect flow from the false lumen. Ideally, depressurization of the false lumen should lead to its collapse and thrombosis, with a concomitant re-expansion of the true lumen. This intriguing idea quickly became the gold standard in the initial management of complicated Type B AD, with both short and mid-term data showing improvements in morbidity and mortality after Thoracic EndoVascular Aortic Repair (TEVAR). Unfortunately, persistent false lumen flow after initial TEVAR is not infrequent, and leaves the aorta vulnerable to aneurysmal degeneration.

21.2 Risk of thoracic endovascular aortic repair failure

Recent data suggests that the long-term benefits of TEVAR in preventing aneurysmal growth may have been overestimated. Several studies discussing growth of the thoracic aorta after TEVAR for acute Type B AD show moderate growth of both the descending thoracic aorta (DTA) and abdominal aorta [1-5]. A portion of this risk is certainly secondary to false lumen patency, which has been shown to predict aortic dilation and aortic-related death in dissection patients [3, 6]. To estimate the risk of aneurysmal degeneration after TEVAR, it is helpful to review some of the landmark dissection trials with existing data on aortic expansion. This data is summarized in Table 21.1.

In 2006, Resch and colleagues reported 1 month follow-up on 74 patients with complicated acute or chronic Type B AD treated with TEVAR [1]. In 14% of their patients, the uncovered aorta distal to their endograft increased in diameter during this short follow-up time. All but one of these patients had persistent flow in the false lumen. Also in 2006, Gaxotte et al. published their findings on aortic remodeling after 50 TEVAR cases [3]. Through close analysis of computed tomography angiography (CTA) at day 8 and 1 year post-operatively, the group

---

Joseph V. Lombardi (lombardi-joseph@CooperHealth.edu)
Cooper Medical School,
Rowan University, Camden, NJ, USA

G. Melissano - R. Chiesa (eds), Aortic Dissection patients true stories and the innovations that saved their lives

made several important observations. In patients with complete false lumen thrombosis, positive remodeling of the aorta occurred, resulting in decreased total aortic and false lumen diameters. When patients had persistent false lumen flow, however, the total aortic diameter increased over time. 57% of patients had persistent thoracic false lumen flow at 1 year. Of patients with abdominal components to their dissection, 88% had persistent abdominal false lumen flow at 1-year imaging. Consequently, both the average true lumen and total aortic diameter of the abdominal aorta increased over time across the group.

In a similar paper by Sobocinski et al., 52 complicated acute Type B AD patients received TEVAR [4]. The total aortic diameter at 1 year increased by >5 mm in the thoracic aorta in 25% of patients, and in the abdominal aorta in 33% of patients, highlighting the magnitude of this late complication.

A summary of the International Registry of Acute Aortic Dissection (IRAD) data in 2013 also revealed increased aortic diameter in 31% of patients 1 year after endograft placement, corroborating the previous study's results [5]. At 5 years, 63% of patients in the IRAD data base had significant aortic growth or new aneurysm formation. This number existed in the face of a 5-year stent graft endoleak rate of less than 14%.

In the Study for the Treatment of complicated Type B Aortic Dissection using Endoluminal repair (STABLE) trial, using a combination treatment of EndoVascular Aneurysm Repair (EVAR) and a bare-metal dissection stent (Provisional Extension To Induce Complete ATtachment, PETTICOAT), persistent false lumen flow was noted in the thoracic aorta in 67.2% of patients and abdominal aorta in 87.9% of patients at 1 year [2]. At 2 years, the number of patients with persistent false lumen flow was 56.5% and 84.8% for thoracic and abdominal aorta respectively. This correlated with 35% of patients presenting with significant growth of thoracic aorta at 2 years, and 47% of patients presenting with significant abdominal aortic growth.

Persistent false lumen flow is likely not the sole determining factor of TEVAR failure. Many patients in the above studies had persistent false lumen flow but no evidence of aneurysmal degeneration at follow-up. It is likely that dilation of the aorta occurs by a more complex mechanism, in which false lumen patency is just one factor. Flow, pressure gradients and number of re-entry tears have been implicated in this process. High-flow secondary entry tears specifically have been identified as a significant risk factor for both persistent false lumen flow and increased aneurysm-related mortality [4]. It is clear, however, that complete thrombosis of the false lumen decreases the risk of aneurysmal degeneration over time.

Table 21.1 Literature studies

Study	Dissections (No.)	Follow-up	Thoracic growth	Abdominal growth
Resch 2006 [1]	74; mixed acute complicated and chronic	1 month	14%	Not reported
Sayer 2008 [7]	76; mixed acute and chronic	1 year	26%	11%
Kang 2011 [8]	76; chronic	34 months	15%	Not reported
Andacheh 2012 [9]	72; chronic	18 months	Not reported	40%
Sobocinski 2013 [4]	52; acute complicated	1 year	25%	33%
Fattori 2013 [5]	276; acute	1 year 5 years	31% 63%	Not reported
Lombardi 2014 [2]	87; mixed acute complicated and chronic	1 year 2 years	29% 35%	29% 47%
Brunkwall 2014 [10]	30; acute uncomplicated	1 year	37%	Not reported

21.3 Interventions

In the setting of a patent false lumen after TEVAR, the first step in management is to localize the source of inflow at the primary entry tear. It is our practice to obtain thin-slice CTA with cardiac gating to reduce motion artifact in the thoracic region, and delayed images to catch late filling throughout the thoracic, visceral and distal aorta. These images and their reconstructions are absolutely necessary for the visualization of small intimal tears and patent lumbar branches. When noninvasive imaging fails to localize a source of false lumen flow, angiography may be necessary with the aid of intravascular ultrasound. In the patient showed in Figure 21.1, CTA suggested an intimal tear in the left common carotid artery, but this area was incompletely visualized. The tear was imaged clearly on angiogram as dynamic observation during the cardiac cycle gives a clearer understanding of re-entry flow. The left carotid was covered with a covered stent. This resulted in complete cessation of false lumen flow (Fig. 21.1) in the thoracic aorta and, ultimately, thrombosis of the vulnerable, aneurysmal aorta.

During secondary procedures, identifying any flow around the proximal edge of the stent graft into the false lumen via the initial entry tear is an important first step. Should this type of leak exist, proximalization of the covered stent is necessary. Depending on anatomy, this may require something as simple as another aortic stentgraft, or as complicated as a proximal debranching procedure followed by repeat TEVAR.

When a proximal seal exists and flow in the false lumen persists, management becomes less clear. Persistent flow into the false lumen requires both ingress and egress. Multiple intimal tears are seen in some acute and many chronic dissections. These tears often involve the visceral aorta and are not easily treated with covered stents. As noted above, secondary intimal tears can be high-flow, and are independent risk factors for aneurysmal degeneration and mortality [4]. Lumbar vessels may provide either ingress or egress, perpetuating the flow caused by secondary tears.

In these complicated scenarios, intervention should have three main goals: 1. to disrupt flow through any patent lumbar arteries communicating with the false lumen, 2. to promote false lumen thrombosis with adjuncts such as embolization, and 3. to cover secondary entry tears should the anatomy allow.

Accessing the false lumen directly is usually required to treat persistent false lumen flow,

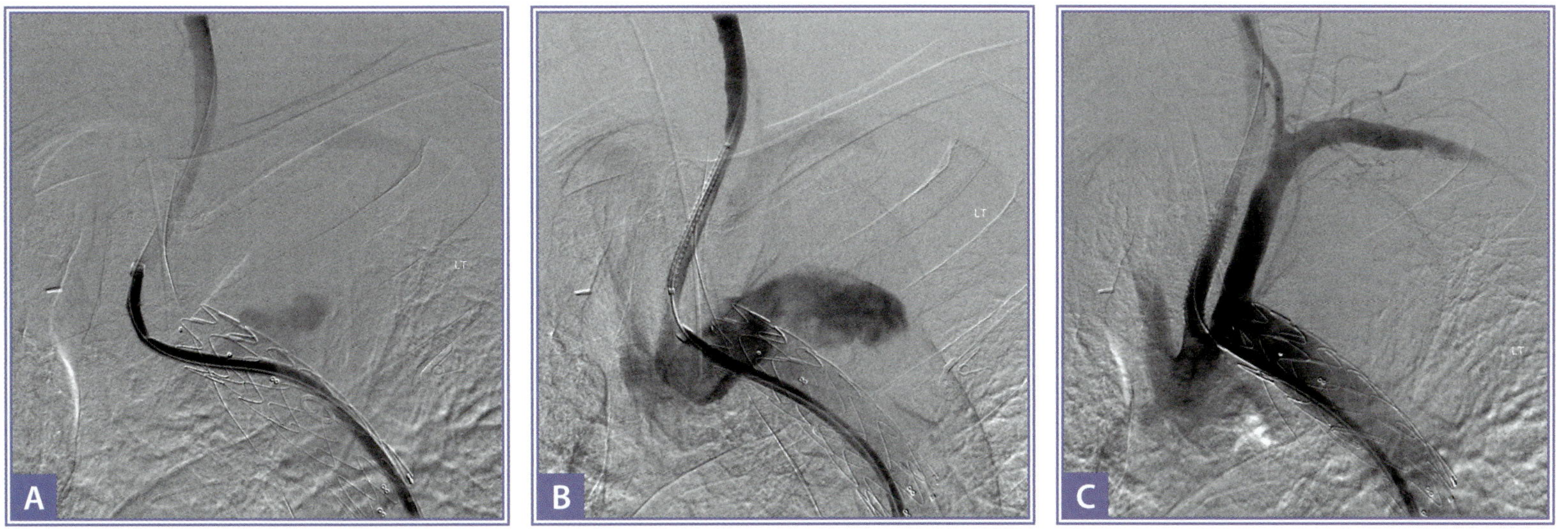

Fig. 21.1 **A-B**, Selective angiogram in the left common carotid artery demonstrates flow of contrast into the false lumen. **C**, Completion angiogram after a covered stent deployed in the left common carotid artery reveals no false lumen flow.

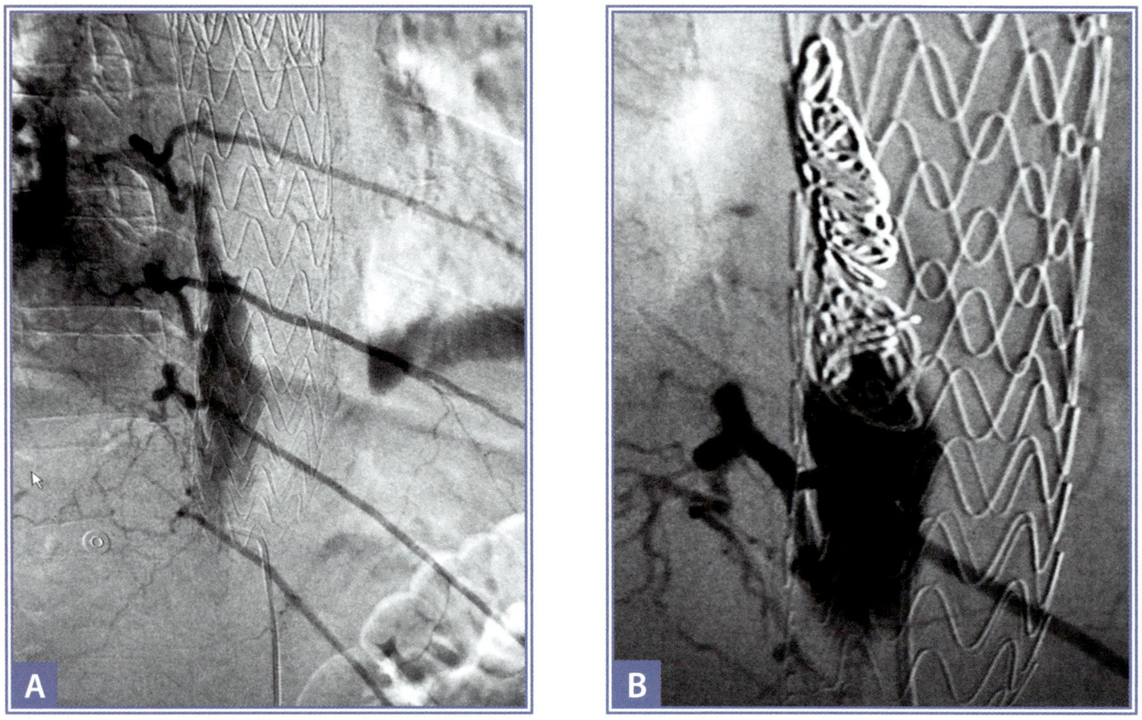

Fig. 21.2 **A**, Angiogram via the false lumen demonstrates four large lumbar egress vessels. **B**, After coiling, only the fourth lumbar remains patent. The false lumen above this level is successfully thrombosed.

where catheter-directed angiography can help identify patent lumbar arteries. A good preoperative CT can serve as a roadmap, but additional contributing vessels are invariably found intraoperatively. These vessels can be accessed individually and embolized with coils prior to treating the false lumen directly. If there are many egress vessels, we plan several staged procedures for embolization in an attempt to avoid complications of spinal cord or visceral ischemia. In these cases, we ensure that our "access-tear" to the false lumen remains uncovered, as this allows an easier planned return and avoids the search for alternative false lumen access. In Figure 21.2 four large egress intercostal arteries are noted on angiography within the false lumen behind a previously placed endograft. Three of the intercostals were covered with coils, resulting in thrombosis of the false lumen at that level. The fourth lumbar was left patent to preserve spinal cord function.

When it is clear there is no communication with visceral, lumbar or intercostal arteries, direct false lumen therapy via coil embolization or gelfoam/thrombin combination can be entertained, particularly if the false lumen flow is stubbornly persistent. Once we are sure that our false lumen therapy has been maximized, we then get aggressive with coverage of all remaining entry tears where appropriate (Fig. 21.3).

Due to the effort and cost needed to treat large, patent false lumens with individual embolic coils, several alternative therapies have been proposed. In the "candy-plug technique," Kölbel and colleagues use a modified thoracic-stent graft to plug the false lumen [11]. The group initially reported using a Zenith® thoracic TX2® device (Cook Medical, Bloomington, IN), but subsequent groups have successfully modified the technique using an Excluder® aortic extender (W.L. Gore & Associates, Flagstaff, AZ) [12]. An iliac occluder device (Zenith® Iliac Plug; Cook Medical) was first reported for use in successful false lumen embolization by Roselli et al. in 2014 [13].

Idrees and colleagues published their experience with 21 false lumen embolizations using covered grafts in 2014 [14]. Their group used mainly iliac plugs for embolization, but also tried

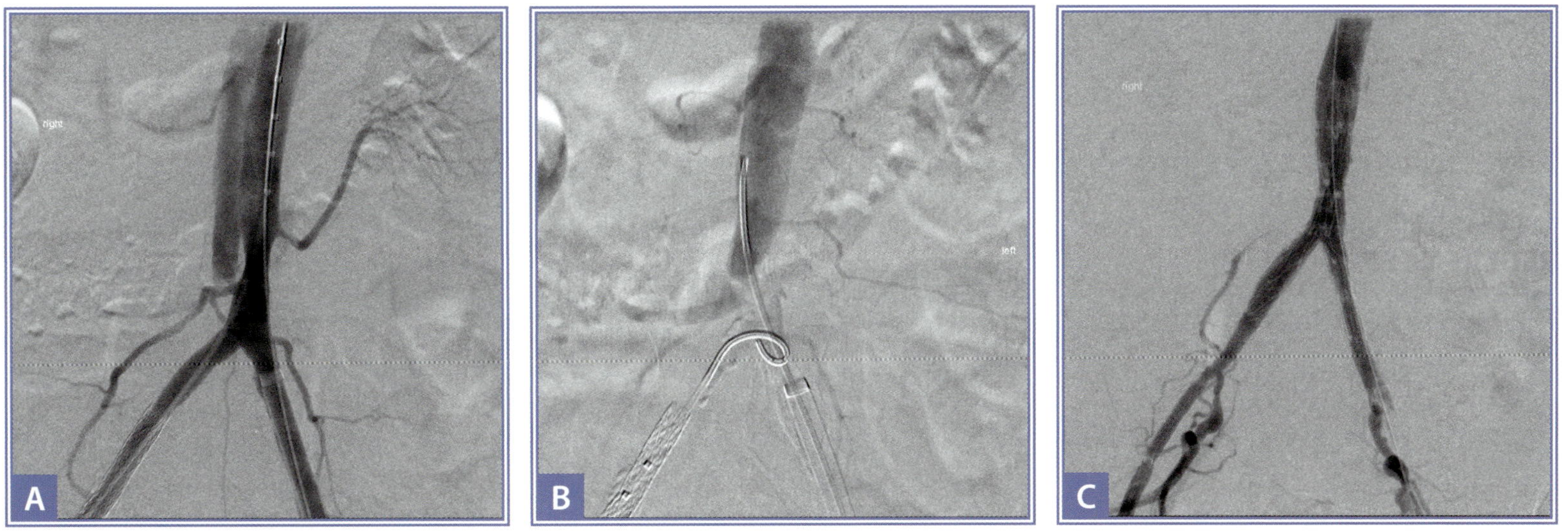

Fig. 21.3 **A**, A patient with a Type B AD and significant false lumen flow in the abdominal aorta after a thoracic endograft was used to cover the proximal entry tear. **B**, Access to the false lumen is obtained and an intravascular occlusion plug deployed into the false lumen to promote embolization. **C**, An endograft is deployed at the bifurcation and successfully covered the entry tear in the distal aorta resulting in cessation of false lumen flow.

nitinol embolization plugs in two patients and an occluded stent graft in one. 71% of patients had complete thrombosis of the false lumen on follow-up imaging.

Stent grafts and iliac occluders can safely be used to promote false lumen thrombosis. Please see Chapter 31 in this text for a more complete discussion of these techniques. Overall, these techniques are effective in occupying space and disrupting flow patterns, but in our practice, planned selective outflow embolization with direct false lumen adjuncts provides a very effective and safe primary mode of false lumen therapy.

Aggressive expansion and disruption of the intimal membrane to equalize pressures between the true and false lumen is a technique that has been successfully used in both acute and chronic dissections. Hofferberth and colleagues first described this technique in acute dissections in 2014 and termed it "Stent-Assisted Balloon-Induced Intimal Disruption and Relamination in Aortic Dissection Repair" or "The STABILISE concept" [15]. In this technique, which is described in more detail in Chapter 27, the distal extent of covered stent-graft is oversized. A bare-metal dissection stent is then used to buttress the aorta distal to the covered portion. Finally, a Coda® balloon (Cook Medical, Bloomington, IN) is used to dilate the over-sized covered stent-graft to approximate the total aortic diameter. This method tears the intima at that level and the resultant, larger true lumen blocks retrograde flow into the thoracic false lumen. Below this level, the result is a uni-luminal aorta.

In chronic dissection, Kölbel et al. described a similar technique [16]. A covered stent-graft is placed in the descending aorta with second, oversized stent-graft used to extend distally. This oversized graft is balloon-dilated to approximate the total aortic diameter. Again, the intimal septum is destroyed. The true lumen at that level blocks retrograde flow into the thoracic false lumen, promoting thrombosis. These newer, alternative techniques provide a potential solution for persistent false lumen flow. More studies are needed to evaluate these procedures for safety and efficacy.

21.4 Conclusion

As our experience with Type B AD has grown, we have come to understand the true nature of this process as a chronic disease in need of long-term management. Newer data is revealing that a significant number of patients will go on to experience aneurysmal degeneration, even after successful TEVAR. Direct management of the false lumen proves to be an effective tool in the effort to control and halt false lumen flow and associated aortic growth. These methods, likely in conjunction with newer techniques, will help us to manage this chronic disease long-term as our patients age after TEVAR.

REFERENCES

1) Resch T, Delle M, Falkenberg M, et al. Remodeling of the thoracic aorta after stent grafting of type B dissection: a Swedish multicenter study. J Cardiovasc Surg 2006; 47(5): 503-8.
2) Lombardi J, Cambria R, Nienaber C, et al. Aortic remodeling after endovascular treatment of complicated type B aortic dissection with the use of a composite device design. J Vasc Surg 2014; 59(6): 1544-54.
3) Gaxotte V, Thony F, Rousseau H, et al. Midterm results of aortic diameter outcomes after thoracic stent-graft implantation for aortic dissection: a multicenter study. J Endovasc Ther 2006; 13(2): 127-38.
4) Sobocinski J, Dias N, Berger L, et al. Endograft repair of complicated acute Type B aortic dissections. Eur J Vasc Endovasc Surg 2013; 45(5): 468-74.
5) Fattori R, Montgomery D, Lovato L, et al. Survival after endovascular therapy in patients with Type B aortic dissection. JACC Cardiovasc Interv 2013; 6(8): 876-82.
6) Akutsu K, Nejima J, Kiuchi K, et al. Effects of the patent false lumen on the long-term outcome of type B acute aortic dissection. Eur J Cardiothorac Surg 2004; 26(2): 359-66.
7) Sayer D, Bratby M, Brooks M, Loftus I, Morgan R, Thompson M. Aortic morphology following endovascular repair of acute and chronic type B aortic dissection: implications for management. Eur J Vasc Endovasc Surg 2008; 36(5): 522-9.
8) Kang W, Greenberg R, Mastracci T, et al. Endovascular repair of complicated chronic distal aortic dissections: Intermediate outcomes and complications. J Thorac Cardiovasc Surg 2011; 142(5): 1074-83.
9) Andacheh I, Donayre C, Othman F, Walot I, Kopchok G, White R. Patient outcomes and thoracic aortic volume and morphologic changes following thoracic endovascular aortic repair in patients with complicated chronic type B aortic dissection. J Vasc Surg 2012; 56(3): 644-650.
10) Brunkwall J, Kasprzak P, Verhoeven E, Heijmen R, Taylor P. Endovascular repair of acute uncomplicated aortic type B dissection promotes aortic remodelling: 1 year results of the ADSORB trial. Eur J Vasc Endovasc Surg 2014; 48(3): 285-91.
11) Kölbel T, Lohrenz C, Kieback A, Diener H, Debus E, Larena-Avellaneda A. Distal false lumen occlusion in aortic dissection with a homemade extra-large vascular plug: the candy-plug technique. J Endovasc Ther 2013; 20(4): 484-9.
12) Ogawa Y, Nishimaki H, Chiba K, et al. Candy-plug technique using an excluder aortic extender for distal occlusion of a large false lumen aneurysm in chronic aortic dissection. J Endovasc Ther 2016; 23(3): 483-6.
13) Roselli E, Idrees J, Reside J, Shafii S. Use of covered stent devices for false lumen embolization in chronic dissection: a novel approach. Ann Thorac Surg 2014; 98(2): 737-9.
14) Idrees J, Roselli E, Shafii S, Reside J, Lytle B. Outcomes after false lumen embolization with covered stent devices in chronic dissection. J Vasc Surg 2014; 60(6): 1507-13.
15) Hofferberth S, Nixon I, Boston R, McLachlan C, Mossop P. Stent-assisted balloon-induced intimal disruption and relamination in aortic dissection repair: The STABILISE concept. J Thorac Cardiovasc Surg 2014; 147(4): 1240-5.
16) Kölbel T, Carpenter S, Lohrenz C, Tsilimparis N, Larena-Avellaneda A, Debus E. Addressing persistent false lumen flow in chronic aortic dissection: the knickerbocker technique. J Endovasc Ther 2014; 21(1): 117-22.

22

Evolution in endovascular treatment of Type B aortic dissection

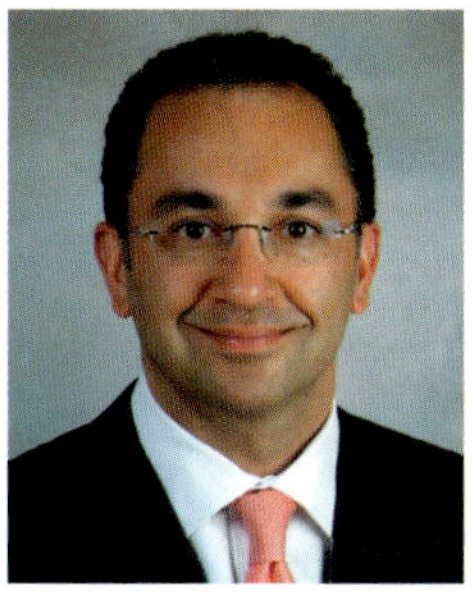

Ali Azizzadeh, Wande B. Pratt, Anthony L. Estrera and Hazim J. Safi

22.1 Introduction

Aortic dissection (AD) represents an increasingly challenging problem, with dynamic pathology, high rates of complications, and considerable risk of fatality if left untreated. It represents the most common aortic emergency, and occurs in three to six persons per 100,000 each year [1-3]. It is further expected that 20-30% of patients will succumb prior to hospital admission [1]. Successful management mandates high clinical suspicion, prompt diagnosis, accurate assessment of aortic and branch vessel involvement, and long-term surveillance and follow up. Although significant improvements in the management of AD have been made since it was first described by Hirst et al. in 1958 [4], consensus guidelines for treatment of Type B AD, where the entry tear originates distal to the left subclavian artery, remain elusive. This chapter will review the evolution of endovascular treatment of Type B AD over the last half century.

22.2 Early descriptions and classifications

Acute AD was first described more than 200 years ago, by Morgagni [5, 6]. According to his recollection, on October 25, 1760, King George II, then age 76, arose at 6 a.m. and called for his chocolate, as per his usual routine. The German valet de chambre heard a noise, which he memorably described as "louder than the royal wind," and then a groan. He ran in and, to his dismay, found the king lying on the floor, having cut his face from the fall. A surgeon was called, but no signs of life were observed. The next day, an autopsy revealed that the pericardium was opened and found to be distended with a pint of coagulated blood. A transverse fissure was noted on the inner side of the ascending aorta, nearly 4-cm long, through which blood had recently passed to form a raised ecchymosis, for which the appearance was interpreted as an aneurysm of the ascending aorta.

Ali Azizzadeh (Ali.Azizzadeh@uth.tmc.edu)
McGovern School at The University of Texas, Health Science Center (UTHealth),
Houston, TX, USA

G. Melissano - R. Chiesa (eds), Aortic Dissection patients true stories and the innovations that saved their lives

Although similar cases were described over the next 40 years, it was not until 1802, when Maunoir [7] uniquely introduced the concept of blood "dissecting throughout the circumference of the aorta." In doing so, he was among the first to distinguish the condition of dissection from that of aortic aneurysm. Despite this characterization, the link to aneurysms persisted, as Laennec – 20 years later – coined the term "dissecting aortic aneurysm" in 1826 [8].

In 1843, Thomas Bevill Peacock provided an elaborate epidemiologic and pathologic account of the condition of dissecting aortic aneurysm, which has since been replaced by the term AD [6]. He collected a total of 19 published cases, and noted that patients with AD were typically older than patients with saccular aneurysms. He described sophisticated experiments in which fluids were injected between the adventitia and tunica media of the aorta. He discovered that a channel tended to re-enter into the original vessel, rather than rupture externally. He ingeniously recognized that dissections arising in the ascending aorta portend a worse prognosis than those originating in the descending aorta. "When the fissures were near the origin of the aorta[...] the extravasated blood readily makes its way into the sac of the pericardium [...] and death is almost instantaneous [...] When the fissures are situated below the arch of the aorta, the blood [...] tends to separate the coats in the lower portion of the vessel and rarely makes it way to its origin; and, thus, the disease [...] may be in no degree accessory to the patients' death."

For many years, the condition of AD remained a post-mortem diagnosis, as the outcome was uniformly fatal. It was not until the introduction of cardiopulmonary bypass in the mid-1950s, when surgical management became a possibility, and helped advance our understand-

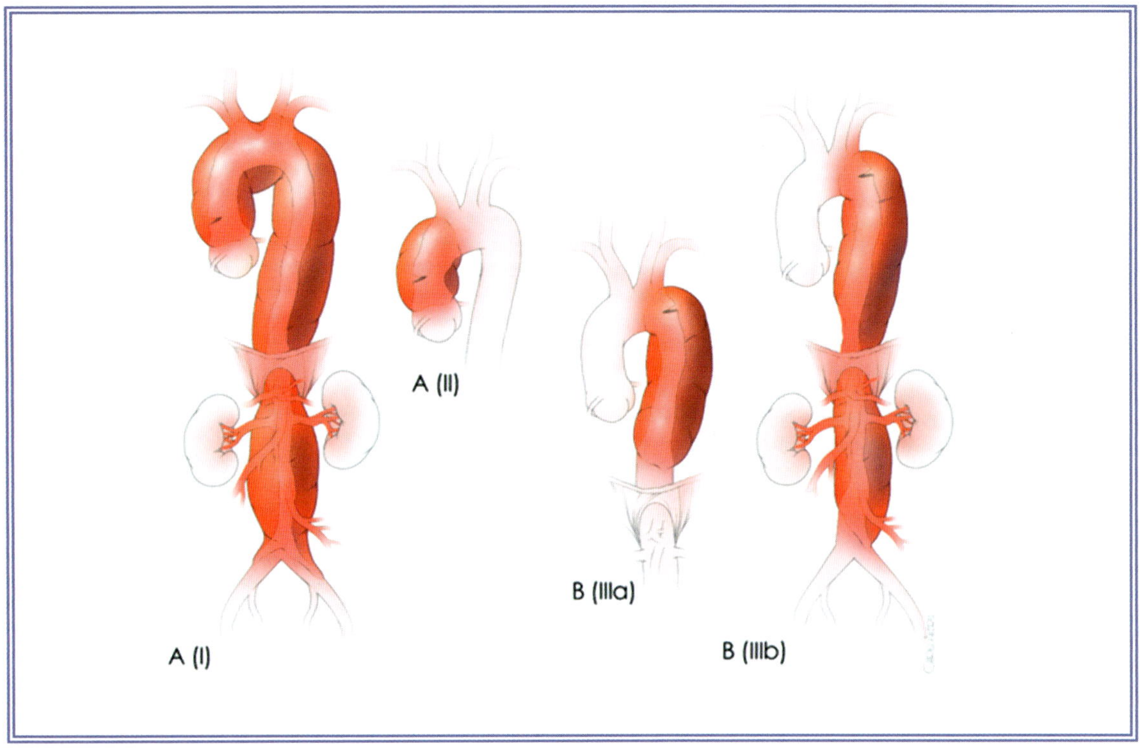

Fig. 22.1 Classifications for aortic dissection. **A**, DeBakey Type I AD are described as those dissections originating in the ascending aorta with further involvement of the descending thoracic and abdominal aorta. Type II AD differ in that they are confined to the ascending aorta. Stanford Type A AD include both DeBakey Types I and II. **B**, DeBakey Type III AD are distinct from the proximal AD, originate at the level of the subclavian artery, and are either entirely confined to the descending thoracic aorta (Type IIIa), or are found to extend to the abdominal aorta (Type IIIb). DeBakey Type IIIa and IIIb AD are collectively classified as Stanford Type B AD.

ing and management of this complex problem. Early attempts at repair included decompression of the false lumen with distal re-entry in the iliac artery, and cellophane wrapping [9, 10]. In 1955, DeBakey reported the first successful operative repair of AD [11]. Ten years later, in 1965, he provided the original classification of AD (Fig. 22.1) [12]. DeBakey Type I AD are described as those dissections originating in the ascending aorta with further involvement of the descending thoracic and abdominal aorta. Type II AD differ in that they are confined to the ascending aorta. Type III AD are distinct from the proximal AD, originate at the level of the subclavian artery, and are either entirely confined to the descending thoracic aorta (Type IIIa), or are found to extend to the abdominal aorta (Type IIIb). Although outcomes for operative repair of dissections in the ascending aorta were encouraging, results in the descending aorta were abysmal, prompting Palmer and Wheat to propose a strategy focused on lowering systolic blood pressure and heart rate [13]. This distinction helped usher in a new, refined classification of AD in 1970. The Stanford classification categorized Type A AD as proximal (DeBakey Types I and II) AD; Stanford Type B AD are described as distal AD (DeBakey Type III) [14]. The Stanford classification is the most widely used description in the literature, and is clinically applicable, as Type A AD generally require primary operative intervention, whereas Type B AD are typically treated medically with operative intervention reserved for malperfusion, rupture, or complications. However, in recent years, the DeBakey classification has re-emerged as a more practical schema as endovascular treatment strategies for treatment of AD dissection have rapidly evolved.

Aortic dissections are further classified according to symptom onset. Historically, acute AD were defined as those dissections that occurred within 14 days of symptom onset; dissections lasting longer than 14 days were defined as chronic AD. More recent nomenclature has introduced subacute dissections as those occurring from 2 to 6 weeks, and chronic dissections lasting longer than 6 weeks [15].

Finally, AD have been stratified based on their natural history and clinical sequelae. Complicated AD include ruptured cases; result in malperfusion of the brain, spinal cord, abdominal viscera, kidneys, or lower limbs; or cause intractable pain, or pain refractory to optimal medical therapy. Complicated dissections represent 25-40% of DeBakey Type III AD, and require urgent or emergent intervention, either by open surgical or endovascular approaches. Uncomplicated AD do not have these complications, and are frequently managed with anti-impulse therapy – frequently beta blockade – titrated to a systolic blood pressure less than 120 mmHg.

22.3 TEVAR trials

Medical management strategies – focused on lowering the systolic blood pressure and heart rate – have remained the standard of care for treatment of uncomplicated acute Type B AD. These strategies have demonstrated favorable historical outcomes, with 30-day mortality approaching 10%, and one-year survival ranging from 70 to 90%. However, these improved outcomes are tempered by results indicating up to 40% of patients will require additional interventions for aneurysmal degeneration or failed medical management, typically within 12 months of symptom onset, and not infrequently within 30 days. Furthermore, 5% of patients will die in the first 30 days, and up to 30% will die within one year [16-23].

In 1999, Dake et al. introduced thoracic endovascular aortic repair (TEVAR) as an alternative treatment option for patients with Type B AD [24]. In contrast to open surgical therapy – in which the dissected septum was removed, the diseased aorta was replaced, and the blood flow was directed into the true lumen – endovascular treatment emerged as a less invasive approach to cover the primary aortic intimal tear and obliterate the false lumen in AD, thereby inducing false lumen thrombosis, and preventing aneurysmal degeneration of the descending thoracic aorta. Initially, TEVAR was reserved for patients with acute AD complicated by malperfusion or rupture, and in select circumstances when open surgery was prohibitive. This strategy was widely adopted, despite a lack of randomized data. TEVAR enthusiasts cited compelling evidence that TEVAR promotes aortic remodeling for complicated Type B AD. Nearly 90% of patients undergoing TEVAR demonstrated thrombosis of the false lumen and a decrease in maximum aortic diameter, even at one year [25]. Similarly, the prospective, multicenter STABLE trial demonstrated a 100% rate of either partial or complete thrombosis of the false lumen in the initial post-procedure imaging study, and a 31% rate of complete thrombosis at one year, compared to 0% at presentation [26].

The role of TEVAR, however, in uncomplicated dissections remained unknown in the early 2000s. The INSTEAD Trial, published in 2009, was the first of its kind to compare medical management and TEVAR for uncomplicated Type B AD [27]. The study randomized 140 patients in stable clinical condition with uncomplicated Type B AD to either a strategy of elective endografting with optimal medical therapy or optimal medical therapy alone. Patients with dissections between 2 and 52 weeks' duration (i.e. subacute and chronic) were eligible for study randomization. Acute Type B AD were excluded.

The study was sponsored by Medtronic (Dublin, Ireland), and all patients randomized to the TEVAR group received Talent stent grafts. The primary endpoint was all-cause mortality at two years; secondary endpoints included aortic-related mortality, disease progression with need for conversion or additional intervention, and aortic remodeling. At two years, there was no difference in all-cause or aortic-related mortality. However, with only 11 deaths, the trial did not achieve the assumption of 28 events necessary to achieve the desired statistical power. The secondary endpoint of disease progression was also similar between the groups. The investigators revealed that aortic remodeling – defined as true-lumen recovery and false-lumen thrombosis – occurred in 91.3% of patients with TEVAR compared to 19.4% of patients who received optimal medical therapy alone ($p < 0.001$). It was this finding that encouraged the investigators to hypothesize that endovascular treatment of Type B AD may have long-term benefits.

These prognostic benefits were examined in the INSTEAD-XL trial, published in 2013 [28]. Long-term follow up – a minimum of five years – was achieved for the original 140 INSTEAD patients, and no patient was lost to follow-up. All-cause mortality, aortic-specific mortality, and disease progression was significantly lower with TEVAR than with optimal medical treatment alone. Further analysis suggested this benefit occurred for all endpoints between two and five years. This landmark contribution demonstrated a long-term survival benefit of TEVAR for uncomplicated Type B AD, and established endovascular treatment as a suitable – and among some groups, a preferred – treatment modality for subacute and/or chronic Type B AD.

The role of TEVAR specifically for acute uncomplicated Type B AD was examined in the ADSORB Trial, published in 2014 [29]. The study randomized 61 patients with acute uncomplicated Type B AD to best medical treatment alone vs. best medical treatment plus thoracic endografting using the GORE® TAG® device (W.L. Gore & Associates, Flagstaff, AZ). Endografting was performed within 48 hours of randomization. The primary endpoint was a composite endpoint, defined as freedom from all of the following: partial or incomplete false lumen thrombosis; aortic dilatation; and aortic rupture. Computed tomography was performed 3 months and 1 year after randomization to assess for aortic remodeling, focusing on maximum diameter of the true and false lumen and the overall aortic diameter. At one-year follow-up, thoracic endografting and best medical therapy performed better than best medical therapy alone, with respect to partial or incomplete false lumen thrombosis, and aortic diameter. Criticisms of the study have focused on its small sample size, underpowered to assess mortality differences; improper use of false lumen thrombosis as a primary endpoint; and its short duration of follow-up.

A recent, nonrandomized, multi-institutional retrospective study compared TEVAR and best medical therapy for 338 patients with acute uncomplicated Type B AD [30]. The authors demonstrated that there were no significant differences in early outcomes, and only 2% of dissections converted to complicated – all of which occurred in the basic medical therapy group. Late outcomes – with the exception of a 9% rate of endoleak – favored the TEVAR group. Rates of aortic dilatation, aortic rupture, aortic-related and all-cause mortality were all significantly lower in the TEVAR group at 5 years. The study demonstrated that TEVAR for uncomplicated Type B AD is feasible in the acute setting with rates of technical and clinical success comparable to those achieved for subacute and chronic dissections. The authors proposed that TEVAR should be considered as an alternative to medical management for acute uncomplicated Type B AD. Indeed, for some, the ADSORB trial and this more recent retrospective study have already expanded the indications for endovascular treatment for Type B AD to include the acute uncomplicated scenarios. Most would agree that these studies highlight the need for a randomized trial for this specific clinical indication.

22.3.1 Endovascular renaissance

There is little doubt that the US Food and Drug Administration's (FDA) approval of thoracic stent grafts – initially in 2005, for descending thoracic aneurysms; again in 2012, for traumatic aortic injury; and then subsequently in 2013, for AD – ushered in a paradigm shift for repair of Type B AD. The current era of treatment of Type B AD favors an endovascular approach over open surgical repair. A recent analysis demonstrated this phenomenon among Medicare beneficiaries across the United States during the last 10 years [31]. The authors found that the overall rate of endovascular repairs rose from 0 to 0.8 per 100,000 persons, and that the increase was most dramatic after 2005, with the introduction of the TEVAR-specific ICD-9 procedural code. In 2000, TEVAR represented 1% of repairs of Type B AD, compared to 27% in 2010. During the same period, rates of open surgical repair declined. Despite these trends, TEVAR patients were more likely to suffer from a number of comorbid conditions, including congestive heart failure, chronic pulmonary disease, diabetes, and renal insufficiency.

Population-based studies demonstrate that TEVAR is utilized for more than one-third of thoracic aortic aneurysms, and this number is rising for AD [32]. Going forward, we will continue to see an explosion in the utilization of endovascular treatments, as the technology improves. Lower profile devices are already under investigation, as are branched devices for deployment in the aortic arch and paravisceral segment. These devices will expand the current indications for endovascular therapies, and increase accessibility of commercial and off-the-shelf devices, particularly for patients who otherwise may not have been offered open repair. It is likely – and probably inevitable – that a growing number of patients with Type B AD will be treated with TEVAR, and that open repair (as observed in abdominal aortic aneurysms) will be reserved for specific patients with more complex anatomic disease at select institutions.

22.4 A case of acute complicated Type B aortic dissection

The following is a case of an acute complicated Type B AD in a 75-year-old woman with hypertension and atrial fibrillation. She presented to an outside hospital with acute onset of severe back and leg pain, and absent pedal pulses. We performed computed tomography, which demonstrated a Stanford Type B (DeBakey Type IIIb) AD with infrarenal aortic occlusion and extension of the dissection to the right common femoral artery (Fig. 22.2). She was transferred to our facility, admitted to the intensive care unit, and subsequently treated with a thoracic endograft.

Following induction of general anesthesia, we circumferentially dissected the right common femoral artery through a transverse groin incision. Gross inspection revealed a dissected common femoral artery. We cannulated the artery with a micropuncture needle and sheath, and

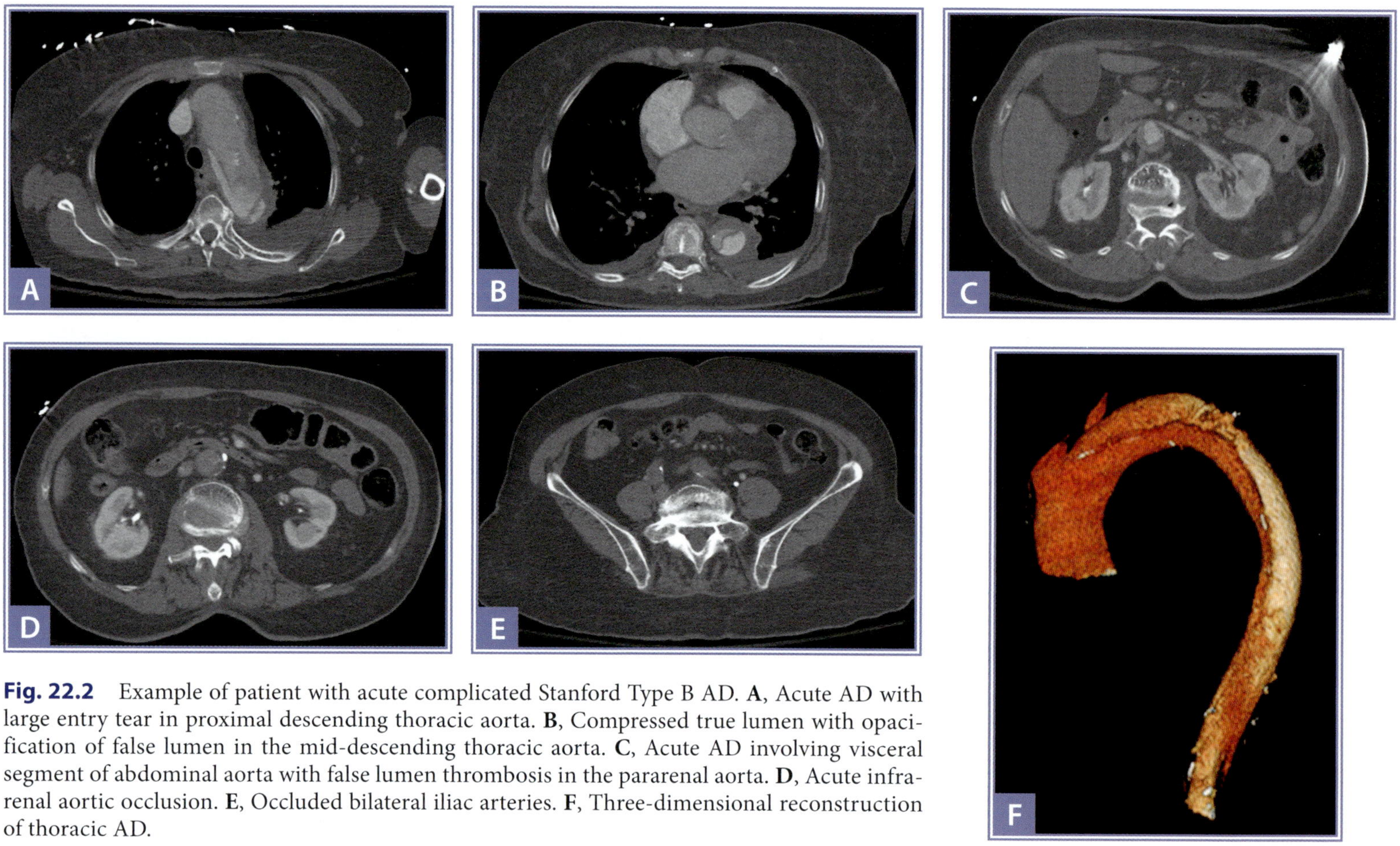

Fig. 22.2 Example of patient with acute complicated Stanford Type B AD. **A**, Acute AD with large entry tear in proximal descending thoracic aorta. **B**, Compressed true lumen with opacification of false lumen in the mid-descending thoracic aorta. **C**, Acute AD involving visceral segment of abdominal aorta with false lumen thrombosis in the pararenal aorta. **D**, Acute infrarenal aortic occlusion. **E**, Occluded bilateral iliac arteries. **F**, Three-dimensional reconstruction of thoracic AD.

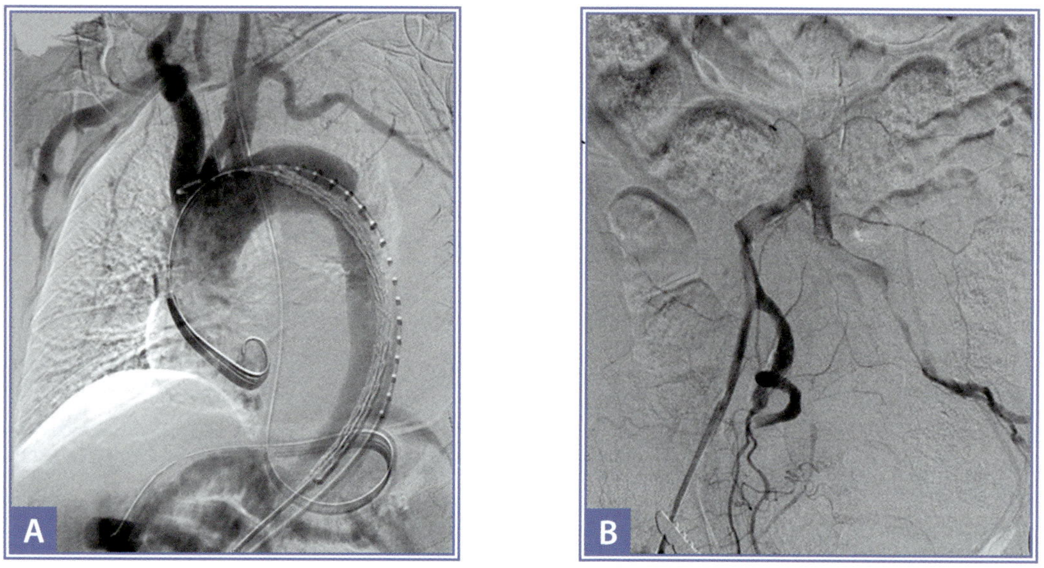

Fig. 22.3 Initial diagnostic angiograms. **A**, Acute AD with primary entry tear in the descending thoracic aorta originating near the takeoff of the left subclavian. **B**, Aortoiliac thrombosis due to a Type B AD.

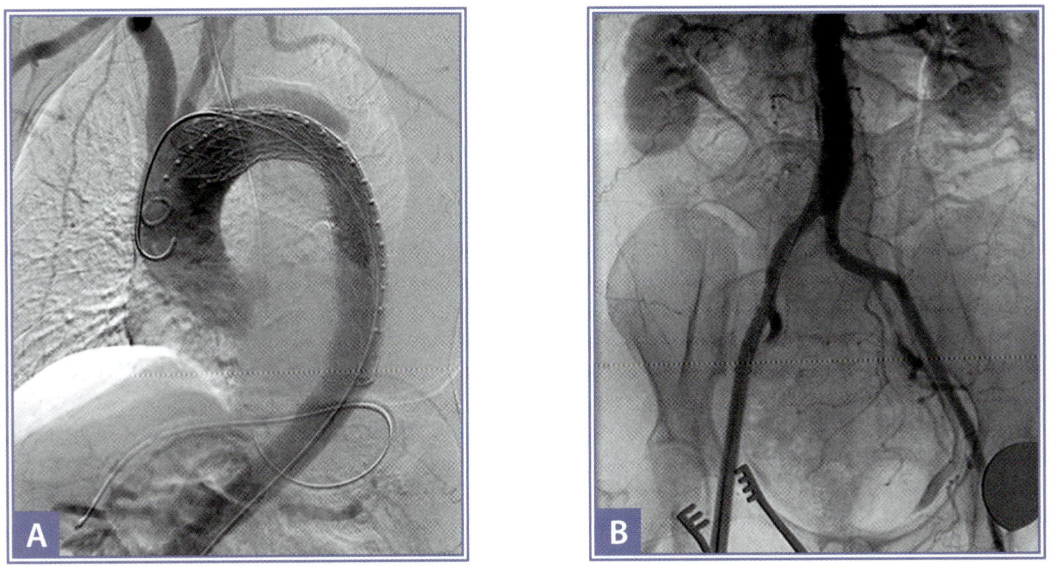

Fig. 22.4 Post-deployment angiograms. **A**, Flow and re-expansion of true lumen in descending thoracic aorta. **B**, Visualization and recanalization of abdominal aorta and bilateral iliac arteries.

performed a retrograde aortoiliac angiogram. This demonstrated extensive aortoiliac thrombus (Fig. 22.3). We traversed the lumen with an angled Glidewire® (Terumo, Somerset, NJ), and confirmed our guidewire was in the true lumen using intravascular ultrasound (IVUS). Interrogation of the aorta revealed a dissection extending from the left subclavian artery (LSCA) to the aortic bifurcation, with a proximal entry tear at the origin of the LSCA. The proximal landing zone was selected, and the neck diameter measured with IVUS. A GORE® TAG® 37-mm x 20-cm stent graft was advanced into the arch. The device was deployed with intentional coverage of the origin of the LSCA in order to achieve a 2-cm proximal seal. Post-deployment arch angiogram demonstrated successful coverage of the proximal entry tear (zones 2 to 5), and minimal flow in the false lumen (Fig. 22.4). Abdominal aortogram similarly demonstrated flow in the bilateral common and external iliac arteries. IVUS confirmed complete re-expansion of the true lumen from the descending thoracic aorta to the iliac arteries.

This case illustrates that when successful, thoracic endovascular aortic repair can re-establish true lumen patency and facilitate aortic remodeling in Type B AD complicated by limb ischemia, visceral and/or renal malperfusion.

22.5 Conclusion

Although once felt to be less morbid than its Type A counterpart, it is now clear that type B AD is not a benign disease. Historically, medical management alone has been the gold standard for its treatment due to more favorable early outcomes compared to open repairs. However, more recent evidence has shown that patients treated medically are at risk for aneurysmal degeneration, aortic rupture, late mortality, and reintervention. As a result, rates of endovascular repair of Type B AD have increased over time, and most rapidly in the United States since the emergence of FDA-approved devices in 2005 (for thoracic aneurysms), and in 2013 (for dissections). This has resulted in a dramatic decrease in perioperative mortality rates for all patients undergoing surgical repair – either open or endovascular. As advancements in technology are made, we can expect the indications for endovascular treatment to broaden, and the short and long-term patient outcomes to improve. Few would disagree that TEVAR has already left an indelible imprint on our treatment strategies for AD. Its legacy will depend on whether we can successfully integrate patient selection with device selection, preserve branch vessel patency, manage intramural hematoma, and evolve our technology for treatment of the ascending aorta.

REFERENCES

1) Olsson C, Thelin S, Ståhle E, et al. Thoracic aortic aneurysm and dissection: increasing prevalence and improved outcomes reported in a nationwide population-based study of more than 14,000 cases from 1987 to 2002. Circulation 2006; 114: 2611-18.
2) Howard D, Banerjee A, Fairhead J, et al. Population-based study of incidence and outcome of acute aortic dissection and premorbid risk factor control: 10-year results from the Oxford Vascular Study. Circulation 2013; 127: 2031-7.
3) Scott AJ, Bicknell CD. Contemporary management of acute type B dissection. Eur J Vasc Endovasc Surg 2016; 51: 452-9.
4) Hirst A, Johns VJ, Krime SJ. Dissecting aneurysm of the aorta: a review of 505 cases. Medicine 1958; 37: 217-79.
5) Morgagni GB. De sedibtus et causis morborum. Ep 26, Art 17 (Ep 48) F 50. Venice; 1761.
6) Leonard JC. Thomas Bevill Peacock and the early history of dissecting aneurysm. BMJ 1979; 2: 260-2.
7) Maunoir JP. Mémoires physiologiques et pratiques sur l'anévrisme et la ligature des artères. Geneva: JJ Paschoud; 1802.
8) Laennec RTH. Traite de l'auscultationt mediate et des maladies des poumons et du coeur. Vol. 2. 2ND Ed Paris: J.-S. Chaude; 1826: 696.
9) Gurin D, Bulmer J, Derby R. Diagnosis and operative relief of arterial obstruction due to this cause. N State J Med 1935; 35: 1200.
10) Abbott OA. Clinical experiences with the application of polythene cellophane upon the aneurysms of the thoracic vessels. J Thorac Surg 1949; 18: 435-61.
11) DeBakey ME, Cooley DA, Creech O Jr. Surgical considerations of dissecting aneurysm of the aorta. Ann Surg 1955; 142: 586-612.
12) DeBakey ME, Henly WS, Cooley DA, et al. Surgical management of dissecting aneurysms of the aorta. J Thorac Cardiovasc Surg 1965; 49: 130-49.
13) Palmer RF, Wheat MW. Treatment of dissecting aneurysms of the aorta. Ann Thorac Surg 1967; 4: 38-52.
14) Daily PO, Trueblood HW, Stinson EB, et al. Management of acute aortic dissections. Ann Thorac Surg 1970; 10: 237-47.
15) VIRTUE Registry Investigators. Mid-term outcomes and aortic remodeling after thoracic endovascular repair for acute, subacute, and chronic aortic dissection: the VIRTUE registry. Eur J Vasc Endovasc Surg 2014; 14: 363-71.
16) Umana JP, Lai DI, Mitchell RS, et al. Is medical therapy still the optimal treatment strategy for patients with acute type B aortic dissections? J Thorac Cardiovasc Surg 2002; 124: 896-910.
17) Suzuki T, Mehta RH, Ince H, et al. Clinical profiles and outcomes of acute type B aortic dissection in the current era: lessons from the International Registry of Aortic Dissection (IRAD). Circulation 2003; 108 Suppl 1: II312-7.
18) Dialetto G, Covino FE, Scognamiglio G, et al. Treatment of type B aortic dissection: endoluminal repair or conventional medical therapy? Eur J Cardio-Thorac Surg 2005; 27: 826-30.
19) Nienaber CA, Zannetti S, Barbieri B, et al. Investigation of stent grafts in patients with type B aortic dissection: design of the INSTEAD trial—a prospective, multicenter, European randomized trial. Am Heart J 2005; 149: 592-99.
20) Estrera AL, Miller CC, Safi HJ, et al. Outcomes of medical management of acute type B aortic dissection. Circulation 2006; 114 Suppl 1: I384-9.
21) Tsai TT, Fattori R, Trimarchi S, et al. Long-term survival in patients presenting with type B acute aortic dissection: insights from the international registry of acute aortic dissection. Circulation 2006; 114: 2226-31.
22) Winnerkvist A, Lockowandt U, Rasmussen E, Radegran K. A prospective study of medically treated acute type B aortic dissection. Eur J Vasc Endovasc Surg 2006; 32: 349-55.
23) Durham CA, Cambria RP, Wang LJ, et al. The natural history of medically managed acute type B aortic dissection. J Vasc Surg 2015; 61: 1192-8.
24) Dake MD, Kato N, Mitchel RS, et al. Endovascular stent-graft placement for the treatment of acute aortic dissection. N Engl J Med 1999; 340: 1546-52.
25) Conrad MF, Crawford RS, Kwolek CJ, et al. Aortic remodeling after endovascular repair of acute complicated type B aortic dissection. J Vasc Surg 2009; 50: 510-7.

26) Lombardi JV, Cambria RP, Nienaber CA, et al. Prospective multicenter clinical trial (STABLE) on the endovascular treatment of complicated type B aortic dissection using a composite device design. J Vasc Surg 2012; 55: 629-40.
27) Nienaber CA, Roussea H, Eggebrecht H, et al. Randomized comparison of strategies for type B aortic dissection: the INvestigation of STEnt Grafts in Aortic Dissection (INSTEAD) Trial. Circulation 2009; 120: 2519-28.
28) Nienaber CA, Kische S, Rousseau H, et al. Endovascular repair of type B aortic dissection: long-term results of the randomized INvestigation of STEnt grafts in Aortic Dissection Trial. Circ Cardiovasc Interv 2013; 6: 407-16.
29) Brunkwall J, Kasprzak P, Verhoeven E, et al. Endovascular repair of acute uncomplicated aortic type B dissection promotes aortic remodeling: 1 year results of the ADSORB trial. Eur J Vasc Endovasc Surg 2014; 48: 285-91.
30) Qin YL, Wang F, Li TX, et al. Endovascular repair compared with medical management of patients with uncomplicated type B acute aortic dissection. J Am Coll Cardiol 2016; 67: 2835-42.
31) Jones DW, Goodney PP, Nolan BW, et al. National trends in utilization, mortality, and survival after repair of type B aortic dissection in the Medicare population. J Vasc Surg 2014; 60: 11-9.
32) Scali ST, Goodney PP, Walsh DB, et al. National trends and regional variation of open and endovascular repair of thoracic and thoracoabdominal aneurysms in contemporary practice. J Vasc Surg 2011; 53: 1499-505.

23

The PETTICOAT technique for endovascular treatment of Type B aortic dissection

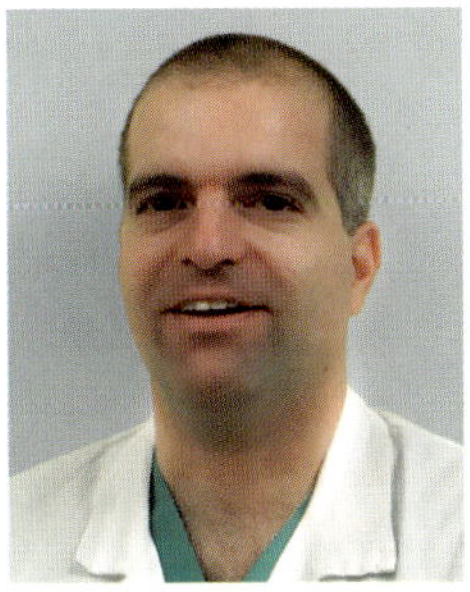

Luca Bertoglio, Germano Melissano, Enrico Rinaldi, Andrea L. Kahlberg, Sthefano Atique Gabriel and Roberto Chiesa

23.1 Introduction

Approximately 25% of patients presenting with acute Type B aortic dissection (AD) meet the definition for complicated status (impending rupture, end-organ malperfusion, refractory hypertension or pain) with an associated higher 30-day mortality rate [1]. An obstruction of flow of one or more aortic side branches is present in one-third of complicated patients who are consequently affected by the so-called "malperfusion syndrome". This syndrome is characterized by a nearly three-fold increased likelihood of in-hospital mortality in acute Type B AD [2]: regardless of the treatment success, the presence of both mesenteric ischemia and limb ischemia has been associated to a poor prognosis [2, 3].

Identifying the mechanisms of branch compromise is a critical step in planning effective treatment strategies. Williams et al. [4] introduced the radiological classification of malperfusion mechanisms based on branch-vessel involvement, identifying two types of obstruction:

- dynamic obstruction (Fig. 23.1): the compressed true lumen (TL) is unable to provide adequate flow because the aortic flap prolapses across the branch-vessel origin covering it like a curtain but without entering into it. Because of the constantly changing position of the intimal flap, particularly in the acute phase, these obstructions can be total or subtotal with persistent or intermittent features. This is the most common mechanism of branch compromise and it is responsible for some 80% of malperfusion syndromes [5];
- static obstruction (Fig. 23.2): the dissection flap intersects or enters the branch-vessel origin propagating into the vessel wall. Typically, flap progression into a branch is tolerated because a distal re-entry develops allowing perfusion of the distal vessel from both the lumens (static malperfusion with re-entry). However, a potential profound malperfusion exists when the false lumen (FL) within the branch does not have a re-entry point in the vessel (static malperfusion with no re-entry). As a result, the FL is a blind cul-de-sac which enlarges and compresses the TL. In all cases of static malperfusion, the obstruction is unlikely to be resolved with the restoration of aortic TL flow alone [6, 7].

Luca Bertoglio (bertoglio.luca@hsr.it)
Scientific Institute Ospedale San Raffaele,
Milan, Italy

G. Melissano - R. Chiesa (eds), Aortic Dissection patients true stories and the innovations that saved their lives

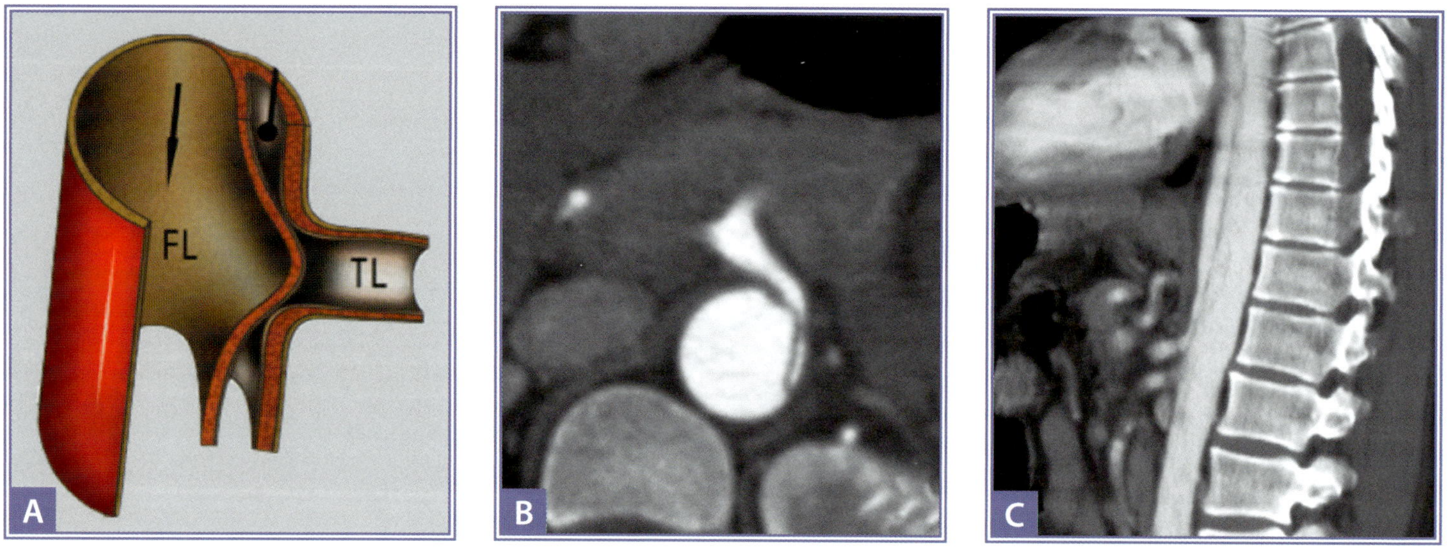

Fig. 23.1 Dynamic malperfusion (**A**): the true lumen (TL) is compressed by the false lumen (FL) and is unable to provide adequate volume flow to the aortic branch. In this example: the axial computed tomography (CT) scan (**B**) demonstrates the collapsed TL due to the FL compression, and the multi-planar reformatting (MPR) view (**C**) shows the extension of the TL collapse to the whole thoracoabdominal aorta.

Nowadays, dynamic obstruction is often managed by means of stent-graft covering of the entry tear, with the following goals [8]:

- covering of the proximal entry tear and creating a seal to stop the flow of blood from entering the FL and prevent the transmission of systemic pressure across the major intimal defect;
- redirecting flow into the TL with FL decompression which may relieve dynamic obstruction of branches supplied by the collapsed TL;
- promoting thrombosis and remodelling of the thoracic FL with the aim of reducing long-term aortic related reinterventions.

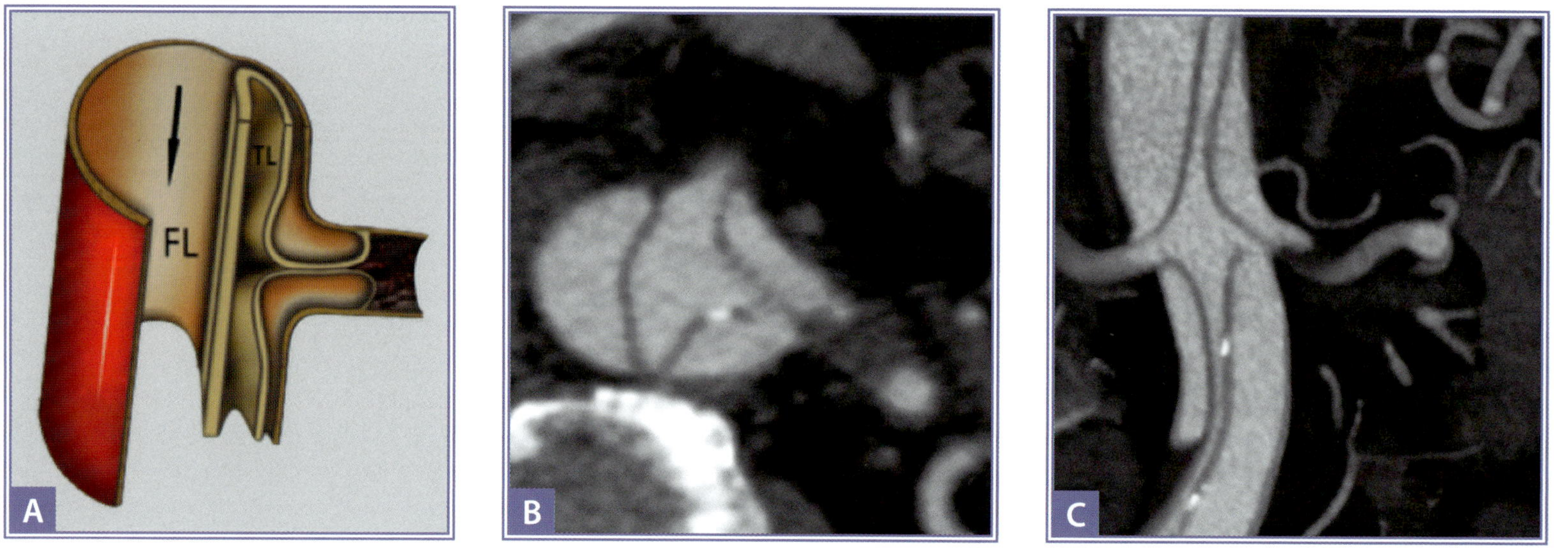

Fig. 23.2 Static malperfusion (**A**): the dissection enters directly and obstructs the ostium of a branch vessel; organ injury can occur as a result of thrombosis or hypoperfusion of the involved vessel. In this example: the axial computed tomography (CT) scan demonstrates the dissection entering into the ostium of the left renal artery (**B**) and the compression of the FL without re-entry causes the partial thrombosis at the ostium of the vessel with end-organ malperfusion (**C**).

Although emergent Thoracic EndoVascular Aortic Repair (TEVAR) for patients with complicated acute Type B AD has shown acceptable 1-year mortality and morbidity (estimated mortality: 10.8%) [9], the fate of the distal thoracoabdominal aorta might remain unaddressed. Distal re-entry tears may sustain distal pressurization of the FL with TL collapse and unsolved dynamic malperfusion. Moreover, the FL may fail to thrombose, thus jeopardizing the aortic remodelling with the consequent risk of an aneurysmal degeneration. Furthermore, the perfusion patterns of visceral and renal branches could change after TEVAR in an unpredictable way leading to persistent or even new malperfusion patterns. For these reasons, additional interventional procedures might be necessary to solve persistent dynamic malperfusion after the initial TEVAR [10].

Some authors have proposed endovascular fenestration alone or in combination with TEVAR aimed at artificially creating a distal abdominal re-entry channel in order to equalize the pressure between the TL and FL [8, 10]. The subsequent FL decompression may relieve TL dynamic obstruction of the aorta and its branch vessels. However, fenestrations may create unpredictable alterations in intimal flap anatomy and flow dynamics. In addition, the effect of fenestration on the long-term outcome of FL expansion in patients with distal dissections is unknown because the FL remains pressurized and therefore at risk of continued progression to aneurysm.

Hence, other solutions have been proposed to solve persistent dynamic malperfusion after TEVAR and to enhance the remodelling of the thoracoabdominal aorta without disrupting the dissection lamellae architecture. Today, aortic scaffolding with bare metal stents, known as the PETTICOAT technique, has been added to the armamentarium of vascular surgeons and it is claimed to improve the short and mid-term results of complicated acute Type B AD.

23.2 The PETTICOAT concept

In 2003, Ito et al. [11] first reported the use of a Gianturco bare Z-stent released in the distal abdominal aorta in order to re-expand a collapsed TL and to solve a visceral dynamic malperfusion. Two years later, Mossop et al. [12] performed a staged endovascular treatment for complicated Type B AD using, first, a standard TEVAR to close the proximal entry tear and, 1 week later, a bare Z-stent deployed in the distal aorta to re-expand the distal collapsed TL. They described the procedure with the acronym of STABLE (Staged ThoracoAbdominal and Branch vesseL Endoluminal repair). In 2006, Nienaber et al. [13] published the first series of 12 patients treated with a proximal TEVAR combined with the use of distal bare stents deployed in the TL in order to help its re-expansion. The authors proposed the acronym of PETTICOAT (Provisional ExTension To Induce COmplete ATtachment) to describe the procedure and, nowadays, this is the term most commonly used to describe it.

The PETTICOAT technique involves the closure of the primary entry tear, performed with standard TEVAR, in order to re-direct blood flow into the TL and depressurize the FL. The expected consequence of the proximal TEVAR is that the thoracic and abdominal TL will tend to expand and the FL to shrink. Usually, thoracic FL thrombosis is obtained at least in the covered stented area and further shrinkage and positive remodelling is achieved. However, in spite of successful deployment of the standard stent graft over the proximal entry tear, the TL distal to the stent graft may fail to dilate satisfactorily with possible persistent dynamic malperfusion. This problem can be addressed by deploying bare metal stents distally to a standard stent graft down into the thoracic and abdominal TL (Fig. 23.3). Not only will the described PETTICOAT technique re-expand the thoracoabdominal TL solving the dynamic malperfusion, but also it will, possibly, address other unmet goals of TEVAR in acute Type B AD.

The intimal lamella distal to a standard TEVAR undergoes continuous movements with each systole and diastole, which keeps the blood in motion in the FL preventing thrombosis occurring at this level. With the introduction of a bare stent beyond the stent graft and down

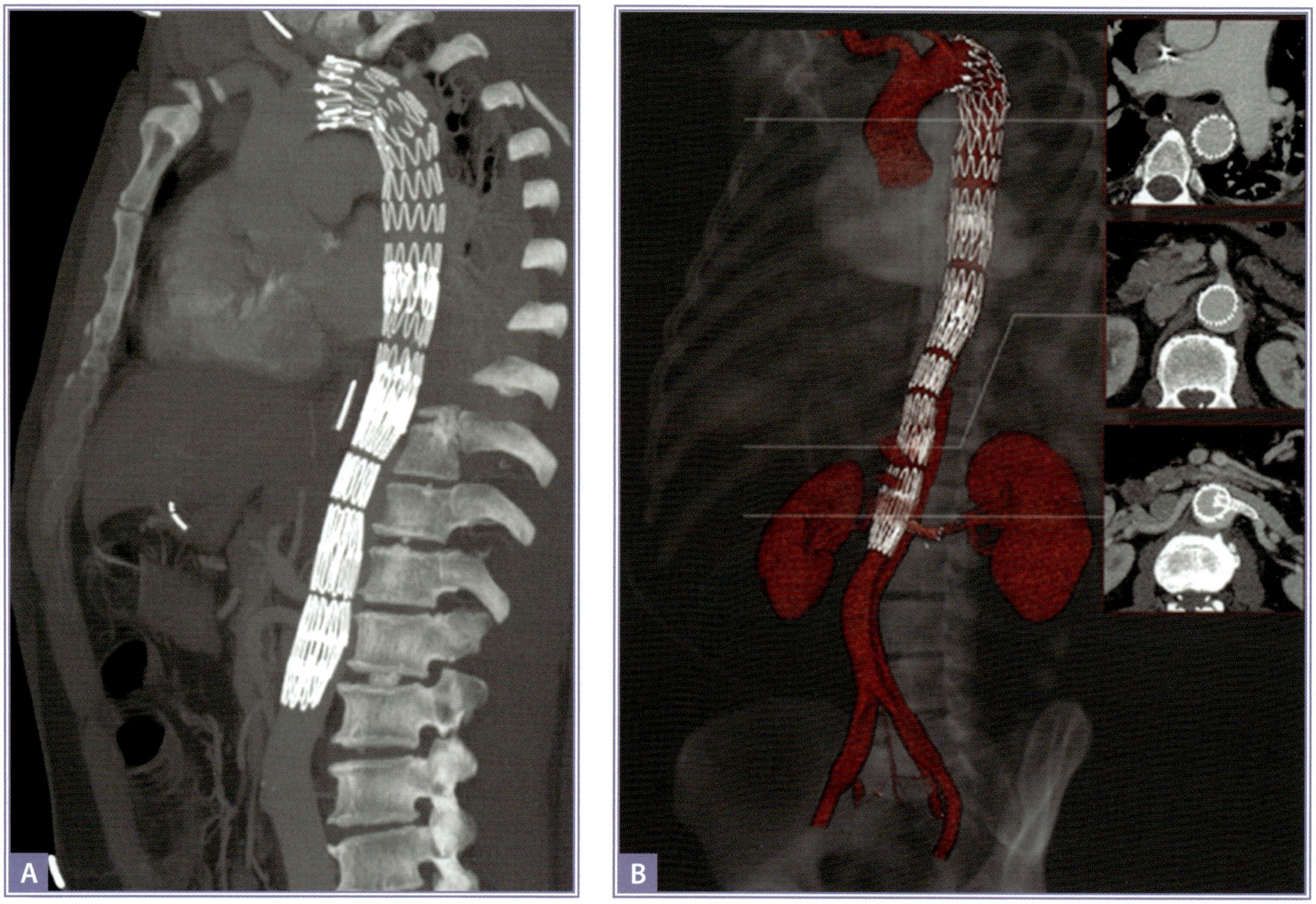

Fig. 23.3 The Zenith® Dissection Endovascular System (ZDES) proposed by Cook (Cook Medical, Bloomington, IN). **A**, The system employed to treat a Type B AD with stent-graft (TX2® graft) coverage of the proximal entry tear and distal extension with two bare stents (Dissection Stent) in order to expand and stabilize the true lumen (TL). **B**, Postoperative angio-CT scan (3D-volume rendering): endovascular treatment of aortic Type B AD with proximal entry tear coverage with a Cook TX2® stent graft and distal extension with two dissection stents (ZDES). Axial scans show exclusion of the thoracic false lumen (FL) and complete re-expansion of the TL in the thoracic and abdominal segments with restoration of perfusion of the right kidney (left renal stenting was performed in this case to perfuse the left renal artery from the re-expanded TL).

to the dissected distal aorta, it is possible both to support the TL and to fix the lamella. The full expansion of the distal TL associated with the stabilization of the dissecting lamella can promote FL thrombosis and remodelling. Moreover, the possibility to use an uncovered stent in the distal thoracic and abdominal aorta reduces the need for extensive aortic coverage with traditional stent grafts, limiting the risk of spinal cord ischemia.

With regard to visceral and renal perfusion, the PETTICOAT technique is helpful not only in solving dynamic malperfusion without interfering with visceral and renal perfusion but also in addressing static obstruction. Static obstruction of aortic branch vessels can persist despite depressurization of the FL and elimination of dynamic obstruction, because of the extension of the FL into branch-vessel ostia. PETTICOAT facilitates subsequent selective stenting of malperfused aortic branches because the expansion of the TL allows realignment of the intimal ostia of dissected branches (Fig. 23.4). The open design of the bare stent mesh allows relatively easy access and cannulation of the aortic branches as well as bridging of the TL to target

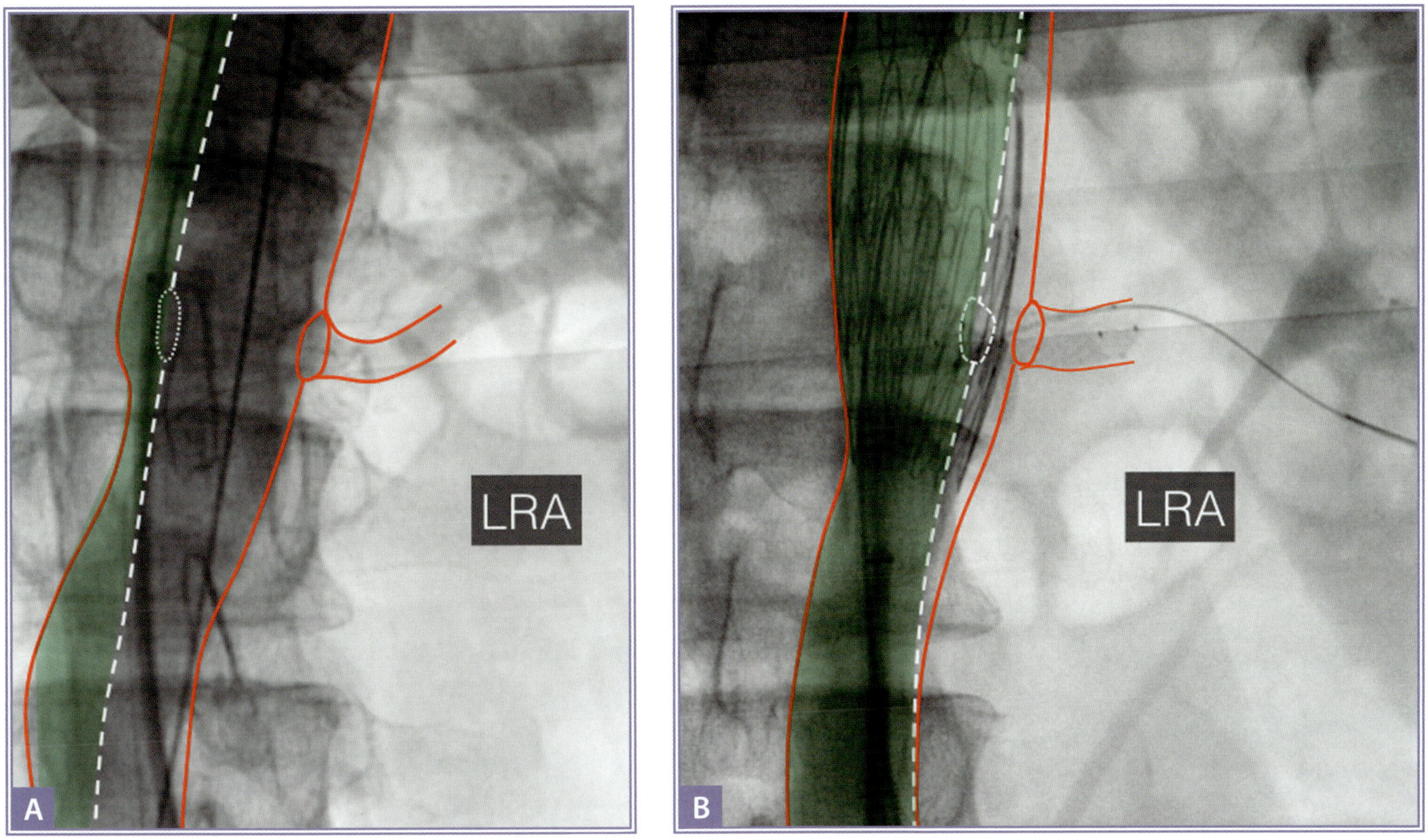

Fig. 23.4 The bare stent-induced true lumen (TL) re-expansion allows realignment of the intimal ostia of dissected branches that could be subsequently stented in order to relieve residual malperfusion. In this case, the left renal artery (LRA) ostium was realigned and then selectively stented with a self-expanding stent. Please note the shorter distance of dissecting lamella (white dotted line) from the renal artery ostium before (**A**) and after (**B**) the deployment of the bare stent into the TL.

vessels with a self-expanding stent (Fig. 23.5). To enhance complete thrombosis of the FL, this bridge stenting can be performed with a covered stent graft if a distal entry tear has to be sealed into the target vessel, as described by Bel et al. [14]. Interestingly, an ex vivo study demonstrated a significant pressure gradient drop (>15 mmHg) across visceral and renal arteries supplied by the FL after PETTICOAT (in 54.5% of cases). These experimental findings might support extensive stenting of visceral or renal vessels arising from the FL after PETTICOAT to reconnect the vessel to the TL and perfectly realign the ostium with the dissecting lamella [15].

Notably, the first published series of PETTICOAT was performed with an off-label use of different self-expanding stents aimed to treat either vena cava or aortic occlusive pathology [13]. In the last decade, new dedicated bare stents have been designed and approved with CE mark to treat AD. The largest series published to date employed two different commercially available stents:

- Zenith® Dissection Endovascular Stent (Cook Medical, Bloomington, IN): this became available in 2005 as a custom-made device. At present, it is commercially distributed with the CE mark obtained in 2010. It is made of very low radial force self-expandable stainless steel Z stents sewn in series. The device is available in two diameters (36 and 46 mm) and three lengths (82, 123 and 164 mm). The delivery system is 20 Fr (outer diameter). Since two diameters of the bare stent component are available (36 mm and 46 mm), the size is chosen according to the diameter of the proximal covered stent graft. A diameter of 36 mm should

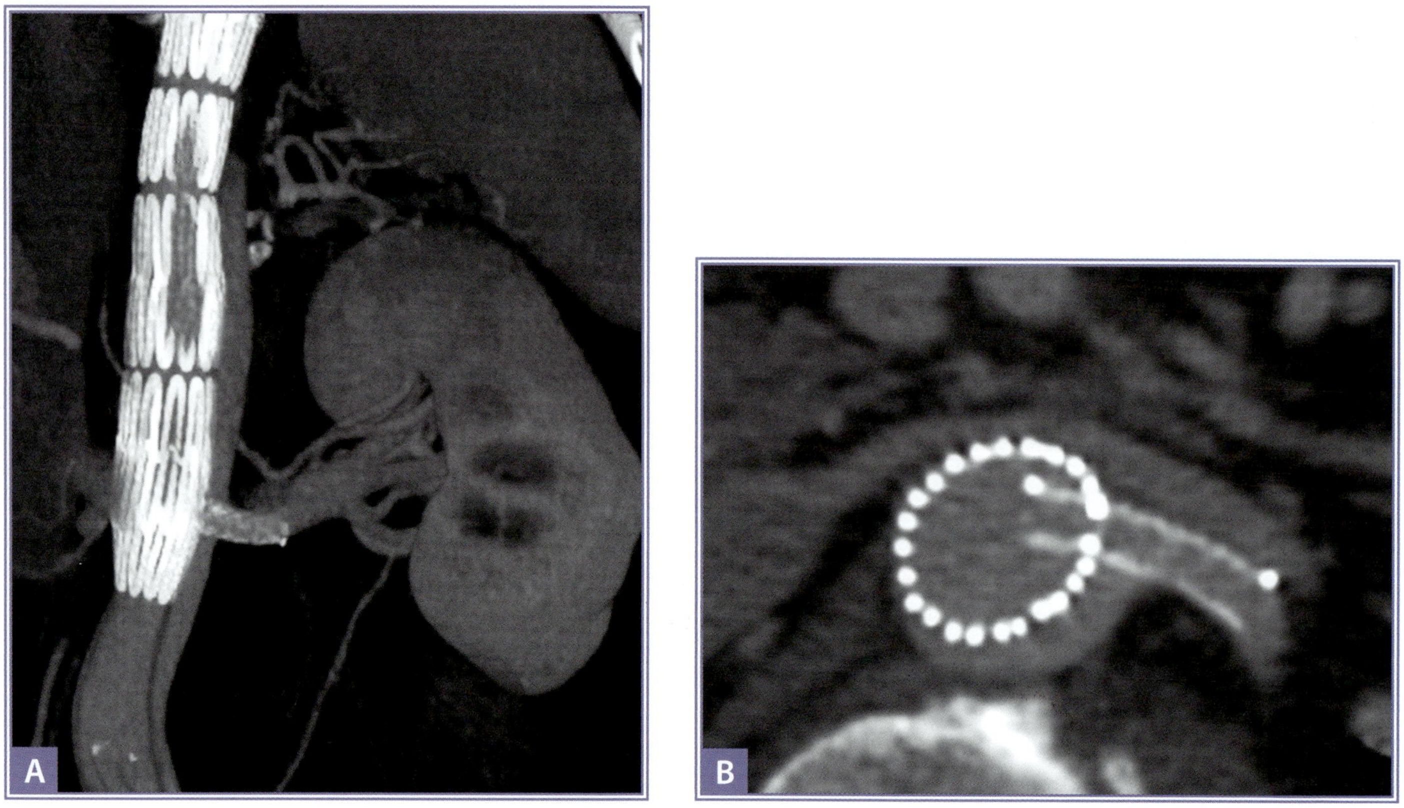

Fig. 23.5 **A**, **B**, Multi-planar reformatting (MPR) of a Zenith® Dissection Endovascular Stent (Cook Medical, Bloomington, IN) deployed to relieve dynamic malperfusion; then the left renal artery was stented through the PETTICOAT to solve residual static malperfusion with a self-expanding stent.

be combined to proximal stent grafts <36 mm, and a diameter of 46 mm to stent grafts >36 mm. The device has been recently modified by the manufacturer with a new configuration. Compared to the previous one, a suture has been added between each peak of the first and second stent of the proximal and distal ends of the device, changing the configuration with a peak-to-peak design. This modification is intended to improve the apposition to the aortic wall by improving the columnar support of the proximal and distal ends of the stent, avoiding the misalignment that might occur during deployment or during inadvertent engagement of the distal loops [16]. A new nitinol version with the same design recently received the CE mark and will soon be commercialized;

- Sinus-XL stent (Optimed, Ettlingen, Germany): this is a self-expanding nitinol stent system. It is commercially distributed with the CE mark obtained in 2007. It has a closed cell design and it is available in different diameters from 16 to 34 mm and different lengths from 30 to 100 mm. The delivery system is 10 Fr (outer diameter).

Anecdotal reports have been published regarding other bare stents, such as the E-xl (JOTEC GmbH, Hechingen, Germany) [17] and the Fortress stent (Curative Medical Devices Inc., Dresden, Germany) [13].

23.3 PETTICOAT literature review

A literature review search was conducted to identify all published studies reporting the combined use of a proximal stent graft with a distal bare metal stent for the management of AD.

Table 23.1 Literature studies

Author [ref]	Year	Study design*	No.	Stanford classification (%)		Malperfusion (%)	Onset (%)		
				Type A	Type B		Acute	Sub-acute	Chronic
Conzelmann et al. [25]	2013	R	13	100%	–	100%	100%	–	–
Hsu et al. [26]	2016	R	9	100%	–	56%	100%	–	–
Nienaber et al. [13]	2006	R	12	16%	84%	0%	16%	42%	42%
Hofferberth et al. [18]	2012	R	40	40%	60%	63%	75%	–	25%
Melissano et al. [19]	2012	P	25	–	100%	20%	20%	52%	28%
Liu et al. [20]	2013	R	33	–	100%	–	100%	–	–
Feng et al. [27]	2013	R	154	–	100%	–	86	–	68
Lombardi et al. [21]	2014	P,T	86	–	100%	65%	64%	36%	–
Alsac et al. [22]	2014	P	15	–	100%	100%	100%	–	–
He et al. [23]	2015	R	35	–	100%	34%	100%	–	–
Kische et al. [24]	2015	P	17	–	100%	71%	71%	29%	–
Overall			439	40 (9.1%)	399 (90.9%)	138 (48.4%)	290 (66.1%)	59 (13.4%)	90 (20.5%)

* R, retrospective; P, prospective; T, prospective trial.

MEDLINE and SCOPUS databases were searched for papers published in English between January 2006 and June 2016, using as keywords: "dissection", "bare stent", "thoracic", "endovascular", and "PETTICOAT". In addition, references to selected studies were screened manually for further identification of relevant studies. Studies were considered for review on the basis of the following criteria: they had to include more than 5 cases, provide full information on the type of dissection treated and the onset of the dissection, as well as report clinical and technical outcomes. Studies containing duplicate (partial or complete) data were excluded and the most recent data coming from the same research group were used. Eleven studies were analysed after literature search (Table 23.1) [13, 18-27].

23.3.1 Short-term results

Notwithstanding 439 patients received a so-called "PETTICOAT" procedure, the materials used, type of dissection treated and time interval from onset of dissection were too heterogeneous to be able to present grouped short-term clinical results. For these reasons, two studies [25, 26] reporting outcomes of 22 PETTICOAT procedures in combination with open surgical repair for Type A AD were excluded. Moreover, two studies [13, 18] presenting cases treated with PETTICOAT for both Type A and B AD were excluded because of the impossibility to extract only the data regarding the treatment of the Type B AD cohort. Finally, three studies were excluded [20, 23, 27] in which a short (<100 mm) bare stent was predeployed into the distal thoracic neck without reaching the visceral and renal artery in order to avoid stent graft-induced distal entry tear.

Table 23.2 Studies reporting the PETTICOAT procedure for acute/sub-cute Type B AD

Outcome	Melissano et al. [19] (2012)	Lombardi et al. [21] (2014)	Alsac et al. [22] (2014)	Kische et al. [24] (2015)	Overall
Patient (no.)	25	86	15	17	143
Device used	ZDES	ZDES	ZDES	ZDES	ZDES
30-day mortality	0 (0%)	4 (4.7%)	0 (0%)	3 (17.6%)	7 (4.9%)
Type I endoleaks	2 (8.0%)	1 (1.2%)	0 (0%)	4 (23.5%)	7 (4.9%)
30-day clinical success	23 (92%)	81 (94.2%)	15 (100%)	10 (58.8%)	129 (90.2%)
Surgical conversion	0 (0%)	0 (0%)	0 (0%)	na	0 (0%)
Retrograde dissection	0 (0%)	7 (8.1%)	0 (0%)	na	7 (5.6%)
Stroke	0 (0%)	6 (7.0%)	1 (6.7%)	na	7 (5.6%)
Any spinal cord ischemia	1 (4.0%)	2 (2.3%)	1 (6.7%)	na	4 (3.2%)
Permanent paraplegia or paraparesis	0 (0%)	1 (1.2%)	0 (0%)	na	1 (0.8%)
Renal failure	5 (25%)	7 (8.1%)	2 (13.3%)	na	14 (11.1%)
Any end-organ resection	0 (0%)	5 (5.8%)	1 (6.7%)	na	6 (4.8%)
1-year survival	92.0%	88.3%	93.3%	80%	–

ZDES, Zenith® Dissection Endovascular Stent; na, not available.

Perioperative (30-day results) of the four remaining papers reporting the PETTICOAT procedure for treatment of Type B AD have been summarized in Table 23.2. All 143 patients were treated with the Zenith® Dissection Endovascular Stent (Cook Medical, Bloomington, IN) for Type B AD either in the acute (89 cases within the first 14 days) or sub-acute phase (54 cases after the first 14 days but before 2 months). The pooled data demonstrated that the procedure is feasible and safe with an overall 30-day mortality rate of 4.9% and a clinical success rate of 90.2%. Notably, 30-day clinical events were recorded in 28.7% of the cases and no different outcomes were recorded between the acute and subacute cases in the two studies presenting data regarding a sub-acute treatment of Type B AD [18-20]. One-year survival ranged from 80 to 93.3%.

23.3.2 TEVAR + PETTICOAT versus TEVAR alone

Six out of the 11 papers proposed a clinical comparison between TEVAR alone (TEVAR) and TEVAR + PETTICOAT (PETTICOAT) in the same dissection setting [18, 23, 24, 26-28]. Although none of these comparative studies were randomized and the decision to employ a distal bare stent was either left to the surgeon or determined by the presence of malperfusion or TL collapse, they do give some insight into the possible benefits of this technique.

Kische et al. [24] did not observe any significant differences in the clinical success rate; however, they did not report separately the morbidity rates in the two different groups.

Hofferberth et al. [18] compared TEVAR versus PETTICOAT in a heterogeneous cohort of patients with both Type A and B AD and with acute and chronic onset, although the incidence of visceral and limb malperfusion in the two groups was similar. No differences were observed in terms of clinical success between the two methods. However, a significantly lower incidence of bowel infarction was recorded (0 vs. 17%) as well as a lower need for late distal aortic reinterventions (0 vs. 19%).

Sobocinsky et al. [28] compared the outcomes of the first 39 patients enrolled in the STABLE trial [21] with 45 cases treated with a standard TEVAR in three European centres for acute complicated Type B AD. No differences were observed within the first year in terms of rupture, conversion, and reintervention rates.

Feng et al. [27] compared 311 cases of simple TEVAR versus 154 cases of modified PETTICOAT (pre-placement of a bare stent in the distal thoracic landing zone) for acute and chronic Type B AD. Despite the fact that the indication of the modified PETTICOAT was a TL collapse and that the bare stent coverage was shorter as well as limited to the thoracic aorta, no significant differences in the peri-operative clinical outcomes were observed between the two arms. However, lesser secondary reinterventions were observed in the PETTICOAT group (3.9% vs. 9.3%). Notably, causes of reintervention in the TEVAR group were related to stent-induced distal re-dissection (0% vs. 2.9%). He et al. [23], in a smaller cohort, obtained the same findings.

Hsu et al. [26] used the PETTICOAT in a subgroup of 9 patients with acute Type A AD after an initial proximal open repair and they did not observe any clinical difference in the perioperative outcomes rate when the comparison was made with a simple TEVAR procedure.

Interestingly, in terms of mid-term survival, no significant differences were observed at 1 year between the TEVAR cohort and the PETTICOAT ones [18, 24, 27].

23.3.3 PETTICOAT and aortic remodelling

The results discussed above justify a selective use of the PETTICOAT technique only in acute TBD complicated by persistent dynamic malperfusion after TEVAR. The lack of evident benefits in terms of short-term survival of the PETTICOAT cohorts does not justify a widespread use of it. However, the analysis of mid-term aortic remodelling of the PETTICOAT series might be helpful in providing valuable insights into other potential benefits of this procedure. Nine out of the 11 papers reported the behaviour of TL and FL after PETTICOAT in the short- or mid-term [13, 18, 19, 21, 23, 24, 26-28]. The different authors proposed either diametric [13, 18, 21, 24, 26-28] or volumetric analysis [19, 23, 28] of thoracic and abdominal lumens and only six studies compared the outcomes with a simple TEVAR control group [18, 23, 24, 26-28].

With regards to TL behaviour, all studies observed that the PETTICOAT technique led to an early significant expansion of the TL not only in the thoracic aorta but also in the distal abdominal aorta if the baseline CT scans were compared to the postprocedural ones. At follow-up, the TL continued to expand significantly in the thoracic aorta, whereas its size remained relatively stable in the abdominal aorta. Interestingly, in the two studies [23, 27] in which a short (<100 mm) bare stent was predeployed only in the distal thoracic aorta in order to prevent distal stent-induced new entry tears, the TL expansion was limited to the stent-grafted thoracic segment with no further expansion in the distal thoracoabdominal aorta. These considerations might be useful in those cases in which a distal TL expansion is necessary to solve dynamic malperfusion.

When the fate of FL is taken into consideration, the data are more heterogeneous. The common finding is that after the procedure both the thoracic and abdominal FL decreased in size significantly due to the redistribution of the lumens in favour of the TL re-expansion. Moreover, a slight increase of the overall thoracoabdominal aorta dimensions was observed after surgery [19, 21, 28]. During follow-up, four studies [18, 19, 21, 24] recorded the same behaviour: the FL continued to decrease in size in the thoracic aorta (usually the stent-grafted area), while the FL in the abdominal aorta remained stable with no shrinkage. Furthermore, two studies, analysing the 2-year follow-up data, observed a tendency towards an increase in the abdominal FL in a small proportion of cases [19, 21]. In those cases, continued pressurization in the FL due to distal entry tears may lead to FL expansion as the aortic wall continues to weaken during follow-up.

A comparative study of the volumetric behaviour of TL and FL in patients enrolled in the STABLE trial [21] versus a cohort of patients who had received a simple TEVAR for compli-

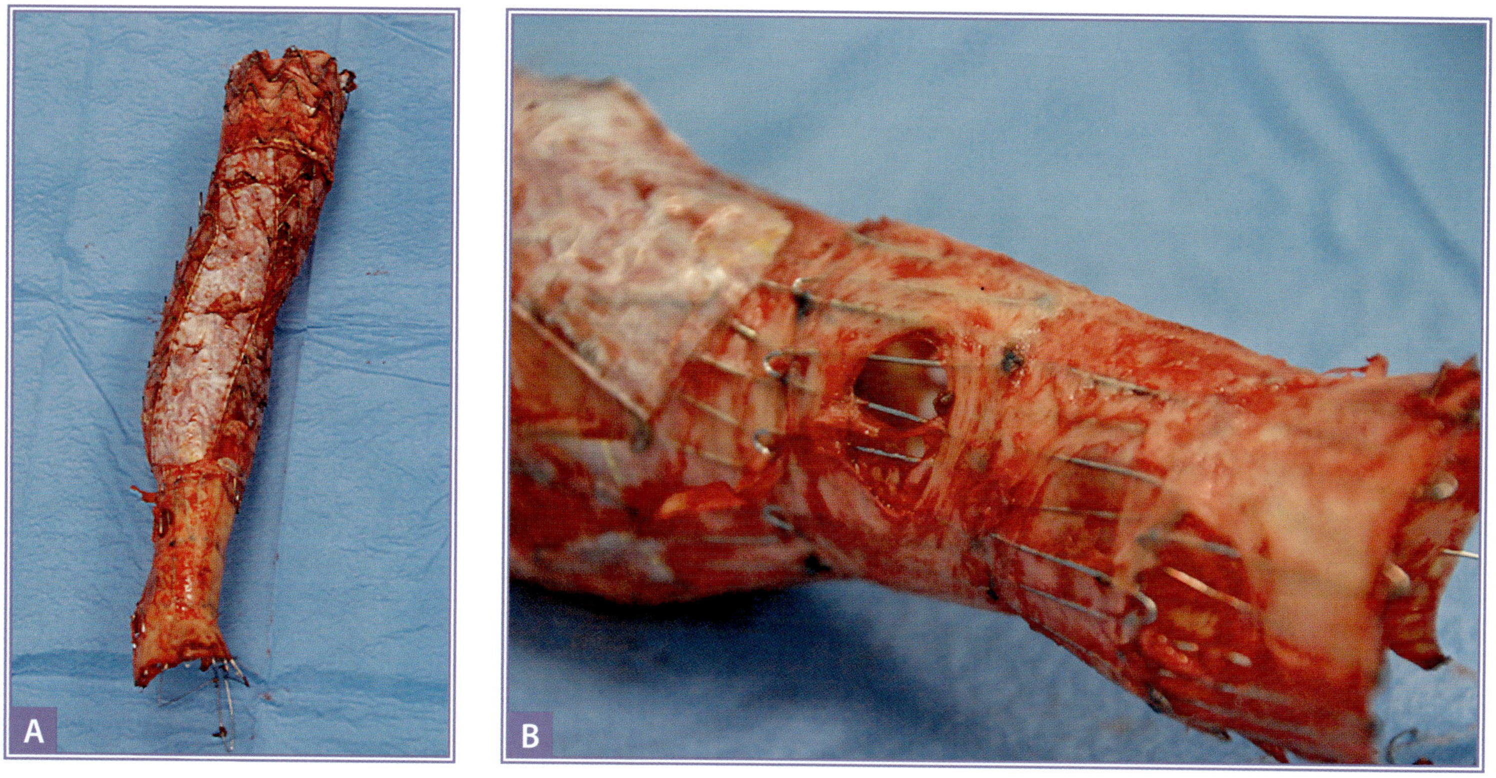

Fig. 23.6 Late open conversion of chronic aneurysmal evolution of distal thoracic and abdominal false lumen in a patient previously treated with the PETTICOAT technique (**A**). The intraoperative examination of the device evidenced full endothelialisation of the distal bare stent with the exception of the ostia of the visceral arteries (**B**).

cated Type B AD has been recently published [28]. Notably, the two groups were largely similar in terms of baseline demographics, medical history, and clinical characteristics. However, there was a trend (though not statistically significant) toward greater stent-graft coverage in the TEVAR group. The overall change in the TL volume was statistically greater in the PETTICOAT group, while the overall change in FL volume was not statistically different (pre-procedure vs. 12 months follow-up). In the abdominal aorta, although the total abdominal aortic size increased similarly in both groups, only the PETTICOAT group had substantial TL expansion postoperatively. In addition, only the PETTICOAT group exhibited a significant reduction in FL volume in the abdominal aorta postoperatively and maintained a net decrease in the average FL volume at 12 months, in contrast to the TEVAR group, although without statistical significance. Therefore, compared with TEVAR alone, the bare-metal dissection stent appeared to improve aortic remodelling in the distal aorta, at least during early follow-up [28]. Recently, Hofferberth et al. [29], in order to enhance the abdominal remodelling, proposed an evolution of the PETTICOAT technique, the So-Called Stent-Assisted Balloon-Induced Intimal Disruption and Relamination STABILISE in AD repair. This procedure aims at the reapposition of the intima lamella to the aortic wall by ballooning the distal bare stent (for details please refer to Chapter 24).

The remodelling data evaluated in this review confirm a clear-cut role of PETTICOAT in acute Type B AD complicated by dynamic malperfusion because this technique enhances the effect of the proximal TEVAR, improving the re-expansion of the TL of the distal thoracoabdominal aorta. However, there is lack of evidence to support a routine employment in Type B AD due to the unproven gain in terms of mid-term survival as well as aortic remodelling of the distal FL.

Moreover, since fenestrated and branched repair has been described with encouraging results in patients with post-dissection thoracoabdominal aneurysms [30-33], the feasibility of such a complex endovascular aortic repair with a previous PETTICOAT has been questioned. The feasibility of fenestrated endografting through a previous PETTICOAT has been demonstrated successfully once in the literature. No major conflict with the struts of the bare dissection stent during catheterization and bridging stent placement were reported [34]. Interestingly, we performed an open standard conversion in two cases of post PETTICOAT chronic aneurysmal evolution of FL (Fig. 23.6). In both cases we noticed a complete re-endothelialisation of the dissection bare stent with the exception of the ostia of the visceral arteries. On the one hand, the presence of a PETTICOAT would seemingly jeopardize a fenestrated procedure by increasing the procedural complexity: the crossing of visceral vessels ostia through the stent struts might be challenging and, as a general rule, the presence of a previous aortic device could reduce the trackability and the rotability of a second endograft [28]. On the other hand, the greater TL in the distal aorta observed in the PETTICOAT cohorts may increase the anatomical feasibility of fenestrated procedures by reducing the excluded cases due to the excessively narrow TLs [28].

23.4 Conclusions

Acute Type B AD complicated by end-organ malperfusion has a substantial augmented risk of 30-day mortality if left untreated. Stent-graft treatment may improve the prognosis of these challenging cases; however, it may fail to completely address residual distal aortic dynamic malperfusion. The combination of proximal standard stent grafting of the proximal entry tear with the deployment of a bare stent in the distal thoracoabdominal aorta, termed the PETTICOAT technique, might be beneficial in solving residual dynamic malperfusion. Analysing the literature data not only confirms that the PETTICOAT technique is safe and feasible but also that it is able to effectively re-expand the TL of the thoracoabdominal dissected aorta, improving end-organ perfusion. However, since there is no evidence of improved mid-term survival as well as positive remodelling of the FL in the distal aorta, when compared to a simple proximal stent grafting, a wide-spread use of the PETTICOAT technique is not justified and it should be limited to cases complicated by dynamic malperfusion.

REFERENCES

1) Patel AY, Eagle KA, Vaishnava P. Acute type B aortic dissection: insights from the International Registry of Acute Aortic Dissection. Ann Cardiothorac Surg 2014; 3: 368-74.
2) Suzuki T, Mehta RH, Ince H, et al. Clinical profiles and outcomes of acute type B aortic dissection in the current era: lessons from the International Registry of Aortic Dissection (IRAD). Circulation 2003; 108 (suppl II): 312-7.
3) Hagan PG, Nienaber CA, Isselbacher EM, et al. The International Registry of Acute Aortic Dissection (IRAD): new insights into an old disease. JAMA 2000; 283: 897-903.
4) Williams DM, LePage MA, Lee DY. The dissected aorta: part I. Early anatomic changes in an in vitro model. Radiology 1997; 203: 23-31.
5) Williams DM, Lee DY, Hamilton BH, et al. The dissected aorta: percutaneous treatment of ischemic complications - Principles and results. J Vasc Interv Radiol 1997; 8: 605-25.
6) Midulla M, Fattori R, Beregi JP, Dake M, Rousseau H. Aortic dissection and malperfusion syndrome: a when, what and how-to guide. Radiol Med 2013; 118: 74-88.
7) Gaxotte V, Cocheteux B, Haulon S, et al. Relationship of intimal flap position to endovascular treatment of malperfusion syndromes in aortic dissection. J Endovasc Ther 2003; 10: 719-27.
8) Swee W, Dake MD. Endovascular management of thoracic dissections. Circulation 2008; 117: 1460-73.
9) White RA, Miller DC, Criado FJ, et al. Report on the results of thoracic endovascular aortic repair for acute, complicated, type B aortic dissection at 30 days and 1 year from a multidisciplinary subcommittee of the Society for Vascular Surgery Outcomes Committee. J Vasc Surg 2011; 53: 1082-90.
10) Fattori R, Botta L, Lovato L, et al. Malperfusion syndrome in type B aortic dissection: role of the endovascular procedures. Acta Chir Belg 2008; 108: 192-7.
11) Ito N, Tsunoda T, Nakamura M, et al. Percutaneous bare Z-stent implantation as an alternative to surgery for acute aortic dissection with visceral ischemia. Catheter Cardiovasc Interv 2003; 58: 95-100.

12) Mossop PJ, McLachlan CS, Amukotuwa SA, Nixon IK. Staged endovascular treatment for complicated type B aortic dissection. Nat Clin Pract Cardiovasc Med 2005; 2: 316-21.
13) Nienaber CA, Kische S, Zeller T, et al. Provisional extension to induce complete attachment after stent-graft placement in type B aortic dissection: the PETTICOAT concept. J Endovasc Ther 2006; 13: 738-46.
14) Bel A, Alsac JM, Baïssas V, Julia P, Fabiani JN. Spot stenting of the tear in type B aortic dissection. Ann Vasc Surg 2013; 27: 671-6.
15) Faure EM, Canaud L, Cathala P, Serres I, Marty-Ané C, Alric P. Assessment of abdominal branch vessel patency after bare-metal stenting of the thoracoabdominal aorta in a human ex vivo model of acute type B aortic dissection. J Vasc Surg 2015; 61: 1299-305.
16) Bertoglio L, Melissano G, Civilini E, Chiesa R. Stent misalignment of the Zenith Dissection Endovascular System. J Vasc Surg 2013; 57: 515-7.
17) Melissano G, Civilini E, Mascia D, Tshomba Y, Bertoglio L, Chiesa R. Clinical use of extra-large self-expanding stents. J Cardiovasc Surg (Torino) 2015; 56: 81-7.
18) Hofferberth SC, Newcomb AE, Yii MY, et al. Combined proximal stent grafting plus distal bare metal stenting for management of aortic dissection: superior to standard endovascular repair? J Thorac Cardiovasc Surg 2012; 144: 956-62.
19) Melissano G, Bertoglio L, Rinaldi E, et al. Volume changes in aortic true and false lumen after the "PETTICOAT" procedure for type B aortic dissection. J Vasc Surg 2012; 55: 641-51.
20) Liu JF, Jiang WL, Lu HT, Li YL, Zhang TH, Yamakawa T. Application of protective stents in endovascular repair of acute complicated Stanford type B aortic dissections. J Endovasc Ther 2013; 20: 210-8.
21) Lombardi JV, Cambria RP, Nienaber CA, et al. Aortic remodeling after endovascular treatment of complicated type B aortic dissection with the use of a composite device design. J Vasc Surg 2014; 59: 1544-54.
22) Alsac JM, Girault A, El Batti S, et al. Experience of the Zenith Dissection Endovascular System in the emergency setting of malperfusion in acute type B dissections. J Vasc Surg 2014; 59: 645-50.
23) He H, Yao K, Nie WP, et al. Modified Petticoat technique with pre-placement of a distal bare stent improves early aortic remodeling after complicated acute stanford type B aortic dissection. Eur J Vasc Endovasc Surg 2015; 50: 450-9.
24) Kische S, D'Ancona G, Belu IC, et al. Perioperative and mid-term results of endovascular management of complicated type B aortic dissection using a proximal thoracic endoprosthesis and selective distal bare stenting. Eur J Cardiothorac Surg 2015; 48: e77-84.
25) Conzelmann LO, Doemland M, Weigang E, et al. Endovascular treatment of symptomatic true-lumen collapse of the downstream aorta after open surgery for acute aortic dissection type A. J Cardiovasc Surg (Torino) 2013; 54: 151-9.
26) Hsu HL, Chen YY, Huang CY, Huang JH, Chen JS. The provisional extension to induce complete attachment (PETTICOAT) technique to promote distal aortic remodelling in repair of acute DeBakey type I aortic dissection: preliminary results. Eur J Cardiothorac Surg 2016; 50: 146-52.
27) Feng J, Lu Q, Zhao Z, et al. Restrictive bare stent for prevention of stent graft-induced distal redissection after thoracic endovascular aortic repair for type B aortic dissection. J Vasc Surg 2013; 57: 44S-52S.
28) Sobocinski J, Lombardi JV, Dias NV, et al. Volume analysis of true and false lumens in acute complicated type B aortic dissections after thoracic endovascular aortic repair with stent grafts alone or with a composite device design. J Vasc Surg 2016; 63: 1216-24.
29) Hofferberth SC, Nixon IK, Boston RC, McLachlan CS, Mossop PJ. Stent-assisted balloon-induced intimal disruption and relamination in aortic dissection repair: the STABILISE concept. J Thorac Cardiovasc Surg 2014; 147: 1240-5.
30) Kitagawa A, Greenberg RK, Eagleton MJ, Mastracci TM, Roselli EE. Fenestrated and branched endovascular aortic repair for chronic type B aortic dissection with thoracoabdominal aneurysms. J Vasc Surg 2013; 58: 625-34.
31) Sobocinski J, Spear R, Tyrrell MR, et al. Chronic dissection - Indications for treatment with branched and fenestrated stent-grafts. J Cardiovasc Surg (Torino) 2014; 55: 505-17.
32) Oikonomou K, Kopp R, Katsargyris A, Pfister K, Verhoeven EL, Kasprzak P. Outcomes of fenestrated/branched endografting in post-dissection thoracoabdominal aortic aneurysms. Eur J Vasc Endovasc Surg 2014; 48: 641-8.
33) Bertoglio L, Marone EM, Civilini E, Cambiaghi T, Mascia D, Chiesa R. Branched stent-grafts deployed in the true and false lumen to exclude a post dissecting thoracoabdominal aneurysm. J Cardiovasc Surg (Torino) 2016; 57: 646-52.
34) Barbante M, Sobocinski J, Maurel B, Azzaoui R, Martin-Gonzalez T, Haulon S. Fenestrated endografting after bare metal dissection stent implantation. J Endovasc Ther 2015; 22: 207-11.

24

The STABILISE concept of eliminating dissection and obtaining a uniluminal aorta

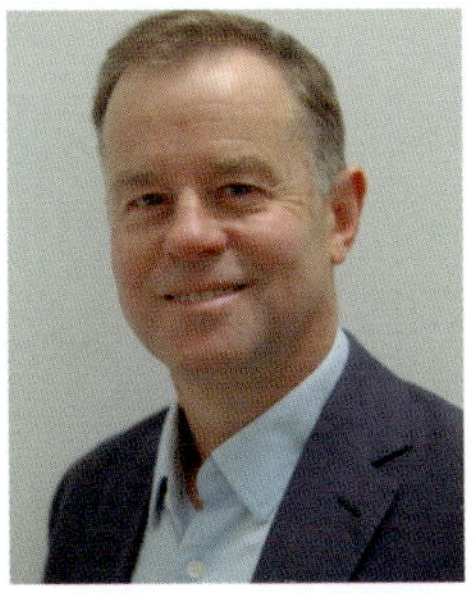

Peter J. Mossop

24.1 Background

Appreciation of the need to repair the entire dissected aorta in the setting of dissection initiated our evolution of the endovascular approach to aortic dissection (AD) in all its forms over a decade ago. Although placement of a proximal endograft to seal the primary entry tear reduces the risk of rupture and leads to shorter-term expansion of the true lumen in the thoracic aorta, the presence of more distal re-entries is not addressed.

This has been demonstrated in a number of studies relating to conventional Thoracic EndoVascular Aortic Repair (TEVAR) for AD [1] and has been confirmed by computation fluid dynamics modeling [2] where the persistence of residual inflows to the false lumen result in ongoing pressurization, turbulence and shear flow. Essentially, the presence of persistent false lumen flow drives possible true lumen under perfusion and dynamic branch compromise and may increase the likelihood of further distal aortic degeneration in the longer term.

With this in mind, the aim of stent-assisted reconstruction beyond a proximal endograft to complete AD repair came about. The primary aims were multiple: to improve short-term outcomes in dissection management by reducing the chance of postoperative malperfusion, particularly for visceral and spinal circulations; to initiate acute and subsequent longer-term remodeling of the true lumen; and in conjunction with ancillary endovascular techniques in a staged fashion, to eliminate false lumen flow. The overarching aim of stent-assisted reconstruction is to achieve improved early and long-term outcomes compared to best medical treatment or TEVAR alone.

24.2 Stent-based reconstruction: staged total aortic and branch vessel reconstruction – STABLE

Staged Total Aortic and Branch vesseL Endovascular repair, known as the STABLE concept, was first described in 2005 [3] (Fig. 24.1A). Although isolated use of stenting for established malperfusion had been reported [4], STABLE introduced the routine and novel use of an

Peter J. Mossop (petermossop@me.com)
St. Vincent's Hospital,
Melbourne, Australia

G. Melissano - R. Chiesa (eds), Aortic Dissection patients true stories and the innovations that saved their lives

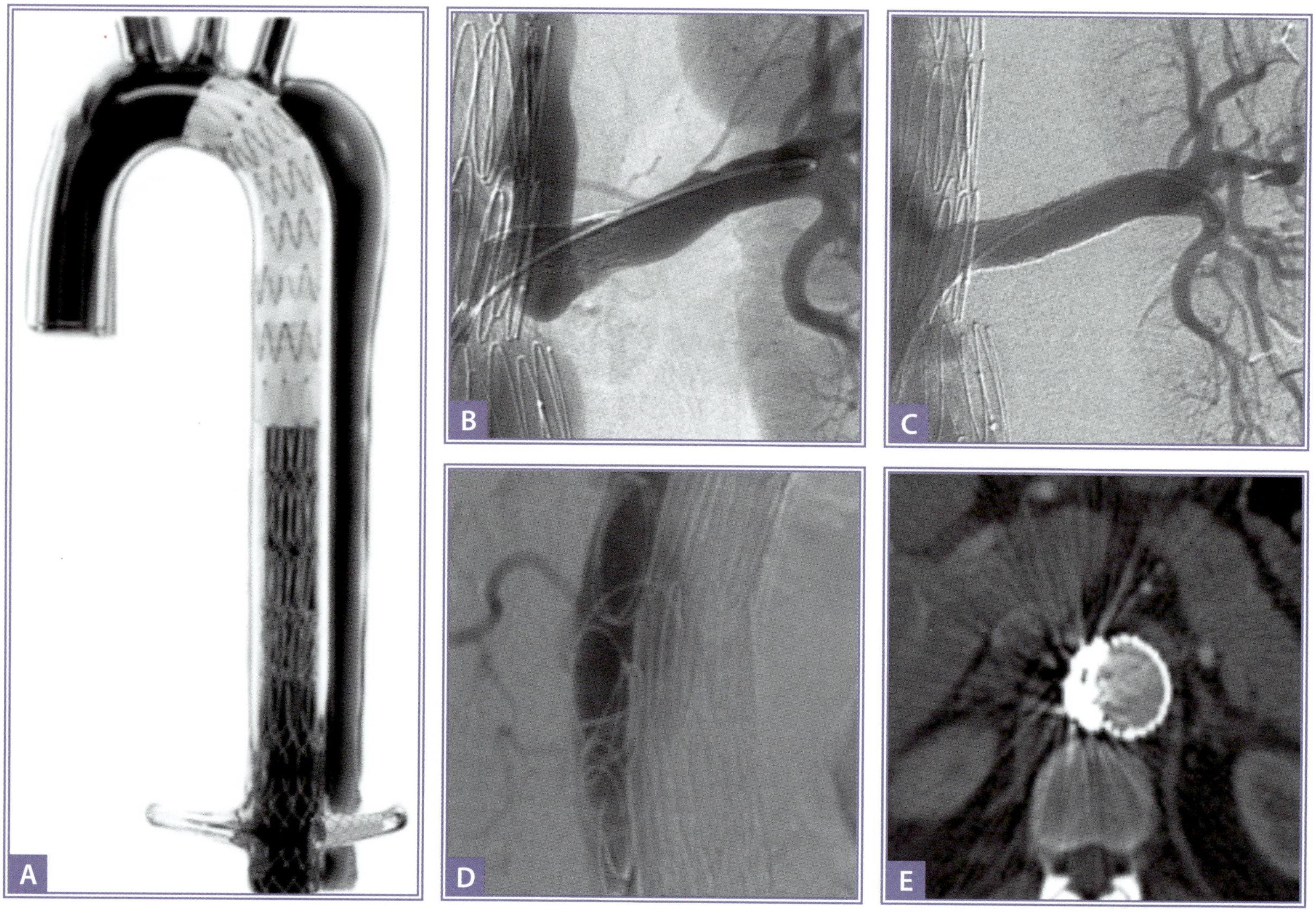

Fig. 24.1 STABLE approach to AD repair. **A**, Proximal TX2® and distal Zenith® Dissection Endovascular Stent (ZDES) reconstruction of true lumen. Note presence of residual false lumen and renal stent bridging stented aortic true lumen to left renal artery. **B**, Digital substraction angiography (DSA) showing re-entry tear at renal origin. **C**, Closure of tear by covered stent reconnection of true lumen to branch lumen. **D**, DSA showing local coil embolization of false lumen to induce thrombosis. **E**, Filling of the false lumen by embolic coils on computed tomography angiography (CTA).

extensive self-expanding, dissection-specific stent scaffold to re-expand the true lumen and reestablish more normal flow dynamics.

Early experience also indicated that endograft and stenting in isolation was insufficient to fully eliminate residual inflows to the false lumen. In fact canine studies almost 20 years ago suggested that in isolation stent based reconstruction for dissection was likely to be inadequate [5]. Hence, in STABLE after initial endograft and stent placement, in conjunction with elimination of any major branch perfusion abnormality or re-entry, a period of follow-up was performed. Any subsequent persistent major entries or any evidence of false lumen growth were treated with a staged intervention. Such procedures were generally preemptive and not indicative of re-interventions for aortic-related complications. When using such techniques to reconstruct the true lumen, it was found that aortic degeneration could be controlled. Hence, STABLE aims to achieve a more robust total aortic repair through application of a staged endovascular approach.

These adjunctive techniques (which were often novel) were an essential element of STABLE and for the endovascular elimination of residual false lumen flow. These techniques included closure of branch vessel re-entries by local covered stenting reconnecting the stented aortic true lumen to the branch true lumen (Fig. 24.1B, C), much in the same way that a fenestrated endograft is connected to a native aortic branch. Selective embolization of the false lumen at the site of re-entries was also found to be a useful adjunctive tool (Fig. 24.1D, E). Our experience of adjunctive embolization, the AFTER (Aortic False lumen Thrombosis by EmbolotheRapy) concept, also represented the first major study examining the use of this approach [6]. We found that AFTER was effective in inducing false lumen thrombosis and arresting growth in 90% of cases where persistent false lumen growth was detected on follow-up after initial reconstruction by STABLE.

24.2.1 Early outcomes

Early outcomes of our experience in the first 31 patients treated using STABLE was encouraging, with low rates of 30-day mortality (3%), stroke (0%), and paraplegia/paresis (0%) [7].

24.2.2 Late outcomes

Survival

At a mean follow-up of 49 months, a cohort of 40 patients undergoing STABLE repair for acute and chronic dissection had an aortic-specific survival of 90% [8]. A further follow-up of 33 patients undergoing stent and endograft-based reconstruction for acute and sub-acute Type B AD demonstrated overall survival of 91% at 97 months (range, 50-154 months), while aortic-specific survival was 94%.

Subsequently to our initial reports a number of case series reported the use of bare-metal stents in the distal thoracoabdominal aorta, with favorable short-term results [9, 10]. The STABLE trail has similarly demonstrated the utility of this approach in the longer term [11]. Survival rates in our own experience using STABLE were higher than similar studies in the literature, with survival rates ranging from 56.3 to 87% at 5 years [12].

Remodeling

Aortic remodeling data (aortic dimensions measured at mid-descending and celiac) have also reflected aortic survival with thoracic and abdominal aortic dimensions remaining stable over longer-term follow-up.

24.2.3 Malperfusion and spinal ischemia

Stent deployment beyond a proximal endograft to cover the lower thoracic and abdominal aorta ensures reperfusion of the true lumen, correction of true lumen collapse and protection against visceral malperfusion. With regard to malperfusion, a further aim of bare stent use was to reduce the chance of spinal cord ischemia by limiting the extent of aortic coverage by endograft and improving direct perfusion of the spinal arteries via the true lumen through correction of distal true lumen collapse. Follow-up angiographic assessment post stent placement often indicated improved direct flow from the aortic true lumen to intercostal and lumbar branches arising from the now much narrowed false lumen. This improved direct flow, combined with a reduction of any pressure gradient down the aortic true lumen, may account for the absence of spinal ischemia in our experience.

24.2.4 Comparison to TEVAR alone

Furthermore, in the first study to compare STABLE treatment to conventional TEVAR alone we demonstrated that the addition of bare-metal scaffolding in the distal thoracoabdominal aorta significantly reduced visceral malperfusion in the acute phase compared with standard endovascular repair [8]. Moreover, this was achieved without increasing periprocedural morbidity or mortality.

24.2.5 STABLE versus composite treatment alone

Significantly, while bare-stenting of the dissection was at core of the STABLE approach, it is considered that the ancillary endovascular repairs were also key in achieving the highest level of false lumen exclusion and hence the greatest likelihood of preventing further aortic degeneration. Unfortunately, the STABLE approach has been confused with the more recently reported PETTICOAT procedure, which promoted the use of a composite technique using proximal endograft and distal stent alone [10]. Composite approaches using self-expanding distal bare stents, while likely to improve collapse of the true lumen, are unlikely to achieve improved false lumen thrombosis in the long term if further interventions to close distal re-entries are not performed. Therefore, a composite approach in isolation is unlikely to achieve best long-term outcome.

24.3 Recreation of the uniluminal aorta: stent assisted balloon induced intimal disruption and relamination – STABILISE

24.3.1 Rationale

Although STABLE has demonstrated the utility of stent-based aortic reconstruction in both acute and chronic dissection, further evolution of the initial approach has occurred over the last decade. The aim was the creation of a more simple, rapid and complete method of repair for acute and potentially chronic dissection, particularly in patients where significant dilatation of the aorta had not yet occurred. While STABILISE (STent Assisted Balloon Induced intimaL dISruption and rElamination) is an evolution of STABLE, rather than leave any residual false lumen complete fenestration and re-apposition of the intimal membrane was proposed [13] (Fig. 24.2). Hence, STABILISE avoids the need to close residual distal re-entries or to actively thrombose the false lumen since no false lumen remains.

The rationale of this approach was again the elimination of haemodynamic drivers of degeneration of the dissected aorta occurring as a result of the false lumen compartment.

This approach is an extension of the long-standing technique of equilibrating pressures within the two compartments of the dissected aorta by localized fenestration either percutaneous or surgical.

24.3.2 Evolution of the technique

Early attempts at stent expansion of the intima had used balloon expandable stents. While feasible, unless multiple devices were used only local expansion of the dissected true lumen could be performed. Our experience with the self-expanding dissection specific stent (Zenith® Dissection Endovascular Stent, Cook Medical, Bloomington, IN), which is available in lengths sufficient to support extensive zones of the dissected aorta, suggested this could enable rapid

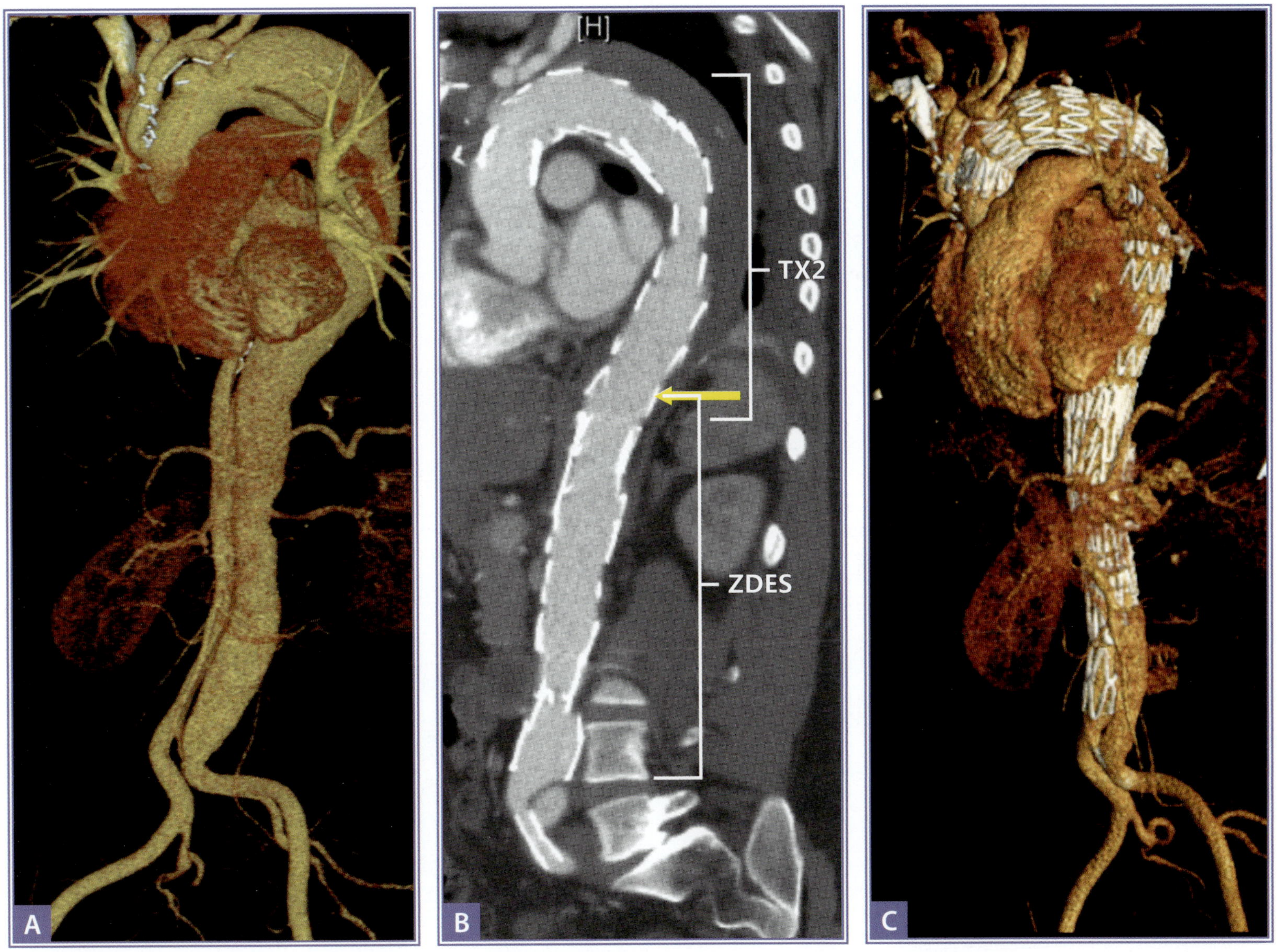

Fig. 24.2 STABILISE concept. **A**, 3D CTA reconstruction of a Type B residual AD (following Type A AD with proximal arch repair). **B**, Oblique view CTA post STABILISE repair with proximal TX2® coverage of superior entry tear and flaring of the distal endograft to aortic wall at thoracoabdominal junction (arrow). Stented fenestration of the remaining dissection flap by bare ZDES obliterates the remaining false lumen. **C**, 5-year follow-up CTA showing stabilization of aortic morphology.

and extensive fenestration and relocation of the intima to the dissected aortic wall using potentially a single device.

However, due to the low radial force of the dissection stent, expansion of the true lumen is usually incomplete (the stent being constrained by the intima) when initially deployed. Hence, in order to achieve complete expansion, balloon assisted fenestration of the stented intimal flap is performed.

24.3.3 Methodology

Unlike STABLE, the STABILISE procedure does not attempt to close residual distal re-entries by branch vessel reconstruction or false lumen embolisation but to disruption of the dissec-

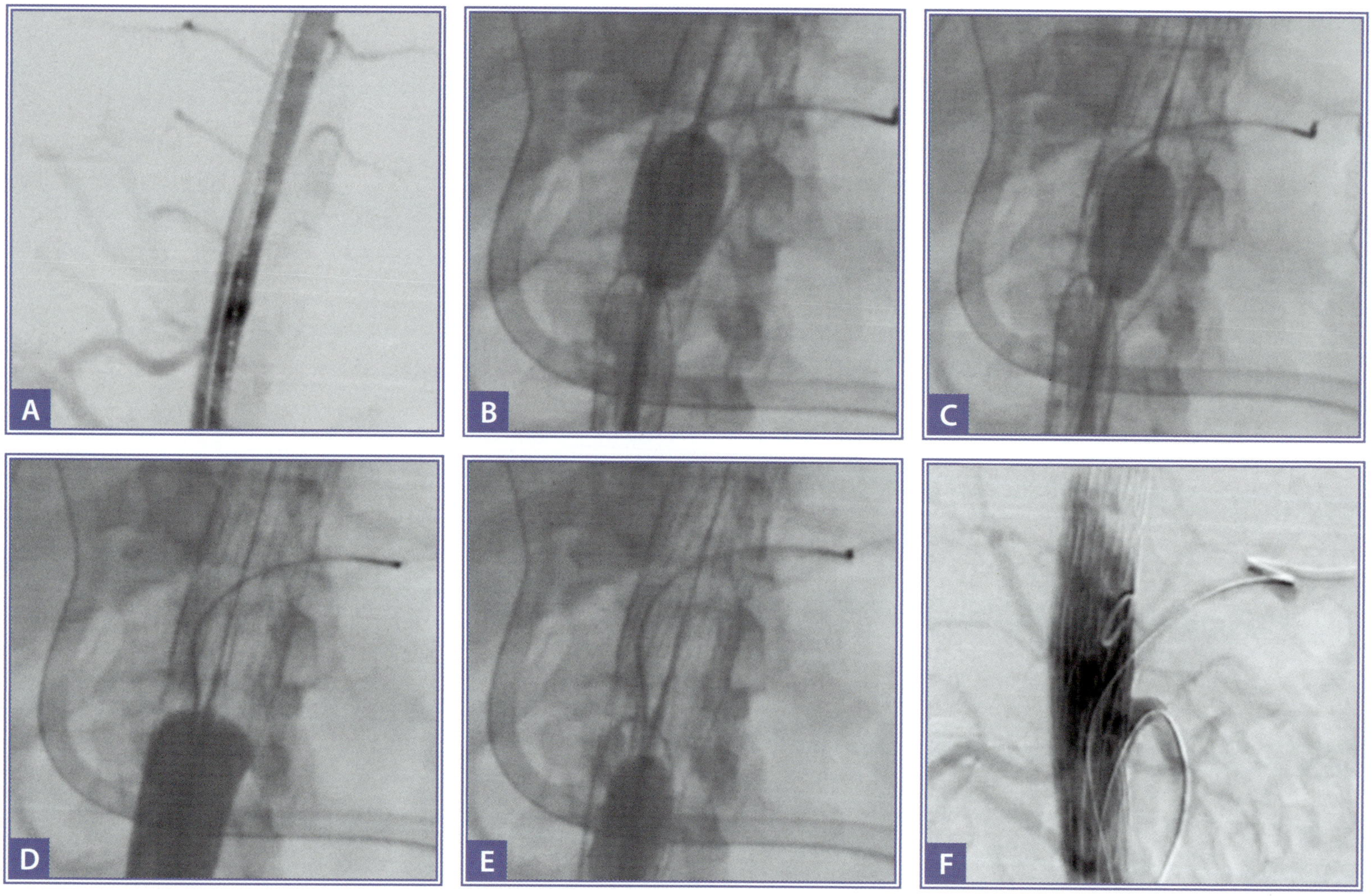

Fig. 24.3 STABILISE repair. **A**, True lumen narrowing distal to proximal endograft. **B**, Bare-metal ZDES supports the distal true lumen while safety wires protect mesenteric vessels (identified to be involved by the dissection lamella). **C**, Balloon dilation of upper stent (note the constrained unexpanded lower stent segments). **D**, **E**, Progressive ZEDS expansion with fenestration of the distal intimal lamella. **F**, Completion angiography post stent expansion and local stenting of a branch origin showing a uniluminal aortic lumen and good branch patency.

tion flap. In this regard the STABILISE approach becomes a more simple and reproducible method of repair for a variety of dissection types.

Baseline computed tomography angiography (CTA) assesses the feasibility of the endovascular procedure, patency, and origin (true or false lumen) of visceral vessels, cerebral circulation, choice of peripheral access site, and sizing of stent grafts. All procedures were performed in a hybrid-operating suite.

Fluoroscopy and transesophageal echocardiography (TEE) were used to guide placement of the proximal Zenith® TX2® (Cook Medical, Bloomington, IN) endograft (length range, 120-150 mm). Endograft sizing is performed to enable an adequate seal within both the proximal neck and coverage is extended to the thoracoabdominal aortic junction or to a distal thoracic landing site where the descending thoracic aorta was preferably 36 mm or less.

Delivery systems are then exchanged, and the Zenith® Dissection Endovascular Stent advanced and deployed, overlapping at least 1 stent body with the proximal endograft. The extent of aortic delamination determines the choice of Zenith® Dissection Endovascular Stent. Combinations of stents ranging from 82 mm to 164 mm length are used to approximate the extent of dissection, and each overlapped by 1 stent body. The extent of bare-metal stenting is determined by the distal extension of the dissection (Fig. 24.3A).

Angiography confirms the extent of the residual false lumen. In cases involving dissected visceral or renal branches that are considered at risk of obstruction at the time of intimal disruption catherization of these branches is performed through the deployed stent with placement of safety guidewires to allow for potential access after dissection stent dilatation (Fig. 24.3B).

Subsequently, a 22 mm Coda® (Cook Medical, Bloomington, IN) or other appropriate balloon catheter was deployed via the dissection stent introducer sheath. After accurate positioning in the lower third of the covered stent graft, the balloon was inflated under fluoroscopic, TEE or intravascular ultrasound (IVUS) guidance within the true lumen of the distal endograft. Balloon expansion within the distal third of the stent graft was undertaken to the point of intimal flap disruption, leading to re-apposition of the intima to the aortic wall. Serial balloon dilatation of the stented true lumen was undertaken in a caudal direction to propagate the intimal tear and simultaneously reposition the intima to the aortic wall throughout the thoracoabdominal aorta (Fig. 24.3C, D, E). Balloon sizing was based on the maximal aortic diameter at each zone undergoing stent expansion. Balloon pressures ranged from 2 to 4 atmospheres with inflation to approximately 80 to 90% of total aortic size to enable intimal disruption without applying pressure to the outer aortic wall.

On completion of balloon angioplasty, angiography confirms adequate seal of the thoracic false lumen assesses false lumen obliteration and branch vessel patency in the thoraco-abdominal aorta (Fig. 24.3F). Any branch requiring additional focal stenting is then treated.

24.3.4 Early and late clinical outcomes

Early and intermediate results of STABILISE were reported in patients having appropriate morphology and undergoing repair of complicated AD. In our experience no intraprocedural complications, no early incidence of stroke, spinal, or visceral ischemia occurred and this continues to be our experience up to date. 30-day mortality using this technique is currently 5% (this mortality being unrelated to the distal STABILISE repair and due to an ascending aortic graft anastomotic dehiscence).

In 35% of patients one or more branch vessels were stented for the presence of either residual irregularity of the lumen or the presence of reduced flow with preexisting dissection involving the branch. However, no instance of branch vessel loss was encountered after dissection stent induced intimal fenestration and re-apposition and no evidence of branch vessel compromise was detected following local branch stent placement. Similarly no late branch vessel loss has occurred.

Survival

In our initial report median follow-up was 18 months (range, 4-54 months). No late adverse events or aortic-related deaths occurred. Complete false lumen obliteration occurred in 90% of patients. Subsequent to our initial report, long-term follow-up of 60 months (median, 33 months) in 21 patients has been achieved. Again no procedural related complications have been reported and currently STABILISE is associated with an aortic-specific survival of 95%.

Aortic remodeling

Long-term follow-up demonstrates a continuation of mid-term trends with stability or positive remodeling of both the thoracic and abdominal total aortic diameters with elimination of the entire false lumen space in up to 90% of treated cases. This was seen to occur either through false lumen thrombosis and remodeling of false lumen within the zone treated by endograft and through stent-supported relamination of the intima to aortic wall more distally (Fig. 24.2).

24.3.5 Discussion

In STABILISE unlike the STABLE concept, balloon expansion within the distal endograft at the thoracoabdominal junction is performed to seal the upstream false lumen while initiating intimal fenestration, which can be propagated more inferiorly. Hence, stent-based re-apposition of intima to the aortic wall has allowed the creation of a uniluminal aorta, mitigating the hemodynamic drivers of false lumen expansion.

Applicability

This approach appears feasible in at least 50% of dissections currently treated by our group, these being largely sub-acute or early chronic dissection; however it has also been used in the hybrid treatment of Type A AD where acute phase stent deployment was followed by staged sub-acute phase stent expansion. Application of the technique has eliminated many of the secondary or staged interventions that have been used to achieve thrombosis of the false lumen using the composite approach of STABLE. Selection does require intervention to be carried out prior to any significant degeneration of the more distal aorta. However, we see this as the ideal time to intervene and eliminate the potential for future degeneration. Further reports have supported the utility of this approach not only in Type B but also in hybrid treatment of Type A AD [14].

Balloon fenestration

Fenestration or disruption of the flap occurs using a balloon of smaller size than the native aorta reduces the risk that the balloon will apply any direct pressure on the outer aortic wall. For this reason a smaller true lumen in which the intima has undergone some degree of thickening and contraction in the axial plane is ideal and this situation is more often seen in the sub-acute phase. In effect as soon as balloon disruption of the intima occurs, the stent is no longer constrained and self expands to reposition the intimal membrane onto the dissected aortic wall and, in doing so, eliminates the false lumen space.

Intraprocedural imaging

Visualization of stent expansion and relationship between the balloon and aortic wall is made using a combination of transesophageal echocardiography, intravascular ultrasound and fluoroscopic screening. Catheterization of the false lumen via a distal entry with introduction of contrast into the false lumen also assists in determining the status of the false lumen space during fenestration. These methods all contribute to the safety of stent expansion.

Stent selection and function

The use of a stent in STABILISE has the purposes of assisting in the fenestration itself, reattaching the intima to the aortic wall (restoring integrity), while also holding the intimal flap stable rather than leaving a mobile structure, which could interfere with branch flow.

Dissection stent sizes range from 36 to 46 mm with the initial intention that some stent oversizing may be acceptable given the low and relatively uniform radial force exhibited by the stent over a range of sizes from under to fully expanded. However, in order to achieve the most optimal stent to aortic surface area coverage (and therefore the most minimal stent strut coverage of branch origins) stent sizing is made with minimal oversizing. Minimizing stent coverage of branch origins also aids in the ability to access branches if needed. Minimal oversizing is also in keeping with a desire to minimize any additional force delivered to the dissected aortic wall by the bare stent.

Branch vessel preservation

Of particular relevance to this technique and its safety is the preservation of branch vessel perfusion post intimal disruption and re-apposition. The potential that branch vessels perfusion may be compromised by the placement of the bare stent or the disruption of the intima is not unreasonable and was of particular concern when pioneering this approach. For example, during this process a re-entry tear or fenestration relating to a branch osteum could undergo slight malpositioning on re-expansion of the intimal lamella. This could compromise branch flow. The dissection stent could also potentially deform a branch origin particularly where the dissection plane propagated into the branch itself.

This scenario of bare stent related compromise of branch flow was recently suggested in an *in vitro* study [15] and has been taken as evidence that such a scenario is likely in clinical use. Unfortunately this *in vitro* study was fundamentally compromised and used dissection stents that were considerably oversized for the vessel utilized. This resulted in complete repositioning of the intima on stent deployment without any intimal fenestration or branch protection on relocation of the intimal flap to aortic wall. This is a situation that does not relate to actual clinical practice in which disruption of the flap is required to fully reposition the intima and, while doing this, branches are protected.

The use of protective guide wire placement is seen as a way to ensure access to all branches that could be compromised by intimal disruption or the relamination of the intima. We have conservatively used this technique and locally stented any branch where possible reduction of flow is detected. This has been easily performed with no evidence that the dissection stent restricts branch access.

Fenestration: eliminating the drivers of degeneration

High levels of long-term aortic specific survival and corresponding evidence of aortic stability using STABILISE are suggestive of the utility of this approach and are consistent with the underlying hypothesis that extensive fenestration of the residual distal AD (after control to the primary entry flow by endograft coverage) – that is the creation of a uniluminal state – will reduce the potential for further distal aortic degeneration. It could be argued that fenestration alone could achieve this aim. In fact, in some cases we have performed, a zone of intima may not be completely apposed to the aortic wall. This results in a gutter of flow outside the stent. However no persistent false lumen compartment is present and the stent ensures the fenestration is held widely open with flow equalization throughout the single aortic lumen.

In the small number of cases where stabilization or positive remodeling of the aorta does not occur, STABILISE does not preclude further intervention. The use of fenestration with dissection stenting does not interfere [16] (in our experience and that of others) with conventional, branched or fenestrated endografts (to address any focal zone of aortic degeneration). In fact the simplification of aortic morphology by elimination of the false lumen may facilitate a more straightforward endograft repair.

24.4 Conclusion

In conclusion, it has been our contention that the false lumen should be considered a continuous single compartment that communicates with the true lumen via intimal fenestrations throughout the dissected aorta. Hence, proximal endograft treatment alone is incomplete in managing dissection in its totality. Stent-assisted reconstruction and intimal disruption eliminating the false lumen and restoring a uniluminal status give us the ability to address the entire AD.

Improved clinical outcomes with high rates of aortic stability, and high aortic specific survival suggest the significant potential value of this approach in AD management. Significantly, the ability to convert the dissected lumen to a uniluminal state offers the prospect of endovascular elimination of AD and with this the enhancement of long-term prognosis.

REFERENCES

1) Eggebrecht H, Nienaber CA, Neuhauser M, et al. Endovascular stent-graft placement in aortic dissection: a meta-analysis. Eur Heart J 2006; 27: 489-98.
2) Chen D, Muller-Eschner M, Kotelis D, et al. A longtitudinal study of type-B aortic dissection and endovascular repair scenarios: computational analyses. Med Eng Phys 2013; 35: 1321-30.
3) Mossop PJ, McLachlan CS, Amukotuwa SA, Nixon IK. Staged endovascular treatment for complicated type B aortic dissection. Nat Clin Pract Cardiovasc Med 2005; 2(6): 316-22.
4) Ito N, Tsunoda T, Nakamura M, et al. Percutaneous bare Z-stent implantation as an alternative to surgery for acute aortic dissection with visceral ischemia. Catheter Cardiovasc Interv 2003; 58(1): 95-100.
5) Kato N, Hirano T, Takeda K, Nakagawa T, Mizumoto T, Yuasa H. Treatment of acute aortic dissections with expandable metallic stents: experimental study. J Vasc Interv Radiol 1994; 5(3): 417-23.
6) Hofferberth SC, Nixon IK, Mossop PJ. Aortic false lumen thrombosis induction by embolotherapy (AFTER) following endovascular repair of aortic dissection. J Endovasc Ther 2012; 19 (4): 538-45.
7) Hofferberth SC, Foley PT, Newcomb AE, et al. Combined proximal endografting with distal bare-metal stenting for management of aortic dissection. Ann Thorac Surg 2012; 93(1): 95-102.
8) Hofferberth SC, Newcomb AE, Yii MY, et al. Combined proximal stent grafting plus distal bare metal stenting for management of aortic dissection: superior to standard endovascular repair? J Thorac Cardiovasc Surg 2012; 144 (4): 956-62.
9) Melissano G, Bertoglio L, Kahlberg A, et al. Evaluation of a new disease-specific endovascular device for type B aortic dissection. J Thorac Cardiovasc Surg 2008; 136(4): 1012-8.
10) Nienaber CA, Kische S, Zeller T, et al. Provisional extension to induce complete attachment after stent-graft placement in type B aortic dissection: the PETTICOAT concept. J Endovasc Ther 2006; 13(6): 738-46.
11) Lombardi JV, Cambria RP, Nienaber CA, et al. Aortic remodeling after endovascular treatment of complicated type B aortic dissection with the use of a composite device design. J Vasc Surg 2014 J; 59(6): 1544-54.
12) Fattori R, Cao P, De Rango P, et al. Interdisciplinary expert consensus document on management of type B aortic dissection. J Am Coll Cardiol 2013; 61(16): 1661-78.
13) Hofferberth SC, Nixon IK, Boston RC, et al. Stent-assisted balloon-induced intimal disruption and relamination in aortic dissection repair: the STABILISE concept. J Thorac Cardiovasc Surg 2014; 147(4): 1240-5.
14) Galvin SD, Perera NK, Matalanis G. Technical aspects of total aortic repair in the surgical management of acute type A aortic dissection. Ann Cardiothorac Surg 2016; 5(3): 248-50.
15) Faure EM, Canaud L, Cathala P, Serres I, Marty-Ané C, Alric P. Assessment of abdominal branch vessel patency after bare-metal stenting of the thoracoabdominal aorta in a human ex vivo model of acute type B aortic dissection. J Vasc Surg 2015; 61(5): 1299-305.
16) Barbante M, Sobocinski J, Maurel B, et al. Fenestrated endografting after bare metal dissection stent implantation. J Endovasc Ther 2015; 22: 207-11.

25

Treatment options for chronic Type B aortic dissection

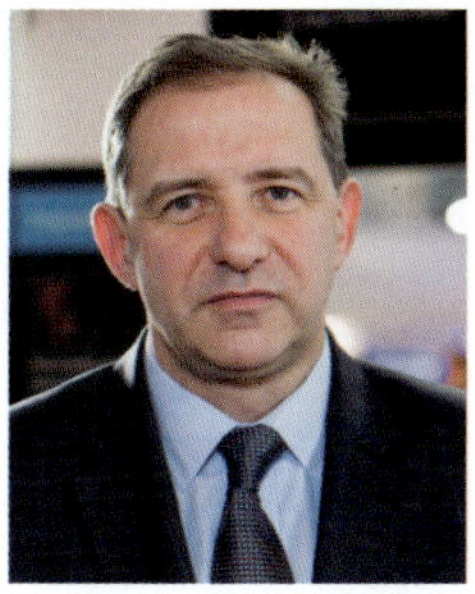

Eric L.G. Verhoeven, Athanasios Katsargyris, Kyriakos Oikonomou, Hozan Mufty and George Kouvelos

25.1 Introduction

Despite major improvements in the management of acute Type B aortic dissection (AD) during the last decade, a proportion of surviving patients will suffer ongoing aortic dilatation. A post-dissection aneurysm is usually the indication for treatment in chronic Type B AD, as other complications such as organ malperfusion rarely occur in the chronic phase following the acute dissection. These post-dissection aneurysms usually represent a serious surgical challenge. They frequently extend to the thoracoabdominal aorta, requiring major open surgery carrying significant mortality and morbidity, including spinal cord ischemia and paraplegia [1].

Standard Thoracic EndoVascular Aortic Repair (TEVAR) is increasingly applied in the treatment of chronic Type B AD, but its efficacy in this setting is doubtful. The dissection flap is usually less compliant in a chronic dissection, and the usual absence of an adequate distal sealing zone makes TEVAR obsolete in most cases [2]. The use of fenestrated and branched stent-grafts (F/BEVAR) to exclude the false lumen completely has been proposed in the last few years, with promising early and mid-term results [3, 4]. Finally, a number of alternative endovascular options have been proposed to induce occlusion of the false lumen in selected patients [5, 6].

This chapter provides an overview of outcomes of post-dissection aneurysm repair with both open and endovascular techniques. The most suitable treatment option depending on patient characteristics is also discussed.

25.2 Open repair

Open surgical repair of post-dissection thoracoabdominal aneurysms is associated with significant perioperative risk, and many patients are unfit for such a major procedure. Current data focusing exclusively on open surgical repair of post-dissection aneurysms are limited to high-volume centers with significant experience in complex open aortic surgery.

Conway et al. reported outcomes on a total of 86 patients with chronic post-dissection aortic aneurysm (descending thoracic, n = 25, thoracoabdominal, n = 61), including eight (9%) patients with rupture [7]. Cardiopulmonary bypass was used in 83 patients (97%) and deep hypothermic arrest in 36 (42%). Hospital mortality was 5.8%. Paraplegia, stroke, and renal

---

Eric L.G. Verhoeven (eric.verhoeven@klinikum-nuernberg.de)
Paracelsus Medical University,
Nuremberg, Germany

G. Melissano - R. Chiesa (eds), Aortic Dissection patients true stories and the innovations that saved their lives

failure requiring permanent hemodialysis were 2.3% each. Univariate predictors of hospital death included redo operations and prolonged pump time (p <0.05). Estimated survival at 1, 5, and 7 years was 92, 83, and 70%, respectively. Freedom from reintervention at 1, 5, and 7 years was 99, 90, and 86%, respectively. The authors concluded that open surgery is a durable option with low mortality. Nevertheless, they suggested that patients who require redo operations or expected prolonged pump time should undergo further evaluation to determine whether endovascular repair would be a better option.

Kouchoukos et al. reported recently their experience on 69 patients with ThoracoAbdominal Aortic Aneurym (TAAA) and chronic dissection that underwent open repair using total cardiopulmonary bypass and hypothermic circulatory arrest [8]. Thirty patients (43%) had Marfan or Loeys-Dietz syndrome, while fifty-three patients (77%) had previous aortic operations. This was a relatively young patient cohort with a mean age of 54±16 years (range, 22-77 years). Thirty-day mortality was 5.8%. Stroke occurred in 3%, and spinal cord ischemia in 6%. Temporary dialysis was required in 4.5% and tracheostomy in 10.6% of the survivors. Estimated survival at 1, 5, and 10 years was 87, 65, and 40%, respectively. Almost 26% of the patients required one or more aortic reintervention during follow-up. Based on these outcomes the authors concluded that open TAAA repair for chronic dissection can be accomplished with acceptable mortality and morbidity and should therefore remain a viable and primary option until long-term efficacy of alternative methods is proven.

A large series with 234 patients was recently published by Fujikawa et al. from Japan [9]. The great majority of operations was performed using left heart bypass. The mean interval between onset of dissection and operation was 61±54 months. Perioperative mortality was 3.9% after descending aortic repair, and 10.2% after TAAA repair. There was no paraplegia after descending repair, while 4.7% of the TAAA repairs resulted in paraplegia. Perioperative stroke was noticed in 3.0%, and cardiac adverse events in 3.8%. Finally, pulmonary complications occurred in 33.3%. Estimated survival and freedom from reintervention at 3 years was 86.7, and 97.0% respectively.

Tian et al. in a systematic review of the literature on open surgical repair for chronic Type B dissection found 19 studies including 970 patients [10]. Pooled perioperative mortality was 11.1%, while stroke, spinal cord ischemia, renal dysfunction, and reoperation for bleeding were 5.9, 4.9, 8.1, and 8.1%, respectively. Late reintervention was needed in 13.3% of patients. Cumulative survival at 3, 5, and 10 years was 74.1, 66.3, and 50.8%, respectively.

Most recently a systematic review including 1081 patients, showed an early mortality ranging between 5.6 and 21.0% for open surgery [11]. Estimated survival at 1 year ranged within 72.0 and 92.0%. Stroke was noted in 0-13.3%, spinal cord ischemia in 0-16.4%, and acute renal failure in 0-33.3% of patients. Recurrent aneurysm formation was reported in 5.8-20.0%, and reintervention was required in 5.8-29.0%.

25.3 Standard thoracic endovascular aortic aneurysm repair

Thoracic EndoVascular Aortic Repair (TEVAR) is an established treatment in acute and subacute Type B AD as it seems to promote false lumen thrombosis and aortic remodeling [12]. The role of TEVAR in the treatment of chronic Type B AD is not well defined.

A recent review with a total of 1397 patients showed an early mortality of 0.0 to 13.7% for TEVAR in chronic Type B AD [11]. Estimated survival at 1 year ranged within 82.9-100.0% and at 5 years within 70.0-88.9%. Stroke was noticed in 0.0-11.8%, spinal cord ischemia in 0.0-12.5%, and acute renal failure in 0.0-34.4%. Early complications included retrograde dissection (0.0-7.1%), malperfusion (1.3-9.4%), cardiac complications (0.0-5.9%) and rupture (0.5-5.0%). Long-term complications included rupture (0.5-7.1%), endoleak (0.0-15.8%) and cardiac complications (5.9-7.1%). Reintervention was required in 4.3-47.4% of the patients among the included series.

Thrumurthy et al., in a systematic review of mid-term outcomes of TEVAR for chronic Type B AD, reported a nearly 90% technical success and 3.2% 30-day mortality rates [2]. However, in the mid-term reintervention rates up to 60% were described, while nearly 10% of patients developed aneurysmal progression of the aorta. In a small study of 76 patients, TEVAR resulted in significantly decreased aortic diameter along the stent-grafted segment, but not in the distal untreated segments [13].

Finally, Mani et al. showed that total false lumen thrombosis occurred in only one third of patients after TEVAR and was more common in dissections confined to the thoracic aorta (83%) than those extended to the abdominal aorta (23%) [14].

Standard TEVAR therefore seems to play only a minor role in the treatment of chronic Type B AD, most probably only for some post-dissection aneurysm limited to the thoracic aorta [15].

25.4 Fenestrated and branched stent-grafts

An endovascular approach using fenestrated and branched stent-grafts (F/BEVAR) has been used in recent years by a few expert centers, in order to achieve complete exclusion of the thoracoabdominal aneurysmal degeneration [3, 4, 16]. Planning of fenestrated and branched stent-grafts is associated with increased challenges in the particular setting of a post-dissection aneurysm. The true lumen is usually narrow. Fenestrations are difficult to plan, as the correct orientation depends on the plasticity of the dissection flap. Branches are often difficult as there is not enough room in the narrow true lumen. Vessels with a downwards sharp take-off may be simpler over a transaxillary access, but this can be limited due to earlier overstenting of the left subclavian artery [17]. Visceral branches originating from the false lumen create additional technical challenges with catheterization. Different techniques have been used to perforate the dissection flap: wires with tips that can be stiffened, the back of a wire, a wire with support of a guiding sheath, or even a transjugular intrahepatic portosystemic shunt (TIPS) needle. Finally, the distal landing zone can be compromised when the dissection extends to the common iliac arteries. Hypogastric artery flow should be preserved to reduce the risk of paraplegia. This can be achieved by adding an iliac branched device (IBD) to the plan, or to land in a dissected common iliac artery with an oversized graft limb and to hope for adequate sealing.

Literature data are still scarce and lack long-term follow-up. Technical feasibility of F/BEVAR for chronic post-dissection aneurysms was first published in 2012 by our group in a limited series of six patients [17]. Kitagawa et al. reported later on the Cleveland Clinic Experience on 30 patients with chronic dissection (15 focal and 15 with thoracoabdominal extent) treated with F/BEVAR [4]. Technical success was achieved in 100% of patients, and perioperative mortality was null. One aortic related death occurred at three months due to progression of a pre-existing untreated arch dissection. No ruptures, cardiac, renal, pulmonary, or spinal cord ischemia complications occurred. No graft compression was noted, despite the initially narrow true lumen dimensions. During a mean follow-up period of 1.7 years aneurysm sac growth was noted in two patients, related to Type II endoleaks, which were treated with translumbar glue embolization. Eight (26.7%) patients (five Type I and three Type III endoleaks) underwent reintervention, with four patients requiring multiple endovascular procedures.

Most recently, the group from Lille published their experience with F/BEVAR for chronic Type B AD in a total of 23 patients [14]. Staged procedures were performed in 14 patients (61%). Seven patients were treated for a dissecting aneurysm involving the aortic arch and 16 patients for a TAAA extension. Technical success was 71% following arch repair and 100% following TAAA repair. The overall 30-day and in-hospital mortality rates were 4.4% (1/23) and 8.7% (2/23), respectively. Major adverse events occurred in 17.4%, including one spinal cord ischemia (TAAA group), one pulmonary embolism (TAAA group), and two early reinterventions in the arch group. During follow-up with a mean duration of 12 months, one patient died of causes unrelated to aneurysm. There were two late reinterventions in the TAAA group to treat endoleaks. There was no target vessel occlusion up to the latest follow-up.

25.4.1 Nuremberg experience

Our experience in the treatment of post-dissection TAAA with F/BEVAR includes 34 patients (29 male, mean age 64.8±9.9 years) treated from October 2010 to December 2015. Part of this experience was published before [12]. All cases were technically successful, but in one case, a retroperitoneal approach was needed for a renal artery catheterization. Two (5.9%) patients died within 30 days postoperatively, one due to multiple organ failure and one due to cardiac decompensation. Perioperative spinal cord ischemia (SCI) occurred in 5 (14.7%) patients.

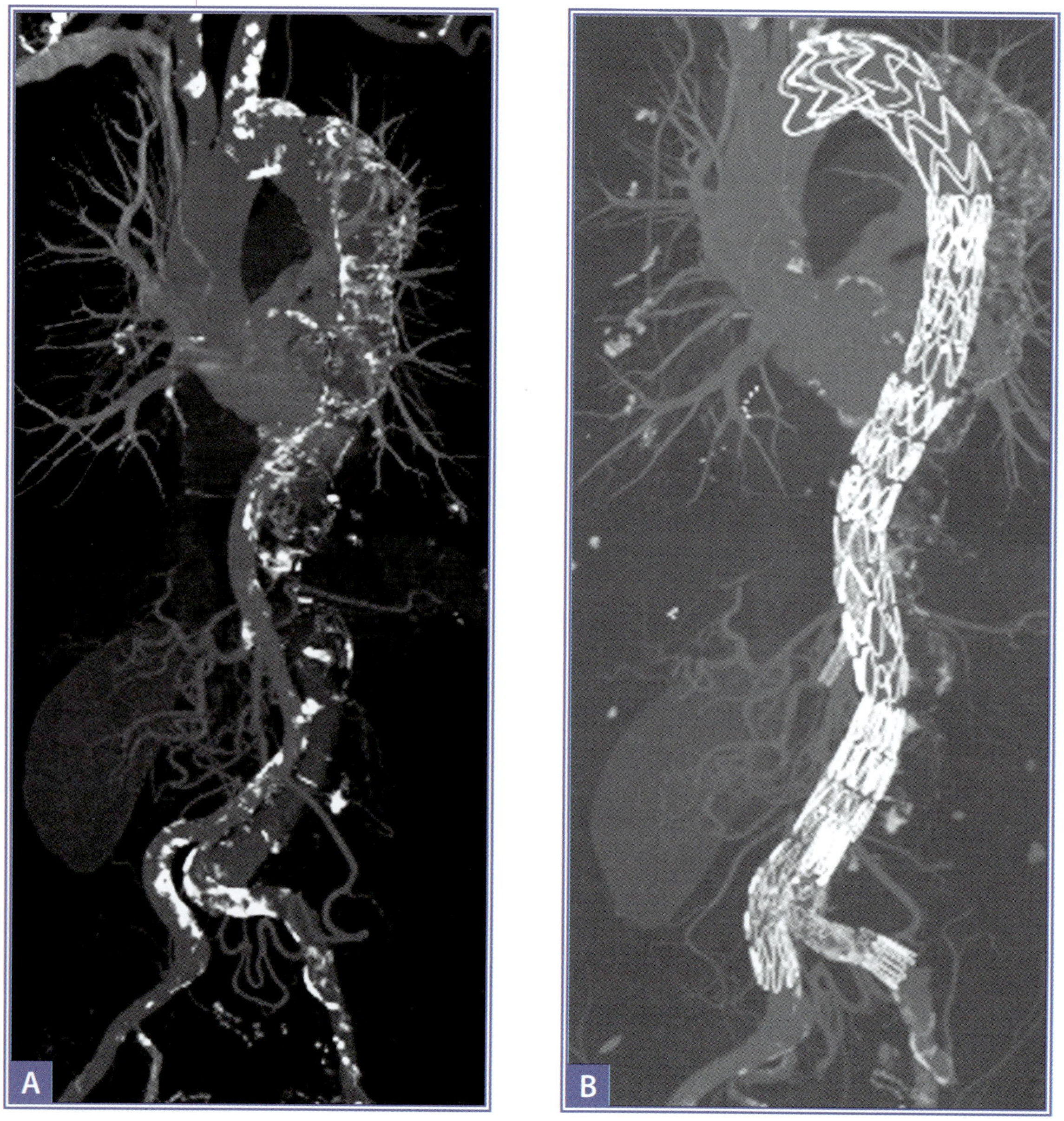

Fig. 25.1 Computed tomography angiography (CTA) of a post-dissection thoracoabdominal aortic aneurysm (**A**). CTA 2 years after endovascular treatment with F/BEVAR showing expansion of the true lumen and shrinkage of the false lumen (**B**).

One (2.9%) patient suffered paraplegia with significant improvement prior to discharge, and four (11.7%) patients suffered transient paraparesis with complete recovery prior to discharge. One (2.9%) additional patient developed late SCI (6 months) with urinary incontinence and lower limb weakness most probably due to regression of a Type II endoleak. He also recovered completely. Mean follow-up was 18.5 months (range 1-66 months). One late death was graft-related and occurred 26 months postoperatively due to an aortoesophageal fistula. Five target vessel occlusions were noticed (3 renal arteries, 1 superior mesenteric artery and 1 celiac trunk) during follow-up. In one case an iliac-renal bypass was carried out. One patient with known occlusion of the contralateral renal artery became dialysis dependent. The remaining three patients were asymptomatic and did not require treatment.

Endoleaks were diagnosed in 17 (50%) patients. These included six (17.6%) Type Ib endoleaks, all from a target vessel. Four (11.7%) patients had a distal Type Ib endoleak from dissected iliac arteries. Six (17.6%) patients had a Type II endoleak. One (2.9%) patient had a Type III endoleak. Reintervention was required in 10 (29.4%) patients. Six (17.6%) patients were treated for Ib endoleak with stent-graft extension into the target vessel or with re-flairing of the existing stent-graft. Other reinterventions included extension with an IBD for distal Type Ib endoleak, one stent-graft extension to the external iliac artery with embolization of the internal iliac for Type Ib endoleak, one coil-embolization of a Type II endoleak and one implantation of a bridging stent-graft for the left renal artery (LRA) presenting with a Type III endoleak. Aneurysm sac regression during follow-up was significant ($p = 0.007$) from 66.5±6.5 mm to 57.4±9.5 mm with a false lumen thrombosis rate of 78% for patients that completed 6 month follow-up (Fig. 25.1).

25.5 Endovascular techniques with occlusion of the false lumen

A small proportion of patients with post-dissection aneurysms develop aneurysmal dilatation in the descending thoracic aorta alone, without major involvement of the abdominal segment. This subgroup of patients may be treated with a less complex endovascular procedure. This can be achieved by using standard TEVAR covering the thoracic aorta down to the celiac artery in combination with techniques to occlude the false lumen. Three options are described below.

25.5.1 False lumen embolization

Embolization of the false lumen at the level of the distal descending thoracic aorta can be achieved by a variety of embolizing agents. The use of cava filters, detachable balloons, thrombin or occlude devices into the false lumen has been reported to achieve successful occlusion of the false lumen. Additional use of coils and cyanoacrylate glue has also been suggested [18]. Idrees et al. recently reported on 21 patients with chronic dissection using iliac occluders to embolize the false lumen [19]. Technical success rate was 100% and false lumen thrombosis was achieved in all patients at a median follow-up of 25 months.

The methods described above however can only address a false lumen with a relatively small diameter. In patients with a larger false lumen diameter, embolization using standard commercially available materials seems obsolete. To occlude larger false lumens at the level of the distal descending thoracic aorta, two new techniques were recently introduced.

25.5.2 The candy-plug technique

Initially this technique was introduced by modifying a Zenith® thoracic TX2® Pro-Form stent graft (Cook Medical, Bloomington, IN) into a large candy-shaped plug by adding a diameter-restricting suture in the middle [6]. The plug was positioned in the false lumen opposing the distal end of the endograft in the true lumen. A large Amplatzer vascular plug was also deployed at the reduced diameter mid-section of the stent-graft to achieve occlusion of the false lumen. The candy-plug was later produced as a custom-made implant with a maximum diameter of 50 mm and a mid-section of 18 mm. Recently the use of a modified Gore® Excluder® (W.L. Gore & Associates, Flagstaff, AZ) aortic extender together with a 16-mm Amplatzer™ vascular plug was also reported in one case [20]. Experience with this technique remains limited.

25.5.3 The knickerbocker technique

The knickerbocker technique describes the use of a large diameter stent-graft in the true lumen, which over-expands and ruptures the dissection membrane into the false lumen, and hopefully achieves occlusion of the false lumen [5]. This is done using custom-made double-tapered stent grafts with a bulbous section in the middle of their length. The knickerbocker-graft is deployed at the intended segment of the aorta with sufficient overlap to the proximal stent-graft and ending proximal to the celiac artery. After deployment, the bulbous section of the stent-graft is dilated with a compliant balloon until the dissection membrane ruptures and the oversized stent-graft expands into the false lumen sealing the false lumen backflow. Clinical experience with this technique is still limited.

25.6 Treatment choice

It is difficult to define which type of procedure is most suitable for a post-dissection aneurysm. Randomized controlled trials could theoretically provide an answer, but are not realizable due to the rarity and complexity of the disease. Comparison of different treatment methods originating from observational studies is biased by patient selection.

Open surgery is often used as a first line treatment for chronic Type B AD, especially for those that extend in the thoracoabdominal aorta. High-volume centers report acceptable outcomes with regard to perioperative mortality and morbidity. Pooled outcomes including experience from smaller centers are less optimistic, with mortality rates of more than 11% [10]. Open surgical repair is a procedure of such a magnitude, that it can only be considered for patients in reasonably good physical condition, and younger healthier patients with connective tissue disease. Results clearly suggest centralization towards larger expert centers.

Standard TEVAR is used liberally for the treatment of acute Type B AD. For chronic Type B AD TEVAR is less useful, mainly due to the frequent involvement of the visceral and abdominal aorta. A complete distal sealing at healthy not dissected aortic wall is rarely possible with standard TEVAR, and its use in chronic Type B AD is associated with high reintervention rates and unsatisfactory aortic remodeling. To our view, standard TEVAR has a role only in the rare cases of chronic dissection limited to the descending thoracic aorta.

For most chronic Type B AD that involve the thoracoabdominal aorta, endovascular treatment requires the use of F/BEVAR to achieve adequate sealing. Our experience along with a few other larger endovascular centers shows that F/BEVAR is feasible in post-dissection TAAA. The technique is associated with additional technical challenges, as discussed above, compared to standard atherosclerotic TAAA, but early and mid-term results are encouraging. To our view F/BEVAR for post-dissection TAAA should be considered as a treatment option, especially for high-risk or previously operated patients with suitable anatomy. Selected patients with connective tissue disease should also be considered for F/BEVAR, provided that endovascular sealing can be obtained within a previous surgical graft.

Endovascular techniques used to trigger false lumen thrombosis are interesting, but up to now scarcely reported. They might be useful in selected patients, when the dissection is mainly located in the thoracic aorta. Nevertheless, available clinical data do not allow for further conclusions.

REFERENCES

1) Schepens MA, Heijmen RH, Ranschaert W, Sonker U, Morshuis WJ. Thoracoabdominal aortic aneurysm repair: results of conventional open surgery. Eur J Vasc Endovasc Surg 2009; 37: 640-5.
2) Thrumurthy SG, Karthikesalingam A, Patterson BO, et al. A systematic review of mid-term outcomes of thoracic endovascular repair (TEVAR) of chronic type B aortic dissection. Eur J Vasc Endovasc Surg 2011; 42: 632-47.
3) Oikonomou K, Kopp R, Katsargyris A, Pfister K, Verhoeven EL, Kasprzak P. Outcomes of fenestrated/branched endografting in post-dissection thoracoabdominal aortic aneurysms. Eur J Vasc Endovasc Surg 2014; 48: 641-8.
4) Kitagawa A, Greenberg RK, Eagleton MJ, Mastracci TM, Roselli EE. Fenestrated and branched endovascular aortic repair for chronic type B aortic dissection with thoracoabdominal aneurysms. J Vasc Surg 2013; 58: 625-34.
5) Kolbel T, Carpenter SW, Lohrenz C, Tsilimparis N, Larena-Avellaneda A, Debus ES. Addressing persistent false lumen flow in chronic aortic dissection: the knickerbocker technique. J Endovasc Ther 2014; 21: 117-22.
6) Kolbel T, Lohrenz C, Kieback A, Diener H, Debus ES, Larena-Avellaneda A. Distal false lumen occlusion in aortic dissection with a homemade extra-large vascular plug: the candy-plug technique. J Endovasc Ther 2013; 20: 484-9.
7) Conway AM, Sadek M, Lugo J, et al. Outcomes of open surgical repair for chronic type B aortic dissections. J Vasc Surg 2014; 59: 1217-23.
8) Kouchoukos NT, Kulik A, Castner CF. Open thoracoabdominal aortic repair for chronic type B dissection. J Thor Cardiovasc Surg 2015; 149: S125-9.
9) Fujikawa T, Yamamoto S, Sekine Y, et al. Operative results and clinical features of chronic stanford type B aortic dissection: examination of 234 patients over 6 years. Eur J Vasc Endovasc Surg 2015; 50: 738-43.
10) Tian DH, De Silva RP, Wang T, Yan TD. Open surgical repair for chronic type B aortic dissection: a systematic review. Ann Cardiothor Surg 2014; 3: 340-50.
11) Kamman AV, de Beaufort HW, van Bogerijen GH, et al. Contemporary management strategies for chronic type B aortic dissections: a systematic review. PloS one 2016; 11: e0154930.
12) Kusagawa H, Shimono T, Ishida M, et al. Changes in false lumen after transluminal stent-graft placement in aortic dissections: six years' experience. Circulation 2005; 111: 2951-7.
13) Kang WC, Greenberg RK, Mastracci TM, et al. Endovascular repair of complicated chronic distal aortic dissections: intermediate outcomes and complications. J Thor Cardiovasc Surg 2011; 142: 1074-83.
14) Mani K, Clough RE, Lyons OT, et al. Predictors of outcome after endovascular repair for chronic type B dissection. Eur J Vasc Endovasc Surg 2012; 43: 386-91.
15) Andacheh ID, Donayre C, Othman F, Walot I, Kopchok G, White R. Patient outcomes and thoracic aortic volume and morphologic changes following thoracic endovascular aortic repair in patients with complicated chronic type B aortic dissection. J Vasc Surg 2012; 56: 644-50.
16) Spear R, Sobocinski J, Settembre N, et al. Early experience of endovascular repair of post-dissection aneurysms involving the thoraco-abdominal aorta and the arch. Eur J Vasc Endovasc Surg 2016; 51: 488-97.
17) Verhoeven EL, Paraskevas KI, Oikonomou K, et al. Fenestrated and branched stent-grafts to treat post-dissection chronic aortic aneurysms after initial treatment in the acute setting. J Endovasc Ther 2012; 19: 343-9.
18) Hofferberth SC, Nixon IK, Mossop PJ. Aortic false lumen thrombosis induction by embolotherapy (AFTER) following endovascular repair of aortic dissection. J Endovasc Ther 2012; 19: 538-45.
19) Idrees J, Roselli EE, Shafii S, Reside J, Lytle BW. Outcomes after false lumen embolization with covered stent devices in chronic dissection. J Vasc Surg 2014; 60: 1507-13.
20) Ogawa Y, Nishimaki H, Chiba K, et al. Candy-plug technique using an excluder aortic extender for distal occlusion of a large false lumen aneurysm in chronic aortic dissection. J Endovasc Ther 2016; 23: 483-6.

26

Maintaining durability following TEVAR for chronic Type B aortic dissection

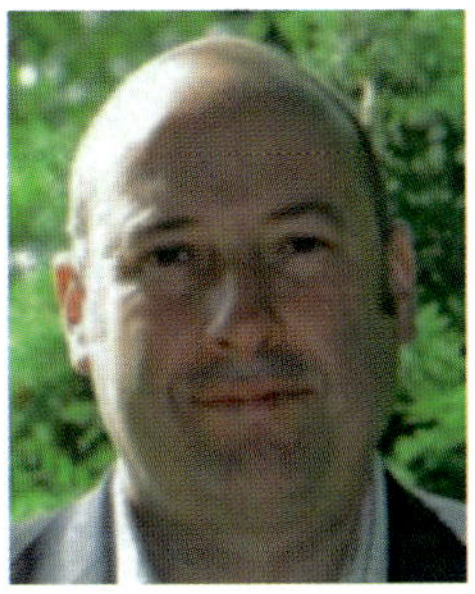

Matt Thompson and Benjamin O. Patterson

26.1 Introduction

Aortic dissection (AD) occurs when there is a tear between the tunica media and tunica intima of the aorta which can propagate in either direction [1]. A Stanford Type B AD occurs when the false aortic lumen arises from an entry tear distal to the left subclavian artery, and can present in either the acute or chronic phase. Patients presenting with an acute, complicated dissection will usually require urgent intervention, as this is by definition a life-threatening condition. In the absence of the need for immediate treatment, the mainstay of treatment is pharmacological blood-pressure reduction to reduce wall stress and prevent aneurysmal dilatation or true lumen compression [1, 2]. If treatment in the sub-acute phase is not undertaken, patients should undergo annual imaging surveillance to detect any late aneurysmal expansion that may necessitate prophylactic surgery to prevent rupture. If the initial dissection event is not reported to a physician or if the correct diagnosis is not ascertained at the time of presentation, the condition will likely go undetected until it is discovered incidentally.

In recent years, Thoracic EndoVascular Aortic Repair (TEVAR) has been increasingly offered as the first line treatment of chronic dissection [3-5]. The aim of this procedure is to seal the entry tear of the dissection, promoting aortic remodelling. Remodelling can be defined as the restoration of the normal anatomy of the aorta by thrombosis and regression of the false lumen with expansion of the true lumen [6, 7]. It is thought that this leads to stabilisation of the aorta and consequently reduces aortic-related death [6, 7]. Patients treated for chronic dissection appear to exhibit less extensive remodelling than those that are treated in the acute phase, and the rates of reintervention reflect this [8, 9]. The reason for this is thought to be that the false lumen becomes less pliable over time, but the overall variation in response to surgery is probably multifactorial (Fig. 26.1) [10]. Identifying factors that are predictive of poor response to treatment may enable measures to be taken to improve long-term outcomes in patients with chronic dissection.

Matt Thompson (matt.thompson@stgeorges.nhs.uk)
St. Georges' Vascular Institute, St. George's Hospital,
London, United Kingdom

G. Melissano - R. Chiesa (eds), Aortic Dissection patients true stories and the innovations that saved their lives

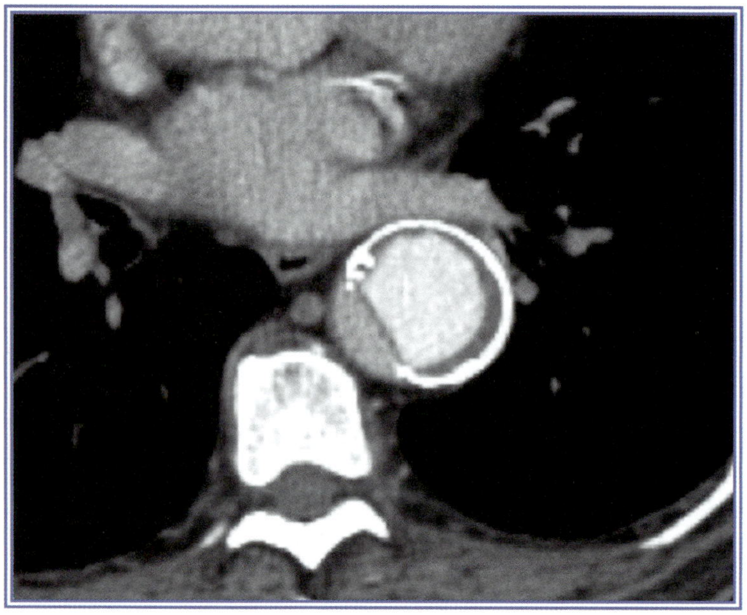

Fig. 26.1 A CT scan of a patient with a chronic Type B AD. Note the rigid, circumferentially calcified appearance of the false lumen.

26.2 Remodelling following TEVAR for chronic dissection is variable

The historical classification of AD as either Type A or Type B is probably an over-simplification given the morphologically heterogeneous nature of the disease. Several other classification systems have been proposed but none has entered widespread clinical use. The variability in remodelling reported in the literature may be related to difference in technical approach to treatment as well as the timing of repair. Poor remodelling or continued degeneration means the observed rate of reintervention in the pooled literature is approximately 20% which equates to 6/100 years of follow-up [11]. Optimising the initial intervention may help to reduce this.

26.3 More extensive aortic coverage seems to promote remodelling

Some experts have advocated extensive aortic coverage when planning the treatment of chronic dissections. The objective of this is to cause direct compression of as much of the false lumen as possible as well as covering the main entry tear, minor fenestrations and more rarely the main re-entry tear. One study reported that if the length of aortic coverage was over 162 mm there was more likely to be complete false lumen thrombosis at three years of follow-up [12]. AD with infrarenal extension (DeBakey IIIb) exhibits less tendency to remodel in some series, and this probably because the main re-entry tear is likely to be to the distal stented segment allowing retrograde perfusion of the false lumen (Fig. 26.2) [10]. A study of purely extent IIIb chronic Type B AD suggested that longer coverage is necessary, as some reinterventions have been linked to patent fenestrations [13]. A recent systematic review noted that distal extension to treat continued distal false lumen perfusion comprised almost half of all aortic reinterventions in patients with chronic dissection [11]. It could be that longer coverage could therefore reduce this rate.

Despite these observations, false lumen thrombosis was achieved in 85% of patients in the INSTEAD (Investigation of STent grafts in Aortic Dissection) trial even though a single stent graft was used in most patients [14, 15], although many of these patients may have been classified as sub-acute dissections rather then "truly" chronic. Other groups have also found length of coverage to be less important [15, 16].

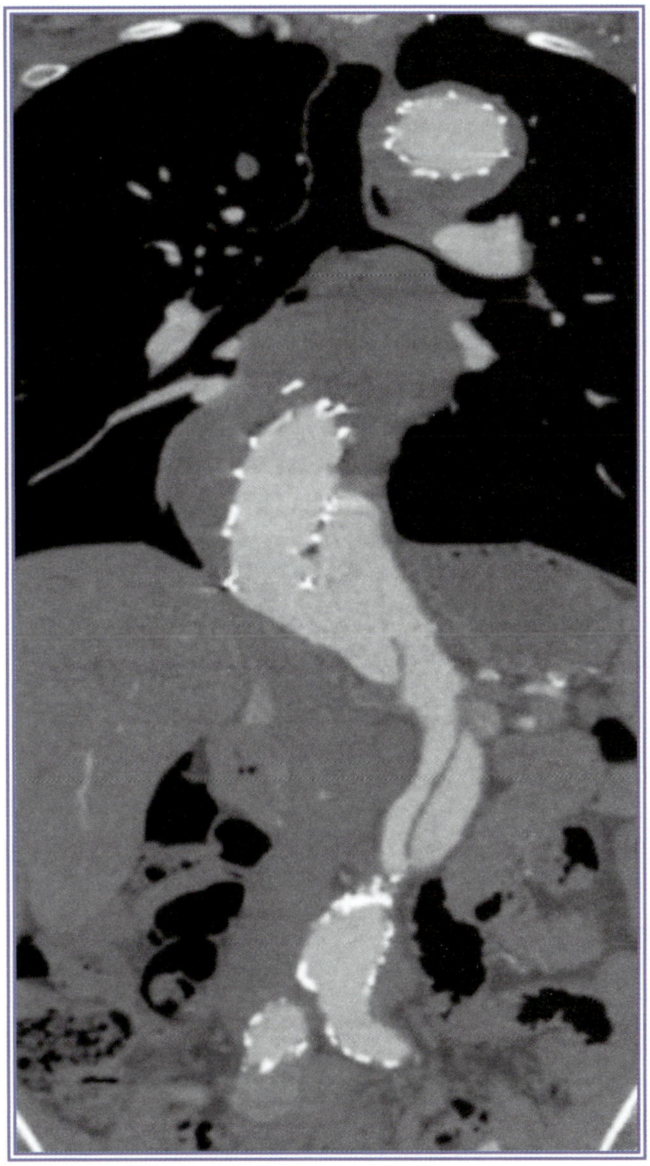

Fig. 26.2 A complex dissection treated with TEVAR. This illustrates that despite long length of coverage treatment of only the thoracic segment will not always guarantee remodelling. This patient will certainly require further treatment to the visceral segment.

26.4 Earlier treatment may lead to better long-term results

The chronological definition of "chronic" dissection varies between different studies [13, 17]. Some would group patients who are 2 weeks from presentation and those who were diagnosed 15 years previously together [16]. The INSTEAD trial intervention arm recruited patients at a mean of 7.5 weeks and a median of 3.5 weeks after the diagnosis [14]. This trial randomised 140 patients with a diagnosis of uncomplicated Type B AD to be treated either by insertion of a endovascular stent graft and best medical therapy (72 patients) or by best medical therapy alone (68 patients), and in the latter group there was a reported 92.6% rate of total false lumen thrombosis. This is far superior to another study that treated patients at a mean of 100 weeks post diagnosis, in which a false lumen thrombosis rate of only 39% was observed [18]. The difference noted between these two groups suggests that the classification of AD into simply "acute" and "chronic" may not be adequate, and that the "sub-acute" classification described in the VIRTUE registry (14-92 days after the acute event) is probably more suitable. This is borne out by the different rate of aortic remodelling seen in the three different groups in this study which also appeared to correlate with mid-term mortality [9].

26.5 Stent-graft induced new entry tears may be underappreciated

Stent-graft induced new entry tears have been noted in patients that have undergone TEVAR, with a significant number requiring urgent reintervention. It is also thought to be the cause of some sudden unexpected deaths in treated patients [19]. This is most likely to be caused by oversizing of the stent-graft at the distal extent of the treated area, with excessive radial force giving rise to trauma to the aortic wall and potentially perforation of the intimal flap [20]. This may be avoided by sizing the stent-graft according to the dimensions of the distal true lumen, and may require the placement of tapered devices. Deploying multiple devices in a reverse order (from distal to proximal) has been suggested to enable to facilitate the correct degree of tapering from proximal to distal aorta [13].

26.6 Branch vessel involvement and fenestrations increase risk of reintervention

The number of aortic branches arising from the true aortic lumen and visible fenestrations in the dissection flap may determine the likelihood of false lumen thrombosis. In one study no patients with one or more branch arising from the false lumen displayed complete false lumen thrombosis, and those with a greater number of patent distal fenestrations were similarly less likely to exhibit aortic remodelling. Those with greater than five fenestrations developed aneurysmal dilatation and required open surgery [13]. These findings have been supported by several other studies which also found a strong correlation between the number of branches coming from the true lumen and remodelling [16, 21]. Acknowledging that the thoracic stent is the first stage of procedure that will eventually require treatment of the visceral aorta is probably most appropriate. The additional risk of major morbidity, including paraplegia, should be accounted for if this course is undertaken.

26.7 Various strategies are emerging to treat ongoing false lumen perfusion

Recently there have been several reports describing active management of persistent flow within the aortic false lumen by attempting embolisation using a variety of means. This can be undertaken if there are features seen on post-operative imaging that suggest that remodelling is unlikely to occur, and may avoid recourse to further invasive surgery in those that may not be fit for this. Commonly this is done using a covered stent, such as an iliac plug, nitinol embolisation plugs or custom made spindle shaped devices that can be easily occluded after placement into the false lumen [22, 23]. Early results are encouraging for these techniques, although further study is required to determine if this is a safe and durable technique.

26.8 Conclusion

TEVAR for chronic AD may be performed with less perioperative morbidity and mortality than invasive open surgical techniques, but reintervention is necessary in a fifth of patients, so regular surveillance and expert medical management are mandatory. Improvements in long-term clinical outcomes may be achieved if predictors of poor outcomes can be identified, although it is difficult to define this given the heterogeneous nature of existing literature. Retrograde flow into the thoracic aortic false lumen accounts for the majority of potentially preventable reinterventions, so a longer length of aortic coverage should be considered in patients with DeBakey IIIb dissections to reduce subsequent reinterventions. Earlier treatment may lead to less reintervention by promoting remodelling, and treatment in the sub-acute phase may be considered in some patients with uncomplicated presentations. Patients with extensive AD with multiple fenestrations and branch vessel involvement in the visceral aorta will often require intervention in this area.

REFERENCES

1) Thrumurthy SG, Karthikesalingam A, Patterson BO, Holt PJE, Thompson MM. The diagnosis and management of aortic dissection. BMJ 2012; 344: d8290.
2) Erbel R, Alfonso F, Boileau C, et al. Diagnosis and management of aortic dissection. Eur Heart J 2001; 22(18): 1642-81.
3) Tefera G, Acher CW, Hoch JR, Mell M, Turnipseed WD. Effectiveness of intensive medical therapy in type B aortic dissection: a single-center experience. J Vasc Surg 2007; 45: 1114-8; discussion 1118-9.
4) Svensson LG, Kouchoukos NT, Miller DC, et al. Expert consensus document on the treatment of descending thoracic aortic disease using endovascular stent-grafts. Ann Thorac Surg 2008; 85: S1-S41.
5) Jones DW, Goodney PP, Nolan BW, et al. National trends in utilization, mortality, and survival after repair of type B aortic dissection in the Medicare population. J Vasc Surg 2014; 60: 11-9.
6) Resch TA, Delle M, Falkenberg M, et al. Remodeling of the thoracic aorta after stent grafting of type B dissection: a Swedish multicenter study. J Cardiovasc Surg (Torino) 2006; 47: 503-8.
7) Patterson B, Holt P, Nienaber C, Cambria R, Fairman R, Thompson M. Aortic pathology determines midterm outcome after endovascular repair of the thoracic aorta: report from the Medtronic Thoracic Endovascular Registry (MOTHER) database. Circulation 2013; 127: 24-32.
8) Kusagawa H, Shimono T, Ishida M, et al. Changes in false lumen after transluminal stent-graft placement in aortic dissections: six years' experience. Circulation 2005; 111: 2951-7.
9) Virtue Registry Investigators. Mid-term outcomes and aortic remodelling after thoracic endovascular repair for acute, subacute, and chronic aortic dissection: the VIRTUE Registry. Eur J Vasc Endovasc Surg 2014; 48: 363-71.
10) Patterson BO, Cobb RJ, Karthikesalingam A, et al. A systematic review of aortic remodeling after endovascular repair of type B aortic dissection: methods and outcomes. Ann Thorac Surg 2014; 97(2): 588-95.
11) Boufi M, Patterson BO, Grima M, et al. A systematic review of reintervention after thoracic endovascular repair for chronic type B dissection. Ann Thorac Surg [accepted].
12) Qing K, Yiu W, Cheng SW. A morphologic study of chronic type B aortic dissections and aneurysms after thoracic endovascular stent grafting. J Vasc Surg 2012; 55: 1268-76.
13) Hughes GC, Ganapathi AM, Keenan JE, et al. Thoracic endovascular aortic repair for chronic DeBakey IIIb aortic dissection. Ann Thorac Surg 2014; 98: 2092-8.
14) Nienaber CA, Rousseau H, Eggebrecht H, et al. Randomized comparison of strategies for type B aortic dissection: the INvestigation of STEnt Grafts in Aortic Dissection (INSTEAD) trial. Circulation 2009; 120: 2519-28.
15) Lee M, Lee DY, Kim MD, et al. Outcomes of endovascular management for complicated chronic type B aortic dissection: effect of the extent of stent graft coverage and anatomic properties of aortic dissection. J Vasc Interv Radiol 2013; 24: 1451-60.
16) Kitamura T, Torii S, Oka N, et al. Key success factors for thoracic endovascular aortic repair for non-acute Stanford type B aortic dissection. Eur J Cardiothorac Surg 2014; 46: 432-7; discussion 437.
17) Nienaber CA, Kische S, Rousseau H, et al. Endovascular repair of type B aortic dissection: long-term results of the randomized investigation of stent grafts in aortic dissection trial. Circ Cardiovasc Interv 2013; 6: 407-16.
18) Kang WC, Greenberg RK, Mastracci TM, et al. Endovascular repair of complicated chronic distal aortic dissections: intermediate outcomes and complications. J Thorac Cardiovasc Surg 2011; 142: 1074-83.
19) Weng SH, Weng CF, Chen WY, et al. Reintervention for distal stent graft-induced new entry after endovascular repair with a stainless steel-based device in aortic dissection. J Vasc Surg 2013; 57: 64-71.
20) Zhang L, Zhou J, Lu Q, Zhao Z, Bao J, Jing Z. Potential risk factors of re-intervention after endovascular repair for type B aortic dissections. Cathet Cardiovasc Intervent 2015; 86(1): E1-E10.
21) Tolenaar JL, Kern JA, Jonker FHW, et al. Predictors of false lumen thrombosis in type B aortic dissection treated with TEVAR. Ann Cardiothorac Surg 2014; 3: 255-63.
22) Idrees J, Roselli EE, Shafii S, Reside J, Lytle BW. Outcomes after false lumen embolization with covered stent devices in chronic dissection. J Vasc Surg 2014; 60: 1507-13.
23) Kölbel T, Lohrenz C, Kieback A, Diener H, Debus ES, Larena-Avellaneda A. Distal false lumen occlusion in aortic dissection with a homemade extra-large vascular plug: the candy-plug technique. J Endovasc Ther 2013; 20: 484-9.

27

Planning endovascular repair of chronic aortic dissections with fenestrated and branched endografts

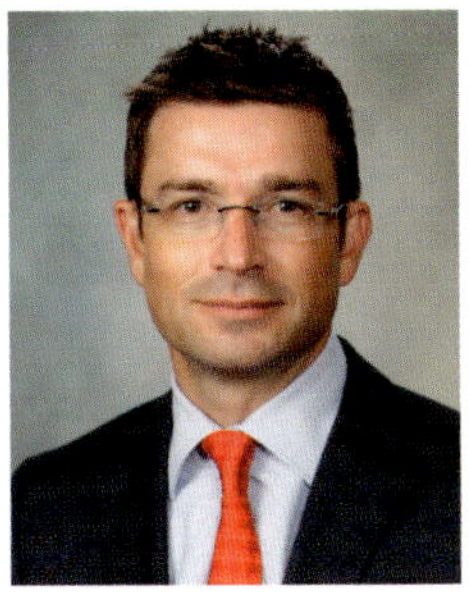

Gustavo S. Oderich, Mauricio S. Ribeiro and Giuliano de A. Sandri

27.1 Introduction

Endovascular aortic repair (EVAR) using fenestrated-branched endografts has been increasingly utilized to treat complex aneurysms affecting the aortic arch and the thoracoabdominal and iliac segments. The ability to incorporate visceral arteries by endovascular means has expanded the indications of EVAR to include patients with extensive chronic aortic dissections that have late aneurysm degeneration [1-14]. Although the clinical experience worldwide is still limited compared to what has been described for degenerative aneurysms, several centers have reported encouraging results with high technical success, and mortality and morbidity that is comparable or superior to open surgical results. Total endovascular repair of chronic dissecting ThoracoAbdominal Aortic Aneurysms (TAAAs) has special anatomical, technical and postoperative particularities. This chapter summarizes some of the key aspects of planning complex endovascular procedures with fenestrated and branched endografts to treat complex TAAAs and chronic dissections.

27.2 Preoperative planning

27.2.1 Clinical history

Patients with chronic TAAA dissections have certain clinical and anatomical pitfalls that deserve special consideration and affect surgical and endovascular planning. Most patients have a history of prior DeBakey Types I or IIIb dissections with involvement of the thoracic and visceral segments (Fig. 27.1). A history of prior ascending aortic repair is frequent in patients with DeBakey I dissection. The average age at presentation is 65 years old, which is approximately 10 years younger than patients who are treated for degenerative TAAAs. Degeneration to TAAA occurs on average 10 years after the initial dissection episode, although this may be affected by current trends to treat uncomplicated dissections by early stent-graft placement.

Gustavo S. Oderich (Oderich.Gustavo@mayo.edu)
Mayo Clinic,
Rochester, MN, USA

G. Melissano - R. Chiesa (eds), Aortic Dissection patients true stories and the innovations that saved their lives

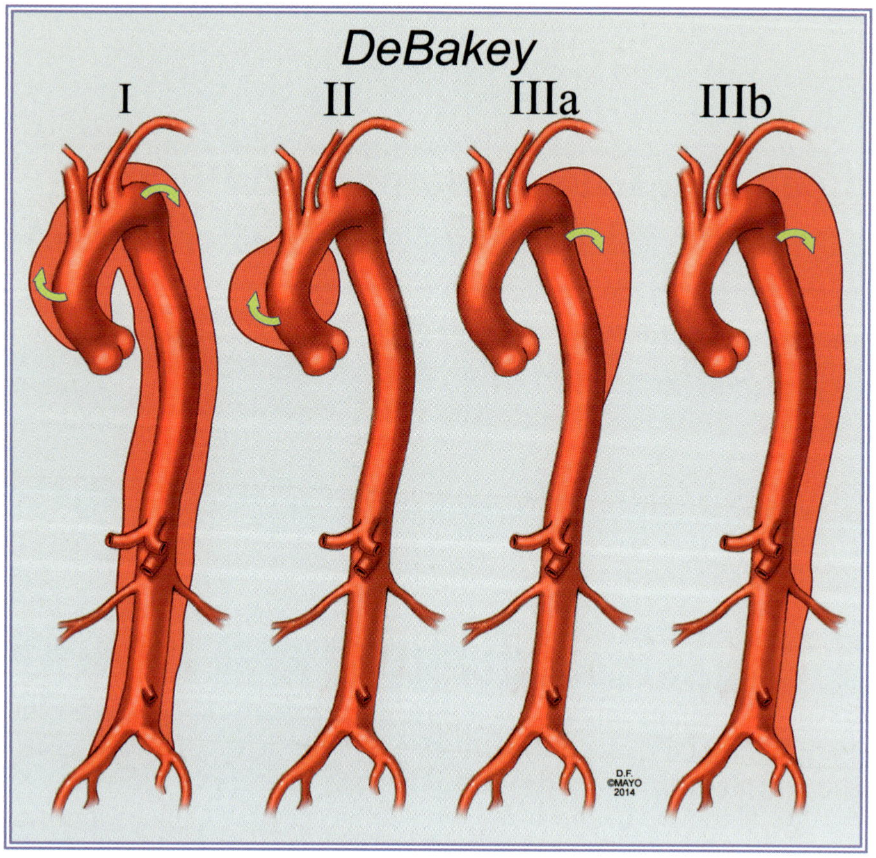

Fig. 27.1 DeBakey classification of aortic dissections (by permission of Mayo Foundation for Medical Education and Research. All rights reserved).

Patients with dissections have higher prevalence of familial disease and should be investigated for genetically triggered aortic disease. The later is particularly frequent if the initial dissection occurs at younger age (<50 years old) or if there is a family history for aneurysm and dissection or clinical features consistent with genetic disorders. Iliac artery involvement is also more frequent, either due to aneurysm or dissection extending beyond the iliac bifurcation.

A review of prior surgical history is of paramount importance. Most patients already underwent some type of open surgical repair or endovascular repair of the thoracic aorta. Repair of the ascending aorta may be coupled with aortic valve repair or coronary bypass grafting. Dimensions of the initial surgical grafts or stent grafts should be noted when selecting landing zones, although a 10-20% natural growth of polyester grafts should be accounted. Presence of a prior left internal mammary artery (LIMA) bypass graft may dictate need to preserve the subclavian artery. For patients who underwent prior thoracic endovascular aortic repair (TEVAR), the type and dimensions of the stent grafts should be noted.

27.2.2 Anatomical review

All patients considered for endovascular repair of chronic TAAA dissections need thorough evaluation of the entire aorta from the arch to the femoral bifurcation with a helical thin-slice computed tomography angiography (CTA). The importance of a thorough imaging evaluation relies on the incidence of concomitant multi-segment disease and the need to assess the arch for access and suitability of landing zones. More often, patients with prior ascending repair have relatively short interposition grafts that are not suitable for landing zone or require an arch procedure (e.g. elephant trunk or arch branch). The non-contrast phase provides valuable information on assessment of calcifications.

The aorta and its branches should be evaluated for stenosis or dilatation on the optimal phase of arterial enhancement. This should be done in a systematic manner, usually relying upon the axial images. Scrolling through the axial images, the aorta is inspected first, followed by each of the main aortic branches, including the supra-aortic trunks, the celiac, superior mesenteric artery (SMA), renals and internal iliac arteries. When pathology is noted and specific measurements are needed, one can rely upon maximum intensity projection (MIP) images and the creation of centerline of flow (CLF) for the assessment of luminal narrowing, and the projection of images perpendicular to the CLF for measurements of the outer wall diameter. The location of the target vessel within true or false lumen should be noted. Importantly, all vessels that have "origin" from the false lumen should have re-entrances in close proximity, unless this has been obliterated by thrombus or remodelling process. The diameter of the intended lumen to be stented (e.g. true lumen in general) should be carefully reviewed, as it has critical role on the selection of type of incorporation (e.g. fenestration vs. branch).

Selecting the seal zone

Disease assessment is performed using surrogates such as changes in diameter or presence of arterial wall abnormalities such as calcium, thrombus, debris or thickening. The vessel wall, in the absence of any pathology, is difficult to accurately quantify on most CT studies. A vessel wall that appears thick or is lined by atherosclerotic debris indicates pathology and should not be selected for sealing zone with few exceptions. Aortic disease moves cranially with progressive involvement of side branches. Therefore, it is not infrequent that very large aneurysms have signs of disease affecting the renal and mesenteric arteries, or the aorta in the chest. In the case of chronic TAAA dissections, the best landing zone is a prior surgical graft or stent graft, when available.

CLF studies provide the greatest amount of information when carefully assessing the aorta. The area of aortic dilatation can be readily identified, compared with adjacent segments, and evaluated for specific vessel involvement. Selection of a healthy proximal and distal sealing zone is the single most important aspect of proper planning to achieve a successful and durable repair. The proximal and distal landing zones must be selected in "normal aortic segments", defined by parallel aortic wall, with minimal or no thrombus or calcification. A minimum length of >2.5 cm is used, although longer lengths are preferred and for chronic TAAA dissections this is usually achieved in prior surgical grafts or stent grafts. Areas that are conic, calcified or thrombus-laden are not considered suitable necks and instead are regarded as part of the aneurysm itself. Longer lengths are needed in tortuous segments, such as in the aortic arch, in patients with familial history of aortic disease, ectasia or thrombus-laden aorta. Because it is critical to assure 360-degree apposition between the stent-graft fabric and aortic wall, the requirement of healthy sealing zone should never be compromised with the idea of planning an "easier" procedure.

Access site

Because chronic TAAA dissections typically have relatively narrow true lumen diameter, the ability to catheterize vessels is more challenging. These patients also often have arch involvement of prior arch repair with elephant trunk technique. Therefore, endovascular repair nearly always requires access via both iliofemoral arteries and one of the brachial arteries. Brachial access is needed when directional down-going branches are used or when fenestrations are planned with preloaded catheters that are intended to be accessed from above. One of the advantages of using brachial access is the ability to perform a staggered partial deployment of the TAAA stent graft, which facilitates catheterization of branches from above. An adequate CTA study should image the iliac arteries and the common femoral artery bifurcation. In patients with chronic dissections, it is critical to evaluate patency of the internal iliac arteries and its involvement by dissection. Patients with small iliac artery diameter, severe calcification, stenosis or occlusion, excessive tortuosity or dissection may need iliofemoral conduits. In these patients, the author preference is to plan a staged conduit whenever possible.

Selection of which side to introduce the main device is dependent upon on a number of factors. These include iliac artery diameter, occlusive disease, tortuosity, prior stents or surgical grafts, and most importantly, the ability to gain access to the true lumen of the dissection. For most operators who are right handed, we favor using the right iliofemoral access for catheterization of the renal branch vessels, whereas the main aortic device is introduced via the left iliofemoral access. If preloaded renal guides are used, then the device is introduced via the right femoral access. For brachial access, most operators select the left side to avoid the arch, but working from the right brachial access is easier and less cumbersome, and may be needed depending on arch anatomy or prior arch repair with elephant trunk technique. Several centers are moving towards routine right brachial artery access.

27.2.3 Device design

Current techniques rely on measurements of lengths and diameters using computed tomography angiography (CTA) and centerline of flow (CLF) analysis. Selection of specific stent design (Fig. 27.2, fenestration vs. branch) and approach (brachial vs. femoral) takes into consideration the extent of aortic disease, location of sealing zones, diameter of the aortic lumen, diameter of true lumen, presence of a re-entrance site, vessel orientation, atherosclerotic debris and quality of access vessels. As a general rule, branches are preferred or ideally suitable to target vessels originating from large aortic lumen, whereas fenestrations were initially designed to

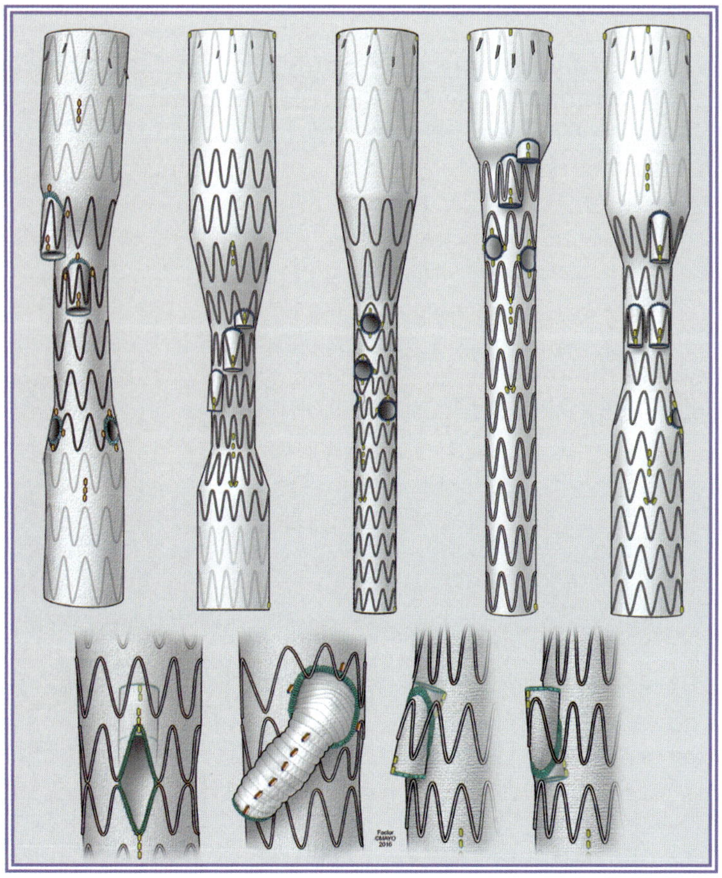

Fig. 27.2 Illustration of patient-specific thoracoabdominal stent-graft designs including combinations of fenestrations and directional branches with tapered segment to accommodate compressed true lumen. Directional branch design includes inner branches, helical branches and internal/external branches with down-going or up-going orientation (by permission of Mayo Foundation for Medical Education and Research. All rights reserved).

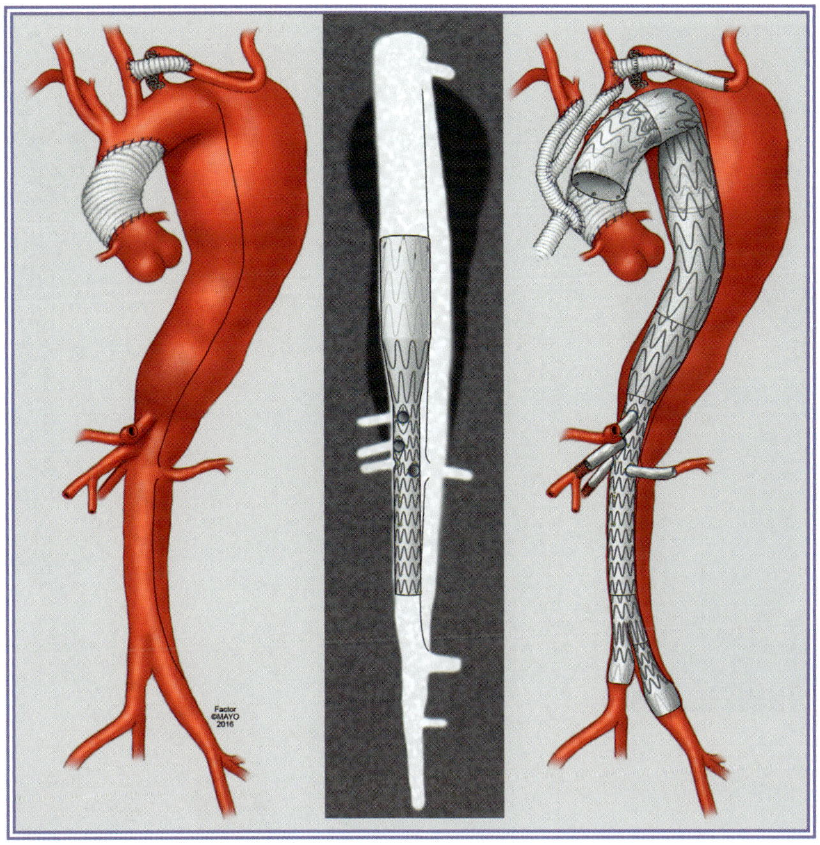

Fig. 27.3 Illustration based on a patient with extensive DeBakey I dissection and history of prior ascending aortic repair. In this case, the visceral arteries were incorporated using a fenestrated thoracoabdominal stent graft with narrow segment (by permission of Mayo Foundation for Medical Education and Research. All rights reserved).

incorporate vessels that originate from narrow aortic segments (Fig. 27.3). As such, for chronic dissections with narrow aortic lumen, fenestrations are often selected from a relatively narrow aortic component (18 to 22 mm). Perhaps one exception is a target vessel that is isolated within the false lumen. In these cases, placement of a fenestration implies that a re-entrance device would be needed to perforate the chronic septum and re-entry the false lumen. If the septum is thickened or partially thrombosed, this may be difficult or impossible (Fig. 27.4). A directional branch with origin from remote location (above or below the target) may be ideal. More recently, Marcelo Ferreira from Brazil has used internal branches with diamond-shaped fenestrations to target vessels in patients with chronic TAAA dissections.

Fenestrations versus branches

Once the sealing zone has been selected based on normal aorta, the next step in the planning is to identify which vessels need incorporation and which specific type of incorporation (fenestration vs. directional branch) will be used. There are three types of fenestrations that can be manufactured: small, large and scallop fenestrations. Small fenestrations have dimensions of 6×6 mm or 6×8 mm, do not have struts crossing the middle of the fenestration and are reinforced by a nitinol ring. Large fenestrations have dimensions of 8, 10 or 12 mm in diameter and may have stent struts crossing the edge or middle of the fenestration, which limits placement of alignment stents. Scallops are openings in the upper edge of the fabric, and are sized as single (10 mm), double (20 mm) or triple (30 mm) wide, with height ranging from 6 to 20 mm in dimension. If a fenestration is selected, the author uses 6×6 mm fenestrations for

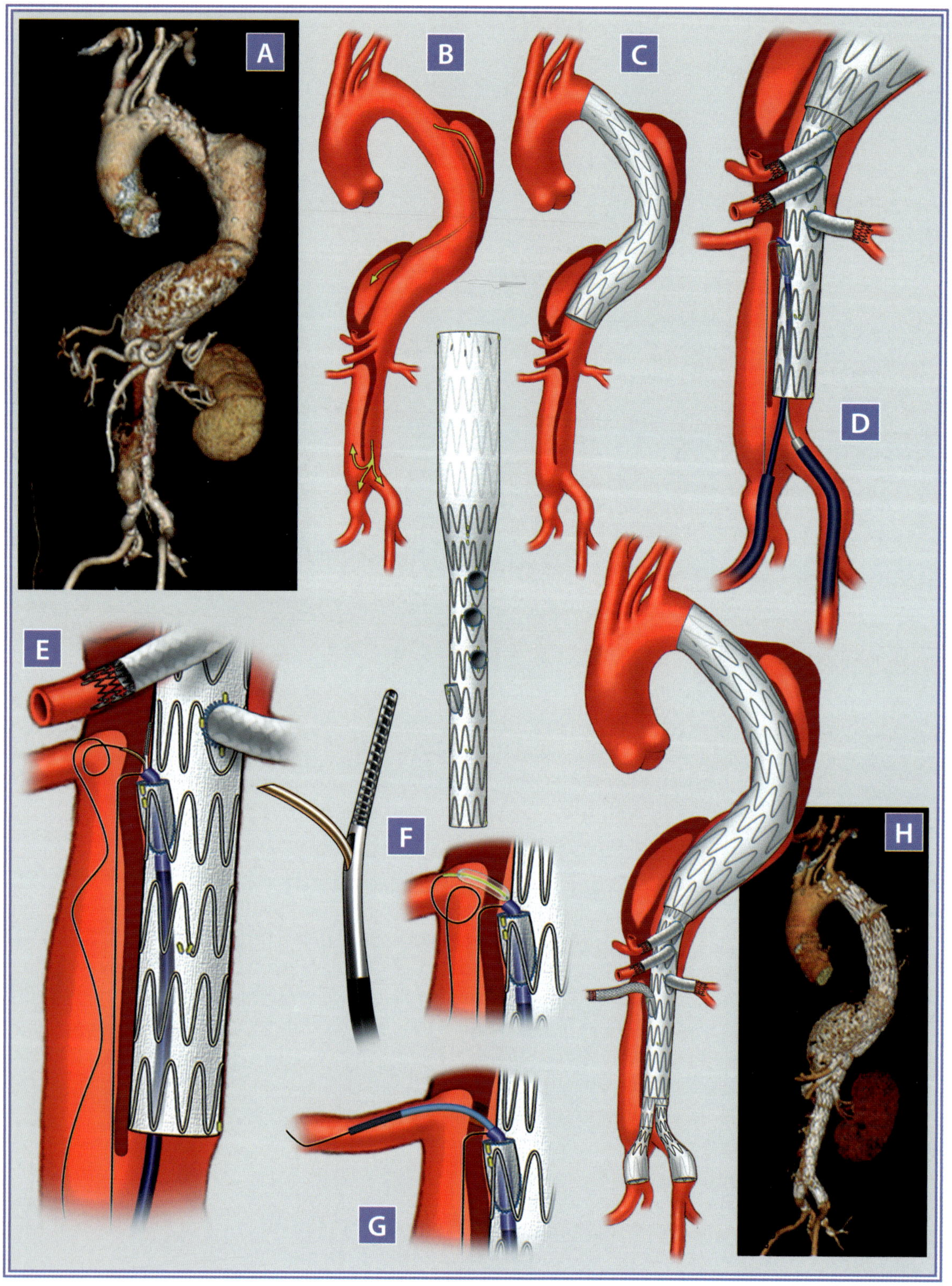

Fig. 27.4 Computed tomography angiography (CTA) of a patient with DeBakey IIIb dissection (**A**). Note that the right renal artery was perfused via the false lumen with re-entrance in the distal abdominal aorta and thickened septum (**B**). Endovascular repair was done using staged TEVAR (**C**), followed by placement of a thoracoabdominal device with three fenestrations and a retrograde branch (**D**). The retrograde branch was accessed via femoral access, allowing use of a reentrance device (**E**) to perforate the septum. The septum fenestration was enlarged using angioplasty balloon (**F**), allowing catheterization of the right renal artery (**G**). The completed repair (**H**) is shown in follow-up CTA (by permission of Mayo Foundation for Medical Education and Research. All rights reserved).

renal arteries and 8×8 mm fenestrations for SMA. In addition, 10×10 mm access scallops may be added for stents designed with preloaded catheters. Directional branches are either 6 or 8 mm in diameter and 18 or 22 mm in length. Branches can be internal, external, down-going or up-going, and can be coupled with diamond-shaped fenestrations to facilitate branch vessel catheterization in narrower aortic segments. As a general rule, if branches are selected, 6 mm branches are used for renal arteries and 8 mm branches for the celiac and SMA.

Fenestrations are selected preferentially for vessels that originate from relatively narrow aortic diameters (<30 mm), which is often the case in patients with narrow true lumen. This is the most frequent type of incorporation in patients with chronic TAAA dissections, although some patients are suited for directional branches. Because patency of renal fenestrations is excellent beyond 5 years with only few occlusions (<3 to 5%), these are particular attractive in patients who have significant chronic kidney disease or a single kidney. Fenestrations are also ideally suited for transversely oriented or up-going vessels.

Branches are preferred in patients who have larger aortic diameters (>30 mm). These have several advantages over fenestrated grafts, notably easier implantation, better alignment with longitudinally oriented or tortuous vessels (e.g. celiac, SMA, down-going renal arteries). However, because branches originate from a narrow segment of graft (with exception of new internal branches with diamond-shaped fenestrations), the repair is often extended higher into the thoracic aorta where the sealing stents are located. This is usually not an issue with chronic dissections, which often require coverage of nearly all thoracic aorta. Ideally, branches should be positioned with the distal edge 1.5 to 2 cm above its intended target vessel to facilitate catheterization (Fig. 27.5). If the vessel has particularly difficult anatomy due to occlusive disease, angulation or tortuosity, longer distances are recommended. Nonetheless, exceedingly long branches (>10 cm) are avoided whenever possible.

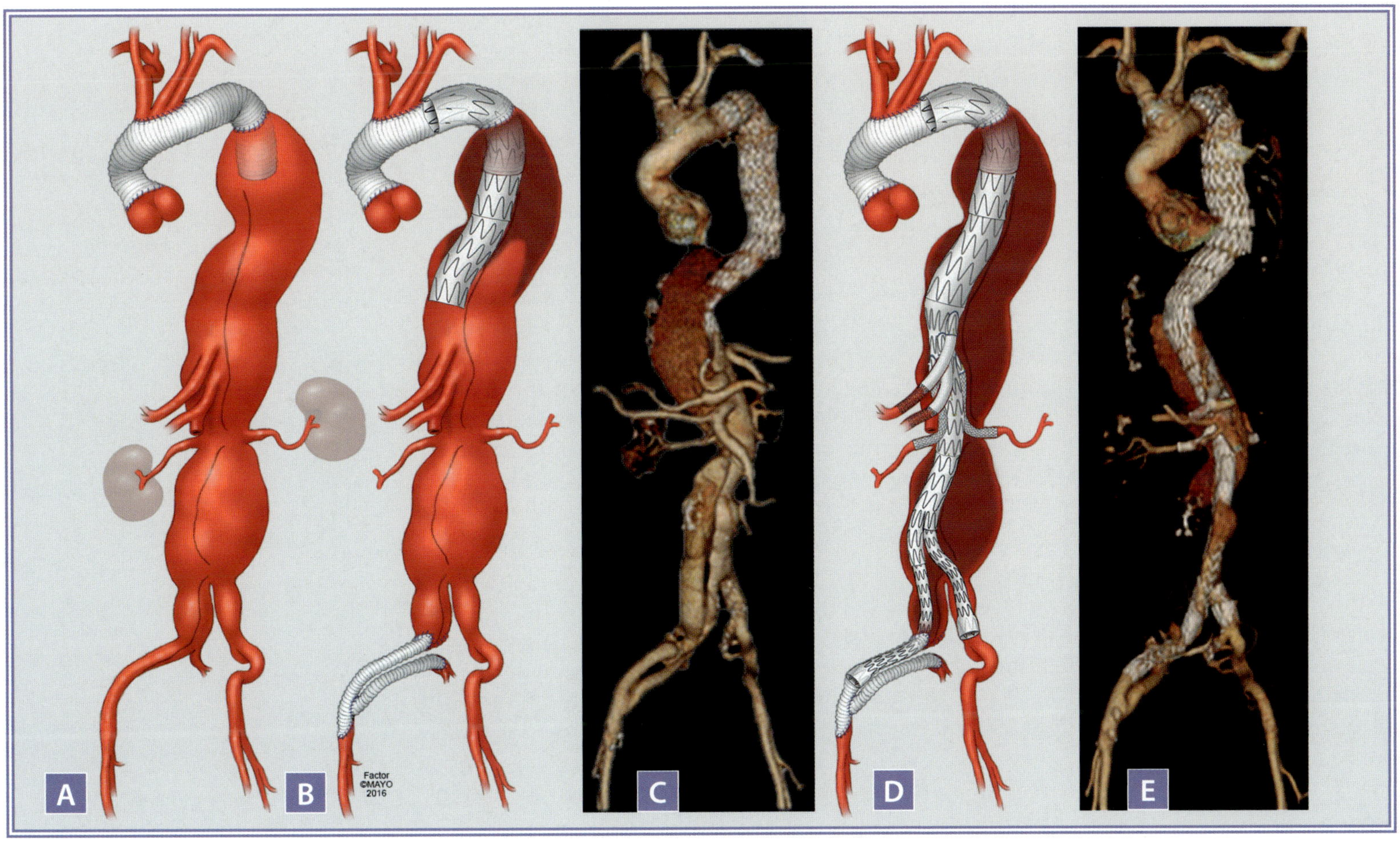

Fig. 27.5 Illustration of a patient treated by elephant trunk procedure (**A**) for extensive thoracoabdominal dissection. The patient was treated in a staged fashion (**B**) with coverage of the proximal thoracic aorta and surgical revascularization of the right internal iliac artery. Computed tomography angiography (CTA) shows thrombosis of the false lumen adjacent to the thoracic stent (**C**). A completion endovascular repair was performed using 4-vessel multibranched stent graft (**D**) with exclusion of the aneurysm and presence of persistent endoleak (**E**) (by permission of Mayo Foundation for Medical Education and Research. All rights reserved).

Graft taper

A feature of patient-specific grafts that can be used to facilitate repair is a tapered graft diameter to facilitate branch vessel catheterization. This is routinely used with branched grafts and is universally adopted by off-the-shelf designs. Traditionally, the taper is placed below the renal arteries and the fenestrations have been based on wider graft diameters to promote apposition between the graft fabric and the aortic wall. In the case of chronic dissections, fenestrations may be needed in a relatively narrow graft diameter (18 to 22 mm).

Adjuncts

Implantation of fenestrated and branched endografts can be a technically demanding procedure, particularly in patients with chronic TAAA dissections. Therefore limiting the number of steps that are needed to complete placement of bridging stents is a priority. This can be done by dividing the procedure between the femoral and brachial segments, and using preloaded systems for each of these. From the brachial approach, preloaded catheters (Fig. 27.6) into the celiac and SMA are added and routed internally to exit via an access scallop placed in the top edge of the graft, or via the top of the graft if there is not an uncovered stent. For the renal arteries, preloaded guidewires allow advancement of guide-catheter sheaths via the delivery system. However, these are long (90 to 110 cm) 6-Fr guide sheaths depending on specific design of the delivery system. Although the need to catheterize the renal fenestrations is eliminated, vessel catheterization and exchanges are made more difficult compared to using a shorter 7-Fr sheath from the femoral approach. For the novel TAMBE (W.L. Gore & Associates, Flagstaff, AZ) stent and the novel Cook Medical (Bloomington, IN) delivery systems, all four vessels can be preloaded with guidewires that are immediately accessible from the brachial approach.

27.2.4 Strategies to prevent spinal cord injury

A standardized protocol to reduce risk of spinal cord injury is applied in all patients undergoing endovascular TAAA repair (Fig. 27.7) [7]. Procedures are performed by a dedicated endovascular team under total intravenous general endotracheal anesthesia using fixed imaging in a hybrid endovascular room. The anesthetic management consists of propofol and fentanyl or sufentanil infusion at the discretion of the anesthesiologist with avoidance of non-depolarizing muscle relaxants. Succinylcholine is used as the muscle relaxant of choice for induction of anesthesia. A predefined standardized protocol was used to prevent spinal cord ischemia (SCI) .

Staged repairs

Staging the repair is recommended whenever possible for all extent I and II TAAAs, and is used selectively for extent III TAAAs (Fig. 27.8). These procedures are typically done at least one week a part. More often there is a 4-6 weeks wait period because of delay in manufacturing patient-specific devices. As part of the staged repair, any cervical debranching or permanent ilio-femoral conduit is done if needed. The proximal sealing zone is selected in the healthy aortic segment in the distal arch (zones 1 to 3) or proximal thoracic aorta (zone 4 or 5). Sealing can also be achieved in a prosthetic graft in patients with prior arch replacement using elephant trunk technique. The author preference is to taper the thoracic graft to a diameter of 30 mm just above the celiac axis, leaving a large distal Ib endoleak at the initial procedure. The distal graft diameter of the proximal thoracic graft should be ideally 30 mm so that the branched graft can be designed with a diameter of 34 mm to sit inside the previously placed graft. Bell-bottom thoracic grafts that flare to 46 or 48 mm have been designed to avoid the distal type Ib endoleak, which is expected and routine with first stage repairs.

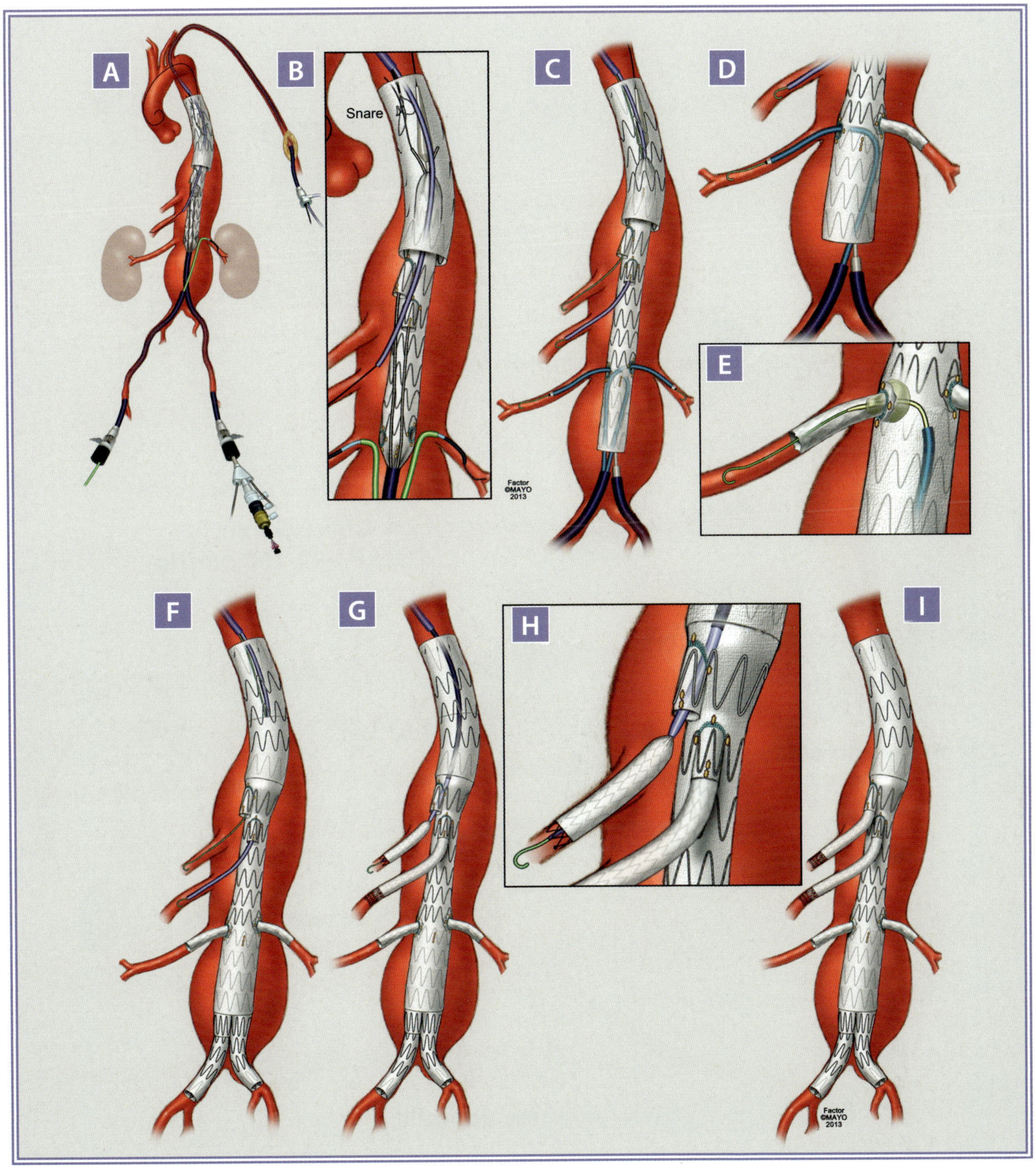

Fig. 27.6 A two branch-two fenestration stent-graft design has been used to treat chronic thoracoabdominal dissections. The procedure is performed usually using bilateral femoral and left brachial approach. A proximal thoracic component is deployed first if needed (**A**). Precatheterization of at least one of the renal arteries is used to locate the target vessels using on-lay computed tomography. The branched component is deployed up to the level of the renal fenestrations (**A**). Using preloaded catheters, guidewires are snared from the brachial approach (**B**), and the celiac axis and superior mesenteric artery (SMA) are catheterized from above. A sheath is typically placed into the SMA (**C**). The device is unsheathed completely (**C**) and the renal fenestrations and renal arteries are catheterized from the femoral approach. Hydrophilic sheaths are advanced into both renal arteries over 0.035-inch Rosen guidewires (**C**). Sequential renal artery stenting is performed using balloon-expandable covered stents (**D**), which are flared using a 10-mm angioplasty balloon (**E**). The bifurcated component and iliac limbs are deployed after placement of the renal stents (**F**). Flow is restored into both lower limbs. The procedure is completed by placement of the SMA and celiac self-expandable stents (**G**). Note that each stent is extended distally with a bare metal self-expandable stent (**H**). Final illustration depicts complete repair (**I**) (by permission of Mayo Foundation for Medical Education and Research. All rights reserved).

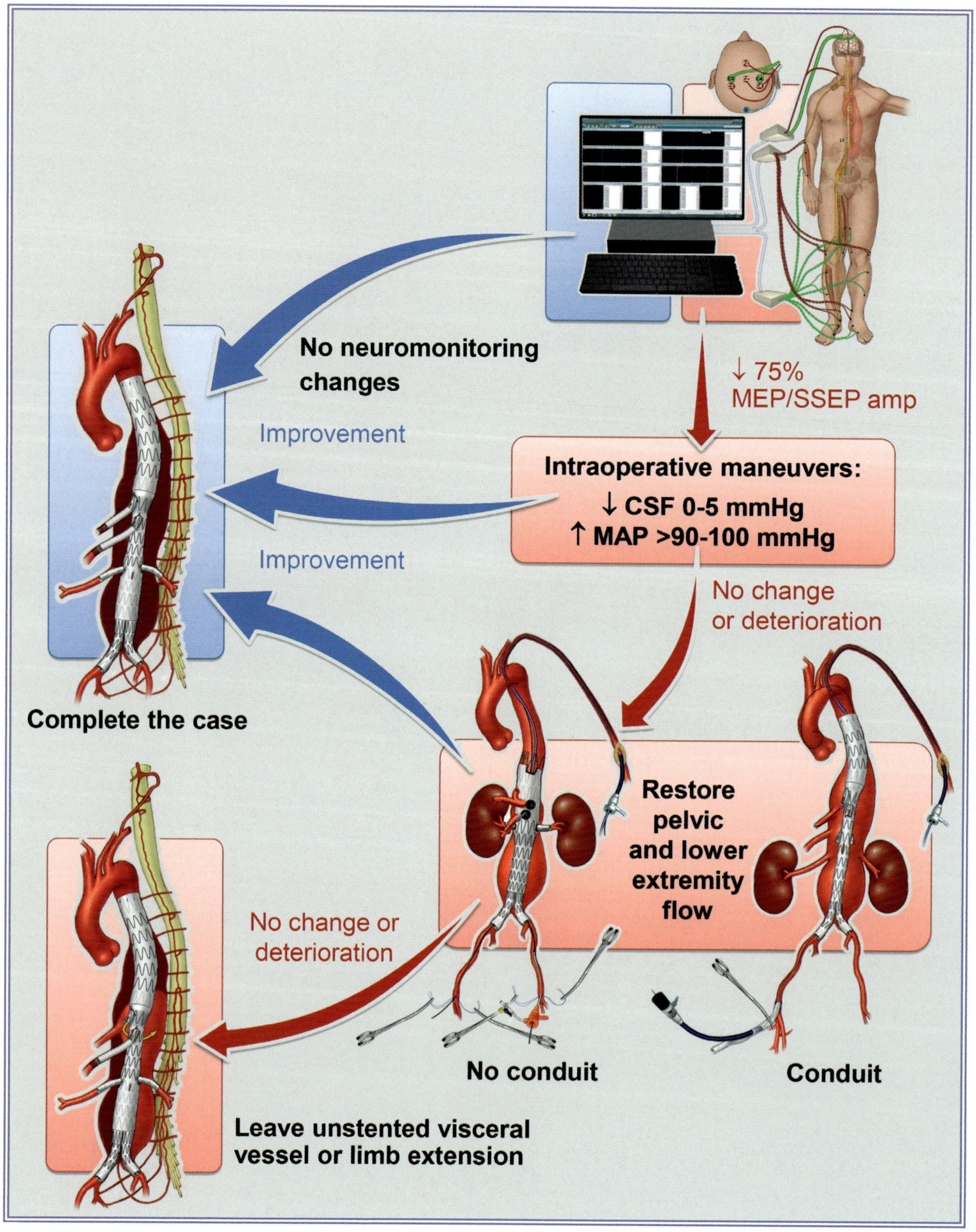

Fig. 27.7 Standardized protocol uses neuromonitoring and standardized maneuvers during thoracoabdominal endovascular repair. For patients with no changes in neuromonitoring, the procedure is completed in standard fashion. Patients with decline in motor evoked potential/somatosensory evoked potential (MEP/SSEP) potentials have intra-operative maneuvers including decrease of cerebrospinal fluid (CSF) pressure to 0-5 mmHg and increase in mean arterial pressure (MAP) goals to 90-100 mmHg. If the changes resolve the procedure is completed. If not, flow is restored to the lower extremities before the aneurysm sac is closed. In patients with reversible MEP changes, the procedure is completed. However, if the changes persist, the sac is left open by either unstented celiac branch or contra-lateral iliac limb.

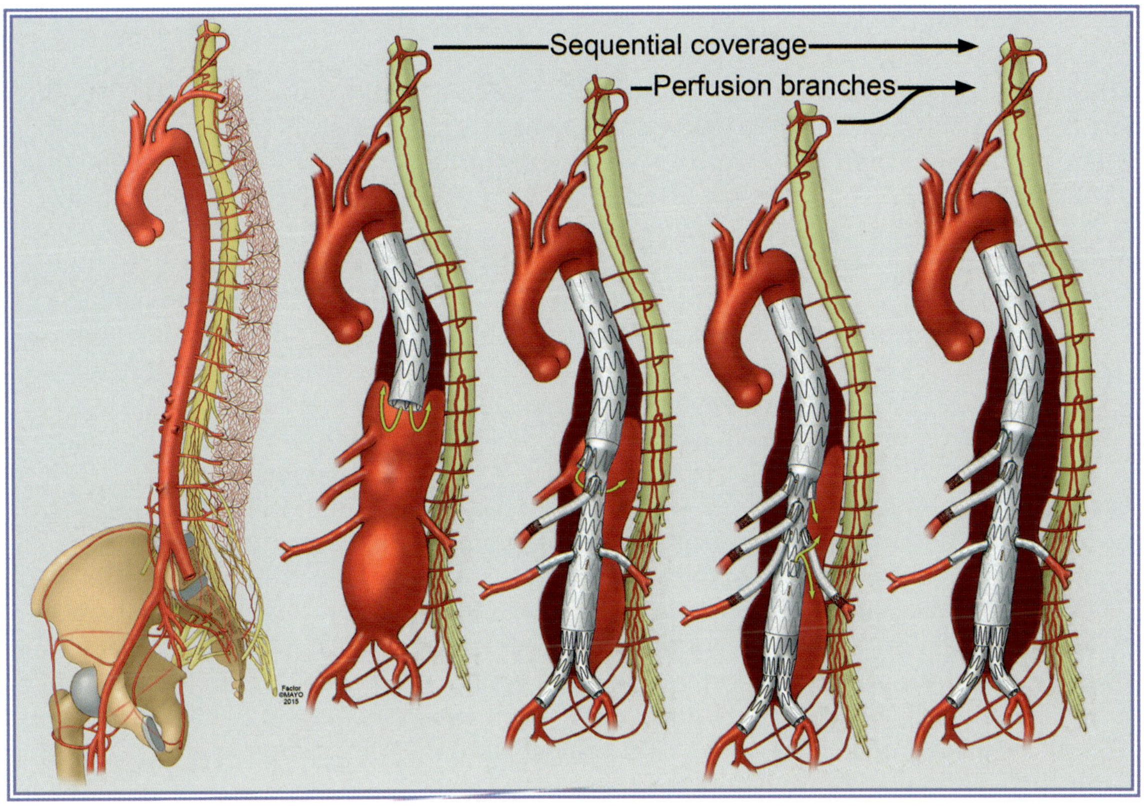

Fig. 27.8 Optimization of the extensive spine collateral network including vertebral, intercostal, lumbar and hypogastric arteries forms the basis for staged endovascular repair of complex aneurysms. Strategies include coverage of the proximal thoracic aorta up to the celiac axis, followed by visceral branch stenting in a second stage. Alternatively the sac can be perfused via perfusion branches or unstented celiac axis or contra-lateral iliac limb (by permission of Mayo Foundation for Medical Education and Research. All rights reserved).

Blood pressure management

Calcium channel blockers and angiotensin-inhibitors are discontinued a week prior to the operation and up to 4-6 weeks after the procedure unless systolic blood pressures are >160 mmHg. Exceptions are patients with severe ischemic heart disease or compensated congestive heart failure, where medications are maintained.

The goal mean arterial pressure (MAP) is targeted at ≥80 mmHg intraoperatively and for the first 72 hours after the operation. Blood pressure goals are titrated according to intraoperative neuromonitoring or postoperative examination. If there are changes in neuromonitoring detected during the operation or neurological changes observed on postoperative physical examination, MAP goals are incrementally raised up to 100 mmHg. In addition, transfusion of blood products is indicated in the first 48 hours after the procedure to keep a target hemoglobin ≥10 mg/dL and normal coagulation profile prior to removal of the spinal drain.

Cerebrospinal fluid drainage

Routine cerebrospinal fluid (CSF) drainage is used in all patients. Spinal fluid pressure is set at a baseline of 10 mmHg. The spinal drain is opened for 15 minutes every hour with a maximum drainage of 20 mL per hour, after which the drain is clamped for the remaining of the hour. A maximum of 150 mL of drainage is accepted for 24 hours. If there are changes in neuromonitoring or neurological exam, CSF pressure is decreased to 5 or 0 mmHg. CSF pressure is raised to 10 mmHg once neuromonitoring or exam improved. Spinal fluid drainage is continued for 24 hours in patients with extent type IV TAAA, and for 48-72 hours in those with extent type I-III TAAAs. The CSF drain is removed in patients who had stable hemodynamics and neurological exam after a 6-hour clamping trial.

Neuromonitoring

Neuromonitoring with continuous motor evoked potential (MEP) and somatosensory evoked potential (SSEP) has been widely applied during open TAAA repair to guide reimplantation of intercostal arteries and to optimize distal aortic perfusion. In contrast to open repair, endovascular incorporation of intercostal arteries is not feasible. Nonetheless, immediate recognition of ischemia using neuromonitoring may allow introduction of maneuvers to optimize spinal cord and lower extremity (LE) perfusion and decrease the rate of SCI. Total intravenous anesthesia is used to allow intraoperative neurophysiological monitoring of MEP and SSEPs. A ≥75% reduction from baseline evoked potential amplitude was considered to be significant. Cadwell Elite machines and Cascade software were used to collect data (Cadwell Industries, Kennewick, WA) by electromyography (EMG) technologists. Electrical charges sent to the motor cortex through C3, C4 scalp electrodes evoke MEP through the motor pathway which are recorded down the cord over multiple muscles in the upper and lower extremities for at least every 10-15 minutes. An upper extremity muscle (extensor digitorum communis) is recorded to help differentiate neurogenic impairment such as spinal and lower limb ischemia from non-specific changes. Bilateral lower extremity muscles are recorded using subdermal EEG electrodes placed in the hamstring, tibialis anterior, and abductor hallucis muscles. In addition, SSEPs consisting of electrical stimulus generated at the ulnar or tibial nerve that travels from the distal extremity were recorded over the neck and scalp. In patients where the lower extremity tibial SSEP are not present at the ankle, subdermal EEG electrodes can be positioned behind the knee. In addition, a compound muscle action potential (CMAP) is performed by stimulating the peroneal nerve and posterior tibialis nerve. The CMAP is important to help differentiate peripheral nerve and spinal cord ischemia.

Limb perfusion

Large transfemoral sheaths are associated with limb and pelvic ischemia (Fig. 27.9A), which may aggravate spinal cord ischemia because of compromised collateral networks. Increasing evidence indicates that minimizing lower limb and pelvic ischemia may improve outcomes of complex endovascular repair including lower risk of paraplegia. This can be done by several adjunctive measures. The superficial femoral artery may be accessed using a small sheath (Fig. 27.9B), which can be connected into the larger transfemoral sheath creating a shunt. However, this technique can be cumbersome and also does not address the occlusion of the internal iliac and profunda femoris arteries, which are the main collateral networks to the spine. Our preference has been to use a temporary iliac artery conduit in patients with small iliac arteries, severe occlusive disease of the aorto-iliac arteries or when technical challenge with prolonged (>2 hours) ischemia time is anticipated. A femoral conduit anastomosed end-to-side to the common femoral artery (Fig. 27.9C) to allow restoration of lower extremity flow. The use of femoral conduit minimizes lower extremity ischemia during visceral branch stenting by allowing the aortic device sheath to be retracted into the conduit. More frequently, we prefer to use total percutaneous femoral approach whenever the common femoral arteries are not calcified and a straightforward case is anticipated. In these cases, the aortic device, renal fenestrated-branches, bifurcated device and iliac limbs are performed using the femoral approach first. Flow is restored into both lower extremities (<2 hours) and the procedure is completed via the left arm by placement of the superior mesenteric and celiac artery stents.

Intraoperative maneuvers

Our protocol uses neuromonitoring to trigger intraoperative maneuvers to optimize spinal cord perfusion. A decrease in MEP/SSEPs triggers introduction of sequential standardized maneuvers as depicted in figure 27.7. These maneuvers include incremental changes in MAP and

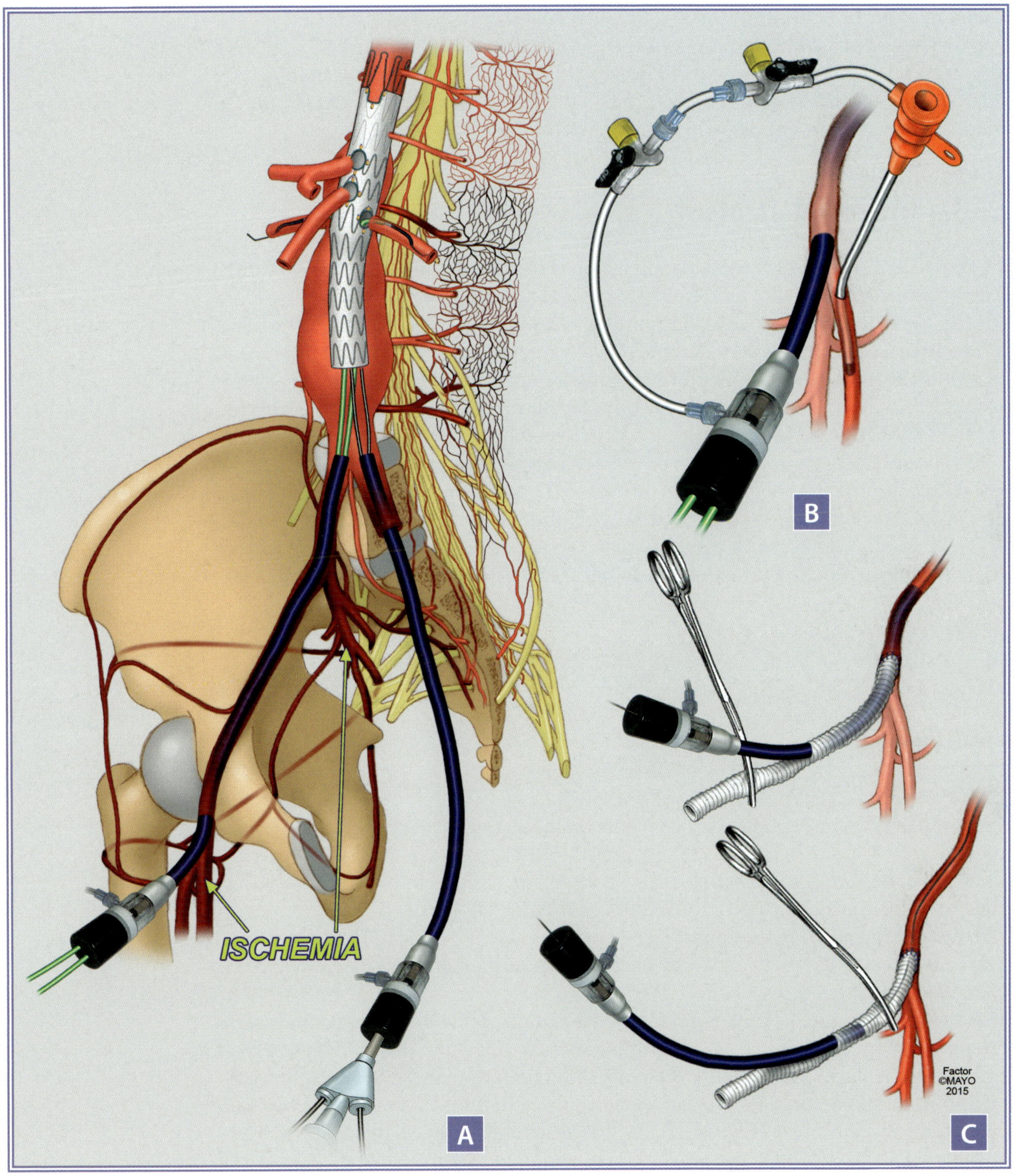

Fig. 27.9 Mechanism of pelvic and lower extremity ischemia due to large transfemoral sheaths (**A**). Use of superficial femoral artery sheath (**B**) and femoral conduits (**C**) to minimize leg ischemia (by permission of Mayo Foundation for Medical Education and Research. All rights reserved).

CSF pressure as previously described. The MAP goals are raised from 80 mmHg up to 100 mmHg with norepinephrine and/or vasopressin infusion along with simultaneous decrease in CSF drain pressure from 10 mmHg to 5 or 0 mmHg. Response to these maneuvers is recorded and the MAP and CSF pressure parameters are readjusted accordingly. In patients with improvement after maneuvers, the procedure is completed in standard fashion. In those with no change or deterioration in neuromonitoring, flow is restored to the pelvis and LEs as fast as possible by changing the sequence of target vessel stenting as depicted in figure 27.7. In patients with normalization of MEP/SSEPs after LE flow is restored, the procedure is completed. If changes persist, the procedure is left incomplete with flow into the sac via the celiac branch or contra-lateral iliac limb whenever possible.

27.3 Postoperative management

Postoperatively, all patients are closely monitored in a closed cardiovascular intensive care unit by a dedicated critical care team. Spinal fluid pressure is set at a baseline of 10 mmHg as previously described. The spinal drain is opened for 15 minutes every hour with a maximum drainage of 20 mL per hour, after which the drain is clamped for the remaining of the hour. Similar adjunctive maneuvers are utilized in the postoperative setting if neurological changes are observed on physical examination. MAP goals are incrementally raised up to 100 mmHg. In addition, transfusion of blood products is performed to keep a target hemoglobin ≥10 mg/dL and normal coagulation profile should the need to reposition or replace a spinal drain be required. CSF pressure is decreased to 5 or 0 mmHg. CSF pressure is raised to 10 mmHg once neuromonitoring or exam improves. Spinal fluid drainage is continued for 24 hours in patients with extent type IV TAAA, and for 48-72 hours in those with extent type I-III TAAAs. The CSF drain is removed in patients who had stable hemodynamics and neurological exam after a 6-hour clamping trial.

27.4 Case scenarios

27.4.1 Large true lumen

Patient with extensive DeBakey I chronic dissection with extent II TAAA on chronic hemodialysis and prior total arch replacement with elephant trunk technique (see Fig. 27.5A). The dissection extended across the origin of the right internal iliac artery, which originated primarily from the false lumen. A first stage procedure was performed using proximal thoracic stent grafts from the elephant trunk to just above the celiac axis (see Fig. 27.5B, C). The right external iliac artery was replaced by iliofemoral graft, with revascularization of the right internal iliac artery. A second stage procedure was performed using off-the-shelf multi-branch stent graft (see Fig. 27.5D, E).

In this case, we elected to place self-expandable stents in both renal arteries, even though the patient was on permanent dialysis. An alternative, which was considered, would be to extent the renal cuffs with stents and occlude the cuffs and renal arteries with plugs. The patient evolved without complications. Follow-up imaging demonstrated a complex endoleak from the SMA and left renal branch (Fig. 27.10A). This was treated by exclusion of the left renal branch using plugs (Fig. 27.10B). The SMA, which was 14 mm diameter and had a large replaced hepatic artery (Fig. 27.10C), was treated by bifurcated parallel stent-graft technique (Fig. 27.10F). A Gore® Viabahn® (W.L. Gore & Associated, Flagstaff, AZ) stent graft was placed in the replaced hepatic artery (Fig. 27.10D) and one in the distal SMA (Fig. 27.10E). Repeat computed tomography angiography showed resolution of the endoleak (Fig. 27.10G).

27.4.2 Narrow true lumen

Patient referred for treatment of enlarging TAAA following a first stage procedure with hemiarch replacement and proximal thoracic stent graft. There was persistent type a endoleak fol-

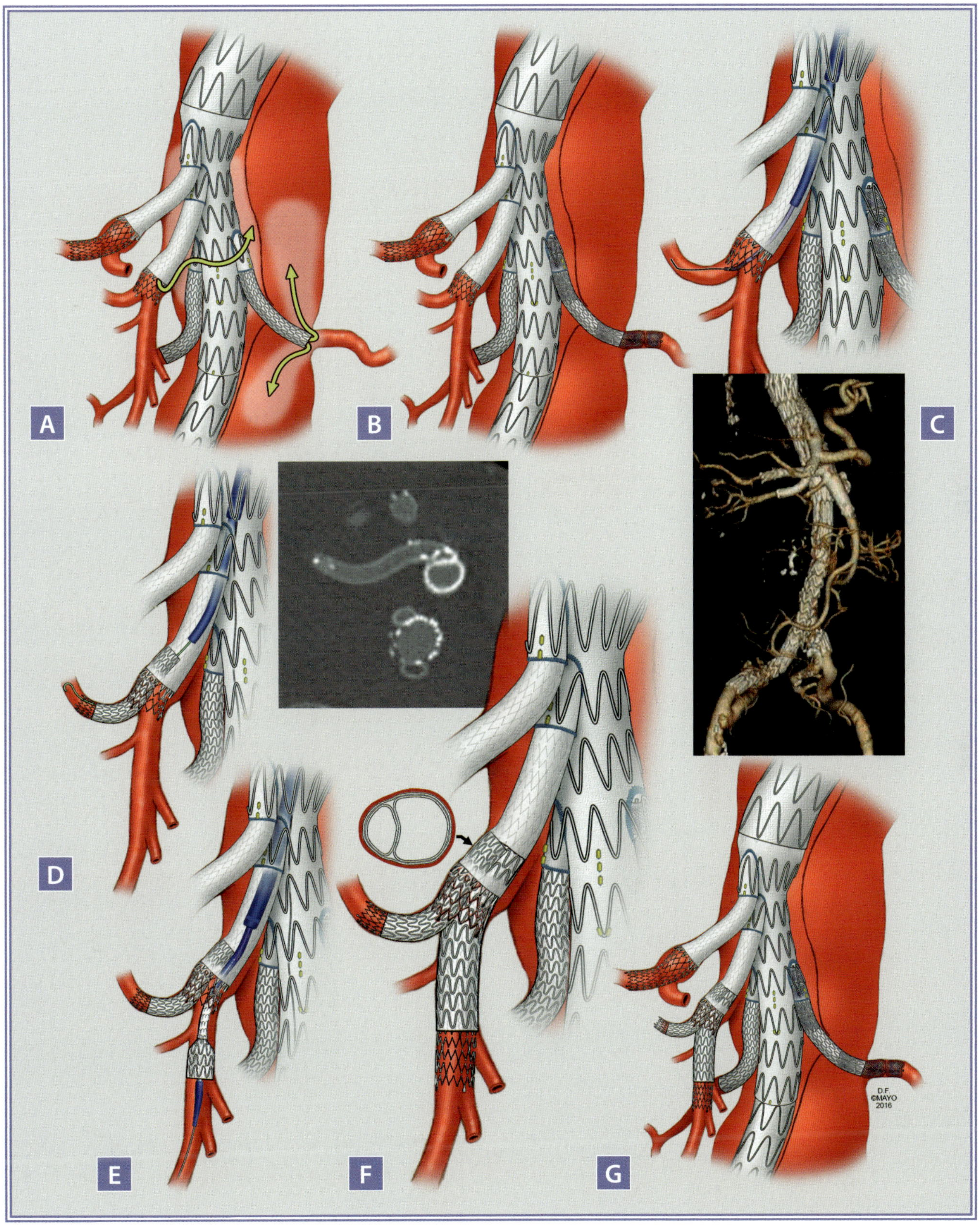

Fig. 27.10 Technique of treatment of multiple endoleaks in a patient on chronic hemodialysis who underwent branched thoracoabdominal repair (**A**). The left renal branch was excluded with Amplatzer plugs (**B**) and the SMA (superior mesenteric artery) branch was extended using parallel technique. After catheterization of a large hepatic artery (**C**), the repair was extended distally using a Gore® Viabahn® into the replaced hepatic artery (**D**) and one into the distal SMA (**E**). Note the parallel stent configuration (**F**) and resolution of the endoleak (**G**) (by permission of Mayo Foundation for Medical Education and Research. All rights reserved).

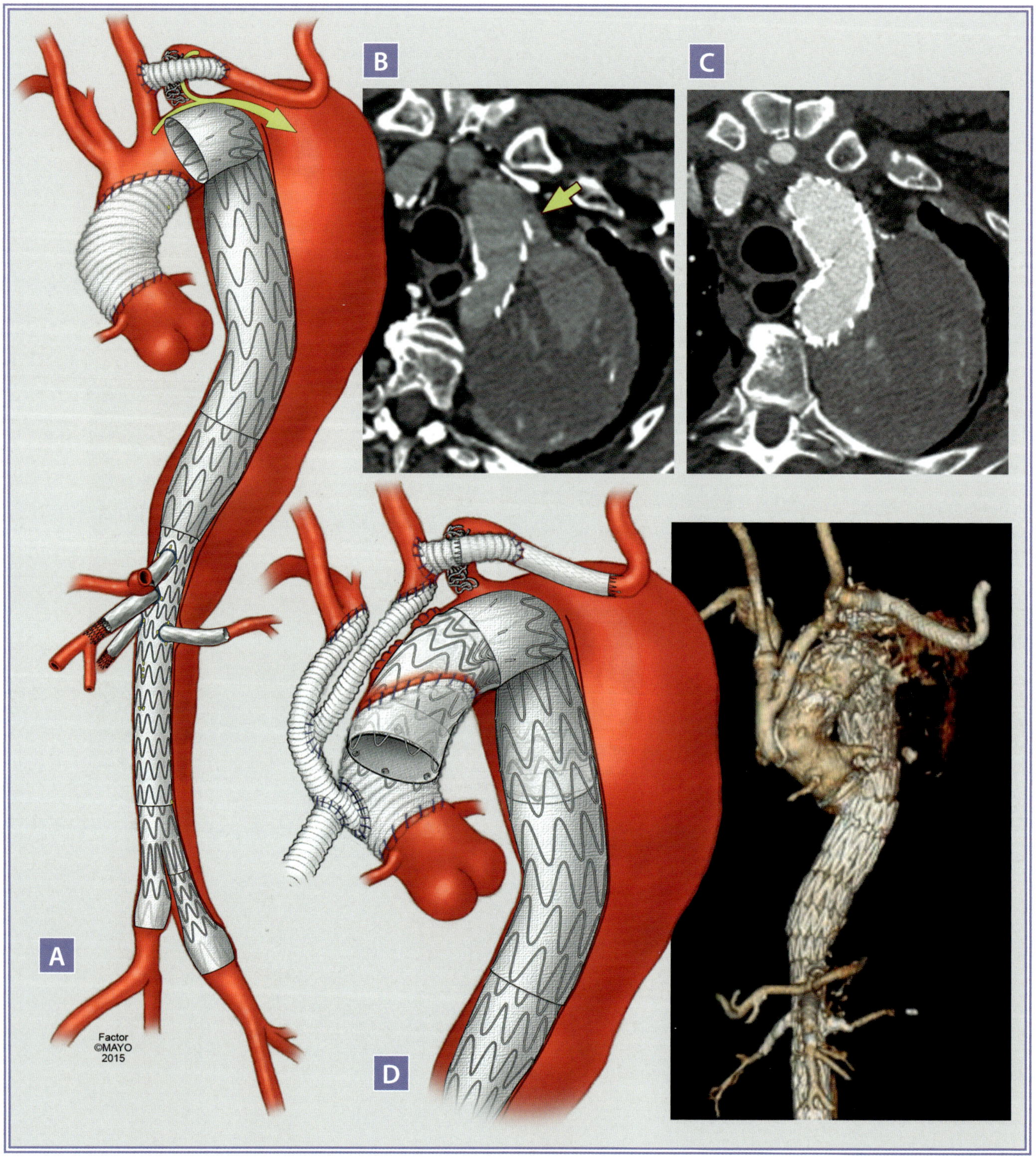

Fig. 27.11 Patient treated for chronic aortic dissection with a proximal type Ia endoleak in the thoracic stent (**A**). Note the axial view of computed tomography angiography depicts lack of apposition between the stent graft and aortic wall, indicative of type Ia endoleak (**B**, arrow). The patient was treated by aortic arch debranching procedure (**D**), with resolution of the proximal endoleak (by permission of Mayo Foundation for Medical Education and Research. All rights reserved).

lowing the proximal thoracic stent graft, but access via the brachial arteries was deemed important because of small true lumen diameter. In this case, a graft was designed with four fenestrations originating from narrow graft diameter (see Fig. 27.3). Following the procedure, CTA demonstrated the proximal type Ia endoleak (Fig. 27.11A, B), which was then treated by median sternotomy and arch debranching with proximal arch stent-graft extension using conformable C-TAG stent graft. Repeat CTA revealed resolution of the type Ia endoleak (Fig. 27.11C, D).

27.4.3 Isolated false lumen vessel

Patient with DeBakey IIIb dissection (see Fig. 27.4A, B). Note that the right renal artery was perfused via the false lumen through a large re-entrance in the distal aorta. The chronic septum was thicken and filled with thrombus at the level of the right renal artery, which was considered difficult for using a re-entrance device. The patient was treated by first stage using proximal thoracic stent graft (see Fig. 27.4C). A device was designed with three fenestrations and a retrograde right renal branch. After placement of stents into the celiac, SMA and left renal artery using brachial approach, the retrograde branch was accessed from the femoral approach (see Fig. 27.4D). An outback re-entrance device was used (see Fig. 27.4E) to perforate the chronic septum in an area where the septum was relatively thin. The re-entrance was enlarged with angioplasty balloon (see Fig. 27.4F), followed by selective catheterization of the right renal artery (see Fig. 27.4G) and stenting (see Fig. 27.4H).

27.4.4 Ruptured aneurysm

Management of ruptured chronic dissections is specially challenging because of inability to stage the procedure, and need to expeditiously establish control of hemorrhage. In this case, the patient presented with ruptured of the thoracic aorta after thoracic endovascular repair three months prior in another institution (Fig. 27.12A, B). The false lumen was pressurized likely due to disruption of the chronic septum below the stent graft (Fig. 27.12C-E). In this case, parallel stent-graft technique was used with a "sandwich" stent into the SMA (Fig. 27.12F) and bilateral renal "periscope" stents (Fig. 27.12G). Repeat CTA reveals complete remodelling of the thoracic aorta (Fig. 27.12H).

27.5 Conclusion

Design of fenestrated and branched endografts continues to evolve. Repairs changed in the last decade with wider applications of fenestrated and branched endografts including patients with chronic dissections and TAAAs. New designs with preloaded catheters and guidewires facilitate the procedure. It is critical that physicians performing these procedures have understanding that aortic disease is progressive, and palliative treatment with aortic endografts needs to be planned to minimize late failures from type I endoleak or migration.

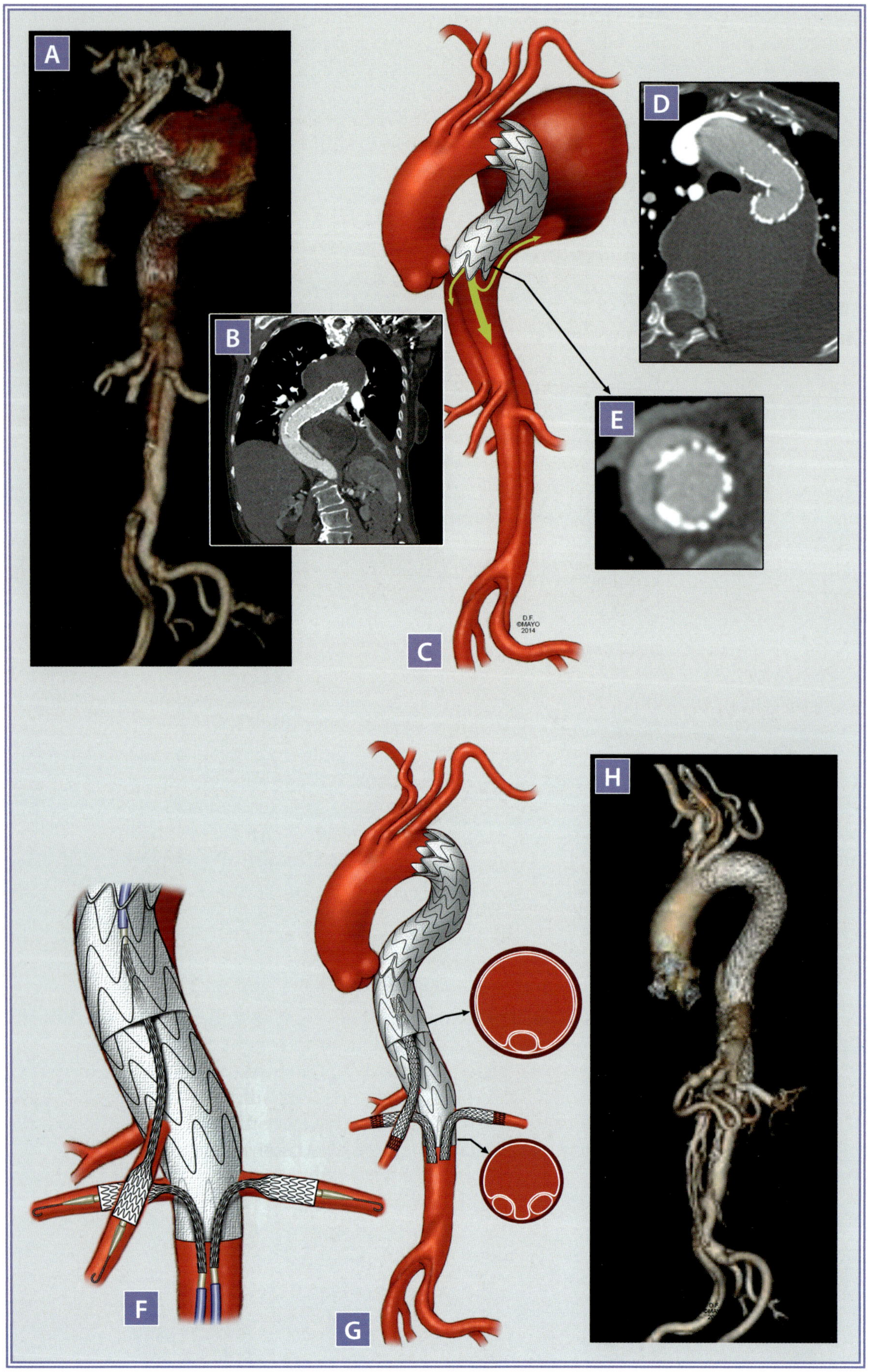

Fig. 27.12 Illustration of patient with complicated dissection (**A**, **B**) following TEVAR (**C**). Computed tomography showed contained rupture (**D**) and tear in the septum (**E**). The patient was treated by placement of sandwich stent graft to the superior mesenteric artery (**F**) and bilateral renal periscope stent grafts (**G**). Repeat computed tomography angiography revealed complete aortic remodelling (**H**) (by permission of Mayo Foundation for Medical Education and Research. All rights reserved).

REFERENCES

1) Oderich GS, Mendes BC, Correa MP. Preloaded guidewires to facilitate endovascular repair of thoracoabdominal aortic aneurysm using a physician-modified branched stent graft. J Vasc Surg 2014; 59(4): 1168-73.
2) Chuter TA, Gordon RL, Reilly LM, Goodman JD, Messina LM. An endovascular system for thoracoabdominal aortic aneurysm repair. J Endovasc Ther 2001; 8: 25-33.
3) Gasper WJ, Reilly LM, Rapp JH, et al. Assessing the anatomic applicability of the multibranched endovascular repair of thoracoabdominal aortic aneurysm technique. J Vasc Surg 2013; 57(6): 1553-8; discussion 1558.
4) Mastracci TM, Greenberg RK, Eagleton MJ, Hernandez AV. Durability of branches in branched and fenestrated endografts. J Vasc Surg 2013; 57(4): 926-33; discussion 933.
5) Verhoeven EL, Tielliu IF, Bos WT, Zeebregts CJ. Present and future of branched stent grafts in thoracoabdominal aortic aneurysm repair: a single-centre experience. Eur J Vasc Endovasc Surg 2009; 38(2): 155-61.
6) Greenberg RK, Lu Q, Roselli EE, et al. Contemporary analysis of descending thoracic and thoracoabdominal aneurysm repair: a comparison of endovascular and open techniques. Circulation 2008; 118(8): 808-17.
7) Banga P, Oderich GS, Reis de Souza L, et al. Neuromonitoring, cerebrospinal fluid drainage, and selective use of iliofemoral conduits to minimize risk of spinal cord injury during complex endovascular aortic repair. J Endovasc Ther 2016; 23: 139-49.
8) Etz CD, Zoli S, Mueller CS, et al. Staged repair significantly reduces paraplegia rate after extensive thoracoabdominal aortic aneurysm repair. J Thorac Cardiovasc Surg 2010; 139(6): 1464-72.
9) Eagleton MJ, Shah SK, Petkovsek D, Mastracci T, Greenberg RK. Collateral bed patency affects outcomes of spinal cord ischemia (SCI) following aortic endografting. J Vasc Surg 2013; 57(5): 28S-9S.
10) Sachs T, Pomposelli F, Hagberg R, et al. Open and endovascular repair of type B aortic dissection in the Nationwide Inpatient Sample. J Vasc Surg 2010; 52(4): 860-6; discussion 6.
11) Kitagawa A, Greenberg RK, Eagleton MJ, Mastracci TM, Roselli EE. Fenestrated and branched endovascular aortic repair for chronic type B aortic dissection with thoracoabdominal aneurysms. J Vasc Surg 2013; 58(3): 625-34.
12) Oikonomou K, Katsargyris A, Ritter W, Spinelli D, Seto Y, Verhoeven EL. Endovascular management of chronic post-dissection aneurysms. Ann Cardiothorac Surg 2014; 3(3): 307-13.
13) Faure EM, Canaud L, Agostini C, et al. Reintervention after thoracic endovascular aortic repair of complicated aortic dissection. J Vasc Surg 2014; 59(2): 327-33.
14) Nozdrzykowski M, Etz CD, Luehr M, et al. Optimal treatment for patients with chronic Stanford type B aortic dissection: endovascularly, surgically or both? Eur J Cardiothorac Surg 2013; 44(3): e165-74; discussion e74.

28

Chronic aortic dissection: how to deal with the false lumen in chronic aortic dissection

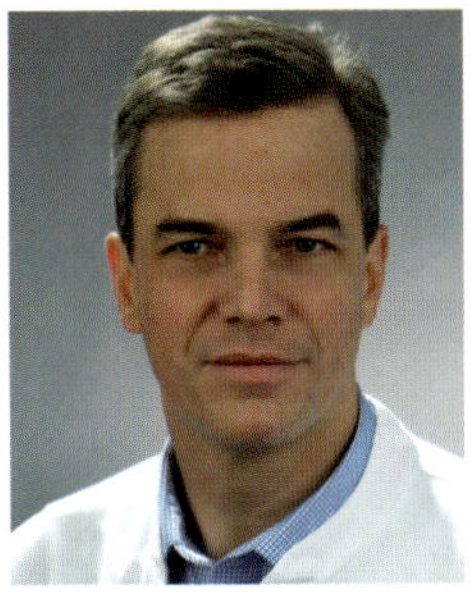

Tilo Kölbel and Fiona Rohlffs

28.1 Introduction

Chronic aortic dissection (AD) is a complex disease that requires individualized treatment concepts, as the pathology is associated with several features making standard Thoracic Endo-Vascular Aortic Repair (TEVAR) procedures barely sufficient. This is, on the one hand, due to the sparse remodelling capacity of the aortic tissue compared to earlier stages of the disease as the aortic wall and the dissection membrane is thickened and more rigid. On the other hand, coverage of the proximal entry tear is not enough to prevent false lumen perfusion, which counts as a main risk factor for the development of hazardous complications as aneurysm formation and death. Treatment strategies in chronic AD should specifically focus on the occlusion of the false lumen to reinforce aortic remodelling. In addition to open surgical treatment, novel endovascular techniques evolved to solve the problem of false lumen backflow. These techniques provide new options and strategies in chronic AD.

28.2 Classification of chronic aortic dissection

Aortic dissection is complex and it is not static but dynamic in time. The disease is divided into an acute, a sub-acute and a chronic stage due to specific characteristics of each period.

Within 14 days of the onset of clinical symptoms, AD is classified as acute. The first two weeks include a vulnerable inflammatory period during which the majority of lethal complications can occur [1].

Usually, AD has not transformed into a stable state after 14 days. The inflammatory response can still be elevated and represent a continued risk for complications. To define a sub-acute state between day 15 and 90 after the onset of symptoms has become common practice. White et al. observed a highly dynamic period 15-30 days after onset of symptoms that could not be considered as stable [2]. Steuer et al. could even show that a subgroup of initially asymptomatic patients had onset of acute complications, especially rapid enlargement of the

Tilo Kölbel (t.koelbel@uke.de)
University Hospital Hamburg-Eppendorf,
Hamburg, Germany

G. Melissano - R. Chiesa (eds), Aortic Dissection patients true stories and the innovations that saved their lives

aorta and end-organ ischemia, within a period of 15-90 days after the initial event, and recommended this unstable period of transition from acute to chronic disease to be considered in future investigations [1]. Lastly, 90 days after onset of symptoms, AD should be classified as chronic.

28.3 The hallmark of chronic aortic dissection

In acute and sub-acute Type B AD multiple studies recommend TEVAR with good results [1-3]. For uncomplicated acute Type B AD 5-year survival is shown to be higher after TEVAR compared to best medical treatment alone. Hence, recommendations for early TEVAR increase also for uncomplicated Type B AD to avoid post-dissection aneurysms (Fig. 28.1) [4].

On the contrary, chronic AD of the aorta poses a specific challenge in regard to efficient therapy. Mostly, the concept of TEVAR with implantation of a tubular stent graft into the thoracic aorta to seal the proximal entry tear and reroute the blood flow into the true lumen alone is not associated with satisfactory results [5]. In literature, the amount of aneurysm formation despite standard TEVAR in a chronic dissection is reported to be 35% [6], mortality is reported to be 36% during 3-year follow-up [7]. This problem affects patients with chronic Type B AD as well as patients with residual dissection after surgical repair of a DeBakey Type I AD or dissection after ascending aortic repair for other pathologies. It is mainly due to the sparse

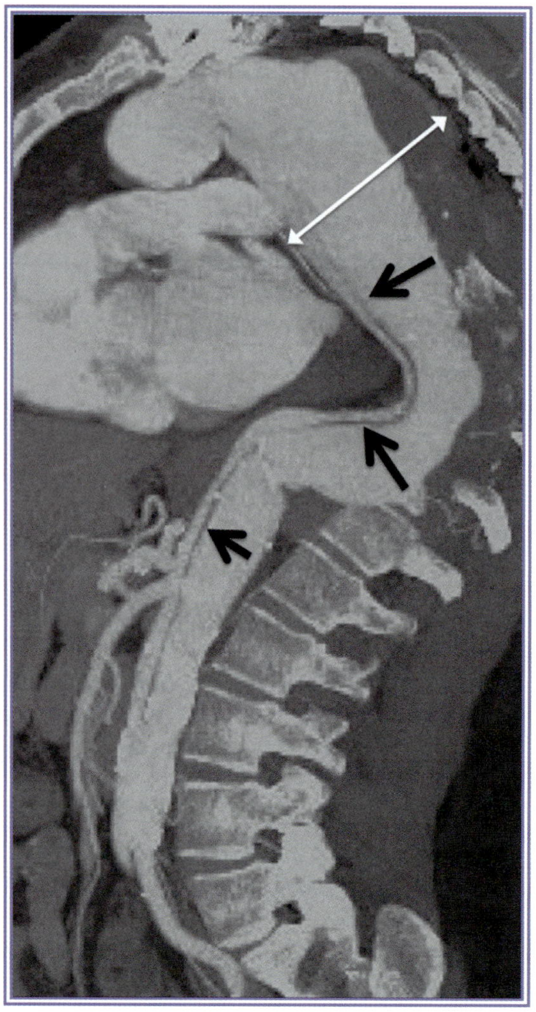

Fig. 28.1 Maximum intensity reconstruction of a chronic Type B AD: the image demonstrates the development of a relevant thoracic false lumen aneurysm of more than 7 cm (white arrow) due to persistent false lumen perfusion in this untreated patient. Therapy for this patient is challenging at this stage due to the small, almost collapsed true lumen (black arrows) and the tissue changes associated with chronic disease.

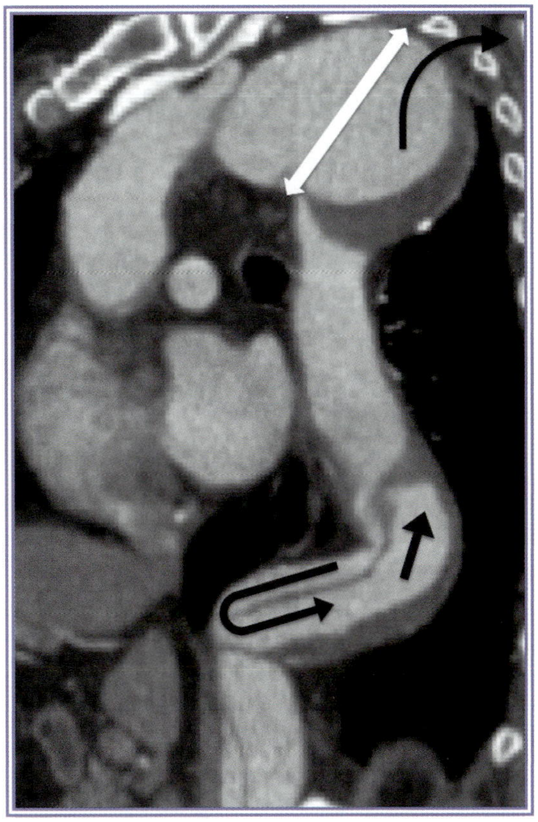

Fig. 28.2 Draft of the concept of persistent false lumen perfusion: retrograde flow in the false lumen arising from distal entry tears with run-of through spinal, bronchial or intercostal arteries from the false lumen at the level of the thoracic aorta (black arrows) leads to pressurization of the false lumen with typical aneurysm formation in the thoracic segment (white arrow). Also sufficient sealing of the proximal entry tear cannot always prevent the development of aneurysms in the long term, but early treatment also in "uncomplicated" acute dissection should be considered to lower the risk of late complications of the disease.

remodelling capacity of the aortic tissue and a rigid and thickened dissection membrane in the chronic state [8].

The most limiting factor for endovascular treatment success in chronic Type B AD is persistent false lumen perfusion. One of the reasons for the persistence of retrograde perfusion in the false lumen also after sealing of the proximal entry tear by TEVAR is the presence of intercostal or spinal run-off arteries arising from the thoracic false lumen in combination with presence of distal entry tears. These arteries supply a continuous backflow with relevant pressure transmission to the thoracic false lumen provoking post-dissection aneurysm formation and leading to potentially deadly complications (Fig. 28.2).

28.4 Treatment indications and strategies

A ruptured false lumen in chronic dissection is one of the most difficult-to-treat complications and all effort should be made to avoid its occurrence. For this reason, guidelines for therapy were made by an international consensus including the following indications for operative treatment in chronic AD [9]:
- rupture or bleeding
- false lumen aneurysm of >5.5-6 cm
- false lumen growth 5 mm/year and more
- malperfusion.

If indicated, treatment should focus on the occlusion of the false lumen. Several approaches from open surgical repair to hybrid techniques are available to achieve this goal. Which approach generally should be chosen – open surgical or endovascular therapy – has not yet been clearly established [10]. As a basic principle, open surgical approaches should be preferred in patients with connective tissue disease as Marfan syndrome, whereas endovascular procedures are more favourable in the older and high risk patients due to less procedural harm.

Irrespective of complete open surgical aortic repair, there are five main principles on how to occlude the false lumen in chronic AD:

- extended aortic coverage combined with visceral debranching (hybrid procedure)
- extended aortic coverage by branched or fenestrated stent grafts
- fenestration of the dissection membrane followed by TEVAR
- embolization of intercostal or bronchial arteries
- direct false lumen occlusion (embolization, new endovascular techniques).

In this article, we give an overview on all these techniques with emphasis on embolization techniques.

28.4.1 Strategies to exclude distal entry tears

Extending aortic coverage distally increases the possibility of entry-tear sealing at the abdominal, especially visceral branch bearing aortic segment. These concepts include:

- hybrid procedures
- fenestrated and branched endovascular aortic repair (F/BEVAR).

Hybrid techniques that represent the fusion of endovascular and open surgical treatment offer a special option for extended distal coverage by performance of a complete visceral debranching of the aorta. This procedure is conducted in advance of deployment of a stent-graft column into the true lumen including the visceral and abdominal segment. However, as shown in a recent multicenter study, significant mortality and morbidity rates of 34% in 30-day follow-up are present for this approach [11].

Fenestrated and branched endovascular aortic repair is another feasible option to seal distal entry tears, although it is challenging especially due to difficulties in maneuvering the fenestrated graft in a small true lumen as commonly present in chronic AD. True lumen expansion cannot be expected immediately due to the adverse tissue changes. Especially in the case of overlapping graft components, requiring more material to fit into the small true lumen, there is a risk for graft-occlusion. Complex stent-graft planning and individualized concepts are required. With this technique long-segment coverage of the aorta is present, which can increase the risk for spinal cord ischemia [12]. Despite these limitations, F/BEVAR is a less invasive method with a favorable course of aneurysm and aortic remodelling if performed in centers with high expertise.

28.4.2 Strategies to deal with a small true lumen or a rigid dissection membrane

Stent-grafting of the true lumen in chronic Type B AD can be difficult. As chronic AD commonly show a small true lumen, rigidity of the dissection membrane and the aortic tissue makes immediate expansion of the true lumen unlikely. This can provoke graft-occlusion especially in case of overlapping graft components. To solve this problem, techniques of false lumen deployment or fenestration of the dissection membrane evolved. In false lumen deployment, the stent graft is placed through the proximal entry tear and redirected into the true lumen through an intentionally preformed endovascular fenestration, most commonly above the celiac trunk [13].

To overcome insufficient distal sealing due to a rigid dissection membrane at the distal landing zone that prohibits complete expansion of the graft to the outer aortic wall, open surgical fenestration of the dissection membrane to create a distal sealing zone can be performed using sternotomy, thoracotomy or laparotomy. This approach was first described by Roselli et al. who performed open fenestration of the descending aorta during a first step elephant trunk procedure through sternotomy-access in 24 patients with Type A AD [14]. This process enabled full expansion of the graft to the adventitia, thereby eliminating retrograde flow into the false lumen. Follow-up of this technique showed good results with 92% survival at 2 years. However, this technique requires open surgical access with aortic cross-clamping.

28.4.3 Techniques to occlude intercostal or bronchial arteries

Continuous backflow to bronchial or intercostal arteries from downstream entry tears with persistent retrograde flow through the false lumen and pressurization of the false lumen is the most likely pathomechanism for late aortic expansion. Following this, direct embolization of bronchial or intercostal arteries arising from the false lumen would be associated with interruption of this continuous flow, thus promoting false lumen thrombosis and aortic remodelling. This strategy is not established in routine clinical practice but might represent a potential approach in the future.

28.4.4 New endovascular techniques to thrombose the false lumen

Complete endovascular fenestration of the dissection membrane using the knickerbocker technique

The knickerbocker technique is a complete endovascular fenestration technique. The concept is based on the dilation of the middle part of a large diameter stent graft that is placed in the true lumen to rupture the dissection membrane. A short bulbous segment of the stent graft is forcefully dilated using a compliant balloon to rupture the dissection membrane and extend the stent-graft to the outer wall of the aorta (Fig. 28.3). Instead of an oversized standard tu-

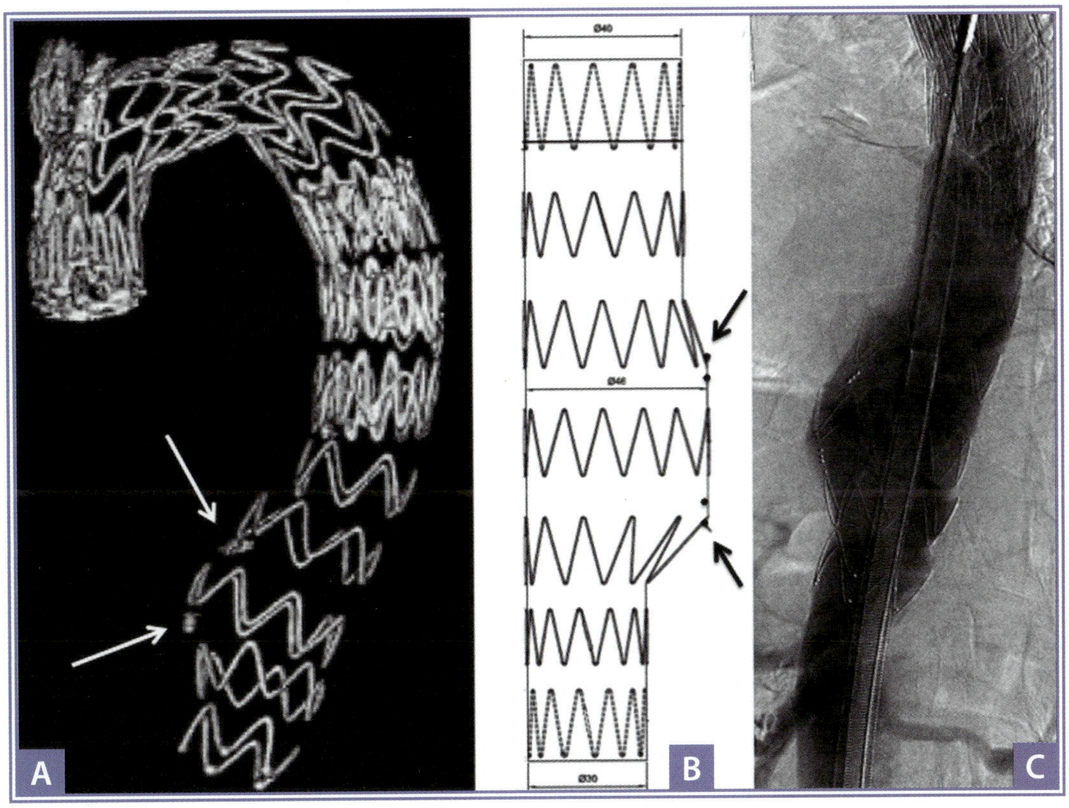

Fig. 28.3 **A**, 3D volume rendering of a knickerbocker stent graft as an extension to the celiac trunk after implantation of a branched aortic arch device. **B**, Draft of the Knickerbocker stent graft. Arrows (white and black) indicate goldmarkers at the bulbous section to adequately orient the graft towards the dissection membrane. This allows controlled rupture of the dissection membrane with sealing of the graft to the outer wall of the aorta. **C**, Final angiography of a deployed knickerbocker stent graft showing the bulbous section without false lumen perfusion above it.

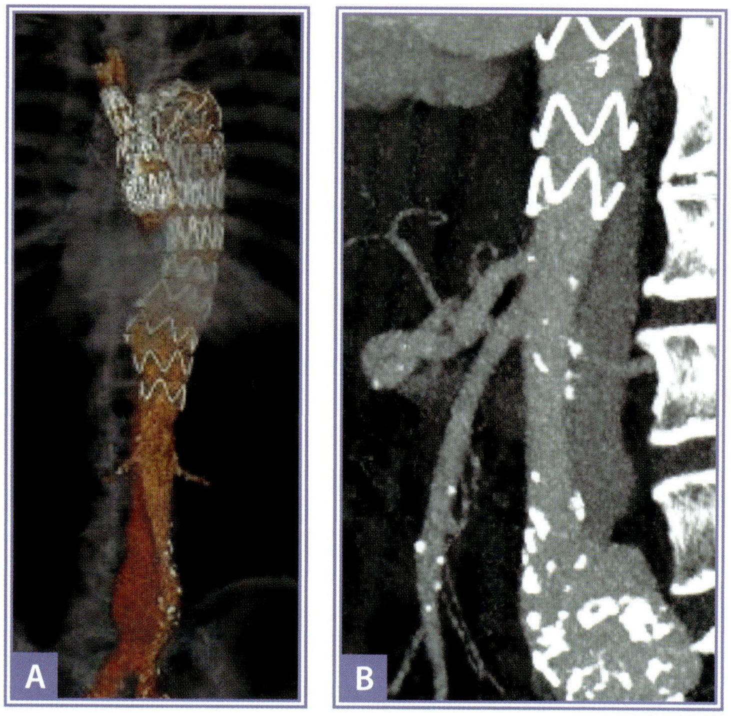

Fig. 28.4 3D volume rendering (**A**) and maximum intensity reconstruction (**B**) of a postoperative CT-scan after deployment of a knickerbocker stent graft. Backflow to the thoracic false lumen is prevented beyond the bulbous section of the graft and false lumen thrombosis can occur.

bular stent graft, a double-tapered graft construction with a bulbous section can be used [15]. After stent-graft placement in the right orientation a compliant balloon is advanced to deploy the bulbous section for septum rupture and false lumen occlusion (Fig. 28.4).

Direct false lumen occlusion using the candy-plug technique

In combination with a stent graft in the true lumen extending to the celiac artery, occlusion of the false lumen can be achieved by placing a large plug into the false lumen itself with

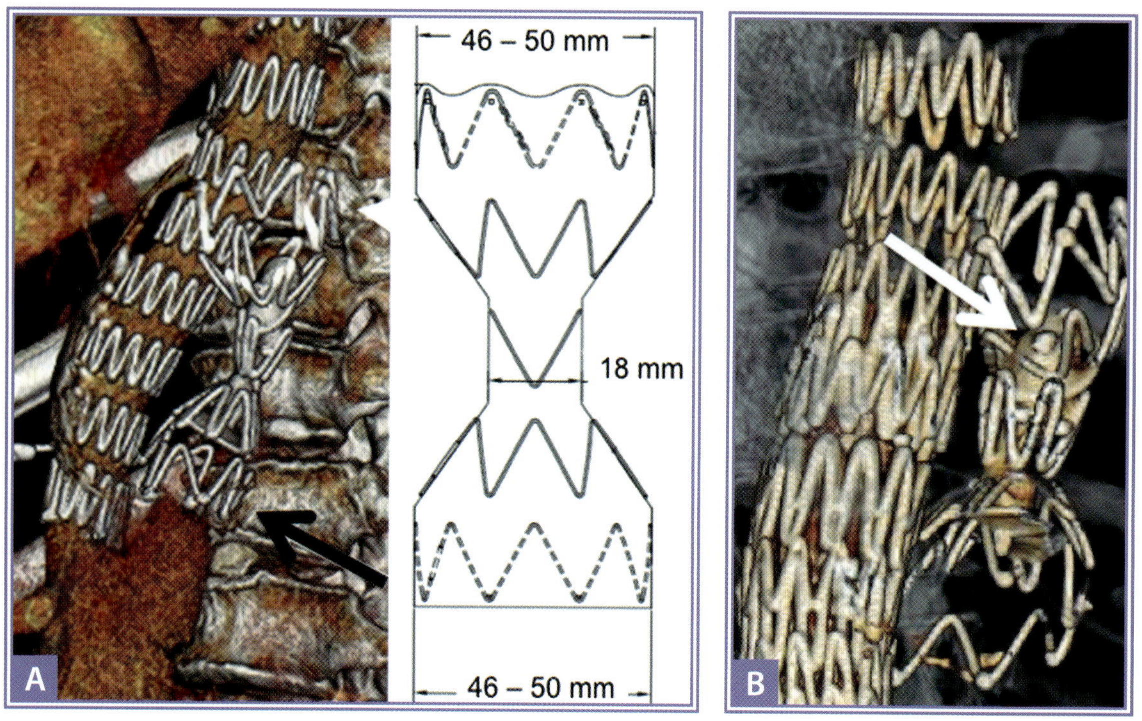

Fig. 28.5 **A**, 3D volume rendering depicting a chronic AD treated with the candy-plug technique. The candy-plug is deployed into the false lumen and positioned parallel to the distal end of the thoracic stent graft in the true lumen above the celiac trunk. Access to the false lumen can be achieved at the iliac, abdominal or visceral level through a distal entry tear of the dissection membrane. The image shows the occlusion of the false lumen with no backflow to the thoracic aneurysm (black arrow). Draft of a candy-plug, which is available as a custom-made device with diameters up to 50 mm. The central narrowing must be occluded by a vascular plug, as shown in figure **B**, white arrow pointing on a Amplatzer™ Vascular Plug Type II (St. Jude Medical, St. Paul, MN).

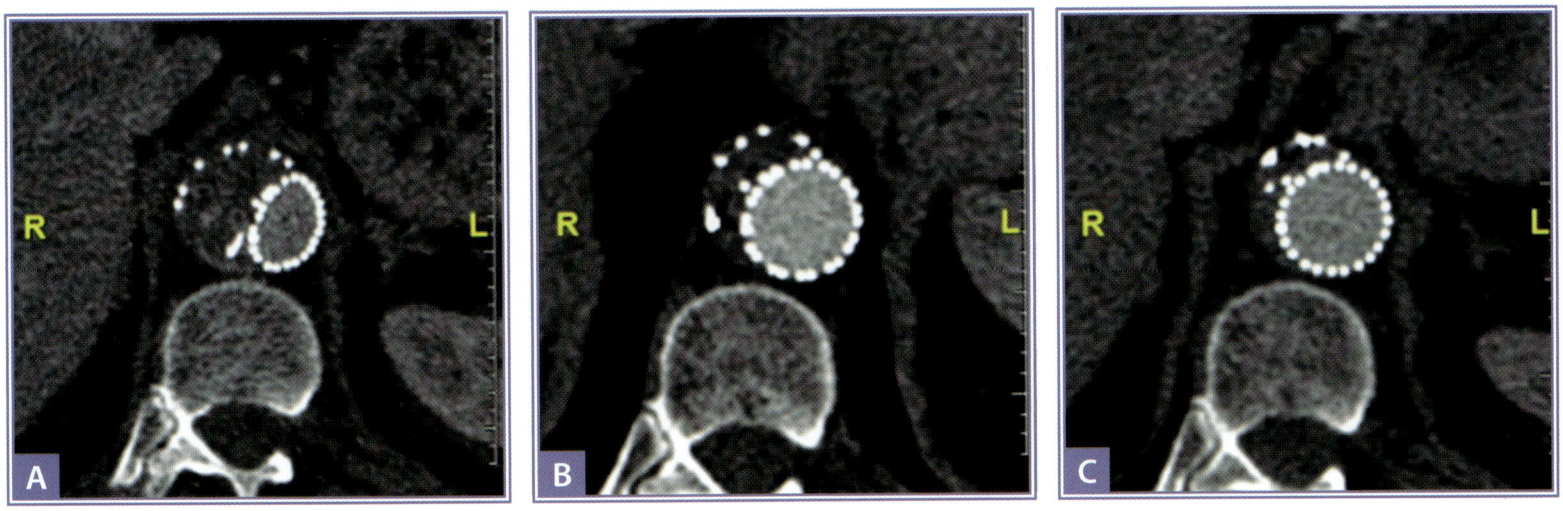

Fig. 28.6 Three-year CT follow-up of a patient with chronic AD treated with the candy-plug technique immediately after the procedure (**A**), 2 years (**B**) and 3 years (**C**) after treatment. The follow-up shows crescent-shaped remodelling and decrease of the plug and the false lumen over the time, allowing the true lumen to expand.

distal alignment to the true lumen stent graft. This strategy was described as the candy-plug technique and is also feasible in patients with large false lumen diameters (Fig. 28.5A). The method was derived from the "cork in the bottle neck" strategy first described by Loubert et al. [16]. The "cork in the bottle neck" report describes two cases where several materials comprising of cava filters, detachable balloons, thrombin and Talent® (Medtronic, Dublin, Ireland) occluders were placed – as a cork – into the false lumen to successfully achieve occlusion. As an extension of this method, a study, which included 31 patients demonstrating additional use of coils and cyanoacrylate glue, was described by Hofferberth et al. [17]. In patients with very large false lumen diameters embolization was not possible, as commercially available materials for arterial embolization were not suitable for the diameters required. So the candy-plug technique evolved to address the problem of large false lumen diameters. It was introduced as an on-table modification of a 42-mm Zenith® thoracic TX2® Pro-Form™ stent graft (Cook Medical, Bloomington, IN) into a candy-shaped plug by adding a diameter-restricting suture [18]. The so called "candy-plug" is now available as a custom-made device (CMD-device) and has a diameter of 46 or 50 mm with a central narrowing of 18 mm to remove the dilator after deployment, which must be occluded using a vascular plug or occluder system (Fig. 28.5B, C). The candy-plug as a CMD-device has yet been used in 20 patients at the University Heart Center Hamburg with good rates of false lumen thrombosis and aortic remodelling (Fig. 28.6).

28.5 Conclusion

Chronic AD needs individual treatment strategies, as the pathology is associated with several features making standard TEVAR procedures barely sufficient. Treatment should aim at the exclusion of the false lumen, since persistent false lumen perfusion counts as one of the most relevant factors for hazardous complications as aneurysm formation and death. The rise of several different treatment strategies to achieve false lumen occlusion demonstrates the need for individualized concepts in this complex disease. As a less invasive, feasible approach, new endovascular strategies as the candy-plug or the knickerbocker technique gain ground in the treatment of chronic AD.

REFERENCES

1) Steuer J, Bjorck M, Mayer D, Wanhainen A, Pfammatter T, Lachat M. Distinction between acute and chronic type B aortic dissection: is there a sub-acute phase? Eur J Vasc Endovasc Surg 2013; 45(6): 627-31.
2) White RA, Miller DC, Criado FJ, et al. Report on the results of thoracic endovascular aortic repair for acute, complicated, type B aortic dissection at 30 days and 1 year from a multidisciplinary subcommittee of the Society for Vascular Surgery Outcomes Committee. J Vasc Surg 2011; 53(4): 1082-90.
3) Nienaber CA, Kische S, Rousseau H, et al. Endovascular repair of type B aortic dissection: long-term results of the randomized investigation of stent grafts in aortic dissection trial. Circ Cardiovasc Interv 2013; 6(4): 407-16.
4) Fattori R, Montgomery D, Lovato L, et al. Survival after endovascular therapy in patients with type B aortic dissection: a report from the International Registry of Acute Aortic Dissection (IRAD). JACC Cardiovasc Interv 2013; 6(8): 876-82.
5) Kölbel T, Tsilimparis N, Wipper S, et al. TEVAR for chronic aortic dissection - Is covering the primary entry tear enough? J Cardiovasc Surg 2014; 55(4): 519-27.
6) Scali ST, Feezor RJ, Chang CK, et al. Efficacy of thoracic endovascular stent repair for chronic type B aortic dissection with aneurysmal degeneration. J Vasc Surg 2013; 58(1): 10-7.
7) Mani K, Clough RE, Lyons OT, et al. Predictors of outcome after endovascular repair for chronic type B dissection. Eur J Vasc Endovasc Surg 2012; 43(4): 386-91.
8) Yang CP, Hsu CP, Chen WY, et al. Aortic remodeling after endovascular repair with stainless steel-based stent graft in acute and chronic type B aortic dissection. J Vasc Surg 2012; 55: 1600-10.
9) Fattori R, Cao P, De Rango P, et al. Interdisciplinary expert consensus document on management of type B aortic dissection. J Am Coll Cardiol 2013; 61(16): 1661-78.
10) Tian DH, De Silva RP, Wang T, Yan TD. Open surgical repair for chronic type B aortic dissection: a systematic review. Ann Cardiothorac Surg 2014; 3(4): 340-50.
11) Idrees J, Roselli EE, Shafii S, Reside J, Lytle BW. Outcomes after false lumen embolization with covered stent devices in chronic dissection. J Vasc Surg 2014; 60(6): 1507-13.
12) Oikonomou K, Kopp R, Katsargyris A, Pfister K, Verhoeven EL, Kasprzak P. Outcomes of fenestrated/branched endografting in post-dissection thoracoabdominal aortic aneurysms. Eur J Vasc Endovasc Surg 2014; 48(6): 641-8.
13) Simring D, Raja J, Morgan-Rowe L, Hague J, Harris PL, Ivancev K. Placement of a branched stent graft into the false lumen of a chronic type B aortic dissection. J Vasc Surg 2011; 54: 1784-7.
14) Roselli EE, Sepulveda E, Pujara AC, Idrees J, Nowicki E. Distal landing zone open fenestration facilitates endovascular elephant trunk completion and false lumen thrombosis. Ann Thorac Surg 2011; 92(6): 2078-84.
15) Kölbel T, Carpenter SW, Lohrenz C, Tsilimparis N, Larena-Avellaneda A, Debus ES. Addressing persistent false lumen flow in chronic aortic dissection: the knickerbocker technique. J Endovasc Ther 2014; 21(1): 117-22.
16) Loubert MC, van der Hulst VP, De Vries C, Bloemendaal K, Vahl AC. How to exclude the dilated false lumen in patients after a type B aortic dissection? The cork in the bottleneck. J Endovasc Ther 2003; 10(2): 244-8.
17) Hofferberth SC, Nixon IK, Mossop PJ. Aortic false lumen thrombosis induction by embolotherapy (AFTER) following endovascular repair of aortic dissection. J Endovasc Ther 2012; 19(4): 538-45.
18) Kölbel T, Lohrenz C, Kieback A, Diener H, Debus ES, Larena-Avellaneda A. Distal false lumen occlusion in aortic dissection with a homemade extra-large vascular plug: the candy-plug technique. J Endovasc Ther 2013; 20(4): 484-9.

29

False lumen embolization in aortic dissection

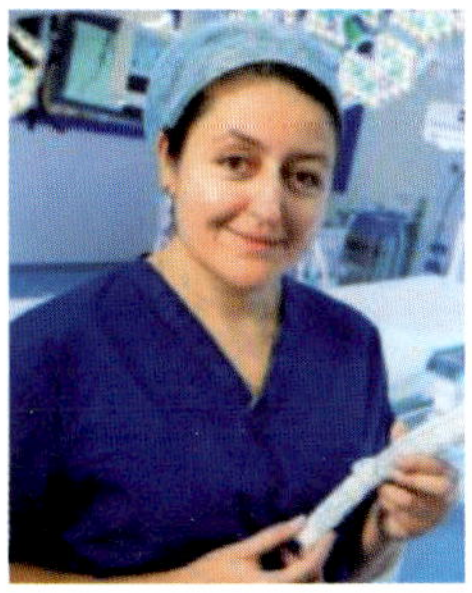

Tara M. Mastracci

Aortic dissection (AD) is one of the most challenging manifestations of aortic disease because of the variability of presentation and the unpredictable course in both the acute and chronic phase. For much of surgical history, the goals of treatment for interventions in AD were aimed at preventing catastrophic events in the acute phase, and repairing aneurysms in the chronic phase. However, recent experience with endovascular intervention in both the acute and chronic phases of the disease has suggested that intervention may change the natural history. This has refocused clinical and research efforts into two simultaneous paths: understanding the predictors of poor outcome or disease progression that causes some patients with AD to continue to have evolving and lethal disease, and role that timing and modality of intervention may have in truncating this course to restore a patients' life curve to that of the age-matched population.

29.1 Our evolving understanding of aortic dissection

Before a thorough discussion can be undertaken about changing the natural history of AD, it is important to establish what we know to be true. Although a number of authors have reported series of AD in the surgical literature over the last 4 decades, these reports have been subject to selection bias because clinical indications for treatment compelled intervention in many cases.

In an early publication from the International Registry of Acute Aortic Dissection (IRAD), the best-known cohort of patients describing both acute and long-term outcomes, the presenting symptoms were described. Abrupt onset (83.8%), sharp pain (68.3%), chest pain (62.9%) and back pain (63.8%) were the most common presenting complaints. And classically, this report describes in-hospital mortality for 31.4% of patients undergoing surgery, and only 10.7% of those who had non-surgical (medical) management [1].

In a more recent update from the same group, in a cohort of 1476 patients with Type B AD, the clinical outcomes in acute presentation remain favourable to medical management, with a 17.2% risk of in-hospital mortality for patients undergoing surgical intervention, and 8.7% for those having non-operative treatment. In this paper, the cohort of patients undergoing endovascular repair is also described, and the in-hospital mortality is documented to be 12.3%

Tara M. Mastracci (tara.mastracci@nhs.net)
The Royal Free London, NHS Foundation Trust,
London, United Kingdom

G. Melissano - R. Chiesa (eds), Aortic Dissection patients true stories and the innovations that saved their lives

[2]. However, if long-term outcomes are considered, the trends seem to favour endovascular intervention: five-year mortality in patients undergoing Thoracic EndoVascular Aortic Repair (TEVAR) for their dissection was 16% in this cohort compared with 29% for those following a non-surgical path [3]. Given the selective treatment strategy for patients enrolled in the IRAD database, namely that clinical judgement prevails and that patients with complications are both more likely to receive intervention and more likely to have aggressive disease, it is difficult to interpret the impact that endovascular intervention would have in all-comers.

With the above example providing a needed caveat, recent studies comparing treatment of the distal aorta in patients with proximal disease have further bolstered interest in preventative endovascular intervention as a means of promoting aortic remodelling or changing the natural history of disease. The primary study that pointed in this direction was written by Pochettino et al. [4]. In this study, 78 patients with Type A AD were treated with either primary ascending aortic repair, or repair including frozen elephant trunk. There was no significant difference in the rate of paraplegia (1/42 in the nonstented group compared with 3/36 in the stented group, p = NS). Subsequent aortic reintervention was informative: 4/36 unstented patients compared with 0/31 stented patients required thoracoabdominal aortic repair (p = 0.083), however 8/31 stented patients required further stenting to induce false lumen obliteration. The unique characteristic of this trial was the focus on false lumen flow as an indicator of success of treatment. Although many authors before Pochettino looked at the role of the false lumen in aortic remodelling, this study provided some substantial evidence of its value in a population that was not biased by events in the distal aorta.

29.2 Interest in false lumen thrombosis

Since the Pochettino study, other authors have also focused on false lumen thrombosis and the impact on long-term outcomes. The most notable study is also the largest randomized

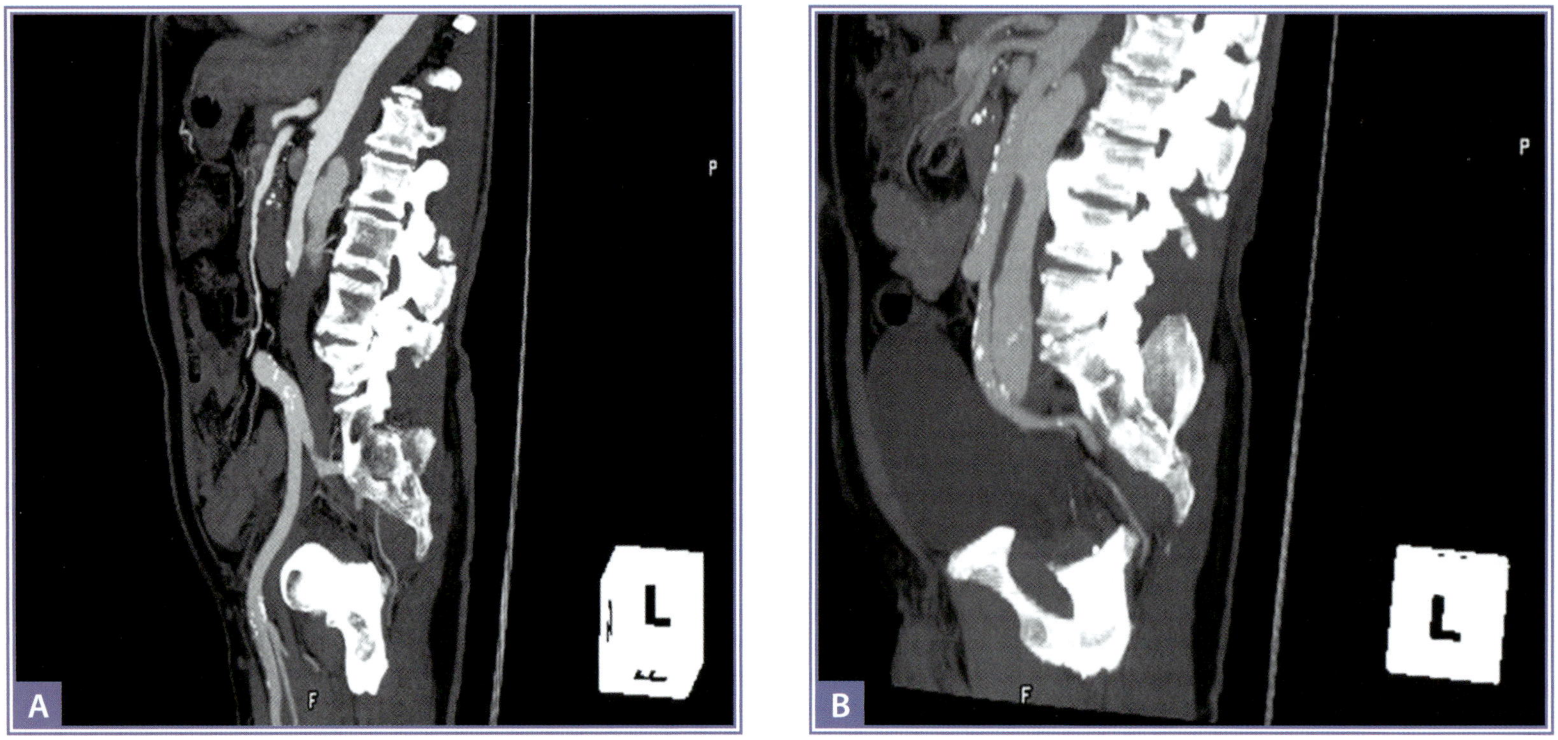

Fig. 29.1 False lumen flow in arterial (**A**) and venous (**B**) phases of the same patient.

Table 29.1 Trials of shunting in aortic dissection reporting false lumen thrombosis

Author	Total false lumen thrombosis	Partial false lumen thrombosis	Rate (%)
Wiedemann (2014)	8/110	25/110	30
Zhu (2015)	24/28	4/28	100
Huang (2015)	69/72	NR	95
Cambria (2015)	20/50	6/50	52
Brunkwall (ADSORB) (2014)		43/61	70
Nienaber (INSTEAD XL) (2013)	48/72	5/72	74

controlled trial of stable Type B AD which published 5-year outcome in 2013 [5]. The INSTEAD XL trial randomized 140 patients to either TEVAR (n = 72) or optimal medical management (n = 68), and at 5 years, found that patients who had undergone TEVAR were more likely to have thrombosis of the false lumen compared with nonstented aortas ($p < 0.0001$). This translated to a smaller false lumen diameter at the level of the stent graft in long-term follow-up, suggesting that the pattern of disease had changed with intervention, putatively by inducing thrombosis of the false lumen. What this, and all other promising studies reporting false lumen thrombosis fail to show, however, is the subsequent decrease in lifetime aortic interventions.

Thrombosis of the false lumen is a difficult phenomenon to image using non-invasive modalities. Depending on the rate of flow of blood into the false lumen, the proximity and size of the entry tears, and the degree of formal thrombus already present, the appearance on both arterial and venous phase computed tomography (CT) scans can be misleading. Figures 29.1A and 29.1B reflect the different appearance of the false lumen in the same patient in two different CT scan phases. Use of magnetic resonance imaging (MRI) to image the false lumen has potential to be more helpful, and in a recent review which provides details beyond the scope of this chapter, the authors describe 3D velocity encoded cine MRI as a modality that may provide more information about the direction of blood flow in the false lumen [6]. Certainly, echocardiography and intravenous ultrasound are also useful in determining the presence of thrombus versus flow in the false lumen, but neither are modalities that can easily be applied to wide surveillance imaging in patients requiring routine assessment of chronic dissections.

The difficulty in visualizing false lumen thrombosis on traditional cross sectional imaging may be the explanation as to why, in modern dissection trials, the rate of false lumen thrombosis is variable. In studies published in the last 2 years, the rate of false lumen thrombosis has ranged from 52% to 100% (Table 29.1). In an earlier systematic review that is likely more representative of the literature, Eggebrecht et al. found that the rate of false lumen thrombosis was 75% of endovascular stent placement for dissection. This was reported after an aggregated mean follow-up of 19 months, in 237 of 600 patients [7]. Thus, recent literature is clearly demonstrating that endovascular intervention may have some role in promoting remodelling of the aorta in areas that are treated, but the heterogeneity of the clinical response could be either due to variable disease characteristics, or inconsistent imaging techniques. Further research is needed to determine the role that each of these factors play in achieving this outcome.

29.3 Proactive false lumen embolization

Despite this ambiguity in the literature, the trend of improved outcomes with false lumen thrombosis has prompted some clinicians to attempt to expedite the process by using a variety of techniques to promote this thrombosis. Early reports included placing occluding devices in the visible entry tears along the septum between the true and false lumen [8]. Although this does have some success, the difficulty in identifying all the micro-tears may be one drawback to this technique.

In most other technique descriptions, interventionalists describe placing thrombogenic materials at the level of the distal stent graft, attempting to isolate only the stented areas of the aorta. This has the dual benefit of augmenting the impact that TEVAR may have on false lumen thrombosis, as well as protecting stray coils from launching into the true lumen and causing misadventure. The material used for embolization is variable. Embolization of the false lumen with coils has also been described with some success [9, 10]. The number of coils needed to achieve occlusion and the timing for this intervention vary depending on the described reports. There is also some concern that the thrombus formed may continue to transmit pressure, thus making this technique less effective. Amplatzer™ (St. Jude Medical, St. Paul, MN) plugs have also been described, but significantly increase the cost of the procedure [11].

The most promising technique described in the literature to date involves placing fabric-lined occlusion devices in the false lumen. This is described using off-the-shelf devices [12] and custom-made "candy-plug" devices [13]. Intuitively, these devices seem more likely to be successful compared with coils because they place a physical barrier between the flow in the false lumen and the isolated area. Anecdotally, clinicians who choose these techniques are describing success, and this is covered in further detail in Chapter 28.

Table 29.2 describes the collective experience with different forms of occlusion in the false lumen that is published in the English literature to date. There is a paucity of long-term follow-up and many case reports which makes it difficult to judge the true effectiveness of the technique. As with other dissection publications, the protocol used for visualizing the false lumen is not well described and leaves room for interpretation if the thrombosis is true, or artefactual.

In the three publications to date which include more than 5 patients, one group describing work with coils and glue and another group describing use of coils alone had a 90% rate and 60% rate, respectively, of stable or increasing sac size over 63 and 11-month follow-up [10, 14]. Thus, although false lumen thrombosis may have been demonstrated, it has failed to promote the remodelling that would prevent further aortic intervention, or worse, aortic catastrophe. In the remaining report [12], where fabric covered occluders were used, there was a 60% rate of complete thrombosis, and the sac size was >5 mm smaller in 52% of patients after 25-month

Table 29.2 Collective experience with different forms of occlusion in the false lumen

Author	Journal/year	Embolic agent	Patients (no.)	Follow-up (months)
Hussain [9]	Annals 2015	Coils and glue	1	NR
Hofferberth [10]	JEVT 2012	Coils, glue, etc.	10	63
Idrees [12]	JVS 2014	Occluders and other things	21	25
Kölbel [15]	JEVT 2016	Coils	2	NR
Kölbel [13]	JEVT 2013	Candy-plug	1	3
Mendes [11]	JEVT 2015	Amplatzer	1	18
Ogawa [16]	JEVT 2016	Candy-plug	1	14
Hager [17]	JVS 2008	Coils and covered stents	1	NR
Smith [18]	EVT 2009	Coils	1	9
Riga [19]	JVIR 2009	Coils and Onyx	1	24
Norberto [14]	JVS 2011	Coils	5	11

follow-up. Although this data is too preliminary to draw definitive conclusions, if a clinician was going to propose embolization of the false lumen, placement of a fabric lined occlusion device may be more likely to be successful than coils or glue alone. However, there is really no justification in the current literature to change practice until groups who have experience in this technique can produce a more definitive outcome data in a larger volume of patients.

29.4 Guiding clinical practice

Every centre with an aortic practice has anecdotal cases of both success and failure using these techniques. At our centre, early adoption of false lumen embolization has provided some perspective on long-term behaviour of the aorta. For example, in one case, where a false lumen occluder was placed with initial success, recent follow-up has shown increased growth in the aneurysm at both the level of the occluder and distal (Fig. 29.2). It is possible that, in AD that involves the entire aorta, false lumen occlusion may not supplant the treatment of the entire aorta with a true lumen intervention, such as open repair or fenestrated stent placement. In other cases, we have favoured using false lumen occlusion if there is a small and defined defect, and if it will not preclude the use of future, more standard and definitive options (Fig. 29.3). This approach has not been tested with prospective trials.

Based on the limited available data in the published literature, it is challenging to know what role false lumen embolization plays in our treatment of AD. Principles that we use at our centre are as follows:

1) true lumen interventions, or proximal placement of thoracic endografts, with an aim to close proximal tears and divert flow from the false lumen are first line in both acute and chronic dissection;

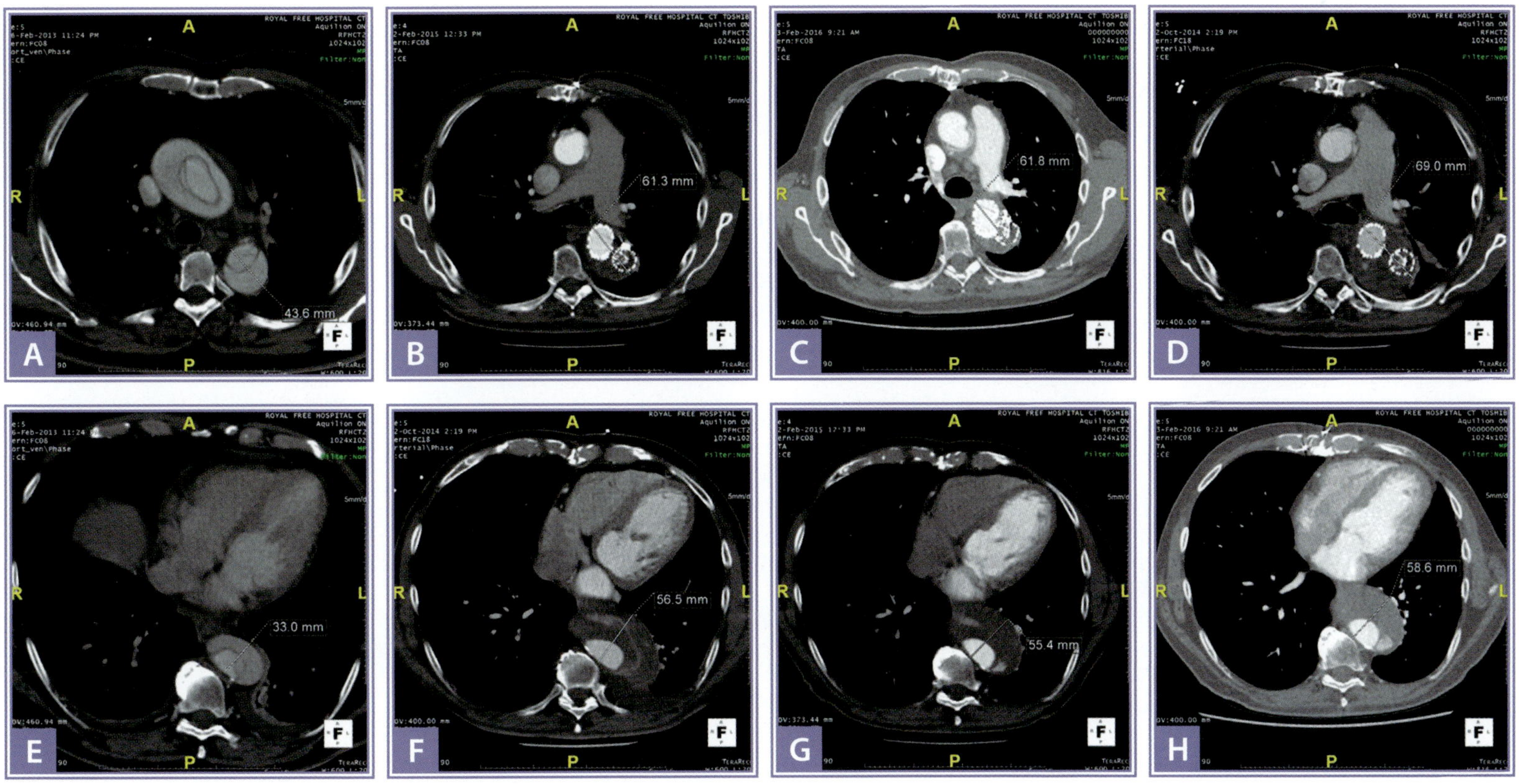

Fig. 29.2 Progression of disease in AD with placement of an occluder device, at the level of the occlusion (**A-D**) and distal to the occlusion (**E-H**).

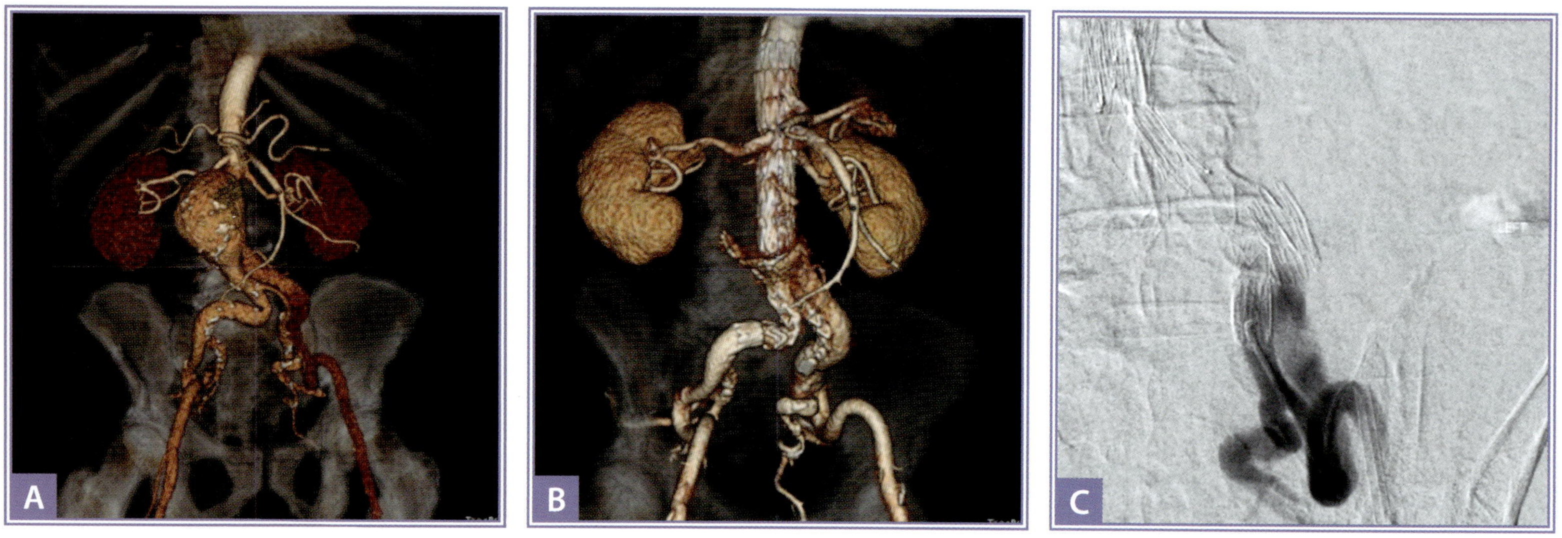

Fig. 29.3 Staged false lumen embolization to prevent spinal injury in patients with complex repair. **A**, Preoperative image of an aneurysm requiring complex repair with dissection of the infrarenal and iliac artery. **B**, Post FEVAR imaging with permissive false lumen flow. **C**, Intraoperative images of device occluding false lumen.

2) failure to halt growth in both stented and unstented regions of dissected aortas usually requires further true lumen intervention, including fenestrated or branched repair;
3) in selected cases where permission of ongoing false lumen flow may improve outcomes by maintaining spinal cord perfusion during the time of the largest intervention, we stage closure of the false lumen. False lumen embolization techniques may be considered if there is a small and well-defined defect, and they do not preclude the use of more definitive options in the future.

29.5 Conclusions

After reviewing the literature, it is clear that the role of false lumen embolization has yet to be defined in the treatment of AD. Future studies looking at the impact on long-term aortic rupture and aortic intervention is needed to warrant adopting this into every day clinical practice.

REFERENCES

1) Hagan PG, Nienaber CA, Isselbacher EM, et al. The International Registry of Acute Aortic Dissection (IRAD): new insights into an old disease. JAMA 2000; 283: 897-903.
2) Pape LA, Awais M, Woznicki EM, et al. Presentation, diagnosis, and outcomes of acute aortic dissection: 17-year trends from the International Registry of Acute Aortic Dissection. J Am Coll Cardiol 2015; 66: 350-8.
3) Patel AY, Eagle KA, Vaishnava P. Acute type B aortic dissection: insights from the International Registry of Acute Aortic Dissection. Ann Cardiothorac Surg 2014; 3: 368-74.
4) Pochettino A, Brinkman WT, Moeller P, et al. Antegrade thoracic stent grafting during repair of acute DeBakey I dissection prevents development of thoracoabdominal aortic aneurysms. Ann Thorac Surg 2009; 88: 482-9; discussion 489-90.
5) Nienaber CA, Kische S, Rousseau H, et al. Endovascular repair of type B aortic dissection: long-term results of the randomized investigation of stent grafts in aortic dissection trial. Circ Cardiovasc Interv 2013; 6: 407-16.
6) Sherrah AG, Grieve SM, Jeremy RW, Bannon PG, Vallely MP, Puranik R. MRI in chronic aortic dissection: a systematic review and future directions. Front Cardiovasc Med 2015; 2: 5.

7) Eggebrecht H, Nienaber CA, Neuhäuser M, et al. Endovascular stent-graft placement in aortic dissection: a meta-analysis. Eur Heart J 2006; 27: 489-98.
8) Falkenberg M, Roos H, Lepore V, Svensson G, Zachrisson K, Henrikson O. Endovascular closure of chronic dissection entries in the aortic arch using the Amplatzer Vascular Plug II as a sealing button. J Endovasc Ther 2016; 23: 378-83.
9) Hussain MA, Lindsay TF, Tan KT, Moloney T. Coil embolization of the false lumen in complicated type B aortic dissection. Ann Vasc Surg 2015; 29(1): 125.e13-17.
10) Hofferberth SC, Nixon IK, Mossop PJ. Aortic false lumen thrombosis induction by embolotherapy (AFTER) following endovascular repair of aortic dissection. J Endovasc Ther 2012; 19: 538-45.
11) Mendes BC, Oderich GS, Erben Y, Reed NR, Pruthi RK. False lumen embolization to treat disseminated intravascular coagulation after thoracic endovascular aortic repair of Type B aortic dissection. J Endovasc Ther 2015; 22: 938-41.
12) Idrees J, Roselli EE, Shafii S, Reside J, Lytle BW. Outcomes after false lumen embolization with covered stent devices in chronic dissection. J Vasc Surg 2014; 60: 1507-13.
13) Kölbel T, Lohrenz C, Kieback A, Diener H, Debus ES, Larena-Avellaneda A. Distal false lumen occlusion in aortic dissection with a homemade extra-large vascular plug: the candy-plug technique. J Endovasc Ther 2013; 20: 484-9.
14) Norberto EM, Gutiérrez VM, Taylor J, Vaquero C. Coil embolization of persistent false lumen after stent graft repair of type B aortic dissection. J Vasc Surg 2011; 54: 201-4.
15) Kölbel T, Tsilimparis N. Commentary: Buttoning up the proximal tear: is a vascular plug the answer to achieving false lumen thrombosis? J Endovasc Ther 2016; 23(2): 384-6.
16) Ogawa Y, Nishimaki H, Chiba K, et al. Candy-plug technique using an excluder aortic extender for distal occlusion of a large false lumen aneurysm in chronic aortic dissection. J Endovasc Ther 2016; 23(3): 483-6.
17) Hager E, Moudgill N, Lipman A, Dimuzio P, Lombardi J. Coil-assisted false lumen thrombosis in complicated chronic type B dissection. J Vasc Surg 2008; 48(2): 465-8.
18) Smith TA, Broker MS, Arko FR. IVUS-directed coil embolization after type b aortic dissection, Endovascular today 2009; 10: 60-3.
19) Riga C, Bicknell C, Jenkins M, Hamady M. Coil embolization of an aneurysmal type B dissection persistent false lumen after visceral hybrid repair. J Vasc Interv Radiol 2009; 20(1): 130-2.

30

Distal stent graft-induced new entry

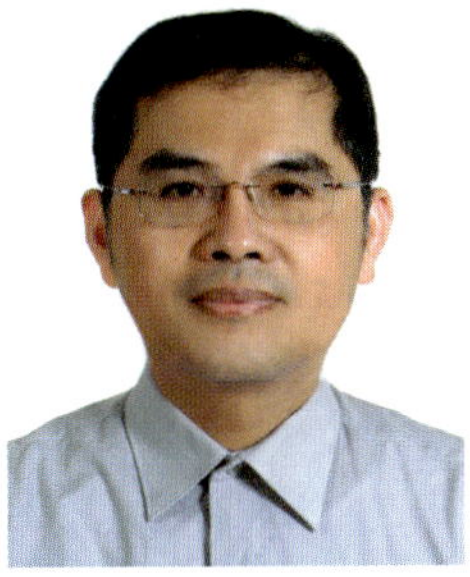

Chun-Che Shih and Hung-Lung Hsu

During the past decades, the treatment of aortic dissection (AD) has greatly evolved after the introduction of Thoracic EndoVascular Aortic Repair (TEVAR). The principle behind this technique is to cover the proximal primary intimal tear of the aorta, to initiate thrombosis of the false lumen, and to re-expand the true lumen. With the advancements of endovascular knowledge and devices, the future prospects on the outcomes of TEVAR are promising and the applications of TEVAR are extensive. However, due to the fact that the distal landing zone of the stent graft is often located in the diseased aorta, the potential intimal injury induced by the endograft still poses a major concern.

Distal Stent Graft-Induced New Entry (DSINE), or stent graft-induced distal redissection (SIDR), defined the complication that is caused by the stent graft when it introduces a new distal intimomedial tear. Reports on events of DSINE or SIDR have increased in numbers throughout literature. A risen widespread discussion on this matter is also growing [1-8]. Distal stent graft-induced injuries are one of the major complications that compromise the long-term durability of endografting and develop into unfavorable outcomes. DSINE may lead to a new patent false lumen, then to aneurysmal degeneration, and eventually, to aortic rupture.

30.1 Incidence, evaluation and diagnosis

Until recently, studies about DSINE were scarce and limited to retrospective evaluation (Table 30.1). The incidence of DSINE varied from study to study [1, 2, 6-11]. Moreover, accurate estimation in terms of events per patient-year was difficult. Of these, Feng et al. reported an incidence of 2.9% in 311 patients treated with standard TEVAR for Type B AD [10]. In our series, Huang et al. showed a much higher incidence of 60% in patients after hybrid arch repair using elephant trunk graft as proximal landing zone for AD [7]. The wide range of incidences may be associated with the differences in patient and device selection. For example, Feng and colleagues used five stent-graft systems to treat Type B AD [10]. Nevertheless, Huang et al. focused on patients undergoing stainless steel based endografting for residual Type A or chronic Type B AD [7]. In addition, a higher incidence was also noted in patients with chronic AD. Our early cohort from 2006 to 2011 revealed an incidence of 18.9% in the acute dissection group but 35.7% in the chronic group during the follow-up period [2]. In another recent

Chun-Che Shih (ccshih@vghtpe.gov.tw)
Taipei Veterans General Hospital,
School of Medicine, National Yang-Ming University, Taipei, Taiwan

G. Melissano - R. Chiesa (eds), Aortic Dissection patients true stories and the innovations that saved their lives

Table 30.1 Summary of studies evaluating the formation of distal stent graft-induced new entry (DSINE)

	Duration	Patients (no.)	DSINE (no.)	Acuity (%)		Stent-graft system	Mean time from initial TEVAR to detection of DSINE (months)	Taper ratio[a] (DSINE vs. Non-DSINE)	Oversizing ratio[b] (DSINE vs. Non-DSINE)
				Acute	Chronic				
Janosi et al. [6]	1999-2010	142	9	41.5	58.5	Nitinol and stainless steel	25.1±24.3	40.9±14.1% vs. 25.36±20.2% $p < 0.05$	95.9±49.3% vs. 55.9±36.2% $p < 0.01$[c]
Dong et al. [1]	2000-2008	650	8	NA	NA	Nitinol and stainless steel	11.0±16.0	NA	NA
Huang et al. [7]	2006-2011	20	12	0	100	Stainless steel	12.6±9.9	30±21% vs. 40±25% $p = 0.90$	4.00±2.96% vs. 1.98±0.66% $p = 0.03$[d]
Li et al. [11]	2009-2013	579	39	66.1	33.9	Nitinol and stainless steel	22.0±17.0	NA	NA

Data are shown as mean ± standard deviation; NA, not available
[a] The ratio between the sizes of the true lumen at the proximal landing zone and that at the distal landing zone before the procedure
[b] The difference between the size of the selected stent graft and that of the true lumen at the presumed level of the distal landing before the procedure
[c] In diameter
[d] In area

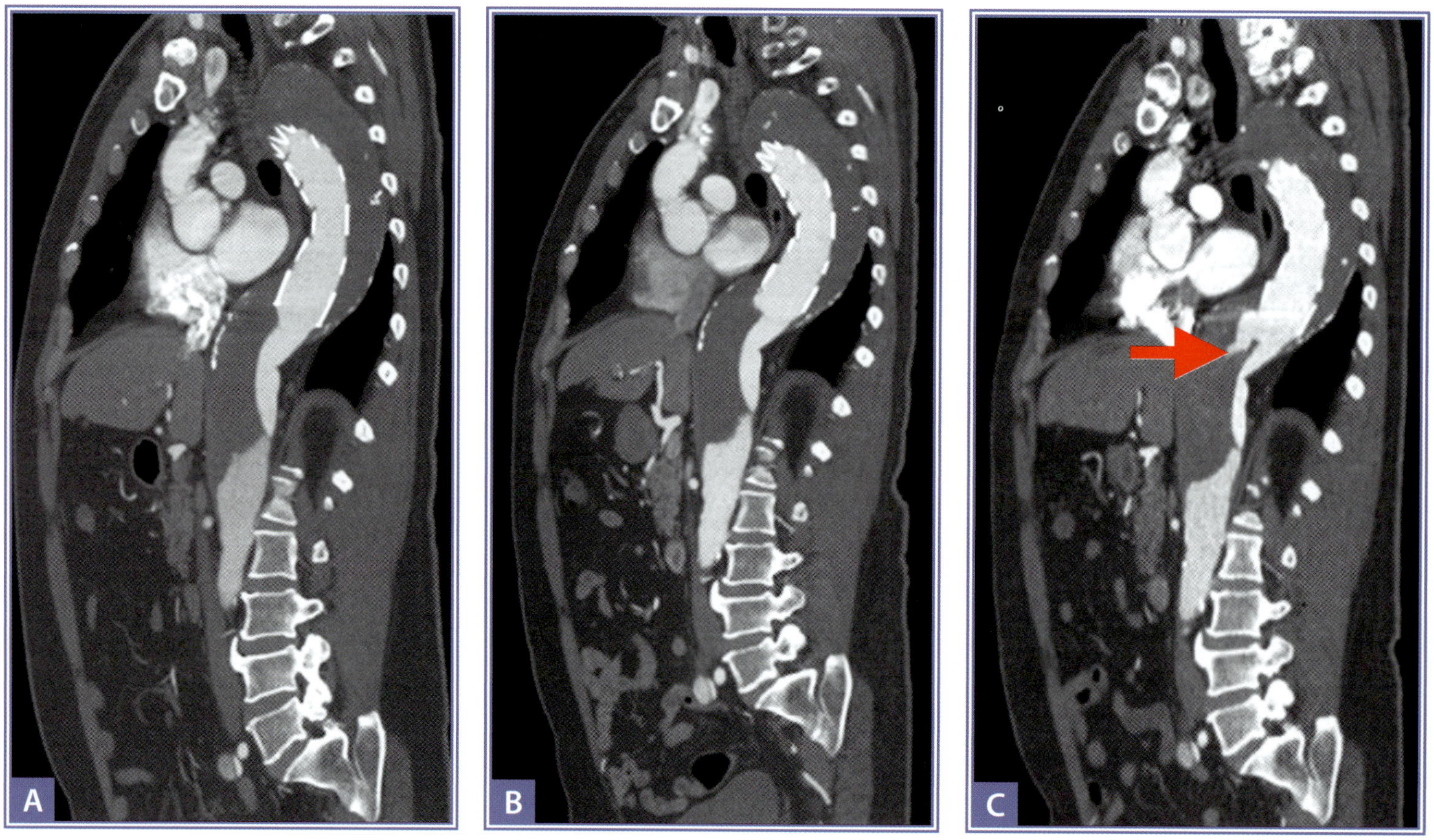

Fig. 30.1 Typical computed tomography (CT) images of distal stent graft-induced new entry (DSINE). **A**, 1 year after initial TEVAR. **B**, 2 years after initial TEVAR. A small outpouching was noted at the distal end of the endograft on the lesser curvature of the aorta. **C**, 2.5 years after initial TEVAR. DSINE (red arrow) with pseudoaneurysm formation.

report made up of 579 patients with Type B AD, the authors also demonstrated a greater incidence in patients with chronic dissection (9.7% vs. 5.2%; $p = 0.042$) [6].

DSINE is usually a late complication after initial endografting. In our study by Yang et al., the average time to onset was 24.8±5.9 months [2]. Other investigators reported that DSINE was detected from 11.0±16.0 months [1] up to 31.5±28.6 months [6] after first TEVAR. These data reflect that the distal stent-related intimal injury slowly evolves into deleterious complication. This insidious process also explains why most patients with DSINE experience no symptoms. In an early report by Dong et al. [1], 6 out of 8 patients with DSINE were asymptomatic upon initial diagnosis. However, if patients with DSINE become symptomatic, recurrent chest pain or back pain is the typical presentation. Other symptoms, such as dyspnea, refractory hypertension, or syncope were also reported.

The diagnosis of DSINE is mainly dependent on computed tomographic angiography (CTA). Magnetic resonance angiography (MRA) may be performed. Dynamic images are provided but MRI will be more time consuming. The most typical image finding of DSINE is the presence of a new intimal erosion with contrast leakage into the false lumen at the distal end of the stent graft (Fig. 30.1).

The mortality rate of DSINE was reported from 11% [10] to 28.6% [1]. Given the substantial mortality and insidious character, long-term follow-up with regular CT protocol is recommended in order to monitor the formation of DSINE.

30.2 Mechanism of distal stent graft-induced new entry development

The potential mechanisms for the development of DSINE are complex. In addition to the natural progression of the aortic disease, aortic wall fragility and stent graft-related factors also play important roles in the formation of DSINE. After placement of the endograft, the aortic pressure and blood flow pass through the less flexible stent graft to the downstream aorta. The pulsatile stimulus from the rigid end of the stent graft against the fragile intimal flap could eventually cause a tear and create a new entry. A computational fluid dynamics study by Karmonik et al. illustrated the changes of the wall shear stress before and after stent graft placement in Type B AD and provided the biomedical imaging model to the stent graft-induced new entry [12]. In the study, a patient with acute Type B AD who underwent endografting was studied by dynamic magnetic resonance imaging pre and post (1 week) TEVAR. The authors demonstrated that high pressure and irregular flow located near the bilateral ends of the stent graft were found. It implied that the intima near the edge of the stent graft endures greater pressure during each cardiac cycle and, imaginably, becomes vulnerable to rupture. Moreover, in chronic dissection, the intimal flap is more fibrotic and less mobile than in the acute phase. The rigid intimal membrane would be less compliant to the expansion of the stent graft and thus carry a higher risk of formation of a new intimal break. This explains why a higher incidence of DSINE was observed in patients treated for chronic AD.

Another important factor for DSINE formation is the distal oversizing or mismatch (the difference between the size of the selected stent graft and that of the true lumen at the presumed level of the distal landing before the procedure) (Fig. 30.2). Feng et al. revealed that the mismatch of the diameter in the distal stent grafting zone was higher (145.4±34.6% vs. 120.3±16.1%, $p < 0.05$) in patients with DSINE [10]. In our series, Huang et al. also demonstrated that the oversizing of the mean diameter (1.48±0.29 cm vs. 1.22±0.15 cm, $p = 0.039$) or the area (2.39±0.85 cm^2 vs. 1.58±0.42 cm^2, $p = 0.031$) at the distal landing zone was greater in the DSINE group [7]. This potential mechanism to DSINE may be associated with the discrepancy of the diameter or area of the true lumen between the proximal and distal thoracic aorta, and its relationship to the size of the chosen stent graft. In AD, the true lumen is usually narrower at the presumed distal landing zone than that at the proximal landing zone. Xu

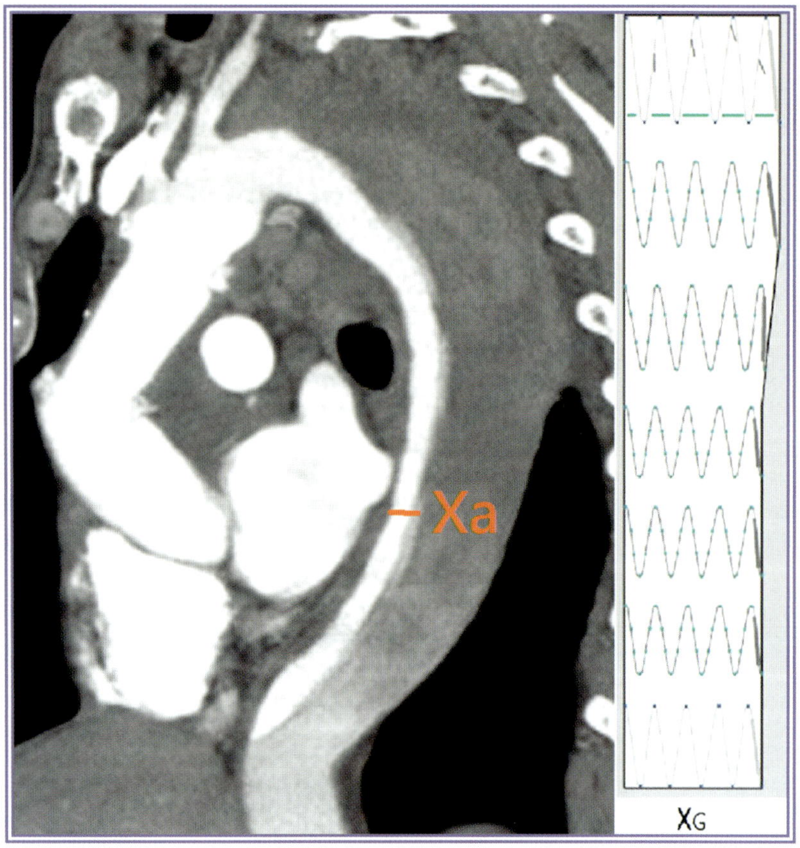

Fig. 30.2 Oversizing ratio = (Xa/XG) – 1. XG, the distal size of the selected stent graft before the procedure; Xa, the size of the true lumen at the presumed level of the distal end of the stent graft before the procedure.

et al. reported the differences in diameter of the true lumen between the aortic arch and the descending aorta in patients with Type B AD [13]. They noted that the diameter in the aortic arch is greater than that in the descending aorta by 22±12% (acute dissection) to 30±11% (chronic dissection). This discrepancy inferred that the diameter of the chosen stent graft according to the proximal landing zone would become substantially oversized at the distal landing part, thus creating an excessive radial force on the dissected intima, and consequently posing a risk to DSINE development. In addition, the preoperative taper ratio (the ratio between the sizes of the true lumen at the proximal landing zone and that at the distal landing zone before the procedure) was noted to be higher in patients with DSINE (40.9±14.1% vs. 25.4±20.2%; $p < 0.05$) [6]. A higher taper ratio means that, during endograft placement, the size of the chosen stent graft planned according to the proximal aortic lumen will become excessively oversized at the distal landing area of aorta, and consequently carry a higher risk for development of DSINE.

Another presumable cause of DSINE is elastic recoil. The tendency of the stent graft to revert to its initial straight form may also induce DSINE. In most TEVAR, the stent graft needs a proximal landing location in the aortic arch and is passively bent to conform to the curvature of the aorta. However, the endograft has the inherent tendency to spring back to its initial straight form. This generates stress along the outer curve of the aorta, which may lead to intimal injury at the distal landing zone and thus the formation of DSINE. To illustrate the tendency of the stent graft to revert to its original straight form, the angle between the distal edge of the stent graft and the continuation of the aortic wall was used to describe the inclination. In a study including 142 patient with Type B AD, the angle was noted to be sharper (149.08±15.09° vs. 166.72±12.47°, $p < 0.005$) in patients with DSINE [6]. From this data, speculations may be made that sharper angles between distal edge of the stent graft and the aortic wall can lead to development of DSINE.

30.3 Prediction and prevention of distal stent graft-induced new entry

Distal Stent Graft-Induced New Entry is not a benevolent event. Its adverse effects are associated with potential life-threatening outcomes. Therefore, prediction and prevention of DSINE are absolutely crucial in TEVAR. On the basis of available studies, oversizing or mismatch is probably the most relevant portending factor. Our published data revealed that a larger oversizing ratio (4.00±2.96 vs. 1.98±0.66, p = 0.031) between the size of the selected stent graft and the true lumen at the presumed distal landing zone is a significant preoperative predictive factor of DSINE [7] (see Fig. 30.1). Worthy of notion, the associated factors were measured by area, not diameter, in this study. The reason for this was that the true lumen in AD is usually elliptical or even crescent in shape. Measuring diameters of an asymmetrical structure is much more complex and much less accurate in estimation and, therefore, not a satisfactory indicator for true lumen measurements. Consequently, the bigger the cross-section area of the selected stent graft is compared to the area of the true lumen of the presumed distal landing zone, i.e. "larger oversizing ratio", the higher the likelihood for DSINE to occur.

Other risk factors for DSINE were reported by Li et al. in a cohort of TEVAR for 579 patients with Type B AD [11], including length of the chosen stent grafts and the timing of stent-graft placement. After a mean follow-up of 47±16 months, they found that stent grafts less than 145 mm in length (odds ratio [OR] 2.268; 95% CI: 1.121-4.587; p = 0.023), and TEVAR performed in the chronic phase (OR 1.935; 95% CI: 1.004-3.731; p = 0.049) were risk factors for DSINE. The results on the length of the stent graft were interpreted to be associated with the leverage of the lesser curvature of the aorta on the endograft. The authors believed that elongating the stent graft in parallel to the straight part of the distal descending aorta would achieve a better conformation and thereby reduce the leverage. The angulation created by the distal edge of the stent graft against the aortic wall will also be minimalized. This is similar to the assumption by an earlier study of Kato et al. [14]. They proposed that the angle between the bottom edge of the stent graft and the aortic wall appears to be a leading factor for the aneurysmal degeneration at the distal end of the graft. Kato et al. [14] also suggested to place several stent grafts until the distal edge of the last endograft is oriented parallel to the aortic wall to avoid DSINE. In our opinion, the leverage effect proposed by Li et al. and the endograft length method proposed by Kato et al. were, in fact, similar to the elastic recoil concept mentioned in the previous paragraph of this topic discussion.

Several preventive techniques have been developed to reduce the formation of DSINE. These procedures are based on three major concepts :

- reducing excessive distal oversizing or mismatch;
- protecting the aortic intima from aortic prosthetic trauma;
- avoiding distal landing in a tortuous portion of the aorta.

To improve oversizing or mismatch ratio at the distal landing zone, endografts with a tapered configuration have been designed. For example, Zenith® TX2® (Cook Medical, Bloomington, IN), Valiant (Medtronic Vascular, Santa Rosa, CA), or Relay® (Bolton Medical, Barcelona, Spain) systems are available commercially nowadays. However, there has been no study published thus far in evaluation of the outcomes of the tapered stent grafts in prevention of DSINE. Alternatively, a bottom-up technique, or the distal small graft-first procedure, is adopted to produce the effect of tapering in diameter or area (Fig. 30.3). In this maneuver, a smaller stent graft is deployed distally, followed by a larger stent graft proximally. This approach had been undertaken at our institution since 2010 when there were no tapered stent grafts available. Our experience in 24 patients with Type B AD showed that both the prestenting and poststenting oversizing ratio, whether in diameter or area, were improved. By using this strategy, the incidence of DSINE was also significantly decreased (36.73% vs. 4.17%, p = 0.004) compared to 49 patients in the control group [9].

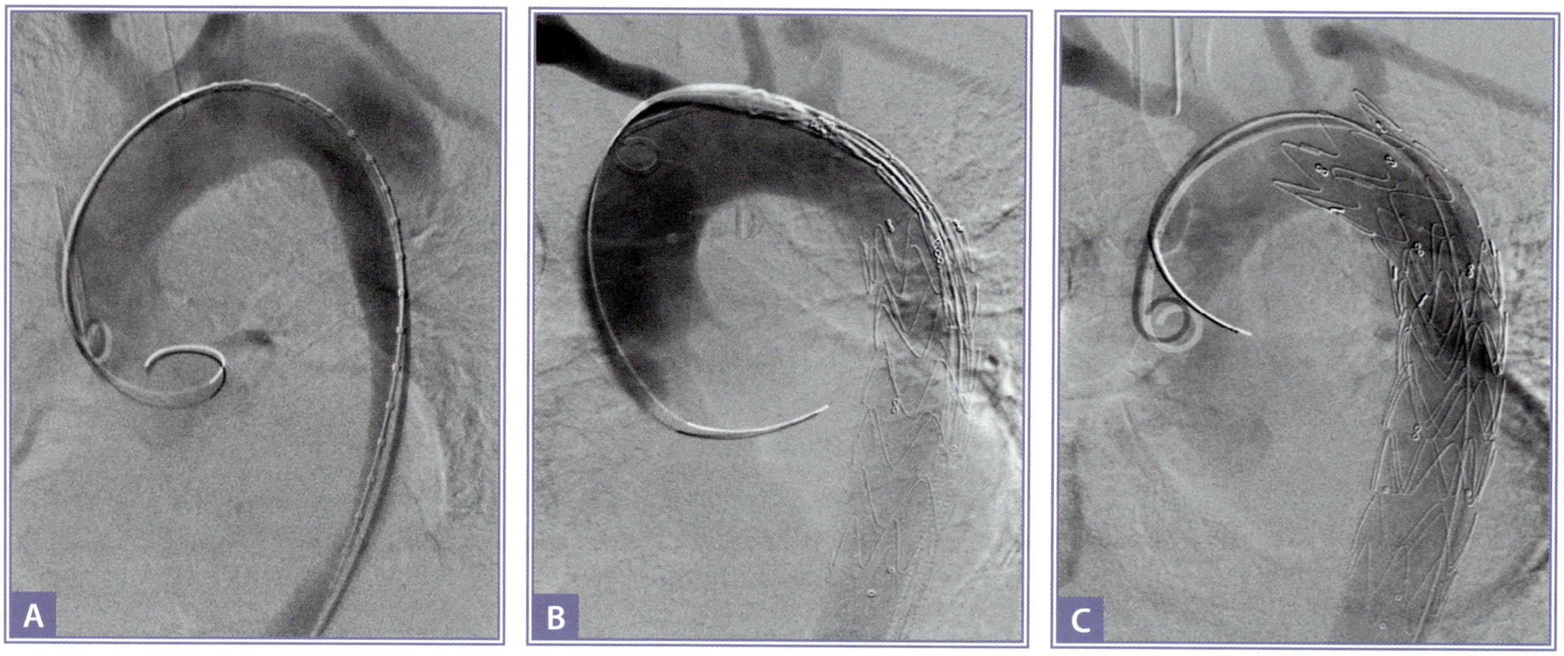

Fig. 30.3 Bottom-up technique or distal small graft-first procedure. **A**, Aortogram and intimal tear located around 2.5 cm distal to the ostium of the left subclavian artery. **B**, Delivery of the proximal larger endograft after deployment of the distal smaller endoprosthesis. **C**, Deployment of the proximal stent graft and exclusion of the intimal tear.

Another method called two-stent graft implantation (TSI) was also proposed to reduce distal oversizing [15]. In contrary to the bottom-up technique, TSI deploys the endoprosthesis consecutively from proximal to distal aorta. After conducting TSI in 72 patients and following up for 10±4 months, TSI provided a mean tapered diameter span of 7.5±1.8 mm and distal oversizing of 11.2±4.1%. There was no DSINE during the follow-up and this favorable result was partly achieved by using a large tapered stent graft in a 10-mm-diameter span as the distal endograft.

Another approach, called the restrictive bare stenting (RBS) technique, was also developed to protect the intima from the excessive radial force of the stent graft at the distal landing zone. This technique involves the placement of a bare stent in the intended distal landing zone of the stent graft, prior to the deployment of the actual stent graft. The bare stent was not oversized and chosen accordingly to the preoperative measurement at the intended distal edge of the stent graft. Feng et al. demonstrated that RBS was associated with a lower incidence of DSINE (0% vs. 2.9%; $p = 0.033$) as was used in 154 patients with Type B AD [10].

Some studies suggested that avoidance of distal landing in a tortuous portion of the aorta or elongation of endografting until the distal end of the last stent graft was aligned parallel to the aortic wall may reduce the stress of the stent graft against the curvature of the aorta [1, 11, 14]. With TSI technique, for example, the deployed length of the stent grafts could be 197.6±20.3 mm. This is another beneficial factor of the TSI method that may play part in reducing the formation of DSINE. Moreover, the PETTICOAT (provisional extension to induce complete attachment) technique may help in reducing the formation of DSINE. This procedure comprises of placing the stent grafts over the primary entry tear proximally, and placing bare metal stents distally to promote true lumen expansion. Previous studies had demonstrated favorable clinical and image outcomes by this technique in management of Type B AD [16, 17]. Our experience with this technique showed another potential benefit in decreasing DSINE. We noticed that only one DSINE occurred in nearly 50 patients of complicated Type B AD who underwent PETTICOAT technique during the follow-up of two years. We postulated that the aortic bare stenting seemingly helps in decreasing the angulation of the aorta at the distal landing area of the stent graft. Further investigation is needed for this proposition to fully determine its value.

30.4 Management of distal stent graft-induced new entry

Upon confirmation of DSINE diagnosis, medical treatment with optimal blood pressure and heart rate control is preferred. Surgical intervention is often needed and close follow-up is mandatory if initial management was conservative treatment. Our indications for re-intervention include: persistent enlargement of the false lumen, contained rupture, pseudoaneurysm formation, malperfusion, or symptomatic presentation. At our institute, the procedures for secondary intervention are performed the same as the standard TEVAR with proper device sizing according to the preceding endografts and true lumen area of presumed distal landing. Nevertheless, paraplegia is a major issue in management of DSINE, because the secondary TEVAR usually involves the lower descending thoracic aorta. To reduce the risk of stent graft-related spinal cord injury, the patency of the left subclavian artery is always preserved either by bypass surgery or endovascular revascularization. The Adamkiewicz arteries localization is attempted by CT preoperatively, and preserved as much as possible during the secondary procedure to reduce the risk of paraplegia. Cerebrospinal fluid (CSF) drainage is set up and relative hypertension (mean arterial pressure between 90 and 100 mmHg) is maintained if the major spinal arteries are planned preoperatively to be sacrificed or if any signs or symptoms related to paraplegia is noted postoperatively.

Our data showed that simple re-endografting seems effective in treating complicated DSINE [8]. Fenestrated or branched endovascular grafts (BEVAR or FEVAR) is an acceptable alternative if the re-intervention involves major branches of the abdominal aorta. Other techniques, such as candy-plug technique [18], may be used in specific situations to avoid extended coverage of the aorta. However, DSINE does recur (Fig. 30.4) and the effectiveness of these managements needs further investigation for validation. Ultimately, open repair or hybrid surgery is indicated when patients are not suitable for sole total endovascular management.

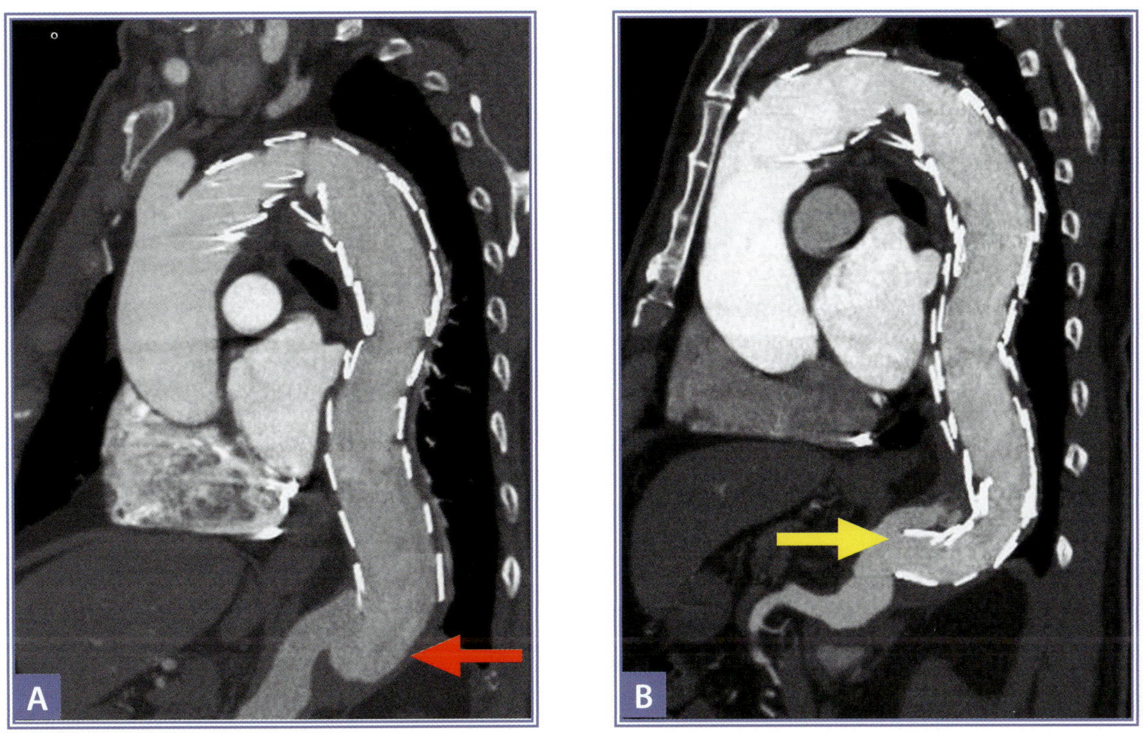

Fig. 30.4 Recurrent DSINE. **A**, First DSINE (red arrow) noted 2 years after initial TEVAR. **B**, Recurrence of DSINE (yellow arrow) at 2 year after secondary TEVAR.

30.5 Conclusion

Distal Stent Graft-Induced New Entry is not rare and is a potentially life-threatening complication of TEVAR. It is related to the stress of the radial force or the elastic recoil of the stent graft on the dissected intima flap. Distal oversizing or mismatch ratio, length of deployed endografts, and/or chronicity of dissection seem predictive of the formation of DSINE. Stent grafts with tapered-diameter design, the bottom-up technique, the two-stent graft implantation, or the restrictive bare stenting can be used to reduce the risk of DSINE. Most of DSINE needs re-intervention. Physicians should be alert to the risks of paraplegia when extended endografting to the lower thoracic aorta is performed. Further investigation is warranted for the effectiveness of the various managements used to prevent or treat DSINE, and long-term follow-up is mandatory to monitor for recurrences.

REFERENCES

1) Dong Z, Fu W, Wang Y, et al. Stent graft-induced new entry after endovascular repair for Stanford type B aortic dissection. J Vasc Surg 2010; 52(6): 1450-7.
2) Yang CP, Hsu CP, Chen WY, et al. Aortic remodeling after endovascular repair with stainless steel-based stent graft in acute and chronic type B aortic dissection. J Vasc Surg 2012; 55(6): 1600-10.
3) Riambau V, Guerrero F, Murillo I, Rivadeneira M, Montana X, Matute P. Stent grafting-related acute type B redissection. Vascular 2008; 16(2): 101-5.
4) Xu SD, Huang FJ, Yang JF, et al. Early and midterm results of thoracic endovascular aortic repair of chronic type B aortic dissection. J Thorac Cardiovasc Surg 2010; 139(6): 1548-53.
5) Hughes GC, Ganapathi AM, Keenan JE, et al. Thoracic endovascular aortic repair for chronic DeBakey IIIb aortic dissection. Ann Thorac Surg 2014; 98(6): 2092-7; discussion 8.
6) Janosi RA, Tsagakis K, Bettin M, et al. Thoracic aortic aneurysm expansion due to late distal stent graft-induced new entry. Catheter Cardiovasc Interv 2015; 85(2): E43-53.
7) Huang CY, Weng SH, Weng CF, et al. Factors predictive of distal stent graft-induced new entry after hybrid arch elephant trunk repair with stainless steel-based device in aortic dissection. J Thorac Cardiovasc Surg 2013; 146(3): 623-30.
8) Weng SH, Weng CF, Chen WY, et al. Reintervention for distal stent graft-induced new entry after endovascular repair with a stainless steel-based device in aortic dissection. J Vasc Surg 2013; 57(1): 64-71.
9) Chen IM, Huang CY, Weng SH, et al. Implantation sequence modification averts distal stent graft-induced new entry after endovascular repair of Stanford type B aortic dissection. J Vasc Surg 2016; 64(2): 281-8.
10) Feng J, Lu Q, Zhao Z, et al. Restrictive bare stent for prevention of stent graft-induced distal redissection after thoracic endovascular aortic repair for type B aortic dissection. J Vasc Surg 2013; 57(2 Suppl): 44S-52S.
11) Li Q, Wang LF, Ma WG, et al. Risk Factors for distal stent graft-induced new entry following endovascular repair of type B aortic dissection. J Thorac Dis 2015; 7(11): 10.
12) Karmonik C, Bismuth J, Davies MG, Shah DJ, Younes HK, Lumsden AB. A computational fluid dynamics study pre- and post-stent graft placement in an acute type B aortic dissection. Vasc Endovascular Surg 2011; 45(2): 157-64.
13) Xu SD, Huang FJ, Du JH, et al. A study of aortic dimension in type B aortic dissection. Interact Cardiovasc Thorac Surg 2008; 7(2): 244-8.
14) Kato N, Shimono T, Hirano T, et al. Midterm results of stent-graft repair of acute and chronic aortic dissection with descending tear: the complication-specific approach. J Thorac Cardiovasc Surg 2002; 124(2): 306-12.
15) Huang X, Huang L, Sun L, et al. Endovascular repair of Stanford B aortic dissection using two stent grafts with different sizes. J Vasc Surg 2015; 62(1): 43-8.
16) Lombardi JV, Cambria RP, Nienaber CA, et al. Prospective multicenter clinical trial (STABLE) on the endovascular treatment of complicated type B aortic dissection using a composite device design. J Vasc Surg 2012; 55(3): 629-40 e2.
17) Alsac JM, Girault A, El Batti S, et al. Experience of the Zenith Dissection Endovascular System in the emergency setting of malperfusion in acute type B dissections. J Vasc Surg 2014; 59(3): 645-50.
18) Kolbel T, Lohrenz C, Kieback A, Diener H, Debus ES, Larena-Avellaneda A. Distal false lumen occlusion in aortic dissection with a homemade extra-large vascular plug: the candy-plug technique. J Endovasc Ther 2013; 20(4): 484-9.

31

Open surgical treatment of chronic Type B aortic dissection (dissecting aneurysms)

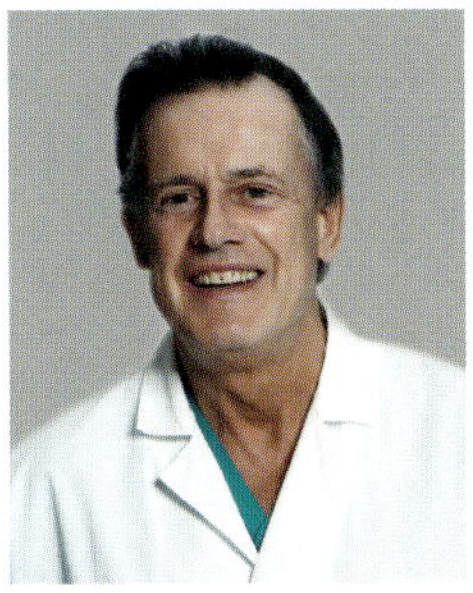

Roberto Chiesa, Germano Melissano, Andrea L. Kahlberg,
Enrico Rinaldi, Sara Spelta, Alessandro Grandi and Domenico Baccellieri

31.1 Introduction

Chronic Type B aortic dissection (AD) is the second most common cause of thoracoabdominal aortic aneurysm (TAAA) development after degenerative etiology. Among patients undergoing surgery for TAAA, up to 24% suffer from chronic dissection [1]. In approximately 20-40% of patients with AD (both types A and B), the descending thoracic and thoracoabdominal aorta may become aneurysmal within 2 to 5 years [2]. The presence of blood flow in the false lumen is the most significant risk factor for an increase in diameter, with aneurysmal degeneration involving the descending thoracic aorta usually starting from the isthmic region and subsequently extending to the abdominal aortic tract or even to the iliac arteries [2].

A dissecting aneurysm can have a similar or faster growth rate compared to a degenerative thoracic aneurysm [3, 4], but its rupture rate is higher [5]. Hence, the indication to surgery for asymptomatic dissecting TAAA is usually considered a diameter ≥5.5 cm, or even lower in the case of associated connective tissue disorders.

Historically, open treatment of dissecting TAAA consisted of graft replacement with reattachment of the main aortic branches by means of the inclusion technique, which was introduced by S.E. Crawford in the 1970s, and mastered by Houston surgeons in the following decades. As open repair of dissecting and degenerative TAAA is known to be associated with significant morbidity and mortality, great efforts have been made in recent decades to improve surgical outcomes, resulting in the current use of a multimodal approach with several surgical and anesthesiological adjuncts, in order to maximize organ protection and prevent end-organ ischemia [6]. In this chapter, we will describe our current strategies used prior, during, and immediately after open surgical treatment of TAAA following chronic Type B AD.

31.2 Preoperative vascular imaging

An accurate preoperative imaging is required in all patients to precisely assess the aortic anatomy, fully evaluate the aortic main branches, and obtain information about the spinal cord

Roberto Chiesa (chiesa.roberto@unisr.it)
Vita-Salute San Raffaele University, Scientific Institute Ospedale San Raffaele,
Milan, Italy

G. Melissano - R. Chiesa (eds), Aortic Dissection patients true stories and the innovations that saved their lives

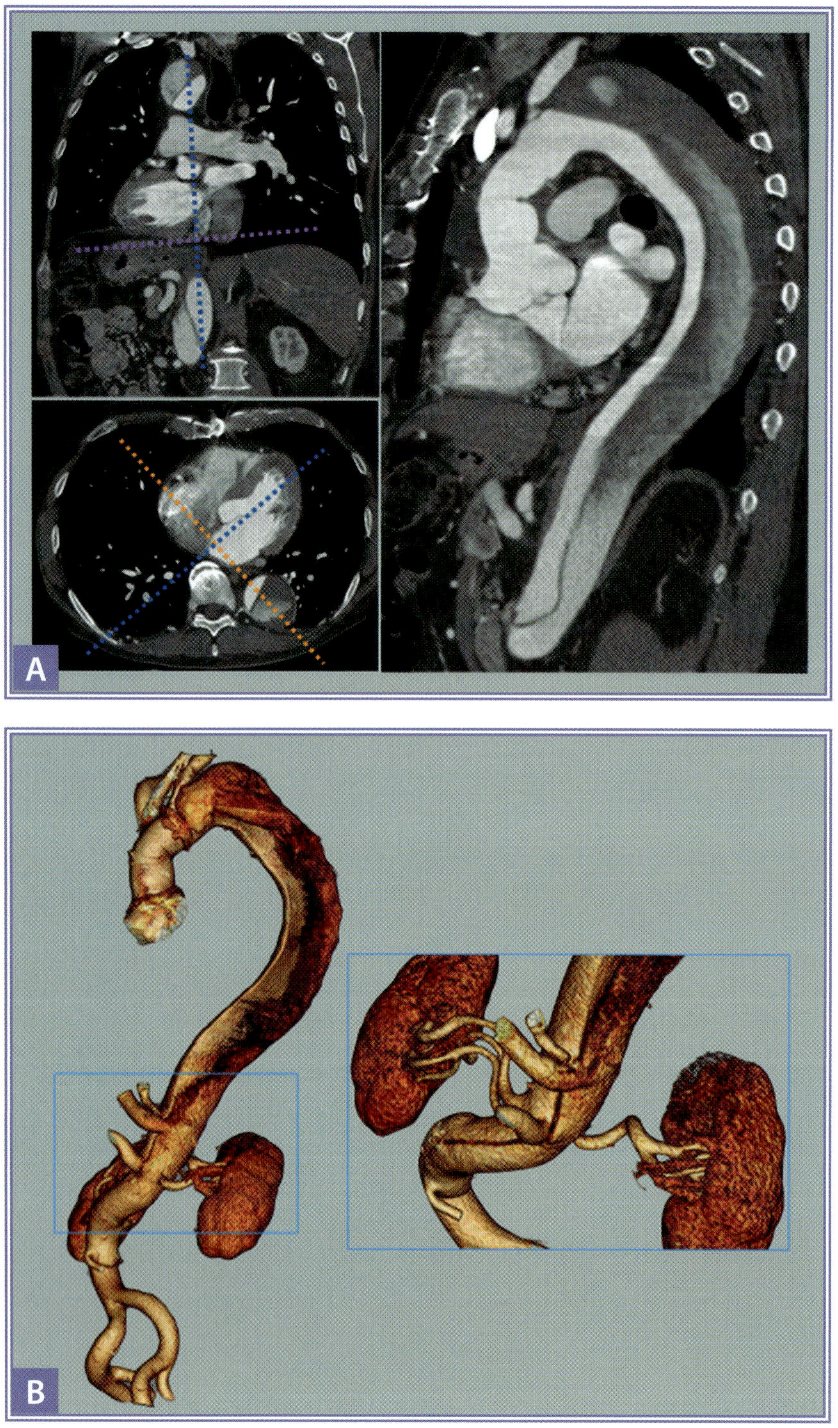

Fig. 31.1 **A**, Thanks to multi-planar reformatting, the curved path of the dilated dissected thoracic aorta is well reproduced and the true and the false lumen are properly visualized. **B**, 3D volume rendering allows to determine the conformation of the entire dissection and the relative position of the visceral and renal vessels, necessary for planning a tailored re-implantation strategy.

vasculature, in order to plan the best surgical strategy tailored to the individual. Provided that there are no specific contraindications, our preoperative imaging protocol includes contrast enhanced computed tomography (CT).

Post-processing of CT images using reformatting software and workstations allows to visualize specific morphologic issues related to AD, needed for a thorough surgical planning. In particular, the aorta and, even more so, the dissecting lamella have a tortuous path, which may be correctly analyzed using oblique multi-planar reformattings (MPRs), as shown in Figure 31.1. Maximum intensity projection (MIP) protocols are usually avoided in the case of dissections, because information on the dissecting lamella and parietal thrombus is lost.

After obtaining an optimal projection of the aorta, the true cross-sectional diameter of the aneurysm is measured and the true and the false lumen are properly visualized, as well as the relationship of the dissection with the major aortic branches, in order to define the extent of the disease. Also, the quality of the aortic wall at the intended clamping sites, the presence, extension, and characteristics of the thrombus, and the number and location of main and secondary tears in the dissecting lamella have to be carefully evaluated.

Special attention must be paid to the quality and relative position of the visceral vessels ostia, in order to plan a tailored preimplantation strategy (e.g. Carrel patch inclusion vs. individual bypass or multi-branched pre-sewn grafts) or prepare associated endovascular maneuvers (e.g. direct stenting or use of sutureless anastomosis).

Finally, preoperative knowledge of the arterial supply to the spinal cord is extremely useful for procedure planning and risk stratification, in order to prevent spinal cord ischemia and subsequent paraparesis or paraplegia (see Chapter 36) [7].

31.3 Patient optimization

An adequate preoperative assessment of the patient's physiologic reserve of cardiac, pulmonary, and renal function, along with an accurate knowledge of the cerebral and spinal cord vascular anatomy are useful for evaluating the operative risk, planning the best operative strategy and taking early additional perioperative precautions.

31.3.1 Cardiac optimization

Preoperative transthoracic echocardiography is a satisfactory non-invasive screening method that evaluates both valvular and biventricular function. Exercise testing or dipyridamole-thallium myocardial scanning identifies regions of the myocardium that are reversibly ischemic, and in patients with a significant history of angina or reduced ejection fraction cardiac catheterization with coronary arteriography is indicated [8].

CT coronary angiography has emerged as a less-invasive method to visualize the coronary arterial anatomy. Multi-detector scanners allow one to obtain images at certain specific phases of the cardiac cycle with the least coronary artery motion, providing information also about the aorta and left ventricular ejection fraction [9].

In patients undergoing thoracic aortic open repair, severe coronary artery occlusive disease is treated with percutaneous transluminal angioplasty prior to aortic surgery. Preoperative coronary stenting is usually accomplished with bare-metal stents, trying to avoid the use of drug-eluting stents requiring prolonged (>6 months) double antiplatelet therapy that in turn increases the risk of perioperative bleeding. Recently, the novel COMBO stent (OrbusNeich, Fort Lauderdale, FL), which combines sirolimus elution with a $CD34^+$ antibody to attract endothelial progenitor cells and thus enhance early endothelialization, is currently under investigation vis-à-vis its potential to reduce double antiplatelet therapy duration from 6 to only 3 months after stent implantation [10]. Its use may be considered in patients needing coronary stenting, who are also affected by large dissecting TAAAs requiring surgical repair in a timely fashion. Nowadays, surgical myocardial revascularization by means of coronary-aortic bypass grafting is limited to selected patients in whom percutaneous transluminal angioplasty would be inappropriate.

31.3.2 Renal optimization

Renal function is a well-established predictor of postoperative outcome [11]. The National Kidney Foundation currently recommends the use of estimated glomerular filtration rate (eGFR) to assess renal function in order to avoid the misclassification of patients on the basis of serum creatinine levels alone [12]. Based on the GFR assessment, chronic kidney disease has been shown to be a strong predictor of death after thoracic aneurysm repair for both open and endovascular procedures, even in patients without clinical evidence of preoperative renal disease [13]. Renal size, corticomedullary ratio, presence of renal cysts, and renal artery anatomy are determined from angio-CT/angio-magnetic resonance (MR) and by ultrasound. Occlusive disease of the renal arteries may be treated during aortic repair, and patients are not rejected as surgical candidates based on impaired renal function only.

Adequate hydration, diuretics administration and premedication with N-acetylcysteine and endovenous bicarbonates may be used in patients with chronic kidney disease to reduce preoperative serum creatinine levels and optimize renal function [14].

31.3.3 Pulmonary optimization

Evaluation of pulmonary function with arterial blood gases and spirometry is performed for all patients undergoing open surgery of the thoracic/thoracoabdominal aorta. In patients with a forced expiratory volume in 1 sec (FEV_1) lower than 1.0 L and a partial pressure of carbon dioxide (PCO_2) higher than 45 mmHg, pulmonary function can be improved by stopping smoking, progressively treating bronchitis by means of steroids and bronchodilators, losing weight and following a general exercise program for a period of 1 to 6 months before operation. However, in patients with very large or symptomatic aortic aneurysms, the operation often cannot be delayed despite their poor pulmonary function. An endovascular approach may be evaluated in these cases, when feasible.

Otorhinolaryngological evaluation by means of fiberoptic nasopharyngoscopy is routinely performed to assess respiratory space, vocal cord motility and possible paralysis that may be due to recurrent laryngeal nerve compression by the false lumen.

31.3.4 Neuropsychological evaluation

A brain CT scan together with a neuropsychological evaluation by an independent neurologist is obtained for all elective patients. Preoperative brain CT scan is evaluated in order to detect possible contraindications to spinal cord fluid drainage. Optimization of psychiatric disorders, and potential pharmacological improvement of mood tone are useful to enhance the patient's compliance in the perioperative period, increasing adherence to medical prescriptions and physical rehabilitation therapy. Preoperative somatosensory evoked potentials (SSEPs) and motor evoked potentials (MEPs) are evaluated to provide the basal peripheral neurological condition for comparison to the intraoperative one, and can drive consequent surgical and anesthesiological maneuvers to decrease spinal cord ischemia risk, such as increasing the spinal fluid drainage rate, blood pressure, volemia, hematocrit, oxygenation, or providing early revascularization of intercostal and iliac arteries [15].

31.4 Surgical strategy

31.4.1 Multisystemic protection strategies

A multimodal anesthesiological approach and complex multisystemic monitoring prior, during, and after dissecting TAAA open repair are of paramount importance, and involve collaboration with many specialists (Fig. 31.2).

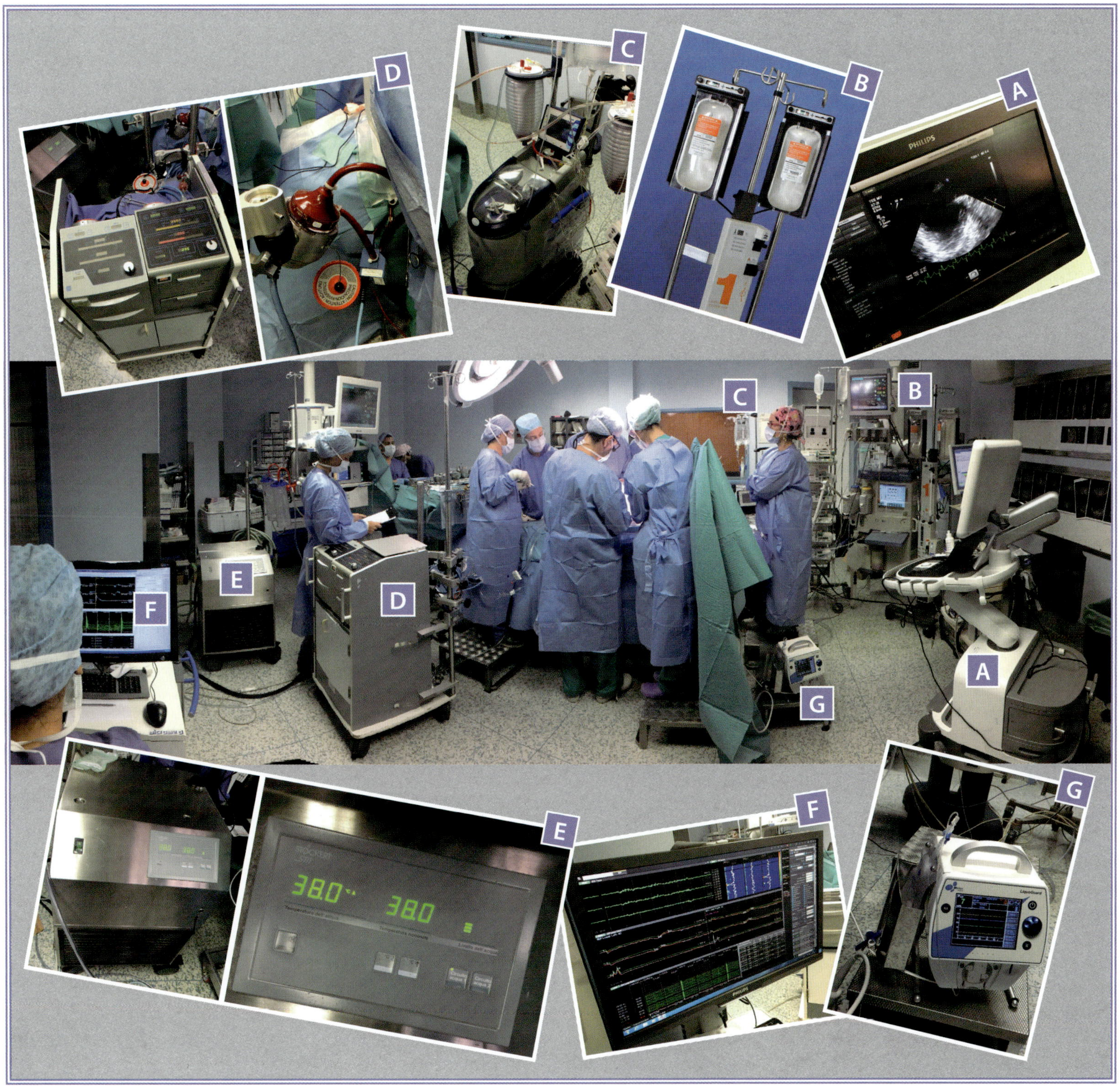

Fig. 31.2 Multidisciplinary approach to TAAA surgery. The cardiovascular anesthesiologist keeps the patient under continuous monitoring and performs transesophageal echocardiography (**A**) in order to evaluate cardiac function during the whole procedure. The anesthesiologist modulates fluid exchange and body temperature with a pressure infusion system and fluid warmer (**B**). Intraoperative blood salvage is performed during TAAA surgery. The cell saver (**C**) is used to recover the blood lost during the procedure and to re-infuse it into the patient. **D**, The perfusionist controls and modulates the left heart bypass performed with Bio-Medicus® Perfusion System (Medtronic, Minneapolis, MN), in agreement with the anesthesiologists. A circulating water mattress with heat exchanger (**E**) is placed under the patient, in order to assist body temperature management. The neurologist checks the motor-evoked and somatosensory-evoked potentials to assess spinal cord integrity (**F**). The LiquoGuard® (Möller Medical, Fulda, Germany) (**G**) allows simultaneous cerebrospinal fluid (CSF) pressure measurements and drainage intraoperatively and during the first 48-72 hours after the surgical procedure.

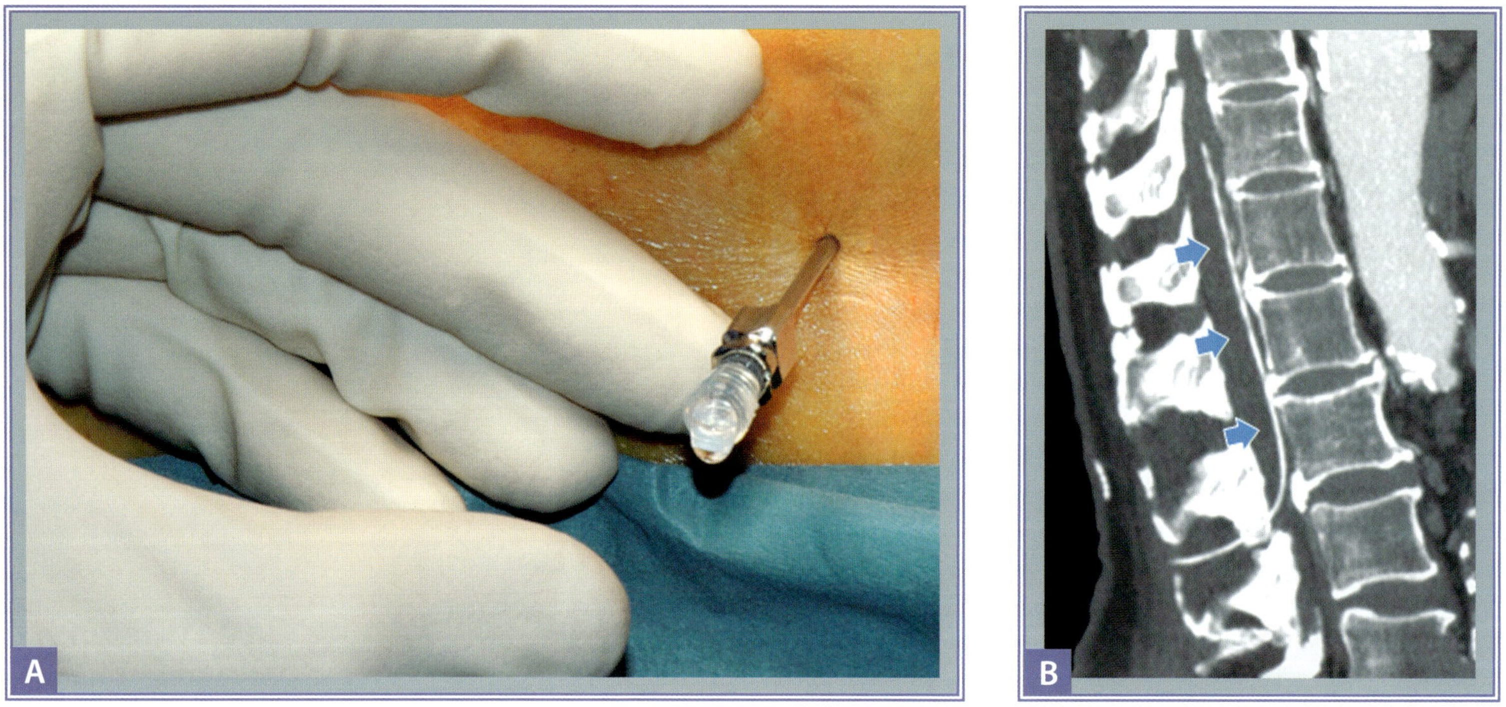

Fig. 31.3 Once the dura mater has been punctured with the introducer needle (**A**), a drainage catheter is inserted 8 to 10 cm beyond the tip of the needle into the subarachnoid space (**B**). After the drain has been secured to the patient, it can be connected to the pressure transducer and baseline measurements can then be made.

Perioperative anesthesiological management is described in detail in Chapter 38. Briefly, blood pressure is monitored invasively through a radial cannula and a femoral cannula that monitors distal perfusion during aortic clamping and left heart bypass (LHBP). In dissecting thoracoabdominal aneurysms, a differential blood pressure between the radial and femoral cannulas is not uncommon: in these cases, it is important to assess the difference at the beginning, and take it into account during the surgical procedure.

Orotracheal intubation is performed using a double-lumen endotracheal tube, in order to maintain a unilateral right ventilation during aortic isolation and reconstruction. Intraoperative transesophageal echocardiography is used to evaluate cardiac function, output and volemia throughout the procedure; in dissections, it is also able to detect if guidewires used for cannulation are correctly placed in the true lumen and can immediately detect a disastrous complication such as retrograde Type A AD after proximal clamping (see Chapter 40).

After anesthesia is induced and prior to surgical incision, the dura mater is punctured with an introducer needle and a standard lumbar CSF drainage catheter (Integra LifeSciences, Plainsboro, NJ) is inserted 8 to 10 cm beyond the tip of the needle into the subarachnoid space for the cerebrospinal fluid (CSF) drainage (Fig. 31.3). The CSF pressure is usually maintained during the first 48-72 hours at 8-10 mmHg using an automatic system (LiquoGuard®, Möller Medical, Fulda, Germany) allowing simultaneously CSF pressure measurements and CSF drainage by a closed system with dual pressure sensors with an electronically controlled peristaltic pump (Fig. 31.2 G).

Intraoperatively, MEP and SSEP monitoring is performed to assess spinal cord integrity, and guide intraoperative strategies to prevent neurologic deficits. Based on decrease or loss of MEPs and SSEPs, intraoperative modifications (spinal fluid drainage, blood pressure, volemia, hematocrit, oxygenation, early revascularization of intercostal and iliac arteries) can be made when necessary.

31.4.2 Surgical technique

The thoracic incision varies in length and level depending on the extent of the aneurysm, but it is usually made between the 5th and 7th intercostal ribs. Section of the rib posteriorly of the rib or, if necessary, its whole resection associated to a gentle and progressive use of the retractor is useful to reduce thoracic wall trauma and fractures; antero-laterally, the incision curves gently as it crosses the costal margin, reducing the risk of tissue necrosis. The pleural space is entered after single right lung ventilation has been initiated. Single-lung ventilation is maintained throughout the aortic replacement.

After the thoracoabdominal incision, a limited circumferential section of the diaphragm is routinely carried out, sparing the phrenic center so as to reduce respiratory weaning time. An involvement of the phrenic center leading to paralysis of the left hemidiaphragm produced by its radial division to the aortic hiatus could contribute significantly to postoperative respiratory failure [16].

Due to the inflammatory reaction in the acute phase of dissection, pleural adhesions are quite common in chronic AD. In these cases it is important to perform a limited tissue dissection to minimize pulmonary bleeding.

Special care must be taken when isolating the proximal aortic neck, which can be encircled using a vessel-loop. The vagus nerve and the origin of the recurrent nerve must be identified, since they can be damaged during isolation of the aortic isthmus and clamping maneuvers. Identification and clipping of some "high" (T1-T6) intercostal arteries can sometimes facilitate the preparation for the proximal anastomosis, thus reducing aortic bleeding. The upper abdominal aortic segment is exposed via a transperitoneal approach; the retroperitoneum is entered lateral to the left colon, and medial visceral rotation is performed so that the left colon, spleen, and left kidney can be retracted anteriorly and to the right. A transperitoneal approach allows direct view of the abdominal organs to evaluate the efficacy of revascularization at the end of aortic repair.

Cross-clamping of the descending thoracic aorta leads to several hemodynamic disturbances, including severe afterload increase and organ ischemia. The technique for distal aortic perfusion with LHBP has proved to be extremely useful during aortic repair [1]. The main rationale for the use of LHBP is the perfusion of distal organs with concomitant reduction of cardiac post-load during clamping of the distal arch/descending thoracic aorta. The basic circuit for LHBP includes an inflow cannula, an inline centrifugal pump without a cardiotomy reservoir or oxygenator, and an outflow cannula. In preparation for LHBP and aortic clamping, to reduce bleeding from the extensive tissue exposure, intravenous heparin is administered (70 IU/kg).

The inflow cannula is placed in the left superior pulmonary vein (20 Fr moldable cannula) to reach the left atrium, and the arterial blood is then reinfused into the femoral artery. In chronic aortic dissections, proximal cannulation of the aorta should be avoided in favor of pulmonary vein cannulation. After left groin cut-down and surgical exposure of the common femoral artery, a percutaneous outflow cannula (14-16 Fr) is placed by means of an over-the-wire technique (.035") and carefully progressed into the non-dissected segment of the left iliac axis (Fig. 31.4). The cannula is then secured with a purse-string suture and the artery is not occluded, allowing distal perfusion of the ipsilateral limb during assisted circulation. A "Y" bifurcation is connected to the circuit and is provided with two occlusion/perfusion catheters (9 Fr) for selective perfusion of the visceral vessels.

In most cases of chronic Type B dissection, proximal aortic clamping is done between the left common carotid artery (LCCA) and the left subclavian artery (LSA), allowing the proximal anastomosis to be performed at a healthy and less fragile aortic site. In a few selected cases, when the location, extent, and severity of disease precludes placement of a proximal aortic clamp distally to the LCCA, hypothermic circulatory arrest is performed to allow proximal anastomosis to be completed.

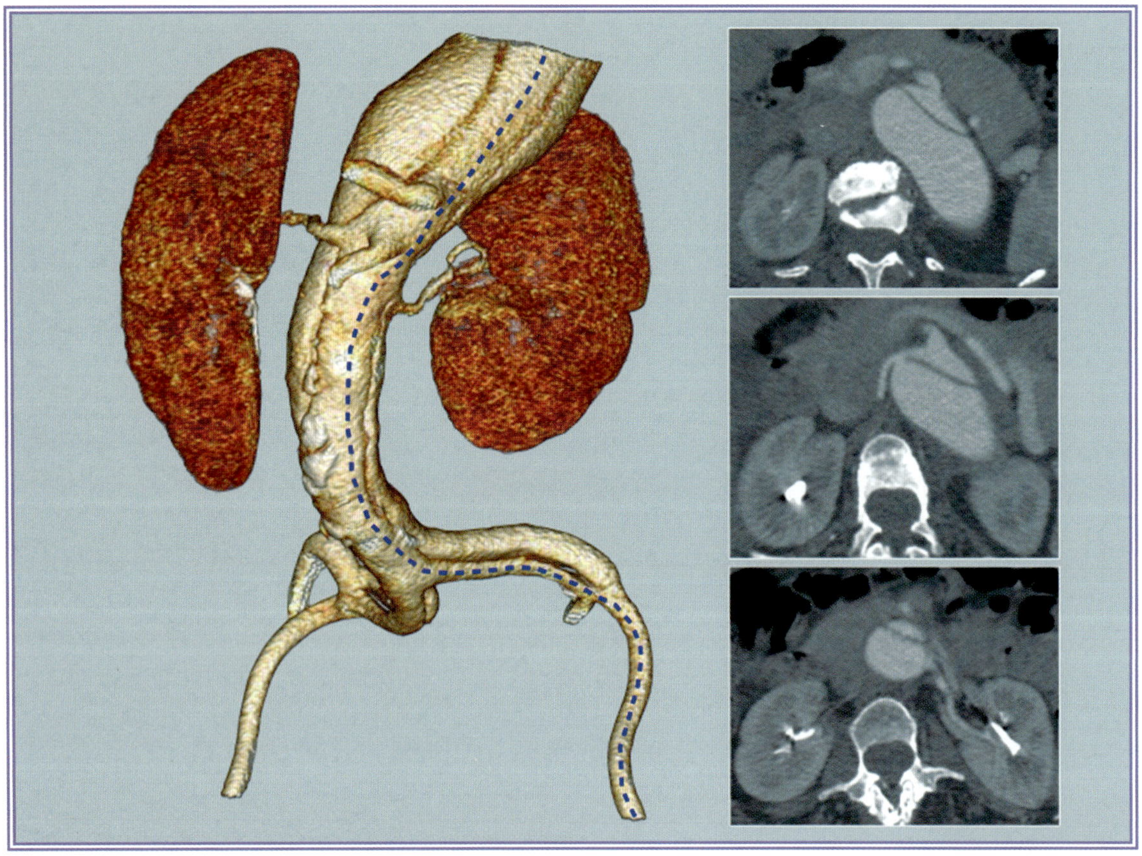

Fig. 31.4 Preoperative evaluation with angio-CT is important to assess the extent to which the dissection has involved the iliac arteries, and the origins of the visceral vessels. The blue line on the 3D volume rendering underlines the partially compressed true lumen; in the axial scans one can distinguish the origins of the visceral and renal vessels from the true and false lumen.

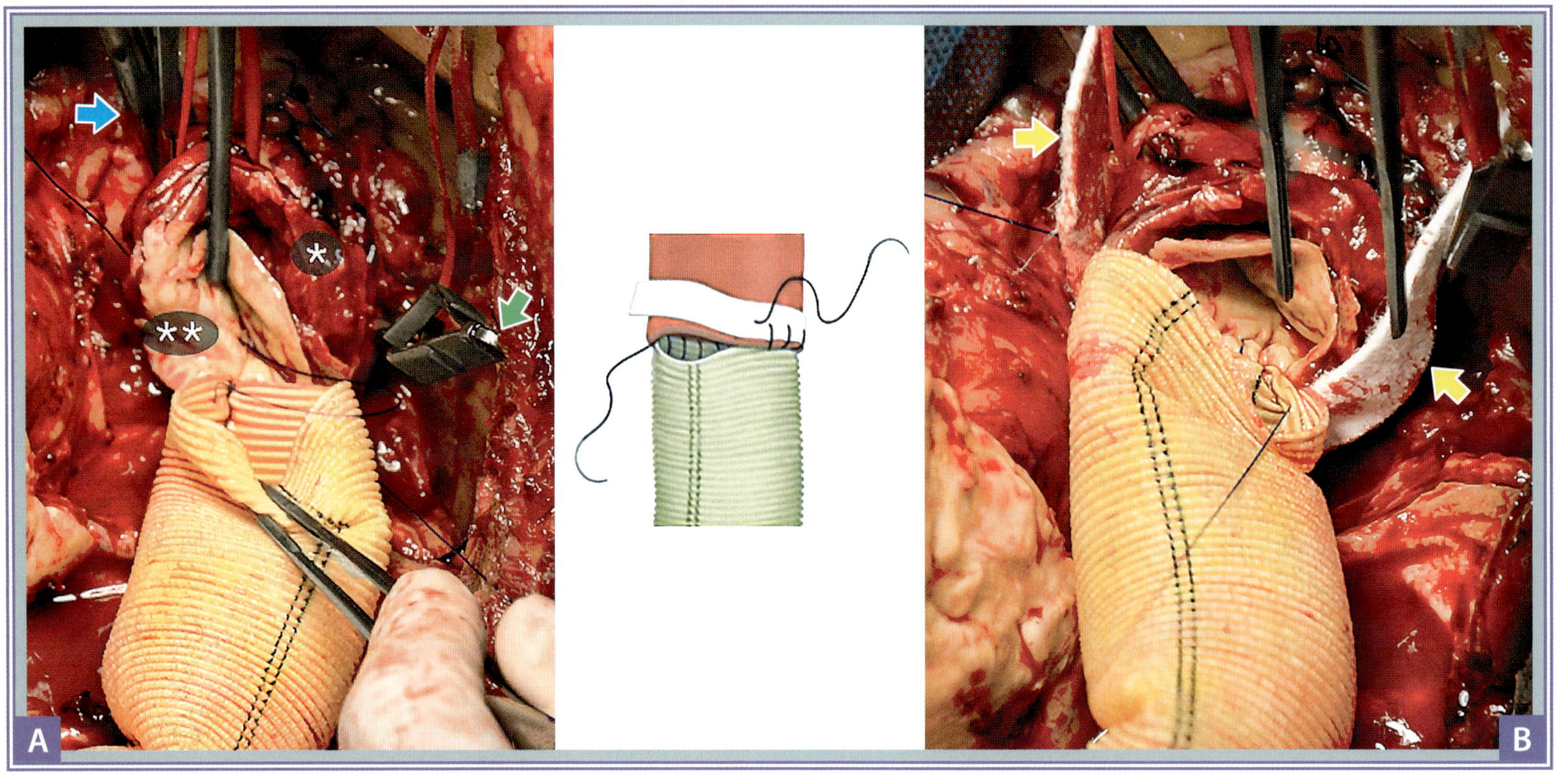

Fig. 31.5 Proximal anastomosis. **A**, The proximal aortic clamp is placed between left common carotid artery (LCCA) and left subclavian artery (LSA) (blue arrow) after the LSA has been selectively clamped (green arrow). The thoracic aorta is completely transected and the false (*) and the true (**) lumen are visualized. **B**, The proximal end of the graft is sutured to the descending thoracic aorta with a 2/0 or 3/0 polypropylene running suture reinforced with a strip of Teflon felt (yellow arrows).

Once the proximal aspect of the TAAA is isolated between clamps, the descending thoracic aorta is transected and separated from the esophagus. The proximal end of the graft is sutured to the descending thoracic aorta, usually using a 2/0 or 3/0 monofilament polypropylene suture in a running fashion. The anastomosis can be reinforced with multiple small Teflon pledgets, with one strip of Teflon felt, or even a double layer of Teflon felt placed inside and outside the aortic wall as a "sandwich" (Fig. 31.5).

The clamp is then removed and reapplied onto the abdominal aorta above the celiac axis (sequential cross-clamping). A longitudinal aortotomy is performed with a complete septotomy. Reimplantation of intercostal arteries to the aortic graft plays a critical role in spinal cord protection. Critical patent segmental arteries from T8 to L2, and/or other specific ones identified by preoperative CT as a candidate source of the Adamkiewicz artery, are temporarily occluded with Pruitt (LeMaitre Vascular, Burlington, MA) catheters to avoid the blood steal phenomenon, then selectively reattached to the graft by means of aortic patch or graft interposition. In dissecting aneurysms, most of the patent intercostal arteries arise from the false lumen. The reimplantation can be technically demanding, and the use of reinforcing Teflon pledgets and strips is often indicated (Fig. 31.6).

When the aneurysmal evolution is limited to the descending thoracic aortic tract, replacement only of the thoracic aorta can be performed with a supradiaphragmatic or supraceliac "double-barrel" distal anastomosis. In this case, the septotomy may be extended distally across the abdominal portion in order to reduce the risk of malperfusion.

In the case of thoracoabdominal dilatation, the distal clamp is moved below the renal arteries and the aneurysm is opened below the diaphragm. Visceral isothermic hematic perfusion

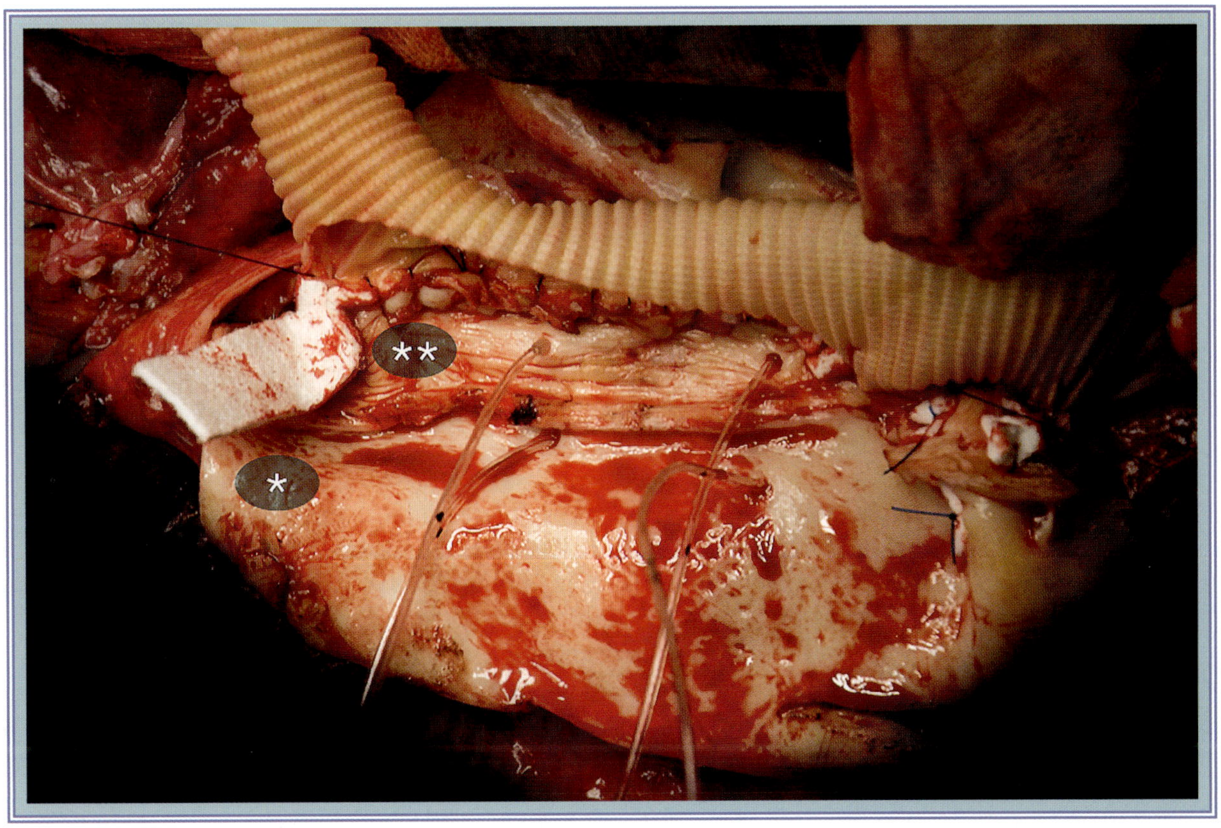

Fig. 31.6 Critical intercostal arteries arising from the false (*) and the true (**) lumen are temporarily occluded with Pruitt catheters and selectively reattached to the graft by an aortic patch or sutured.

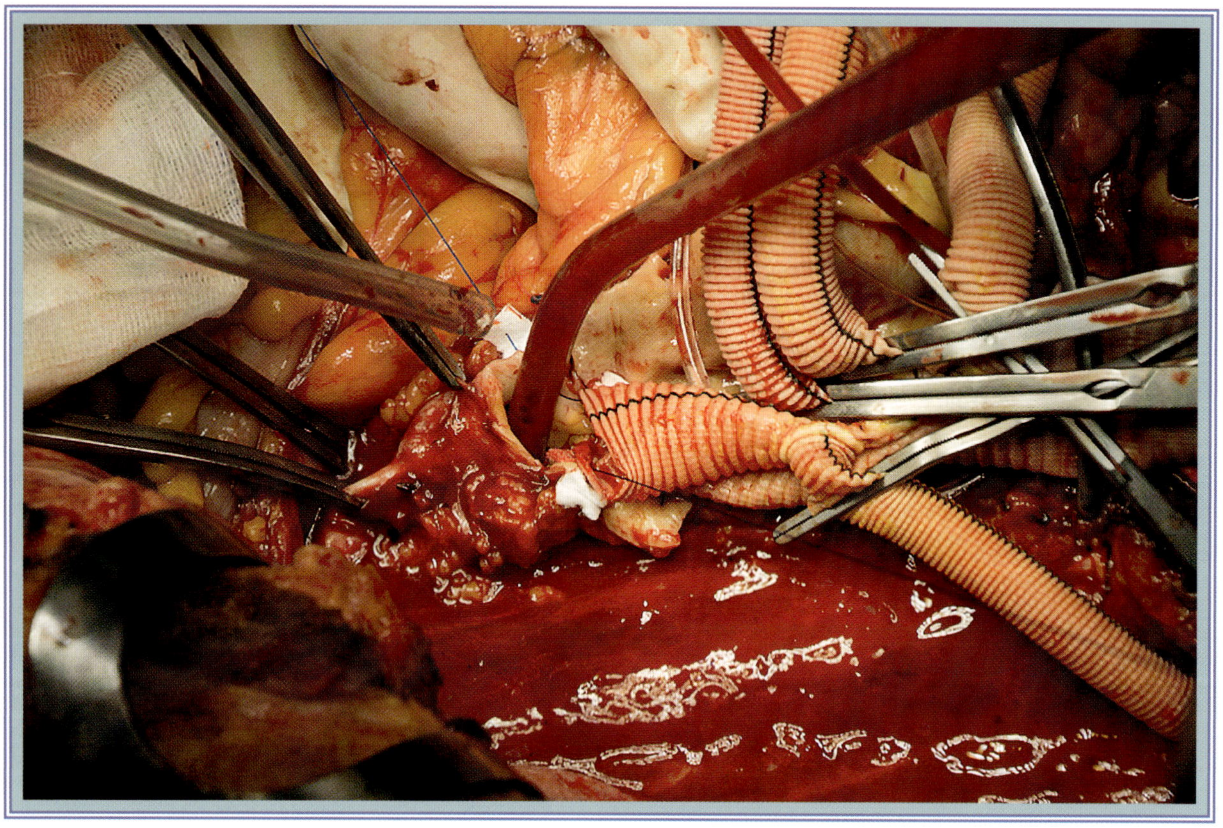

Fig. 31.7 Distal anastomosis. In the case of a multi-branched aortic graft, the distal anastomosis is performed before reattachment of the visceral and renal vessels in order to restore first the antegrade flow to the iliac and hypogastric arteries. During this period, visceral perfusion is maintained by the left heart by pass (LHBP).

is then maintained by the pump with irrigation-perfusion catheters of the same size (9 Fr) inserted selectively into the celiac trunk and the superior mesenteric artery. Selective cold perfusion of the renal arteries is performed with Custodiol (histidine-tryptophan-ketoglutarate, Essential Pharmaceuticals, Ewing, NJ) [17]. Special attention must be paid when inserting the cannula in a visceral vessel that might be involved by the dissection. For reimplantation of the visceral arteries, a side cut is tailored in the graft, and the celiac trunk, superior mesenteric artery, and renal arteries are reattached by means of a Carrel patch. If the dissecting lamella involves the origin of the visceral vessels it must be carefully removed at this time. In some cases, a direct stenting of the vessel ostia could also be useful. The Carrel patch is usually limited to not more than three vessels to avoid large aortic wall islands, which are known to be at risk of further aneurysmal degeneration in time [18].

The remaining vessels to be reimplanted, in particular the left renal artery, are usually reattached separately by a 6-8 mm Dacron graft interposition or using the Gore® Hybrid Vascular Graft (W. L. Gore and Associates, Flagstaff, AZ) for a distal "sutureless anastomosis" (Fig. 31.7). This ePTFE graft is composed of a distal section, radially supported by a nitinol self-expandable stent that allows for a sutureless anastomosis and prevents kink [19].

After reattaching the vessels included in the Carrel patch, we prefer to restore first the antegrade flow to the iliac and hypogastric arteries by completing the distal anastomosis (Fig. 31.8), and then reattach the remaining renovisceral vessels (mainly the left renal artery), provided that an adequate cold perfusion can be maintained throughout the procedure. After unclamping and renal reperfusion, indigotindisulfonate sodium (40 mg) is administered intravenously, and its urine excretion is verified thereafter.

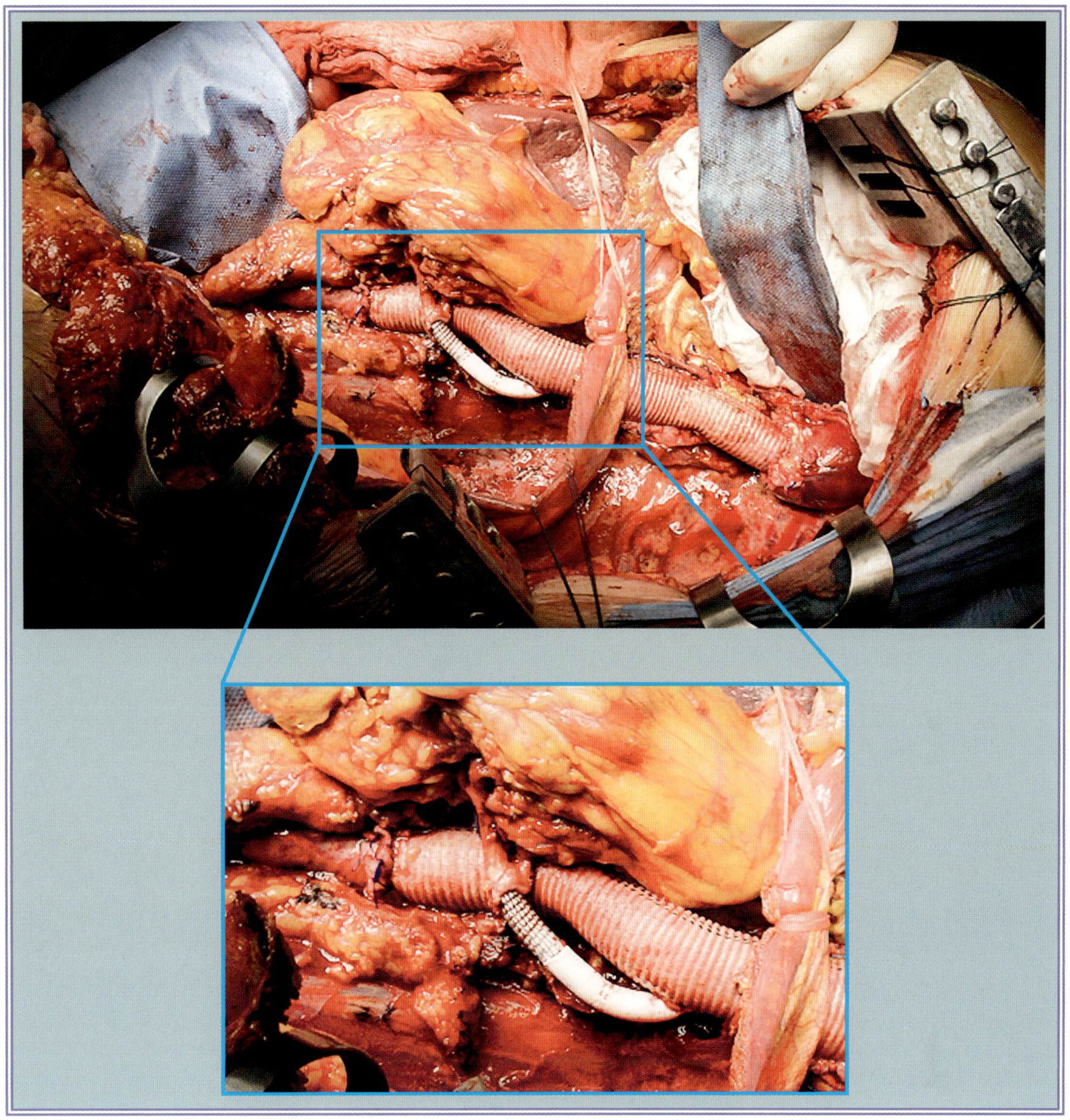

Fig. 31.8 Thoracoabdominal aortic aneurysm surgical repair with reimplantation of the celiac trunk, superior mesenteric artery and right renal artery in a Carrel patch; the left renal artery is subsequently reattached separately by a 8 mm Gore® Hybrid Vascular Graft.

31.4.3 Multi-branched grafts

The reimplantation of a large amount of native aorta in the inclusion technique for TAAA repair carries the risk of subsequent recurrent aneurysm formation [18]. Techniques proposed to reduce the incidence of visceral aortic patch degeneration include routine exclusion of the left renal artery from the Carrel patch, or single-vessel reattachments using commercially available pre-sewn multi-branched aortic grafts. These individual anastomoses can be safely accomplished, especially in the case of increased distance between the visceral vessel ostia (i.e. when the visceral segment of the aorta is involved by severe aneurysmal degeneration). If vessels originate close together, the use of a multi-branched graft may be technically demanding. In this case, a separate extended exposure of the visceral vessel is performed, with transection of each artery at its origin, and end-to-end anastomoses with the graft branches. Additionally, in order to reduce the amount of native aorta included in our repair, a pre-sewn multi-branched graft is always preferred in patients with connective tissue disorders (Fig. 31.9).

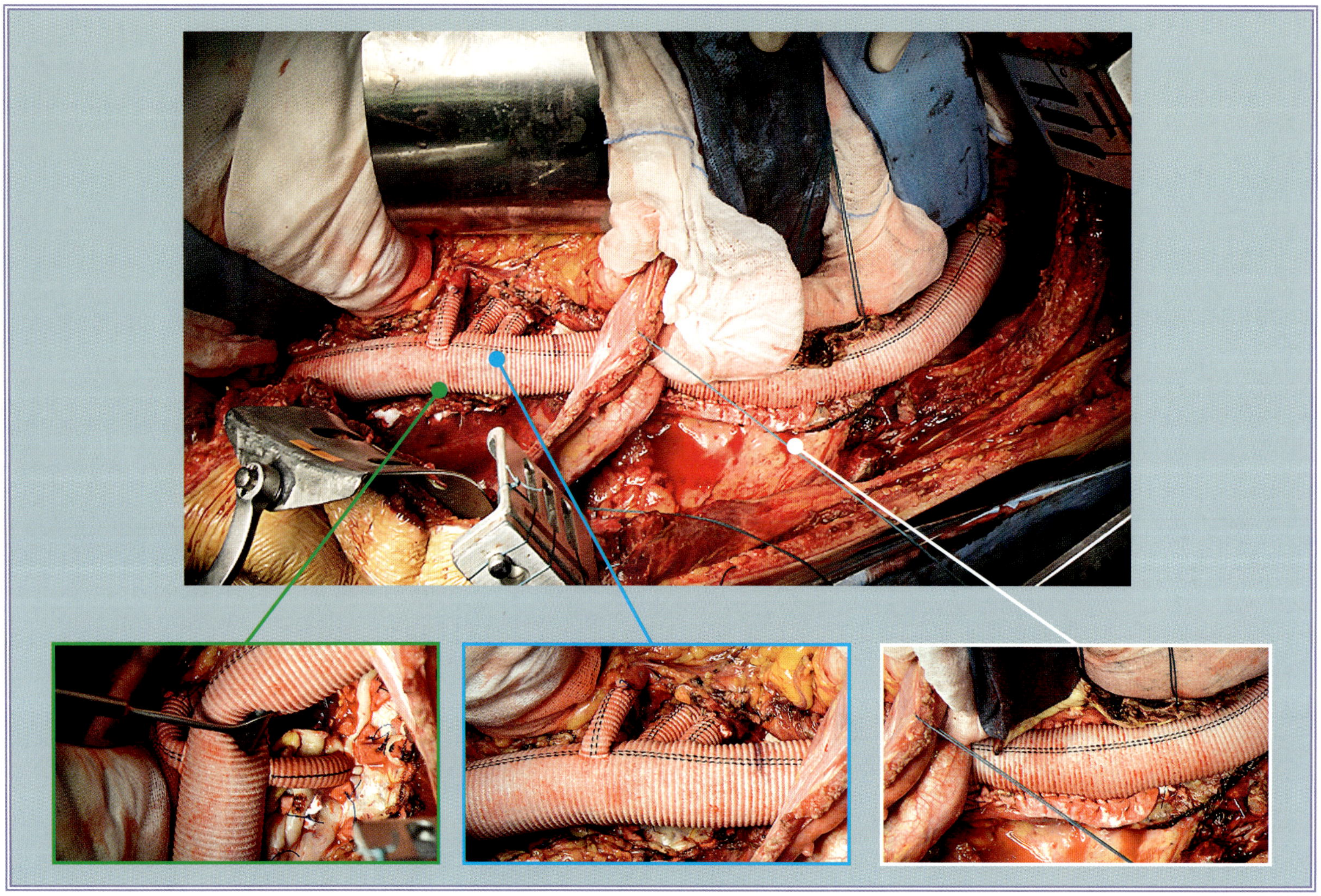

Fig. 31.9 Dissecting TAAA surgical repair. The intercostal arteries are reattached to the graft by means of an aortic patch using a Teflon felt strip to reinforce the suture (white box). The celiac trunk, superior mesenteric artery and left renal artery are reattached separately using the pre-sewn branches (blue box). The right renal artery is also reattached to the graft using a dedicated single-branch graft (green box).

31.4.4 End of procedure

After unclamping, the entire aortic repair is inspected, and all the pulses of the aortic branches exposed are palpated also after de-rotation of the abdominal viscera. Any bleeding, kinking or torsion of the aortic branches is carefully checked. Urine output is monitored regularly.

The atrial and femoral cannula are removed; the purse string sutures are tied and reinforced. Protamine is then given, and lab tests, including thromboelastometry (ROTEM®, TEM group, Basel, Switzerland), are conducted to check for any coagulopathy that has to be reversed (see Chapter 38).

The diaphragmatic pillars are approximated to reshape the aortic hiatus, and the left hemidiaphragm is sutured with a running polypropylene suture. A closed-suction abdominal drain is positioned along the repaired aorta in the left retroperitoneal space and two chest tubes are placed in the postero-apical and basal space. The abdominal and thoracic walls are sutured in standard fashion.

31.5 Specific strategies in patients with previous TEVAR

Due to the increasing number of Thoracic Endovascular Aortic Repair (TEVAR) procedures that have taken place over the last few decades, a specific section must be dedicated to the management of Type B AD in patients with previous TEVAR, who in time often require conversion to open surgical repair of the thoracic or thoracoabdominal aorta.

The most common situation for TEVAR failure requiring conversion to open surgery is that of false lumen enlargement leading to aneurysmal degeneration, and subsequent rupture. This is mainly due to false lumen reperfusion and re-pressurization, caused by unsuccessful exclusion of the proximal entry tear (i.e. Type Ia endoleak, or late migration), or distal reperfusion from abdominal re-entry tears (even after successful coverage of the proximal entry tear).

Typically, the first therapeutic option in this scenario is endovascular relining, by means of proximal or distal extension with covered endografts, false lumen obliteration with custom-made devices, or thoracoabdominal total endovascular repair with fenestrated and branched endografts. However, in selected cases, conversion to open surgery may be chosen, entailing total or partial endograft removal (Fig. 31.10). In addition, surgical conversion is preferred in most cases of endograft infection, in young and fit patients, and in cases of associated connective tissue disorders.

Although open repair techniques for thoracoabdominal dissecting aneurysm repair in the case of previous TEVAR are generally the same as those earlier described in this chapter, the following topics deserve a special attention:

- exposure of the thoracic aorta;
- location and techniques for proximal clamping;

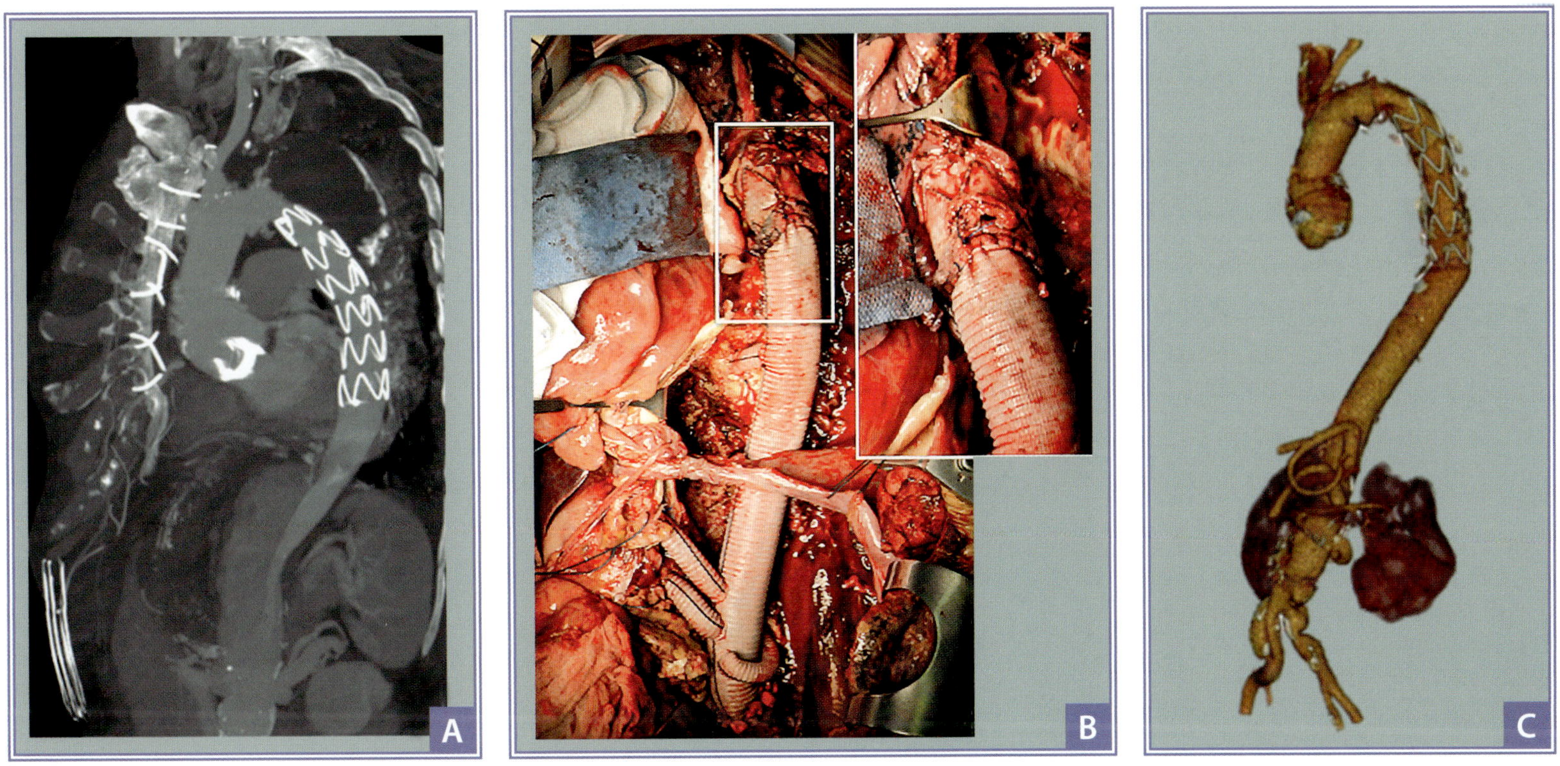

Fig. 31.10 **A**, Preoperative angio-CT. Dissecting TAAA in a Marfan patient with previous ascending aorta and aortic valve replacement and frozen elephant trunk. **B**, Surgical repair with a multi-branched graft and selective reattachment of visceral and renal vessels. In this case, the proximal end of the graft is sutured to the distal end of the previous stent graft using a 2/0 monofilament polypropylene running suture. **C**, Postoperative angio-CT 3D volume rendering.

- techniques for endograft removal;
- graft-to-endograft anastomosis characteristics;
- intercostal and visceral arteries management.

In the case of previous TEVAR, an inflammatory reaction is commonly observed involving the aortic wall and surrounding structures. This is usually associated with intraoperative findings such as tight left pulmonary adhesions, a fibrous reaction involving the heart and left pulmonary veins, vagus nerve, left recurrent laryngeal nerve and/or the thoracic duct. Special care needs to be employed in accessing the left pleural space, in the pulmonary vein cannulation, and in the thoracic aorta exposure, with a cautious progressive dissection of the tissues, which sometimes requires collaboration between the cardiac and the thoracic surgeon.

Proximal aortic cross-clamping is achieved at the level of the previous proximal endovascular neck in most cases. Consequently, the proximal metal struts of the endograft may be clamped together with the aortic wall, possibly requiring the use of atraumatic clamps with sponge rubber inserts. In the case of planned total endograft explantation, a "strut-free" proximal portion of the aorta (usually involving the distal arch) has to be exposed, generally requiring delicate retraction of the vagus and left recurrent laryngeal nerve, resection of the ligamentum arteriosum, exposure of the LCCA and LSA, and aortic cross-clamp placement between these two vessels.

Total endograft removal may be deemed necessary in cases of suspected prosthetic infection, device rupture or collapse, or complete loss of proximal sealing by means of major migration. However, total excision of the endograft is considered a dangerous maneuver in most cases, due to the risk of aortic wall damage by metal struts, hooks and barbs during device rip-out. This may also lead to retrograde dissection of the arch and the ascending aorta. Moreover, the residual aortic wall after endograft removal often appears extremely fragile, perhaps due to the chronic wall ischemia caused by the prolonged radial force exerted by the stent graft. Finally, complete endograft removal requires aortic cross-clamping proximally to the endovascular device, mostly at the level of aortic arch branches, or even hypothermic circulatory arrest.

In the majority of cases, the conversion to open aortic surgical replacement may be accomplished following only a partial explantation of the endograft. In this case, an intraoperative evaluation of the re-entry tears by transesophageal echocardiography can be useful to guide the level of proximal clamp placement. From a technical point of view, after cross-clamping, endograft and aortic transection is performed. This type of incision allows to obtain a section of the aorta that contains both the endograft into the true lumen, and the septum as well as the false lumen. Resection of the stent graft is always accomplished at the level of the fabric to reduce the risk that the cut stent struts may damage the surgical graft or the suture line. If the stent struts have to be cut, special attention has to be paid to avoid direct impingement of the leftover spikes on the new aortic tube-graft.

The "graft-to-endograft" anastomosis is then performed by including within the vascular suture the previous stent graft and the outer aortic wall; in these cases a "three-layer technique" is suggested in order to reinforce the anastomosis using Teflon felt all around the aorta (Fig. 31.11). Particular attention is needed concerning the metal stent spikes at the level of the anastomosis, which must be pushed inside the graft lumen with each running suture stitch.

Intercostal arteries in the stented zone in patients with previous TEVAR are usually totally thrombosed or the aortic wall is inadequate to allow the replanting. Critical intercostal arteries at the level of T8-T12 might be found distally and are thus reimplanted.

The distal clamp is sequentially moved to the distal abdominal aorta or iliac arteries. After extending the aortotomy, septotomy, visceral perfusion and reimplantation of the arteries is performed with the same techniques as previously described. If the dissection has extended into a vessel origin, separate reimplantation (with or without graft interposition) is recommended. If the dissection involves the iliac or femoral arteries, bifurcated reconstructions are suggested.

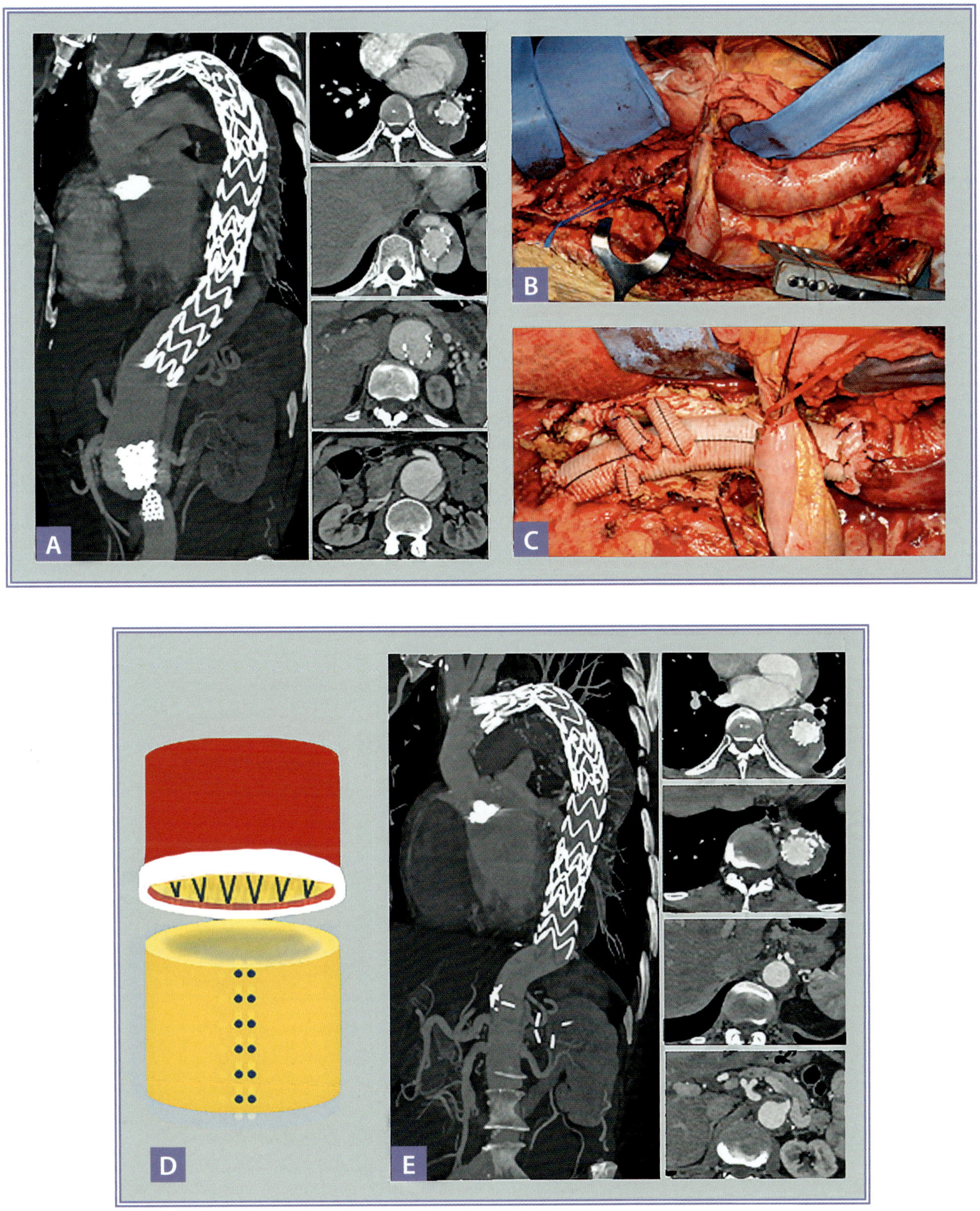

Fig. 31.11 **A**, Preoperative angio-CT. Marfan patient with previous ascending aorta and aortic valve replacement and TEVAR. The distal thoracic and the visceral aorta are progressively enlarged causing a dissecting TAAA. A balloon-expandable stent had also been placed previously at another institution in order to re-expand the true lumen. **B**, Surgical exposure of the dissecting TAAA. **C**, The stent graft and the aorta are transected 5 cm above the diaphragm and a multi-branched graft is used with selective reattachment of the visceral and renal vessels. **D**, Included in the proximal anastomosis are the partially preserved stent graft, the aortic wall and a Teflon felt strip. **E**, Postoperative angio-CT. Complete exclusion of the thoracic part of the aneurysm with surgical replacement of the visceral aorta and selective reimplantation of the visceral and renal vessels.

31.6 Early postoperative management

The main focus of the immediate postoperative management after thoracoabdominal aortic repair in the Intensive Care Unit (ICU) is aimed at early detection of any possible neurological and cardiovascular complication, to promptly institute prophylactic or therapeutic interventions.

As soon as normal body temperature is reached, the patient is allowed to temporarily wake up even if prolonged ventilation support is still required. If spinal cord or brain damage is suspected, CT imaging is immediately performed to exclude intracerebral bleeding or spinal cord compression by an intradural hematoma. Brain MRI is used to detect early any ischemic or embolic lesions; if none are detected, brain CT scan may be repeated 24-48 hours after the event. In the case of paraparesis or paraplegia, mean arterial pressure is kept above 90 mmHg, cerebrospinal fluid is drained in order to lower the cerebrospinal fluid pressure below 10 mmHg, and methylprednisolone (1 g in bolus, then 4 g over 24 hours in continuous perfusion) and 18% mannitol (5 mg/kg four times a day) are administered. MRI of the spinal cord is electively performed to confirm the diagnosis and identify lesion location and extension.

If signs of lower-limb, renal, or visceral malperfusion develop in the postoperative period, immediate diagnostic measures must be performed to assess organ blood supply and to appropriately plan surgical revascularization procedures. For a precise visualization of visceral organ perfusion, emergency digital subtraction angiography or angio-CT scanning is performed.

In uncomplicated cases, drainage tubes are removed at 36 to 48 hours postoperatively, while the intrathecal catheter for cerebrospinal fluid drainage is usually stopped after 48 hours, and then removed after 72 hours if no clinical signs of spinal cord ischemia have occurred.

A prolonged period of several days of mechanical ventilation is not unusual, especially after emergency operations, in patients with intraoperative abundant bleeding, and after longer periods of circulatory arrest. Recent studies suggest the use of noninvasive ventilation (NIV) after TAAA open surgery, also in a prophylactic fashion, in order to reduce postoperative acute respiratory failure (ARF) [20]. The benefit of perioperative NIV was demonstrated in a recent systematic review and meta-analysis of randomized trials, both for patients with established ARF as well as for those without ARF but with a high risk of common postoperative pulmonary complications [21].

In patients with severe chronic kidney disease, transient temporary hemodialysis may be needed early after surgery.

31.7 Conclusions

Open surgical repair is still considered the best therapeutic option in most patients affected by chronic Type B AD with aneurysmal evolution, especially those with associated connective tissue disorders. Recent results from our institution and from the literature confirm that surgical outcomes of dissecting TAAA open repair have improved significantly over the last decades, thanks to technical evolution, especially in the area of organ protection. However, despite adjunctive strategies, morbidity and mortality rates are still not negligible. Patient selection has to be based on a careful preoperative assessment and risk evaluation. Surgical repair of dissecting TAAA requires a multidisciplinary approach, usually in high-volume centers. If all specialists involved constantly update and refine their techniques in order to prevent perioperative complications, the outcomes of open surgery for dissecting TAAA will likely continue to improve still further in the coming future.

REFERENCES

1) Coselli JS, Bozinovski J, LeMaire SA. Open surgical repair of 2286 thoracoabdominal aortic aneurysms. Ann Thorac Surg 2007; 83: S862-4.
2) Huynh TT, Porat EE, Miller CC 3rd, et al. The effect of aortic dissection on outcome in descending thoracic and thoracoabdominal aortic aneurysm repair. Semin Vasc Surg 2002; 15: 108-15.
3) Bonser RS, Pagano D, Lewis ME, et al. Clinical and patho-anatomical factors affecting expansion of thoracic aortic aneurysms. Heart 2000; 84: 277-83.
4) Coady MA, Rizzo JA, Hammond GL, et al. What is the appropriate size criterion for resection of thoracic aortic aneurysms? J Thorac Cardiovasc Surg 1997; 113: 476-91.
5) Juvonen T, Ergin MA, Galla JD, et al. Risk factors for rupture of chronic type B dissections. J Thorac Cardiovasc Surg 1999; 117: 776-86.
6) Chiesa R. New frontiers in thoracic and thoracoabdominal aortic repair. J Cardiovasc Surg (Torino) 2015; 56(5): 685.
7) Melissano G, Civilini E, Bertoglio L, et al. Angio-CT imaging of the spinal cord vascularisation: a pictorial essay. Eur J Vasc Endovasc Surg 2009; 39: 436-40.
8) Kieffer E, Chiche L, Baron JF, et al. Coronary and carotid artery disease in patients with degenerative aneurysm of the descending thoracic or thoracoabdominal aorta: prevalence and impact on operative mortality. Ann Vasc Surg 2002; 16: 679-84.
9) Spagnolo P, Giglio M. Role of cardiac CT in assessment of patients with thoraco-abdominal aortic aneurysm. In: Chiesa R, Zangrillo A, Alfieri O, Melissano G, Coselli JS. Aortic surgery and anesthesia "How to do it" IV. Berlin: Springer; 2011.
10) Camaro C, Damen SA, Brouwer MA, et al. Randomized evaluation of short-term dual antiplatelet therapy in patients with acute coronary syndrome treated with the COMBO dual therapy stent: rationale and design of the REDUCE trial. Am Heart J 2016; 178: 37-44.
11) Huynh TT, van Eps RG, Miller CC 3rd, et al. Glomerular filtration rate is superior to serum creatinine for prediction of mortality after thoracoabdominal aortic surgery. J Vasc Surg 2005; 42(2): 206-12.
12) Stevens LA, Coresh J, Greene T, et al. Assessing kidney function - Measured and estimated glomerular filtration rate. N Engl J Med 2006; 354: 2473-83.
13) Mills JL Sr, Duong ST, Leon LR Jr, et al. Comparison of the effects of open and endovascular aortic aneurysm repair on long-term renal function using chronic kidney disease staging based on glomerular filtration rate. J Vasc Surg 2008; 47: 1141-9.
14) Ftouh S, Lewington A. Acute Kidney Injury Guideline Development Group convened by the National Clinical Guidelines Centre and commissioned by the National Institute for Health and Care Excellence, in association with The Royal College of Physicians' Clini. Prevention, detection and management of acute kidney injury: concise guideline. Clin Med (Lond) 2014; 14(1): 61-5.
15) Melissano G, Bertoglio L, Mascia D, et al. Spinal cord ischemia is multifactorial: what is the best protocol? J Cardiovasc Surg (Torino) 2016; 57(2): 191-201.
16) Engle J, Safi HJ, Miller CC 3rd, et al. The impact of diaphragm management on prolonged ventilator support after thoracoabdominal aortic repair. J Vasc Surg 1999; 29: 150-6.
17) Tshomba Y, Kahlberg A, Melissano G, et al. Comparison of renal perfusion solutions during thoracoabdominal aortic aneurysm repair. J Vasc Surg 2014; 59(3): 623-33.
18) Tshomba Y, Melissano G, Civilini E, Setacci F, Chiesa R. Fate of the visceral aortic patch after thoracoabdominal aortic repair. Eur J Vasc Endovasc Surg 2005; 29(4): 383-9.
19) Chiesa R, Kahlberg A, Mascia D, et al. Use of a novel hybrid vascular graft for sutureless revascularization of the renal arteries during open thoracoabdominal aortic aneurysm repair. J Vasc Surg 2014; 60(3): 622-30.
20) Cabrini L, Landoni G. Non-invasive ventilation and survival rates: the more, the better. A plea against its underuse. Minerva Anestesiol 2016; 82(6): 611-5.
21) Olper L, Corbetta D, Cabrini L, et al. Effects of noninvasive ventilation on reintubation rate: a systematic review and meta-analysis of randomised studies of patients undergoing cardiothoracic surgery. Crit Care Resusc 2013; 15: 220-7.

32

Use of deep hypothermic circulatory arrest for Type B dissecting aneurysm

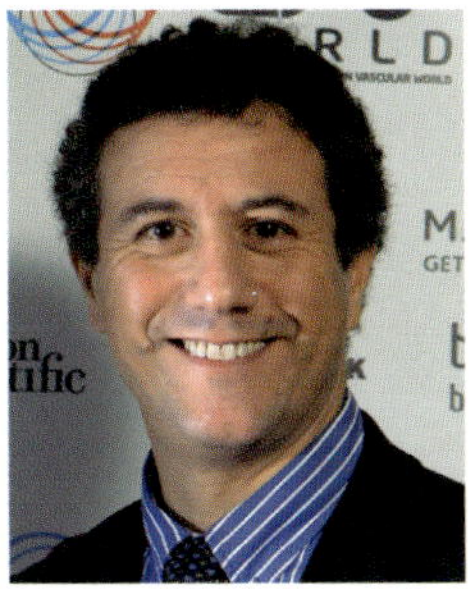

Laurent Chiche, Thibault Couture, Philippe Tresson, Julien Gaudric, Fabien Koskas and Edouard Kieffer(†)

The usefulness of elective Deep Hypothermic Circulatory Arrest (DHCA) in the management of descending thoracic or thoracoabdominal aneurysms has been established by Crawford et al. [1] in 1987. Subsequently, the potential benefits of DHCA in technically complex thoracoabdominal aortic aneurysms operated through left thoracotomy were demonstrated by several series [2-5], including one from our institution. These benefits included easier proximal aortic control, ability to treat the aortic arch simultaneously and better organ and spinal cord protection. In none of these series, the technical issues encountered during dissecting thoracoabdominal aneurysm repair were specifically described. In 1989 however, Caramutti et al. [6] reported the first series of ten patients in whom DHCA was systematically used during Type B aortic dissection (AD) repair.

This chapter aims to describe the technique, indications and results of DHCA in the management of Type B dissecting thoracic and thoracoabdominal aneurysms.

32.1 Surgical technique

We use a standard, simplified technique modified from that of Crawford et al. [1]. All patients receive conventional monitoring lines and a double-lumen endotracheal tube. Rectal and esophageal temperatures are monitored routinely. Transesophageal echocardiography is inserted before mobilizing the patient from supine to right lateral position. The pelvis is rotated to the left in order to allow access to the left femoral vessels. A cell-saver device is used in all patients. No cooling blankets or head ice packs are used. Intraoperative electroencephalography is not performed in our institution.

Laurent Chiche (laurent.chiche@aphp.fr)
Hôpital Universitaire Pitié-Salpêtrière,
Paris, France
(†) In memoriam

G. Melissano - R. Chiesa (eds), Aortic Dissection patients true stories and the innovations that saved their lives

32.1.1 Surgical approach

Left posterolateral thoracotomy is performed in patients undergoing replacement of the proximal descending thoracic aorta. The chest is entered through the fifth or sixth intercostal space, often extended by cutting the posterior neck of the sixth rib and the anterior chondral insertion of the rib.

In patients undergoing repair of the whole descending thoracic aorta, the approach is converted into a thoraco-phrenolaparotomy by extending the cutaneous incision in an oblique way until the anterior midline of the abdomen is reached. The distal descending thoracic aorta is then exposed once the diaphragm is entirely or partially divided in a circumferential fashion and the crux of the muscle is divided longitudinally.

Patients in whom replacement of the whole thoracic and thoracoabdominal aorta is planned are approached by a combination of a left posterolateral thoracotomy through the sixth intercostal space, a total division of the diaphragm in a circumferential fashion and a pararectal vertical retroperitoneal lombotomy extended towards the groin with an italic S shape. Complete medial visceral rotation is performed behind the left kidney. The pericardium is opened vertically in front of the phrenic nerve.

32.1.2 Cardiopulmonary bypass

Left femoral vessels are isolated in the groin and heparin is given systematically. It is essential to reach an optimal outflow in the cardiopulmonary bypass (CPB). Venous drainage is usually obtained by inserting a special 28Fr cannula or a Bio-Medicus® (Medtronic, Minneapolis, MN) 21Fr venous cannula from the left femoral vein to the right atrium. Proper positioning of the distal tip of the cannula is checked by transesophageal echocardiography. Alternatively, cannulation of the right atrium may be obtained through the left renal vein or through the inferior vena cava. Cannulation of the left pulmonary artery may also be used in selected cases. The site of arterial cannulation should be selected to avoid malperfusion of visceral branches of the aorta and, after the cardiac arrest occurs, of arteries to the brain and coronary arteries. Whenever possible, we cannulate the left femoral artery with a straight arterial cannula (16 to 22Fr) connected to a Y arterial line for dual perfusion and rewarming of the upper part of the body. In case of a sudden lowering of radial arterial blood pressure when cardiac arrest occurs, we advocate the insertion of an additional cannula through the ascending aorta, the supra-aortic vessels or the apex of the left ventricle.

In patients presenting an occlusion of the abdominal aorta by the dissection, it may be useful to start the operation with a prosthetic replacement of the abdominal aorta. Depending on the distal extension of the dissection, the limbs of the graft are anastomosed to the iliac or to the femoral arteries. The intimal flap at the level of the renal arteries or above them should be fenestrated. A side prosthesis prior reattached to the principal graft is cannulated and perfused to allow an optimal perfusion of the visceral arteries, of the lower limbs and of the two lumens of the descending thoracic aorta.

A Bio-Medicus® centrifugal pump and heat exchanger are used. Cooling starts immediately after cannulation and full-flow CPB. We lower the temperature by approximately 1 °C every 3 minutes. During this cooling period, we anastomose a 10 mm side-branch graft to the main aortic graft for later proximal perfusion and rewarming of the upper body. Ventricular fibrillation usually occurs between 26 and 30 °C. Lung ventilation is stopped and left ventricular venting is performed through the apex of the left ventricle with a special venting needle or with a 12Fr venous cannula.

The level of hypothermia varies according to predictable issues during the confection of the proximal anastomosis. A temperature of 20 °C is usually low enough to allow confection of the proximal aorto-prosthetic anastomosis. Mean duration of CPB may thus be limited. When technical issues are predictable regarding the proximal control and anastomosis, we advocate to reach 18 °C or sometimes 15 °C in order to obtain up to 45 minutes under DHCA to manage with the proximal anastomosis.

32.1.3 Proximal anastomosis

During the period of cooling, any attempt of proximal aortic control, division of the ligamentum arteriosum or aortic isthmus isolation should be avoided. It is also advocated to avoid any control or mobilization of the pneumogastric or laryngeal nerves, which are often included in a dense and inflammatory fibrosis. In acute dissections, the adventitial aortic layer is often extremely fragile and thin. In chronic dissections, the volume of the dissecting aneurysm sometimes precludes any possibility of proximal control and carries a high risk of intraoperative rupture. The occurrence of an aortic rupture or of a pulmonary artery injury during this maneuver may lead to interrupt the CPB prematurely while cerebral and myocardial protections are still not optimal.

Once the desired level of hypothermia is reached, CPB is stopped and the patient is placed in the head-down position. The patient is exsanguinated through the venous line into a reservoir and all lines are subsequently closed. The mid or distal portion of the descending thoracic aorta is clamped to avoid exsanguination from the lower part of the body. It is not only useless but also dangerous to clamp the aortic arch or its branches. The pneumogastric and laryngeal nerves are then exposed and freed and the ligamentum arteriosum is divided. The aorta is opened longitudinally below the origin of the left subclavian artery up to the distal aortic clamp. Usually, the opening of the aorta directly leads into the external lumen of the dissection. The intimal flap separating the true and the false lumen is analyzed looking for the entry tear, often located 2 or 3 cm distal to the origin of the left subclavian artery or directly close to it. The intimal flap is then opened longitudinally, thus giving a wide exposure of the inner part of the distal aortic arch. The ostia of the supra-aortic trunks are inspected from the true lumen. Back bleeding from upper intercostal arteries is controlled by selective 2/0 polypropylene stitches. The aorta is completely transected in the healthiest segment, close to the origin of the subclavian artery. Most of the times, the dissecting process spares this section area. This allows mobilization of the distal aortic arch and proper exposure of the posterior wall of the aorta in order to avoid any esophageal or laryngeal nerve injury during the confection of the proximal anastomosis. Proximal aorto-prosthetic anastomosis is then performed with polypropylene running sutures and Teflon felt strip to strengthen fragile tissues. Biological glue is frequently used as an adjunct for anastomotic reinforcement.

Retrograde extension towards the aortic arch is usually partial and limited to the posterior and sometimes superior wall of the arch (Fig. 32.1). In this case, the proximal anastomosis may be oblique in order to treat the largest part of the dissected aorta, end-to-end on the posterior arch transected between the left carotid and the left subclavian arteries, or less frequently end-to-end just below the level of the subclavian artery. In that case, the aorta should be first reinforced by a double internal and external Teflon felt strip completed with biological glue.

After completion of the proximal anastomosis, a 24-Fr straight arterial cannula is inserted and secured tightly in the side-branch tube graft prior attached to the main graft. This cannula is connected to the Y arterial line. The proximal segment of the prosthesis is filled with saline solution, clamped and vented and the CPB is resumed for the upper part of the body (Fig. 32.2). Rewarming is started immediately. Any proximal suture leaks are repaired with interrupted sutures. A short interruption of the CPB may be useful to achieve these sutures without additional risks of tearing the aortic wall. Distal aortic perfusion is not resumed to take advantage of hypothermia of the lower part of the body during distal aortic (including spinal cord and visceral arterial) reconstruction.

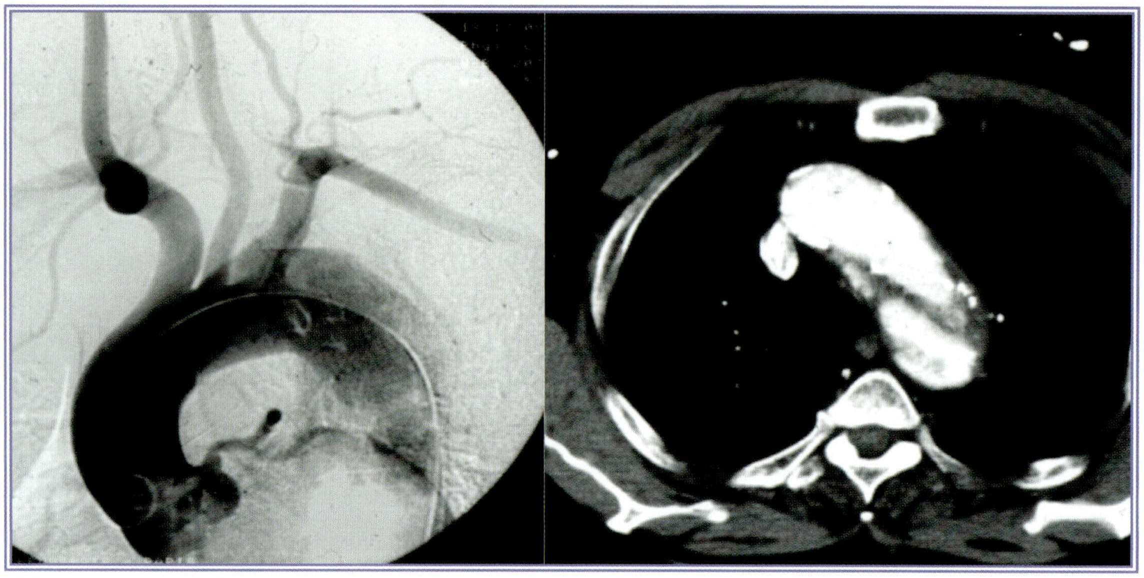

Fig. 32.1 Retrograde extension on the aortic arch of a Type B AD that should be treated using a longer time of circulatory arrest under deeper hypothermia.

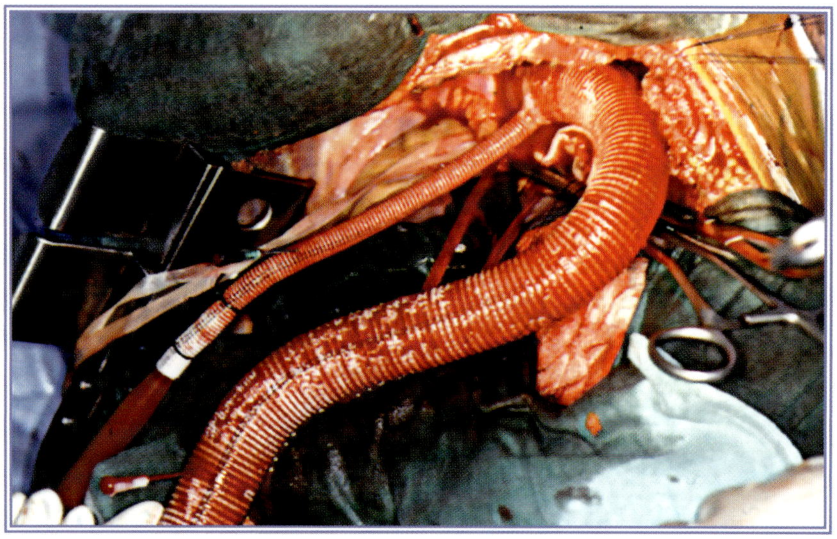

Fig. 32.2 Rewarming of the upper part of the body through the side arm of the main prosthesis after completion of the proximal anastomosis.

32.1.4 Distal anastomosis

The level of distal anastomosis is variable. In rare cases of acute symptomatic dissections treated emergently, we advocate to replace the smallest length of dissected aorta as possible in order to minimize the risk of spinal cord ischemic injury.

Before elective repair of chronic dissecting aneurysm, we advocate spinal cord arteriography or scannography before selective reimplantation of critical arteries [7]. Despite frequent fragility of the aortic wall, it is usually possible to reattach the critical intercostal arteries to the

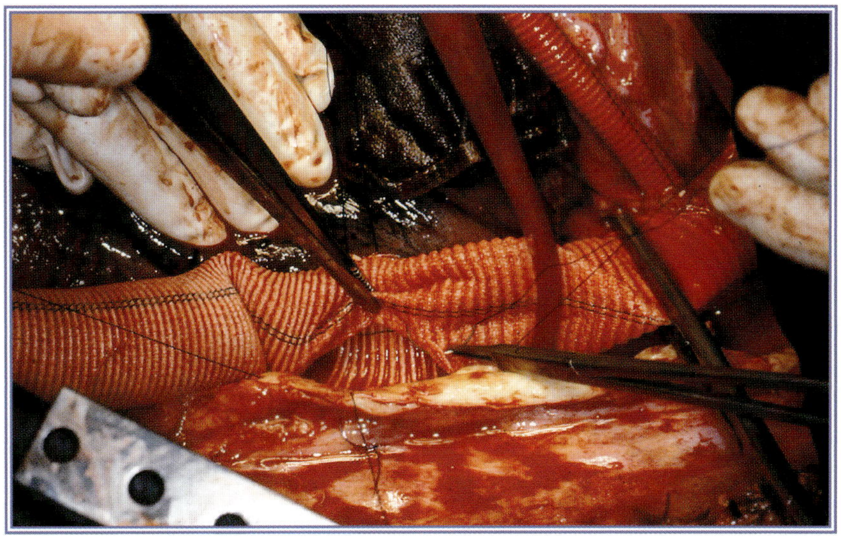

Fig. 32.3 Reattachment of critical intercostal arteries to the main graft. The thoracic and lower part of the body remains under hypothermia, providing an optimal spinal cord and visceral protection, while the upper part of the body is already perfused and rewarmed through the side arm of the main prosthesis.

prosthesis in a side-to-end fashion or to include those critical arteries in the distal prostheto-aortic anastomosis.

The distal anastomosis is performed in an open fashion. The distal aortic clamp is released after the patient has been placed in the head-up position to fill with blood the lower part of the body. The distal aorta is transected below the level of the distal clamp to avoid leaving a potential intimal injury at the level of the anastomosis.

In the vast majority of acute dissection cases, the distal aorta is not enlarged, its walls are flexible and the blood perfusion to the collaterals originating from the false lumen is not definitely organized. It is then often possible to fix the aortic wall with a double Teflon felt strip reinforced with biological glue. The distal anastomosis is directly performed on this reinforced wall. Distal reperfusion is reinstituted by removing the femoral clamp and the prosthesis is vented through a needle inserted at the middle part of the prosthesis just below the proximal clamp located at the middle part of the prosthesis. Additional interrupted sutures on the distal aorta require a short interruption of distal aortic perfusion.

When the aortic repair is extended to the abdominal aorta, a direct reimplantation of visceral arteries, digestive and renals, is necessary, either by an oblique prostheto-aortic anastomosis, or by direct end-to-side reimplantation. Thereafter, the main prosthesis is anastomosed to the distal aorta or to the iliac arteries. In dissecting thoracoabdominal aneurysm operations, reattachment of the intercostal (Fig. 32.3) and visceral arteries is then performed with sequential blood flow restoration to the spinal cord, to the visceral circulation, and finally to the lower extremities.

32.1.5 End of the operation

Rewarming of the upper part of the body usually begins once the proximal anastomosis is completed or once the intercostal arteries are reattached and perfused. Rewarming is accelerated by the presence of two arterial lines (the proximal one into the side arm of the prosthesis and the distal one in the femoral artery). Rewarming to 36 °C is performed by full CBP, low thermic gradients, and raising the patient's temperature by no more than 1 °C every 3 minutes. During rewarming, all the anastomoses are checked. Cardiac defibrillation is often obtained spontaneously. If necessary, a direct electric shock is given at an esophageal temperature of around 32 °C.

CPB is stopped when the rectal temperature reaches 36 °C, cardiac function is satisfactory as assessed by transesophageal echocardiography, and all spinal and visceral reconstructions have been performed. Decannulation is performed and reversal of the heparin is achieved with protamin injection. Blood components are given after decannulation as required by operative bleeding and laboratory data. The prosthesis is covered by suturing the edges of the aortic parietal wall or by a piece of autologous pericardium. Closure of the thoracic or thoracoabdominal approach is performed as usual.

32.2 Current indications of deep hypothermic circulatory arrest in Type B aortic dissection repair

Indications of DHCA in Type B AD rely on technical and spinal cord protection considerations.

32.2.1 Technical indications

In our experience as in most published series, treatment and prevention of technical problems represent the main indication for using DHCA. Our anatomical or technical indications include the following situations:

- patients with huge dissecting aneurysms of the proximal portion of the descending thoracic aorta (Fig. 32.4) or with previous reconstruction of the transverse aortic arch. In these cases, DHCA drastically simplifies the procedure while avoiding trans-sternal extension of the approach to the right chest;
- patients with spontaneous aortic rupture unless hemodynamic unstability calls for an immediate thoracotomy and reconstruction using a "clamp and sew" technique. In these cases, CPB is instituted from the left femoral vessels and circulatory arrest is induced before entering the chest, with the aim to avoid exsanguination before proximal aortic control is gained;
- intraoperative aortic or pulmonary artery rupture during surgical exposure of the proximal aorta. In these cases, DHCA may be induced by a single femoral cannulation while the bleeding is usually controlled by digital compression. This situation highlights one of the potential advantages of DHCA over a simple left atriofemoral shunt;

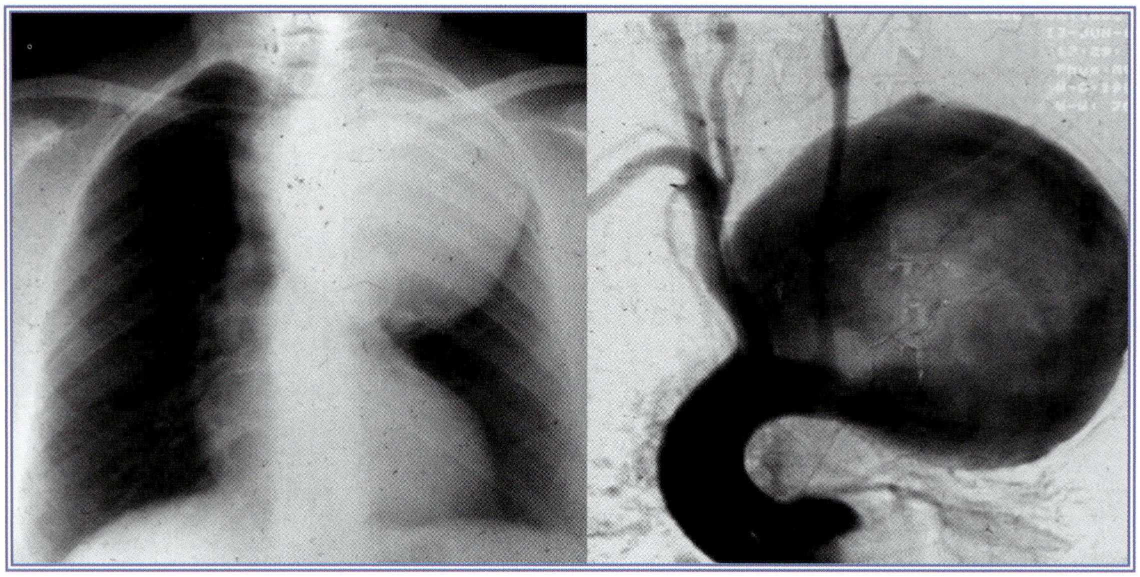

Fig. 32.4 Huge dissecting aneurysm of the proximal descending aorta requiring the use of DHCA.

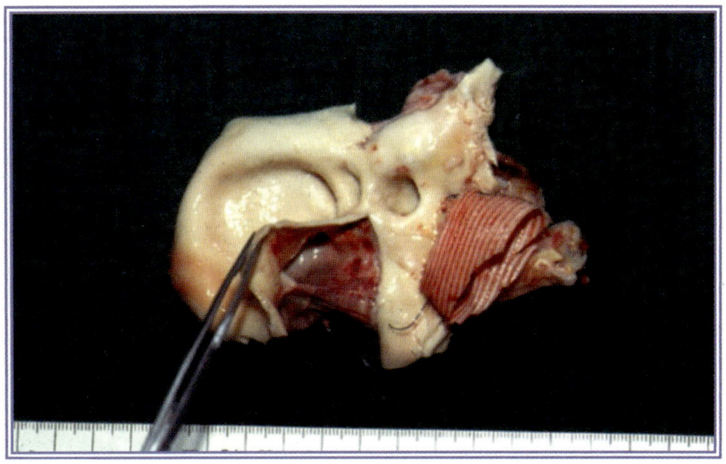

Fig. 32.5 Post-mortem specimen of the aortic arch after surgical repair of a thoracic AD. The forceps indicates the entry tear of a lethal retrograde dissection caused by cross-clamping of the aorta between the left common and the subclavian arteries.

- retrograde involvement of the aortic arch by the dissection needing a proximal control and clamping at the level of the left common carotid artery or of the innominate artery. In these cases, DHCA is the only technique that safely allows an interruption of blood flow to the supra-aortic trunks under left thoracotomy. DHCA is also useful for treating chronic dissection of the descending thoracic aorta in patients with previous sternotomy and repair of a Type A AD leaving a dissected wall at the level of the aortic arch;
- our most frequent indication of DHCA concerns the fear of clamping a deemed fragile aorta, even in a non dissected segment. We consider that this is always the case in patients with Marfan syndrome, in young patients, in patients with a familial history of AD or aneurysms. Cross-clamping of fragile aortas may sometimes be responsible for an intimal or an intimo-medial rupture which entails a risk of intra- or postoperative rupture or retrograde dissection of the proximal aorta and a risk of late anastomotic pseudoaneurysm. Although in rare cases it could be possible to successfully treat such dramatic complication by rapid institution of DHCA [8], the outcome is usually lethal (Fig. 32.5). For this reason, we concur with Caramutti et al. [6] in advocating the routine use of DHCA to perform the proximal anastomosis in the management of all cases of Type B AD;
- redo surgery is also a good indication of DHCA which entails significant technical difficulties during both the surgical approach and aortic reconstruction, especially given that duration of visceral and spinal cord ischemia is usually unpredictable.

32.2.2 Spinal cord protection

The interest of DHCA for spinal cord protection during thoracic and thoracoabdominal aneurysms repair has been underlined by Guilmet et al. as early as 1981 [9].

Our indications of DHCA for spinal cord (or visceral) protection are:

- cases in which imaging techniques failed to demonstrate the localization of critical arteries to the spinal cord, Adamkiewicz artery and also dorsal superior artery. In these cases, DHCA allows to reattach multiple patent intercostal/lumbar arteries into the prosthesis without being feared about the duration of ischemia;
- cases in which we can anticipate technical difficulties which preclude sequential clamping such as an Adamkiewicz artery originating at the level of L1 or L2, or huge aneurysms. During these situations, it is not possible to cross clamp the aorta while the intercostal arteries have been reimplanted;
- in most cases of redo surgery, when the duration of spinal cord or visceral ischemia cannot be estimated.

32.3 Results

The safety and efficacy of DHCA for the management of thoracic or thoracoabdominal AD has been confirmed by several series. However, many series in the literature have reported their global results for thoracic and thoracoabdominal aortic disease without analyzing separately the subgroup of patients with acute or chronic Type B AD.

Tables 32.1 and 32.2 [10-16] report modern results of DHCA use for thoracic or thoracoabdominal aortic aneurysm repair. Four series representing 270 patients [10-13], including one historical series from our institution, are focused on treatment of Type B dissecting aneurysms or complications. The three remaining series report the global results of DHCA in 246 patients including 149 with Type B AD. The localization of aortic repair was thoracic in around 42% and thoracoabdominal in 58%. Several attitudes towards prevention of spinal cord complications were described. They included systematic reattachment of patent or large intercostal or lumbar arteries originating from a critical segment of the aorta (mainly below T6 or T7), and selective reattachment of intercostal or lumbar arteries based on preoperative

Table 32.1 Series of patients with thoracic or thoracoabdominal aortic diseases, including more than 50% of aortic dissections, operated with the use of DHCA

Author [ref]	Year	DHCA patients (no.)	AD no. (%)	Mean age (y)	Connective disorders (%)	DTA/TAA (DHCA pts) (%)
Kouchoukos et al. [10]	2015	69	69 (100)	54±16	43	0/100
Andersen et al. [11]	2014	32	32 (100)	51.5	28.1	28/72
Corvera et al. [12]	2012	93	93 (100)	60±14	NA	29/71
Kieffer et al. [13]	2002	76	76 (100)	57.1±11.9	NA	42.1/57.9
Yoo et al. [14]	2014	79	40 (50.6)	52.4±13.3	NA	57/43
Coselli et al. [15]	2008	111	74 (67)	61.4±13.1	NA	75/25
Misfeld et al. [16]	2008	56	35 (62.5)	55±16	19.6	66.1/33.9

DHCA, Deep Hypothermic Circulatory Arrest; AD, aortic dissection; DTA, descending thoracic aorta; NA, not available; pts, patients; TAA, thoracoabdominal aorta.

Table 32.2 Main results from series of patients with thoracic or thoracoabdominal aortic diseases, including more than 50% of aortic dissections, operated with the use of DHCA

Author [ref]	CPB time (min)	DHCA time (min)	Mortality 30 days/in-hospital (%)	Stroke (%)	SCI (%)	Permanent dialysis (%)	Late survival (%)
Kouchoukos et al. [10]	197.1±43.4	30.8±11.0	5.8/8.7	3	6	0.0	87 (1 y), 65 (5 y), 40 (10 y)
Andersen et al. [11]	199.8	17	6.25/NA	15.6	9.4	0.0	DTA: 89 (5 y); TAA: 87 (1 y), 75 (5 y)
Corvera et al. [12]	254±83	28.5±12.9	NA/2.2	1.1	3.3	0.0	93 (1 y), 79 (5 y), 61 (10 y)
Kieffer et al. [13]	191.7±45.5	29.0±8.8	11.8/NA	NA	5.6	NA	NA
Yoo et al. [14]	220	NA	12.7/12.7	7.6 *	1.3	NA	NA
Coselli et al. [15]	137.7±46.2	39.7±16.2	21/27	9	1.0	2.5	NA
Misfeld et al. [16]	NA	NA	5.4/NA	NA	3.6	NA	78 (5 y)

CPB, cardiopulmonary bypass; DHCA, Deep Hypothermic Circulatory Arrest; SCI, spinal cord ischemia; DTA, descending thoracic aorta; TAA, thoracoabdominal aorta; NA, not available.
* TIA + Stroke

imaging assessment or on perioperative measures of motor or somatosensory evoked potentials. Cerebrospinal fluid drainage was performed either systematically or selectively according to the level and extent of aortic repair or to the perioperative results of motor or sensitive evoked potentials. We advocate systematic preoperative assessment of spinal cord vasculature, systematic spinal fluid drainage and reattachment of critical intercostal or lumbar arteries to the main aortic graft.

Mean CPB time was approximately 200 minutes. In their series, Coselli et al. [15] reported a significantly lower CPB duration (137.7±46.2 min), mainly because the aortic replacement was limited to the thoracic segment in almost 75% of cases. The extent of aortic repair, which should potentially include spinal cord and visceral simultaneous revascularization, is a determining factor of CPB duration as the patient's weight and the deepness of hypothermia are.

Mean DHCA time was around 30 minutes in most series. Those precious minutes should include several important steps of the aortic repair. First, the aortotomy opens both the false and the true lumens, which are inspected looking for the entry tear. Backflow from upper intercostal arteries is controlled by selective stitches. Then the proximal anastomotic site is prepared and reinforced with Teflon felt stripes and biological glue if needed. Potential need for posterior aortic arch repair should be anticipated because it requires a longer duration of DHCA and subsequently a deeper hypothermia. Final surgical steps during the DHCA period concern the confection of the prostheto-aortic anastomosis and its quality control before reperfusion and rewarming of the upper part of the body.

The series by Coselli et al. [15] has a substantial in-hospital mortality rate (27%), probably explained by a large number of emergency procedures. From other series, DHCA appears to be a safe method, which provides a 2.2 to 12.7% in-hospital mortality rate in often really complex cases of extended aortic replacement. Spinal cord protection appears also optimal with a mean spinal cord ischemia rate of 4.3% only, although 58% of patients underwent an extended thoracoabdominal repair. Permanent dialysis is quite infrequent, most cases of postoperative renal failures being cured after a transitional renal supply.

32.4 Conclusion

Deep Hypotermic Circulatory Arrest has become for many teams a safe and well-regulated technique of Type B dissecting aneurysm repair. Treatment and prevention of technical problems have been its major indications in the recent literature.

The most obvious advantages of DHCA are that it drastically limits the amount of aortic control necessary and allows operation in a dry and exsanguinated field. DHCA provides a relatively good protection against visceral and spinal cord ischemia in extensive thoracoabdominal dissecting aneurysm repair. Conversely, the technique has several important drawbacks, including long CPB times, with an increased risk of hemorrhagic and pulmonary complications. According to us and although our trend is to use it widely in AD repair, indications of DHCA should remain selective, based on anatomical considerations or on spinal cord and visceral protection.

REFERENCES

1) Crawford ES, Coselli JS, Safi HJ. Partial cardiopulmonary bypass, hypothermic circulatory arrest, and posterolateral exposure for thoracic aortic aneurysm operation. J Thorac Cardiovasc Surg 1987; 94: 824-7.
2) Kieffer E, Koskas F, Walden R, et al. Hypothermic circulatory arrest for thoracic aneurysmectomy through left-sided thoracotomy. J Vasc Surg 1994; 19: 457-64.
3) Grabenwoger M, Erlich M, Simon P, et al. Thoracoabdominal aneurysm repair: spinal cord protection using profound hypothermia and circulatory arrest. J Cardiovasc Surg 1994; 9: 679-84.

4) Safi HJ, Miller CC, Subramanian MH, et al. Thoracic and thoracoabdominal aortic aneurysm repair using cardiopulmonary bypass, profound hypothermia, and circulatory arrest via left side of the chest incision. J Vasc Surg 1998; 28: 591-8.
5) Carrel TP, Berdat PA, Robe J, et al. Outcome of thoracoabdominal aortic operations using deep hypothermia and distal exsanguination. Ann Thorac Surg 2000; 69: 692-5.
6) Caramutti VM, Dantur JM, Favaloro MR, et al. Deep hypothermia and circulatory arrest as an elective technique in the treatment of type B dissecting aneurysm of the aorta. J Card Surg 1989; 4: 206-15.
7) Kieffer E, Fukui S, Chiras J, et al. Spinal cord arteriography: a safe adjunct before descending thoracic or thoracoabdominal aortic aneurysmectomy. J Vasc Surg 2002; 35: 262-8.
8) Graham JM, Stinnett DM. Operative management of acute aortic arch dissection using profound hypothermia and circulatory arrest. Ann Thorac Surg 1987; 44: 192-8.
9) Guilmet D, Mosier J, Richard T, et al. Chirurgie des anévrysmes thoraciques et thoraco-abdominaux intéressant l'artère d'Adamkiewicz : intérêt de l'hypothermie profonde. Nouv Presse Med 1981; 10: 3303-6.
10) Kouchoukos NT, Kulik A, Castner CF. Open thoracoabdominal aortic repair for chronic type B dissection. J Thorac Cardiovasc Surg 2015; 149: S125-9.
11) Andersen ND, Keenan JE, Ganapathi AM, et al. Current management and outcome of chronic type B aortic dissection: results with open and endovascular repair since the advent of thoracic endografting. Ann Cardiothorac Surg 2014; 3: 264-74.
12) Corvera JS, Fehrenbacher JW. Open repair of chronic aortic dissections using deep hypothermia and circulatory arrest. Ann Thorac Surg 2012; 94: 78-83.
13) Kieffer E, Chiche L, Koskas F, et al. Traitement des dissections aortiques de type B : arrêt circulatoire en hypothermie profonde. In: Kieffer E, Fabiani JN, eds., Chirurgie des Dissections Aortiques. Paris: Editions AERCV; 2002: 217-29.
14) Yoo JS, Kim JB, Joo Y, et al. Deep hypothermic circulatory arrest versus non-deep hypothermic beating heart strategy in descending thoracic or thoracoabdominal aortic surgery. Eur J Cardiothorac Surg 2014; 46: 678-84.
15) Coselli JS, Bozinovski J, Cheung C. Hypothermic circulatory arrest: safety and efficacy in the operative treatment of descending and thoracoabdominal aortic aneurysms. Ann Thorac Surg 2008; 85: 956-64.
16) Misfeld M, Sievers HH, Hadlak M, et al. Rate of paraplegia and mortality in elective descending and thoracoabdominal aortic repair in the modern surgical era. Thorac Cardiovasc Surg 2008; 56: 342-7.

33

Hybrid treatment of aortic dissection with or without endograft false lumen intentional placement

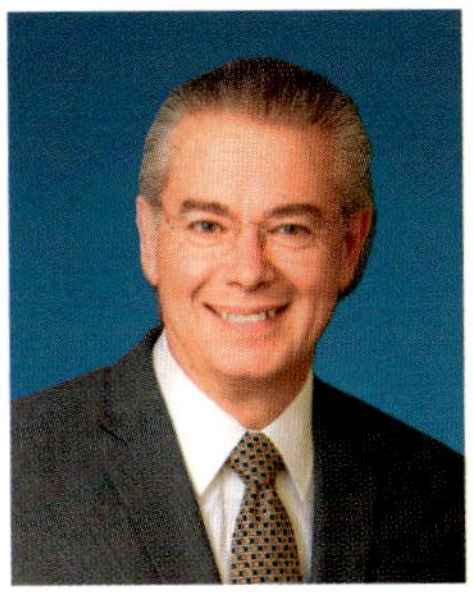

William J. Quinones-Baldrich and Taimur Saleem

33.1 Introduction

Aortic dissection (AD) is perhaps the most complex pathology within vascular disease. General guidelines are helpful in recommending management but most cases are unique requiring specific tailoring when intervention is necessary. Additionally, restoring most, if not all, flow through the true lumen has been the goal of surgical or endovascular treatment. This chapter will focus on the hybrid (combined surgical and endovascular) approaches for the management of AD. It will also present the alternative of False Lumen Intentional Placement (FLIP) of the endovascular component in specific cases.

Aortic dissection is a life threatening condition with multiple acute and chronic sequelae. Mortality can be attributed to aortic rupture, aneurysmal degeneration, aortic insufficiency, malperfusion syndromes, valvular dysfunction and cardiac tamponade [1]. Without treatment, patients with acute Type A AD die at a rate of 1-2% per hour during the first 24 hours [2].

33.2 Management of aortic dissections

Traditionally, Stanford Type A AD and complicated Stanford Type B AD have been managed with operative intervention while medical management has been advocated for the treatment of uncomplicated Stanford Type B AD. In all types of AD, optimal blood pressure control primarily using intravenous beta-blockade and pain control remains paramount.

The goals of operative therapy are to approximate the aortic wall layers, restore true lumen flow, provide hemodynamic stabilization, reverse end-organ ischemia and prevent future aortic dilatation through aortic remodelling. If aneurysmal degeneration exists in the setting of chronic AD, then replacement or stent-graft exclusion of the aneurysmal segment is performed [3, 4]. Management of AD can, however, be challenging when several important bra-

William J. Quinones-Baldrich (wquinones@mednet.ucla.edu)
UCLA Medical Center,
Los Angeles, CA, USA

G. Melissano - R. Chiesa (eds), Aortic Dissection patients true stories and the innovations that saved their lives

chiocephalic or visceral arteries originate from different lumens. Under such circumstances, thrombosis of the false lumen may actually disrupt blood flow to vital organs and structures and result in devastating complications such as paraplegia, cerebrovascular insults, bowel ischemia and renal failure [3].

As more minimally invasive techniques in the past few years have been championed and subsequently widely adopted in many surgical specialties, management of AD has undergone a paradigm shift. Despite advances in anesthetic management, circulatory dynamics and graft designs, open aortic surgery is still associated with considerable morbidity and mortality [5]. Zoli et al. described a series of 104 patients with open repair of descending chronic AD between 1994 and 2007 and reported a mortality of about 10%. Additional morbidity due to cerebrovascular accidents, renal failure and tracheostomy was also described [6]. Morbidity with open repair of acute dissections has been reported to be higher when compared to open intervention for chronic AD. Thirty-day mortality for open operative repair of ascending AD has been reported to be between 10-35% at experienced centers. Open surgical repair may also require the use of single lung ventilation, left heart bypass and hypothermia – advanced maneuvers that present their own set of challenges [7-9].

Use of endovascular techniques in the management of Type B AD has, therefore, gained popularity and its expansion to other complex aortic pathologies, including Type A AD, has also been explored. When applicable, this technique is particularly appealing in patients who have had prior open surgery such as patients with prior history of sternotomy or thoracotomy or who have prohibitive risk factors for open surgery. In one series, the operative mortality from Thoracic EndoVascular Aortic Repair (TEVAR) for AD was reported to be 5%; however, reintervention was also required in up to 22% patients. The mortality seen in the TEVAR series represents a significant improvement over open procedures [10]. Technical success rates for TEVAR for acute Type B AD and chronic Type B AD have been reported to be between 93.3 to 100% and 77.6 to 100% respectively [4].

33.3 Hybrid repair of aortic dissection

Open aortic surgery remains an important part of the contemporary management of AD, particularly in the chronic stage. Treatment often needs to be individualized to patient's comorbidities, disease pathology and anatomy. In selected patients with complex AD, a hybrid approach incorporating both endovascular and open surgical techniques often offers the best possible treatment strategy. In addition, a hybrid approach offers the opportunity to perform a staged procedure depending on patient demographics and extent of the aortic pathology. Furthermore, the open surgical part of the procedure offers pliability and durability while providing an opportunity to provide an optimum landing zone for endografting which would not exist otherwise.

For patients with concomitant aortic arch and proximal descending aortic arch pathology, the elephant trunk (ET) technique was introduced in Germany by Dr. Hans-Georg Borst in 1982 whereby, in the second stage of the operation, the descending aortic graft could be anastomosed to the pre-existing ET. To simplify this further, the technique of frozen elephant trunk (FET) evolved as a combination of the ET technique and endovascular stent grafting whereby the aortic arch is surgically replaced in conjunction with endograft stenting (antegrade or retrograde) of the descending thoracic aorta [4, 11]. The FET may potentially be performed as a single-stage operation [11]. Using the FET technique, Shrestha et al. demonstrated an improvement in survival with lower in-hospital mortality when compared to the ET technique. A length of about 10 cm has been considered adequate for the FET beyond the left subclavian artery [11].

In a series published by Liu et al., 56 patients who underwent hybrid aortic arch repair without deep hypothermic circulatory arrest for DeBakey Type I dissection were described.

Results were overall favorable with an in-hospital mortality of 3.6%. Three patients had Type Ia endoleak during the operation while 1 patient had a Type II endoleak 5 days after the operation. False lumen complete thrombosis was observed in 94% patients at level of pulmonary bifurcation, 68% patients at the level of the diaphragm and 36% patients at the level of the superior mesenteric artery [12]. In another series by Martin et al., heterogeneous arch pathologies including AD were studied in a sample of 55 patients. The overall extra-anatomic graft patency was 99%. Importantly, the overall rate of aortic reintervention was 18% at 1 year, 21% at 2 years and 36% at 5 years [13]. A similar high rate of reintervention (24%) was reported by Faure et al. [14].

Kang et al. performed a retrospective comparison of hybrid endovascular repair and open surgical repair for aortic arch pathology (n = 55). There was no statistical difference between the two groups in terms of perioperative mortality, stroke or overall survival. More reinterventions were needed in the hybrid group [15].

For dissections involving the thoracoabdominal aorta, a variety of renovisceral debranching procedures can be performed resolving malperfusion and at the same time establish a suitable landing zone for endograft stent placement. It provides an opportunity to treat patients who are not candidates for open or totally endovascular approaches. In a series of 30 patients with complex thoracoabdominal aortic pathology, the 30-day and 1-year primary graft patency of renovisceral grafts was 97.3% and 95.3% respectively [16, 17]. Chiesa et al. have recommended careful follow up of these visceral bypasses as complications have been described [17]. Bypassing the visceral arteries from the ascending aorta has also been described in the literature with use of partial clamping. This can avoid the use of extensive thoracoabdominal incisions, cardiopulmonary bypass and deep hypothermia [18, 19].

33.4 False lumen intentional placement: the concept

The traditional goals of intervention for AD have been to direct blood flow to the true lumen, restrict blood flow to the false lumen by closing fenestrations within the two, eventually inducing thrombosis of the false lumen and aortic remodelling. In the past, surgical treatment of acute and sub-acute Type B AD consisted of short segment replacement of the proximal descending aorta with distal fenestration maintaining flow to both lumens. On occasion, when all visceral vessels originated from the true lumen, the distal anastomosis was done obliterating the false lumen and directing all flow to the true lumen. Persistent flow to the false lumen through more distal fenestrations was not uncommon which can lead to aneurysm dilation of the aorta distal to the repair. Such was the situation of a 51-year-old patient who presented to us with chest and back pain, enlarging thoracoabdominal aneurysm, and severe hypertension from malperfusion of the renal arteries (Figs. 33.1, 33.2). Using a hybrid approach, infrarenal aortic replacement with septectomy of the proximal infrarenal aorta created a potential landing zone for staged repair of the AD (Fig. 33.3). Abdominal retrograde de-branching was then performed not only to allow placement of an endograft across the visceral segment but also to resolve malperfusion of the affected visceral vessels now providing retrograde flow (Fig. 33.4) while also preserving flow through a separate graft to a pair of lumbar arteries. During the second endovascular stage one week later, given the small size of the true lumen, and the presence of a proximal descending thoracic graft (proximal landing zone) and a distal graft, the false lumen was used as the route for the endovascular prosthesis. In reality, given the anatomy, it made no difference which lumen was used except the true lumen would restrict expansion of the endograft. This case was reported in 2009 as part of our series of hybrid repairs of aortic pathology and represents the first case of false lumen intentional placement (Fig. 33.5) [20]. Three-year follow-up is shown in Figure 33.6. Since then, two additional cases of the use of the false lumen for the endovascular repair of AD have been reported, one being unintentional [21, 22].

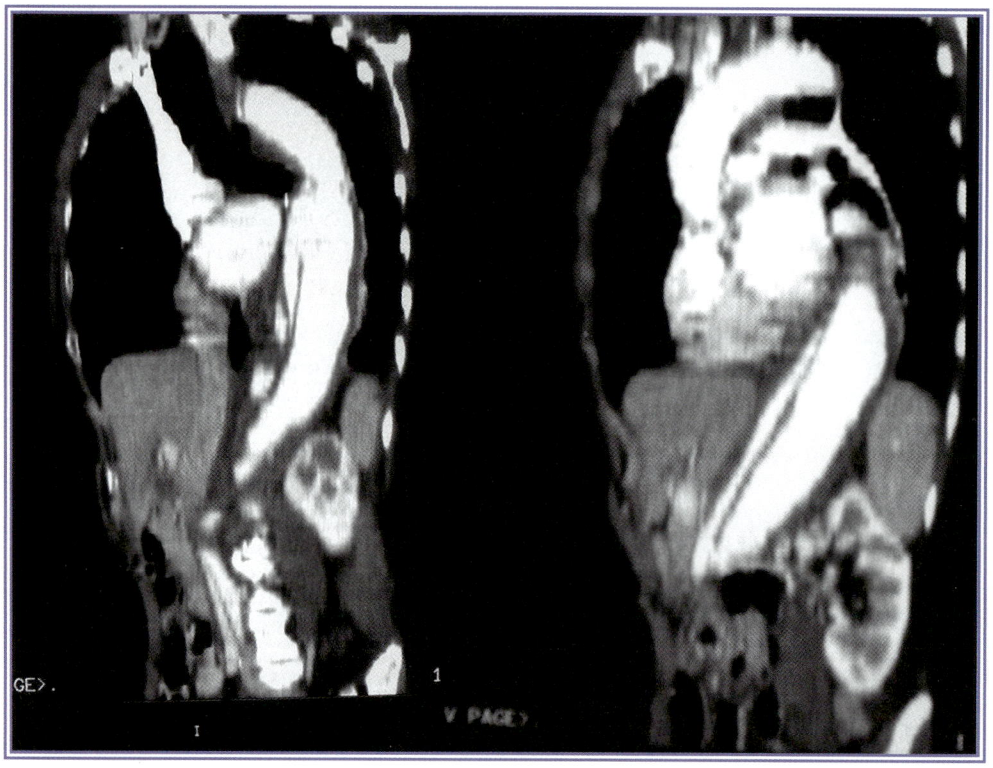

Fig. 33.1 51-year-old patient with AD and enlarging thoracoabdominal aneurysm.

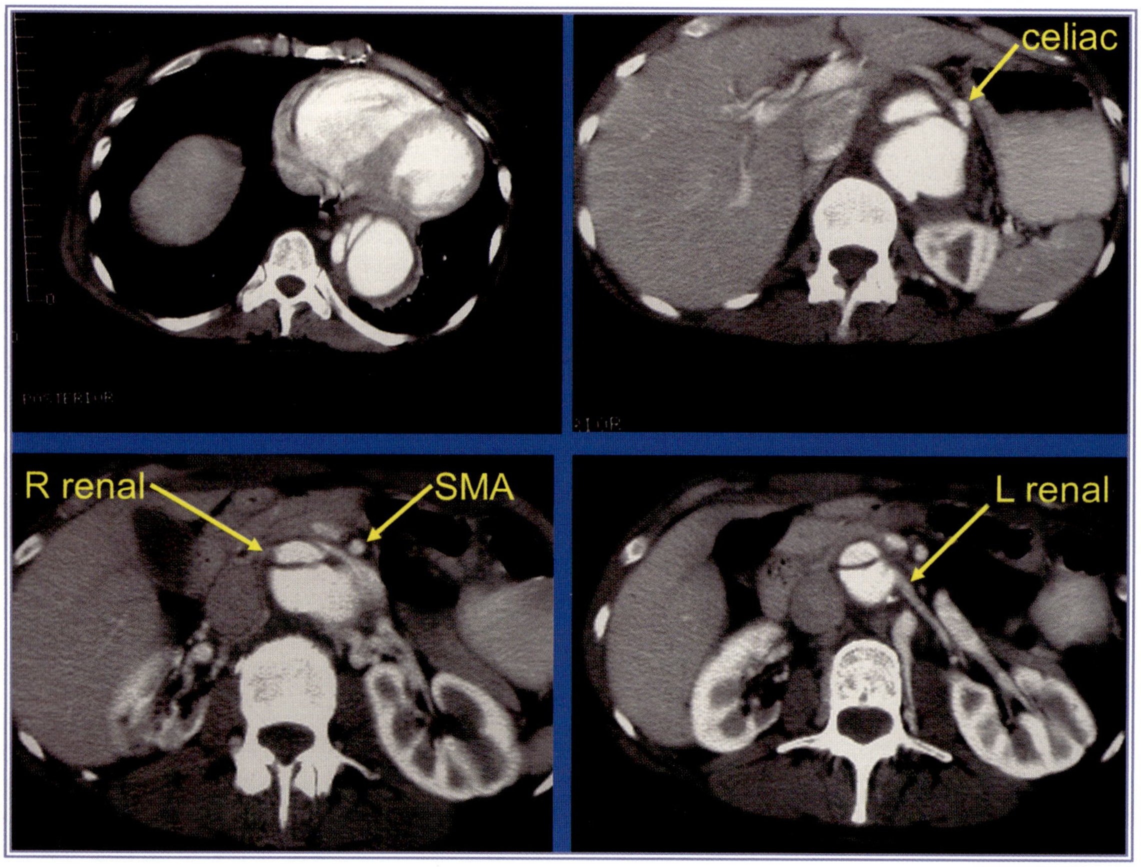

Fig. 33.2 Demonstration of origin of superior mesenteric artery (SMA), celiac, right (R) and left (L) renal arteries from different lumens in the same patient.

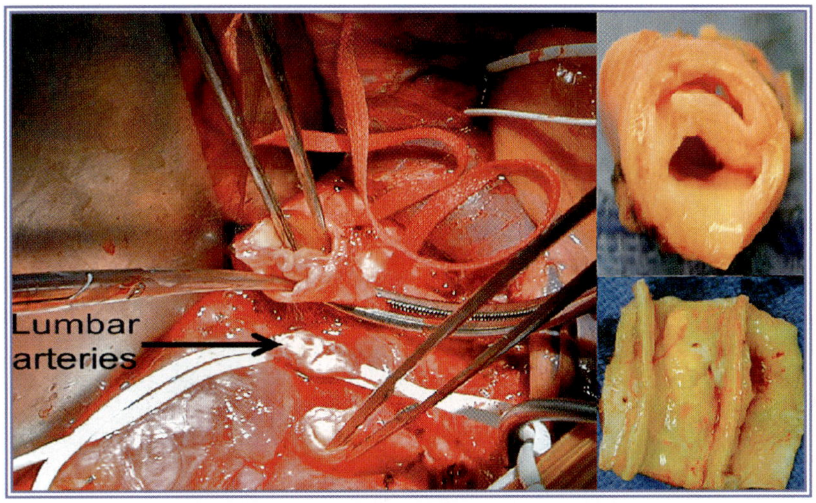

Fig. 33.3 Septectomy of the proximal infrarenal aorta in a patient with AD. Of note, the lumbar arteries are preserved.

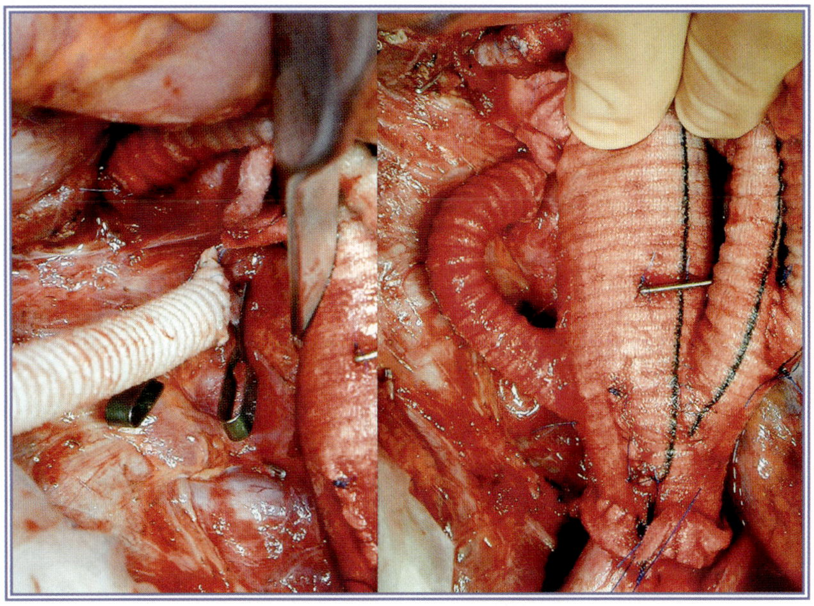

Fig. 33.4 Abdominal retrograde de-branching with 6 mm Dacron graft anastomosed to the lumbar arteries.

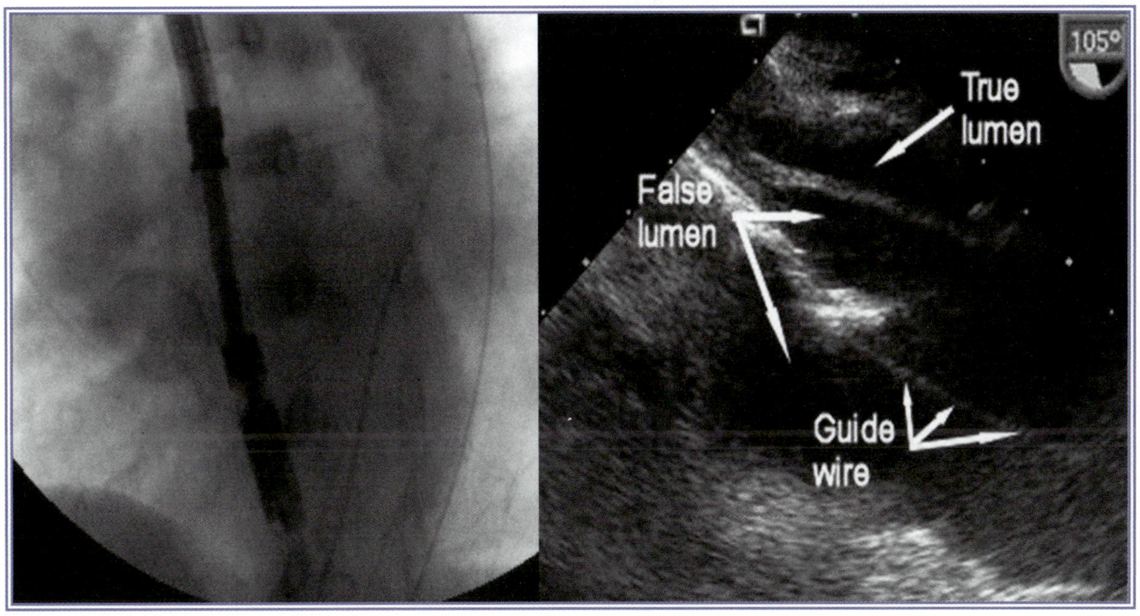

Fig. 33.5 Transesophageal echocardiography demonstrating true and false lumens in a patient with AD. Guidewires seen in the false lumen which was used as a route for endovascular prosthesis. Reproduced from [20], with permission.

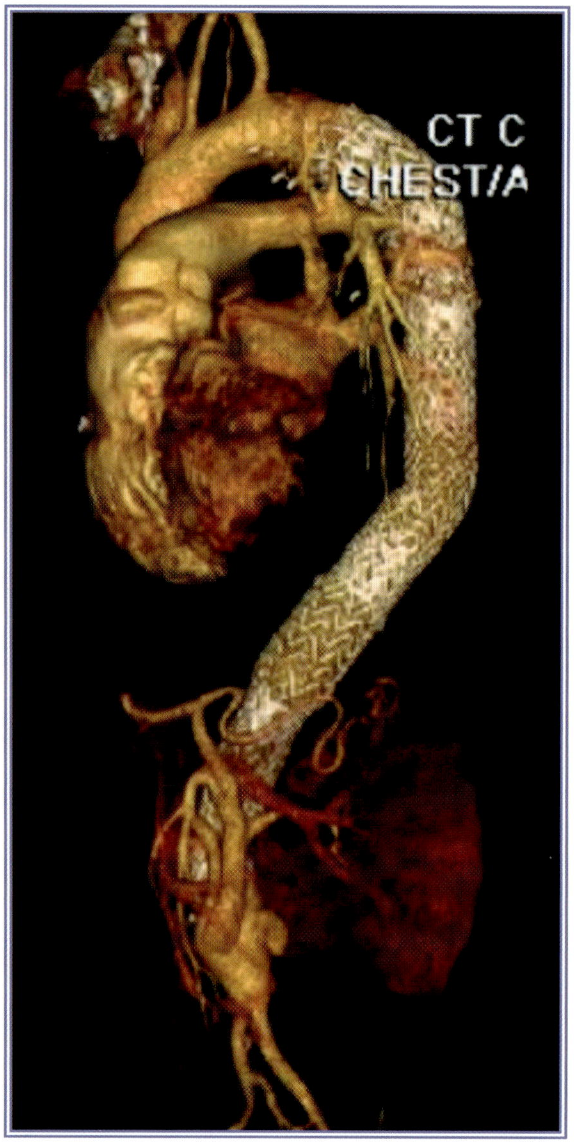

Fig. 33.6 CT reconstruction at follow-up of patient with false lumen intentional placement of endovascular prosthesis in repair of AD.

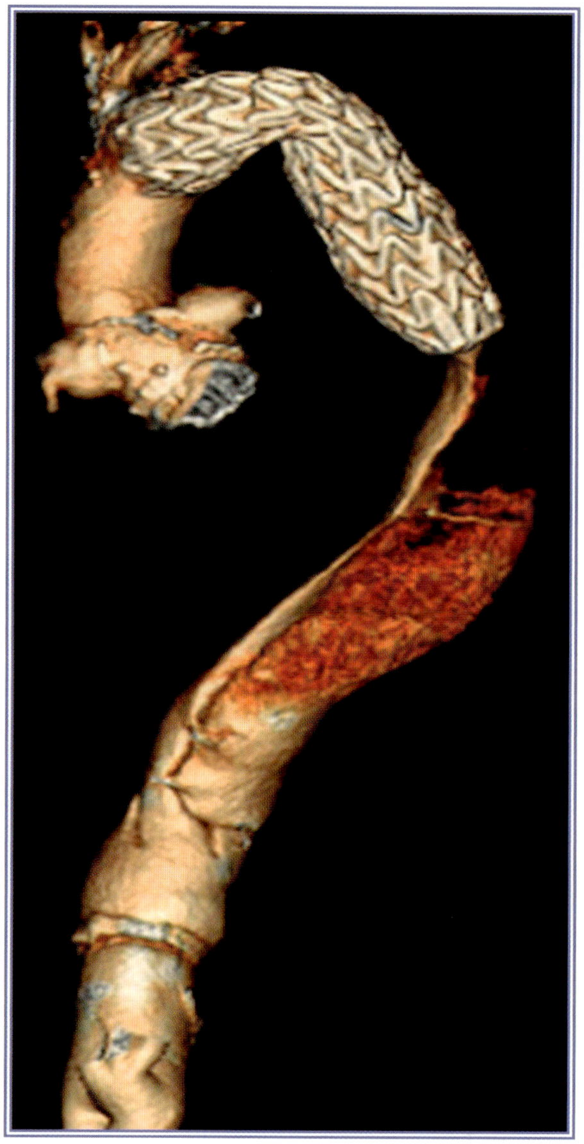

Fig. 33.7 CT reconstruction showing restrictive true lumen in the chronic stage of AD in a patient.

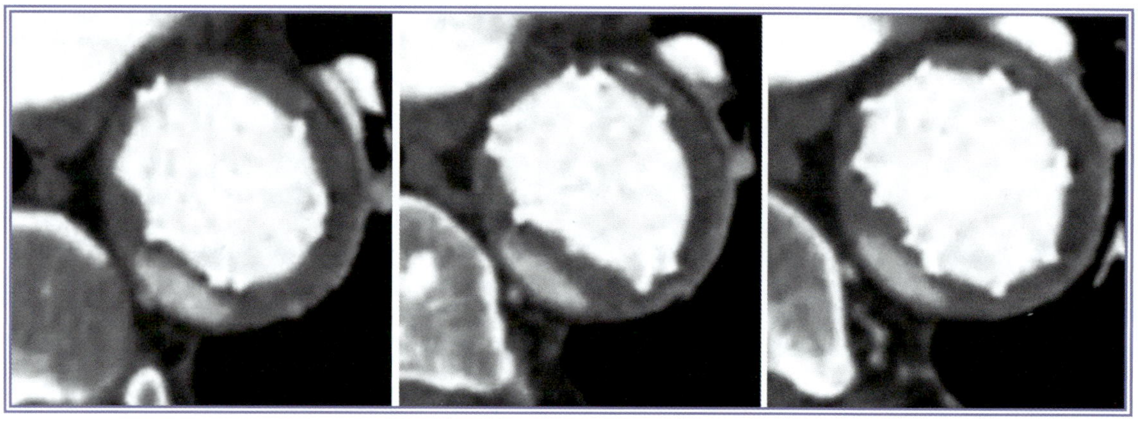

Fig. 33.8 False lumen intentional placement of endovascular prosthesis with demonstration of persistent flow in the true lumen through distal fenestrations.

The rationale for using the false lumen as the route for placement of an endovascular graft in an AD is based on several factors. The true lumen is smaller in almost all AD and particularly in the chronic stage can be very restrictive (Fig. 33.7). The false lumen will most often allow full expansion of the endograft. The false lumen is the weaker part of the dissected aorta and is responsible for aneurysmal dilation and rupture. Placement of the endograft in the false lumen protects the most vulnerable part of the aorta and has the best chance of thrombosing the false lumen outside of the endograft, a goal of all interventions for dissection. Persistent flow in the true lumen seems a lesser concern as it is unlikely to become aneurysmal and or rupture. In fact, in one of our cases continued flow in the true lumen after FLIP is the result of distal fenestrations supplying intercostal arteries likely contributing to spinal cord perfusion (Fig. 33.8).

33.5 Anatomic requirements for false lumen intentional placement

Use of the false lumen for placement of the endovascular component for hybrid treatment of AD requires a proximal seal zone perfused by the true lumen. This can be the normal undissected proximal aorta, a proximal surgical graft, or an elephant trunk placed during aortic arch replacement for Type A dissection. However, in all instances, access from the false lumen to the proximal landing zone in the true lumen is essential. This must be assessed with intravascular ultrasound (IVUS) or transesophageal echocardiography or both (see Fig. 33.5). We have used the proximal tear (fenestration) to go from the false lumen to the landing zone proximal aorta in one of our FLIP cases (Fig. 33.9).

The distal landing zone can initially be the distal false lumen in a staged repair. In such instance, the visceral vessels must be perfused by either the false lumen (very rare) or as a second stage after the infrarenal replacement with septectomy and aortic visceral de-branching. A third stage completes the repair with total endografting in of the entire dissected aorta joining the proximal endograft with the infrarenal surgical graft (see Fig. 33.6).

Therefore, FLIP of an endograft during staged repair of AD can only be done in specific circumstances given the anatomic requirements. It is, however, an attractive alternative with specific advantages over the traditional approach. Long-term follow-up is needed before embarking on a treatment algorithm that would have as a goal creating the necessary requirements to be able to use the false lumen as the conduit for repairs of AD.

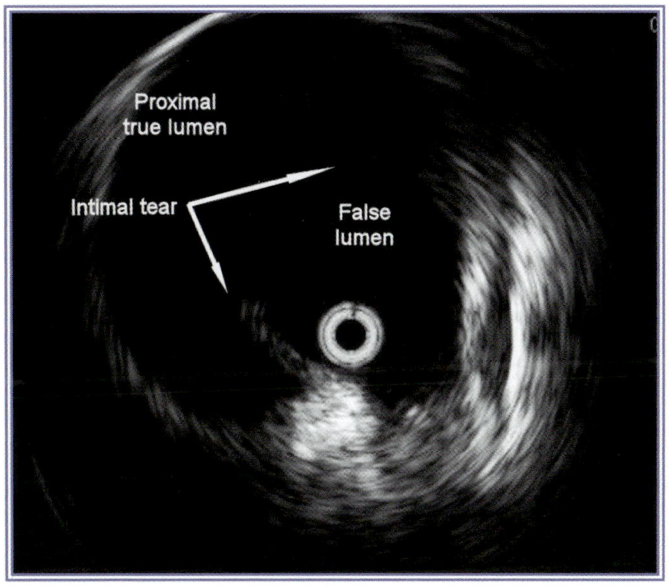

Fig. 33.9 Intravascular ultrasound (IVUS) study with IVUS catheter seen in false lumen. In this patient, proximal fenestration was used to go from the false lumen to the landing zone proximal aorta to perform false lumen intentional placement.

REFERENCES

1) Melvinsdottir IH, Lund SH, Agnarsson BA, et al. The incidence and mortality of acute thoracic aortic dissection: results from a whole nation study. Eur J Cardiothorac Surg 2016; Pii: ezw235 [Epub ahead of print]
2) Hagan PG, Nienaber CA, Isselbacher EM, et al. The International Registry of Acute Aortic Dissection (IRAD): new insights into an old disease. JAMA 2000; 283: 897-903.
3) Urbanski PP, Bougioukakis P, Deja MA, et al. Open aortic arch surgery in chronic dissection with visceral arteries originating from different lumens. Eur J Cardiothorac Surg 2016; 49: 1382-90.
4) Nauta FJ, Trimarchi S, Kamman AV, et al. Update in the management of type B aortic dissection. Vasc Med 2016; 21: 251-63.
5) Benrashid E, Wang H, Keenan JE, et al. Evolving practice pattern changes and outcomes in the era of hybrid aortic arch repair. J Vasc Surg 2016; 63: 323-31.
6) Zoli S, Etz CD, Roder F, et al. Long-term survival after open repair of chronic distal aortic dissection. Ann Thorac Surg 2010; 89: 1458-66.
7) Pansini S, Gagliardotto PV, Pompei E, et al. Early and late risk factors in surgical treatment of acute type A aortic dissection. Ann Thorac Surg 1998; 66: 779-84.
8) Erbel R, Alfonso F, Boileau C, et al. Diagnosis and management of aortic dissection. Eur Heart J 2001; 22: 1642-81.
9) Svensson LG, Kouchoukos NT, Miller DC, et al. Society of Thoracic Surgeons Endovascular Surgery Task Force. Expert consensus document on the treatment of descending thoracic aortic disease using endovascular stent-grafts. Ann Thorac Surg 2008; 85: 1-41.
10) Roselli EE. Thoracic endovascular aortic repair versus open surgery for type-B chronic dissection. J Thorac Cardiovasc Surg 2015; 149: S163-7.
11) Shrestha M, Beckmann E, Krueger H, et al. The elephant trunk is freezing: the Hannover experience. J Thorac Cardiovasc Surg 2015; 149: 1286-93.
12) Liu P, Chang Q, Qian X, et al. Early and mid-term results after hybrid total arch repair of DeBakey type I dissection without deep hypothermic circulatory arrest. Interact Cardiovasc Thorac Surg 2016; 23(4): 608-15.
13) Martin G, Riga C, Gibbs R, et al. Short and long term results of hybrid arch and proximal descending thoracic aortic repair: a benchmark for new technologies. J Endovasc Ther 2016; 23(5): 783-90.
14) Faure EM, Canaud L, Marty-Ane C, et al. Hybrid aortic arch repair for dissecting aneurysm. J Thorac Cardovasc Surg 2016; 152: 162-8.
15) Kang WC, Ko YG, Shin EK, et al. Comparison of hybrid endovascular and open surgical repair for proximal aortic arch diseases. Int J Cardiol 2016; 203: 975-9.
16) Gkremoutis A, Schmandra T, Meyn M, et al. Hybrid approach to emergent and urgent treatment of complex thoracoabdominal aortic pathology. Eur J Vasc Endovasc Surg 2014; 48: 407-13.
17) Chiesa R, Tshomba Y, Logaldo D, et al. Possible graft-related complications in visceral debranching for hybrid B dissection repair. Ann Cardiothorac Surg 2014; 3: 393-9.
18) Abdulamit T, Mangialardi N, Petrosyan A, et al. Aortic debranching from the ascending aorta: a novel surgical approach for extended TAAA and chronic type B dissections in high risk patients. J Cardiovasc Surg (Torino) 2012; 53: 345-53.
19) Brueck M, Heidt MC, Szente-Varga M, et al. Hybrid treatment for complex aortic problems combining surgery and stenting in the integrated operating theatre. J Interv Cardiol 2006; 19: 539-43.
20) Quinones-Baldrich W, Jiminez JC, DeRubertis B, et al. Combined endovascular and surgical approach (CESA) to thoracoabdominal aortic pathology: a 10-year experience. J Vasc Surg 2009; 49: 1125-34.
21) Simring D, Raja J, Morgan-Rowe L, et al. Placement of a branched stent graft into the false lumen of a chronic type B aortic dissection. J Vasc Surg 2011; 54: 1784-7.
22) Watanabe Y, Kuratani T, Shirakawa Y, et al. Hybrid endovascular repair of a dissecting thoracoabdominal aortic aneurysm with stent graft implantation through the false lumen. J Vasc Surg 2014; 59: 264-7.

34

The sandwich technique in Type B aortic dissection

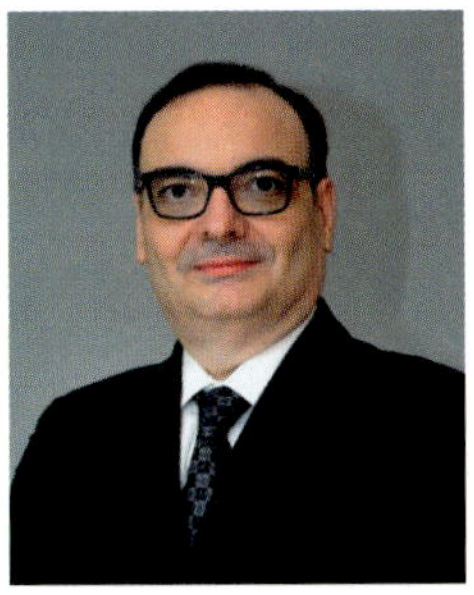

Armando C. Lobato and Luciana Camacho-Lobato

34.1 Introduction

Acute aortic dissection (AD) is a life-threatening cardiovascular disease associated with considerable morbidity and mortality [1-3]. Patients with acute Type B AD, defined by the absence of false lumen propagation in the ascending aorta, have better survival than those with involvement of the ascending aorta (Type A) [4, 5]. Thoracic EndoVascular Aortic Repair (TEVAR) was introduced as an alternative treatment option for patients with acute Type B AD complicated by retrograde dissection, critical limb ischemia, contained rupture, or visceral malperfusion syndrome [6-8].

TEVAR in addition to optimal medical treatment is associated with improved 5-year survival and adverse event rates for an uncomplicated acute Type B AD in the first randomized comparison trial between elective endovascular surgery and best medical treatment [9].

Usually, uncomplicated patients are managed with optimal medical therapy alone. However, long-term outcomes remain sobering because of aneurysmal expansion of the false lumen and late complications [10-12].

Huptas et al. [13] reported that TEVAR for Type B AD results in a significant increase in true-lumen and a decrease in false-lumen volumes, not only acutely but also over time, due to continued remodelling processes primarily in the thoracic aorta, with little or no impact on abdominal aortic volumes.

For stable survivors of Type B AD, benefits of TEVAR begin to show after 2 years of follow-up. Landmarking at 2 years of follow-up was selected a priori in anticipation of events both before and after 2 years [14]. Nevertheless, with landmark analysis, findings become observational because some confounders may not be accounted for, and early events may be omitted, thus rendering the analysis susceptible to time point – specific results and loss of power.

Suzuki et al. [15] reported that real world 5-year cumulative mortality of Type B AD is 28% with β-blockers, and 25% with calcium antagonists compared with 33-36% without those drugs.

Nienaber et al. [9] reported that although preemptive TEVAR was associated with an excess early mortality (attributable to peri-procedural hazards), the procedure turned beneficial at 5 years of follow-up with a number needed to treat of 13. Thus, INSTEAD-XL corroborates recent observational evidence, suggesting long-term beneficial results of TEVAR in sub-acute

Armando C. Lobato (aclobato@icve.com.br)
ICVE - Instituto de Cirurgia Vascular e Endovascular,
São Paulo, Brazil

G. Melissano - R. Chiesa (eds), Aortic Dissection patients true stories and the innovations that saved their lives

and chronic dissection. With safer procedures attributable to improve operator skills and better technology, TEVAR may emerge as first-line therapy of Type B AD; the attempt to heal and remodel dissected aorta may replace the current complication-specific strategy. Moreover, INSTEAD-XL suggests medical management and surveillance were associated with failure to prevent late complications, such as expansion, rupture, and late crossover/conversion to emergent TEVAR, conveying a higher aorta-specific mortality. The notion of uncomplicated Type B AD may in fact be a misnomer and should be reconsidered because the need for late repair of critical expansion and progression of dissection is common.

Chimney graft allows for the endovascular repair of juxtarenal and Types IV and V thoracoabdominal aortic aneurysms (TAAA) in a simple and straightforward way. The main indications comprise urgent settings such as Type I endoleak (EVAR in short neck) and symptomatic and/or expanding Types IV and V TAAA [16-25].

Chimney graft is not applicable to Types I, II, and III TAAA, or to Type B AD with progressive expansion at the visceral arteries level. We have developed the sandwich technique (ST) to address these aneurysms and dissection that cannot be repaired by chimney graft.

34.2 Technique

34.2.1 Access selection

The access selection and destination for Type B AD with TAAA repair depends on the number of vessels undergoing revascularization as follows:

- four-vessel revascularization – left open subclavian artery access is the preferred access and should be made available with a 28-cm-long, 20-Fr sheath and two 90-cm-long, 7 and 8Fr sheaths placed inside it to allow for two-vessel cannulation (one visceral artery and one renal artery). In addition, proceed with the percutaneous right brachial artery approach using a 90-cm-long, 8-Fr sheath to cannulate another visceral artery with a percutaneous contralateral retrograde femoral artery approach. Femoral access can be open or percutaneous based on the surgeon's discretion. We usually opt for open access on one side to make it easy to deliver the endoprosthesis and for percutaneous access on the other to cannulate one of the renal arteries with a 65-cm-long, 7-Fr sheath;
- three-vessel revascularization – the approach for three-vessel revascularization uses the same accesses previously described for four-vessel revascularization, but one femoral approach (11-cm-long 5-Fr sheath) should be used for angiographic purposes only;
- two-vessel revascularization – spare the right brachial artery access and save one femoral approach for angiographic purposes only, as previously mentioned.

34.2.2 Procedural logistics

The procedure for Type B AD with TAAA repair includes the following four steps to be undertaken in the order listed. Shuffling the steps may make the procedure cumbersome. Suggested overlapping measures and changes in device length may increase the risk for endoleak or occlusion.

Step 1

Address the thoracic part of the aneurysm. Insert the thoracic aortic stent graft through a femoral approach and deploy it on the full thoracic extension of the aneurysm, leaving its distal end 10 to 20 mm above the celiac axis (Fig. 34.1A).

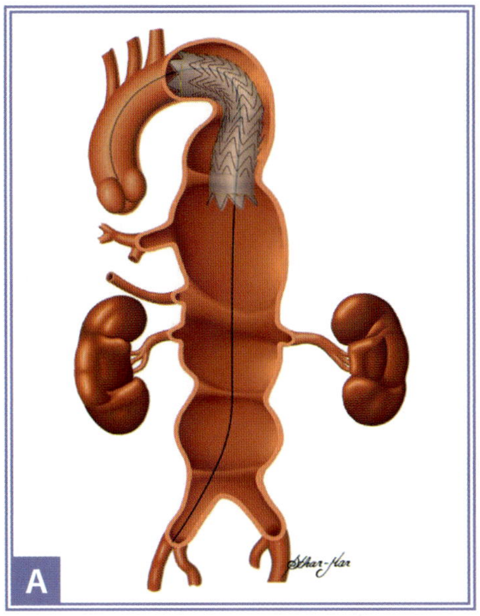

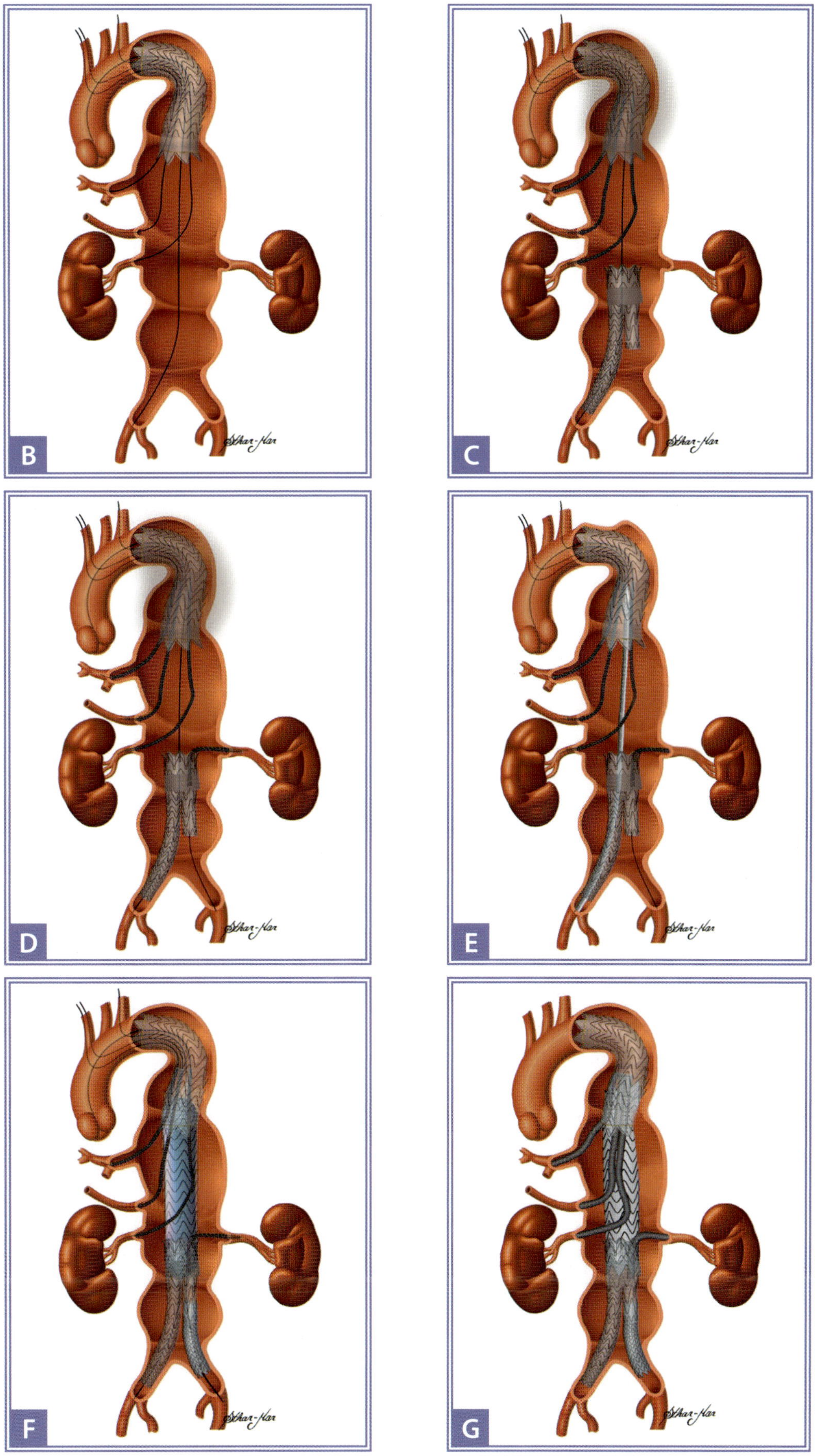

Fig. 34.1 Schematic description of the different steps to be followed when performing a TAAA endovascular repair with the sandwich technique, as explained in the text.

Step 2

Treat the visceral arteries. Cannulate the visceral arteries using a stiff 0.035-inch hydrophilic guidewire and 5-Fr catheters with vertebral, multipurpose tip curves at least 125-cm long. After cannulation, the stiff hydrophilic guidewire is exchanged for an extra stiff, 0.035-inch guidewire with a floppy tip no longer than 20 mm, and then position the introducer 20 mm inside the target visceral vessel (Fig. 34.1B).

Step 3

Treat the remaining segment of the aneurysm. For Type I TAAA, insert the thoracic stent graft through the femoral access site. For Types II, III, and IV TAAA, a bifurcated stent graft is deployed followed by the insertion of Self-Expanding Covered Stent (SECS) into the one renal artery (Fig. 34.1C, D). A thoracic stent graft is then positioned to treat the remaining segment of the aneurysm (Fig. 34.1E). The aortic stent graft should be deployed 1 cm below the proximal end of the SECS to obtain at least a 5 cm overlapping (between the thoracic endoprostheses and SECS), followed by aortic stent-graft accommodation with a latex balloon (Fig. 34.1F).

Step 4

Deploy the SECS (the suggested diameter is 1 mm larger than the target visceral vessel lumen) (Fig. 34.1G), followed by a bare self-expandable stent inside them (same diameter and length of the SECS) to avoid kinking and future occlusion. The suggested lengths of the SECS are 10 cm for celiac trunk and superior mesenteric artery, 15 cm for antegrade renal arteries revascularization, and 5 cm for retrograde renal artery revascularization. Dilatation of the SECS with an angioplasty balloon is performed only when lumen compression is greater than 50%. The distal stent graft must be larger than the proximal stent graft. A 30% oversizing of the sandwich stent graft is recommended to enable two-to four-vessel endorevascularization.

34.3 Results

From January 2000 to June 2016, 168 consecutive patients submitted to TEVAR for Type B AD in our institution. We developed the ST in October 2008 and since then have performed elective stent-graft placement in 15 patients with a stable clinical condition. There has been no operative death, with a 24-month cumulative survival rate of 80%. No neurological adverse events occurred during the follow-up. Finally, aortic remodelling (with true-lumen recovery and thoracic false-lumen thrombosis) occurred in 66.6% of patients.

We will present two cases of Type B AD with progressive expansion at the descending thoracic aorta including the visceral arteries.

Case 1 – A 61-year-old male with sub-acute Type B AD associated with right common iliac artery true lumen subocclusion (Fig. 34.2A) underwent a ST with endorevascularization of all visceral arteries, both renal arteries and the right common iliac artery patency restoration with a SEC (Fig. 34.2B).

Case 2 – A 55-year-old female with sub-acute Type B AD associated with left renal occlusion (Fig. 34.3A). She underwent a ST with endorevascularization of the celiac axis, superior mesenteric artery, and right renal artery. Angio-CT (1 month) showed a good result (false-lumen seal and visceral arteries patent) (Fig. 34.3B).

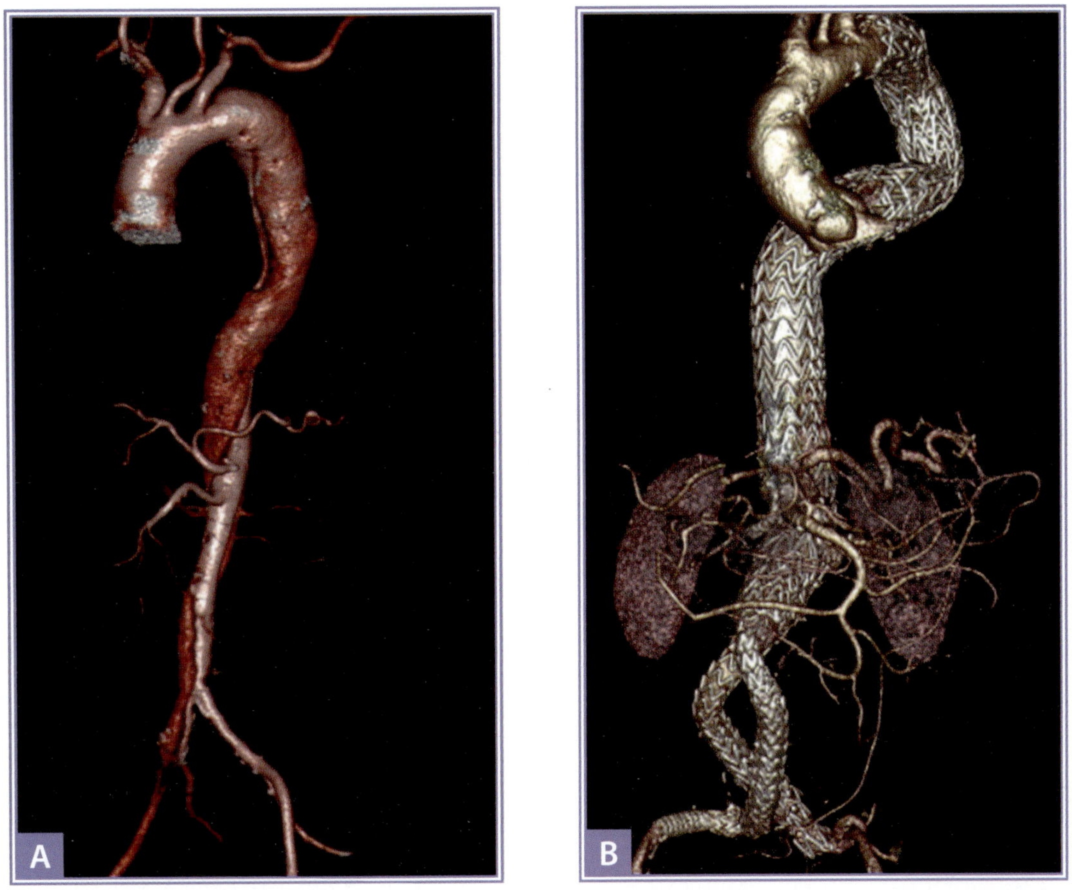

Fig. 34.2 Case 1. **A**, Preoperative approach of a subacute Type B AD associated with a common iliac artery true lumen subocclusion. **B**, Final result of the sandwich technique.

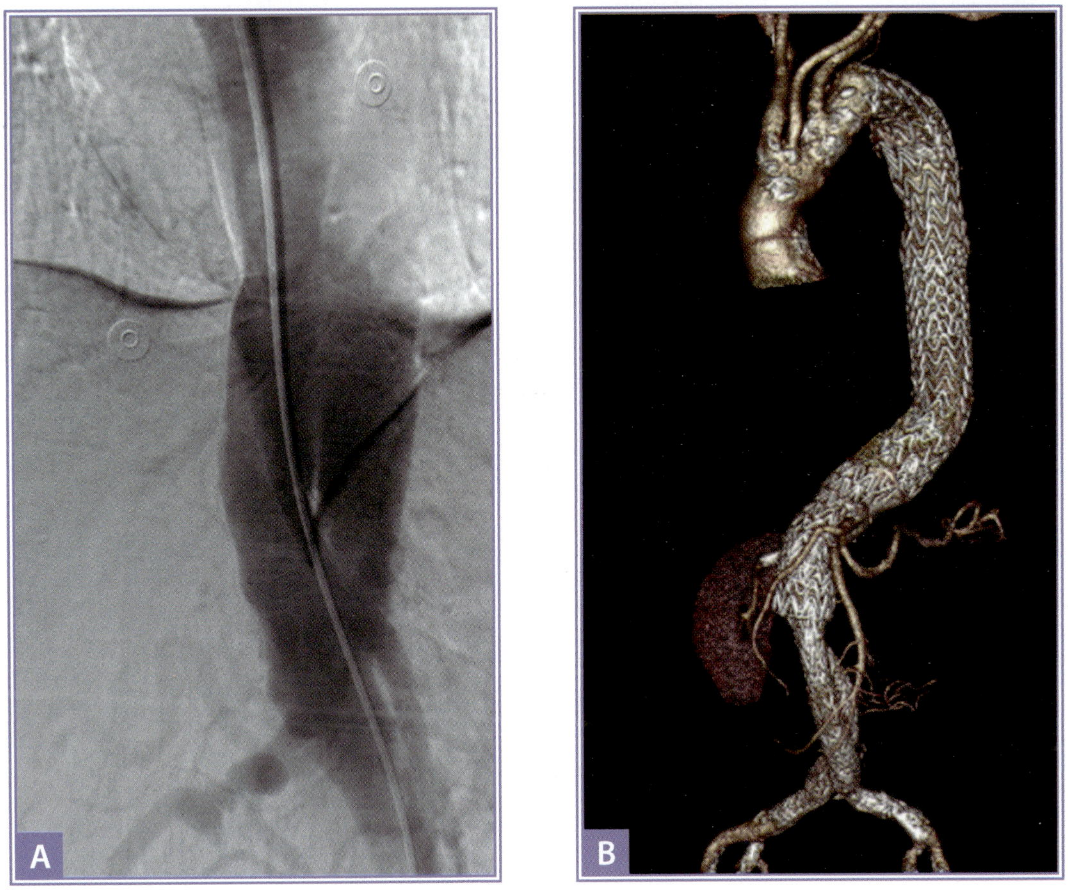

Fig. 34.3 Case 2. **A**, Angiography of a Type B AD with left renal occlusion. **B**, Appearance after endovascular repair with the sandwich technique.

34.4 Conclusion

In comparison to side-branch graft, ST is a feasible, cheap alternative employing ready-to-use endoprosthesis to maintain visceral revascularization in Type B AD.

34.5 Summary

Acute AD is a life-threatening cardiovascular disease associated with considerable morbidity and mortality. Patients with acute Type B AD, defined by the presence of false lumen propagation in the descending aorta, have better survival compared with dissections involving the ascending aorta (Type A). Thoracic EndoVascular Aortic Repair (TEVAR) was introduced as an alternative treatment option for patients with acute Type B AD complicated by retrograde dissection, critical limb ischemia, contained rupture, or visceral malperfusion syndrome. TEVAR is currently indicated for Type B AD only in patients who fail to respond to medical management and with progressive expansion or late malperfusion. Chimney graft allows endovascular repair of juxtarenal and Types IV and V ThoracoAbdominal Aortic Aneurysms (TAAAs) in a simple and straightforward way. The main indications comprise urgent settings such as Type I endoleak (EVAR in short neck) and symptomatic and/or expanding Types IV and V TAAA. Chimney graft is not applicable to Types I, II and III TAAA, or to Type B AD with progressive expansion at the level of the visceral arteries. We developed the Sandwich Technique (ST) to address these aneurysms and dissections that cannot be repaired by chimney graft. From January 2000 to June 2016, in our institution, 168 consecutive patients were submitted to TEVAR for Type B AD. Since the introduction of the ST, we have performed elective stent-graft placement in 15 patients with a stable clinical condition. There was no operative death, and a 24-month cumulative survival rate of 80%. No neurological adverse events occurred during the follow-up. Finally, aortic remodelling with true-lumen recovery and thoracic false-lumen thrombosis occurred in 66.6% of patients. In comparison to side-branch graft, the ST is a feasible, low-cost alternative employing ready-to-use endoprosthesis to maintain visceral revascularization in Types I, II, and III thoracoabdominal aneurysms.

REFERENCES

1) Hagan PG, Nienaber CA, Isselbacher EM, et al. The International Registry of Acute Aortic Dissection (IRAD): new insights into an old disease. JAMA 2000; 283: 897-903.
2) Roberts CS, Roberts WC. Aortic dissection with the entrance tear in the descending thoracic aorta. Analysis of 40 necropsy patients. Ann Surg 1991; 213: 356-68.
3) Suzuki T, Mehta RH, Ince H, et al. Clinical profiles and outcomes of acute type B aortic dissection in the current era: lessons from the International Registry of Aortic Dissection (IRAD). Circulation 2003; 108(Suppl 1): II312-17.
4) DeBakey ME, Beall AC Jr, Cooley DA, et al. Dissecting aneurysms of the aorta. Surg Clin North Am 1966; 46: 1045-55.
5) Daily PO, Trueblood HW, Stinson EB, et al. Management of acute aortic dissections. Ann Thorac Surg 1970; 10: 237-47.
6) Dake MD, Kato N, Mitchell RS, et al. Endovascular stent-graft placement for the treatment of acute aortic dissection. N Engl J Med 1999; 340: 1546-52.
7) Nienaber CA, Fattori R, Lund G, et al. Nonsurgical reconstruction of thoracic aortic dissection by stent-graft placement. N Engl J Med 1999; 340: 1539-45.
8) Mukherjee D, Eagle KA. Aortic dissection: an update. Curr Probl Cardiol 2005; 30: 287-325.
9) Nienaber CA, Kische S, Rousseau H, et al. Endovascular repair of type B aortic dissection: long-term results of the randomized investigation of stent grafts in aortic dissection trial. Circ Cardiovasc Interv 2013; 6(4): 407-16.
10) Tsai TT, Fattori R, Trimarchi S, et al. International Registry of Acute Aortic Dissection. Long-term survival

in patients presenting with type B acute aortic dissection: insights from the International Registry of Acute Aortic Dissection. Circulation 2006; 114: 2226-31.

11) Svensson LG, Kouchoukos NT, Miller DC, et al. Expert consensus document on the treatment of descending thoracic aortic disease using endovascular stentgrafts. Ann Thorac Surg 2008; 85(Suppl 1): S1-S41.
12) Erbel R, Alfonso F, Boileau C, et al. Task Force on Aortic Dissection, European Society of Cardiology. Diagnosis and management of aortic dissections. Eur Heart J 2001; 22: 1642-81.
13) Huptas S, Mehta RH, Kühl H, et al. Aortic remodeling in type B aortic dissection: effects of endovascular stent-graft repair and medical treatment on true and false lumen volumes. J Endovasc Ther 2009; 16: 28-38.
14) Nienaber CA, Rousseau H, Eggebrecht H, et al. Randomized comparison of strategies for type B aortic dissection: the INvestigation of STEnt Grafts in Aortic Dissection (INSTEAD) trial. Circulation 2009; 120: 2519-28.
15) Suzuki T, Isselbacher EM, Nienaber CA, et al. Type-selective benefits of medications in treatment of acute aortic dissection (from the International Registry of Acute Aortic Dissection [IRAD]). Am J Cardiol 2012; 109: 122-7.
16) Ohrlander T, Sonesson B, Ivancev K, et al. The chimney graft: a technique for preserving or rescuing aortic branch vessels in stent-graft sealing zones. J Endovasc Ther 2008; 15: 427-32.
17) Hiramoto JS, Chang CK, Reilly LM, et al. Outcome of renal stenting for renal artery coverage during endovascular aortic aneurysm repair. J Vasc Surg 2009; 49: 1100-6.
18) Hiramoto JS, Schneider DB, Reilly LM, et al. A double-barrel stent-graft for endovascular repair of the aortic arch. J Endovasc Ther 2006; 13: 72-6.
19) Baldwin ZK, Chuter TA, Hiramoto JS, et al. Double-barrel technique for preservation of aortic arch branches during thoracic endovascular aortic repair. Ann Vasc Surg 2008; 22: 703-9.
20) Baldwin ZK, Chuter TA, Hiramoto JS, et al. Double-barrel technique for endovascular exclusion of an aortic arch aneurysm without sternotomy. J Endovasc Ther 2008; 15: 161-5.
21) Criado FJ. Chimney grafts and bare stents: aortic branch preservation revisited. J Endovasc Ther 2007; 14: 823-4.
22) Lobato AC, Camacho-Lobato L. Endovascular treatment of complex aortic aneurysms using the sandwich technique. J Endovasc Ther 2012; 19: 691-706.
23) Lobato AC, Camacho-Lobato L. A new technique to enhance endovascular thoracoabdominal aortic aneurysm therapy: the sandwich procedure. Semin Vasc Surg 2012; 25: 153-160.
24) Lobato AC, Camacho-Lobato L. Sandwich techniques for complex aortoiliac and thoracoabdominal aortic aneurysms. Endovascular Today 2016; 15(3).
25) Lobato AC, Camacho-Lobato L. The sandwich technique to treat complex aortoiliac or isolated iliac aneurysms: Results of midterm follow-up. J Vasc Surg 2013; 57: 23-34.

35

Spinal cord vascularization

Germano Melissano, Roberto Chiesa, Christian Etz and Randall B. Griepp

This chapter is the joint effort of two groups with a profound interest in spinal cord vasculature and how it is related to ischemic complications after aortic procedures. These groups have pursued two different lines of research stressing, on one side, the importance of the anterior spinal artery and its segmental feeders (in particular, the arteria radicularis magna) and how they can be visualized with different imaging modalities, and, on the other side, the importance of the paraspinal collateral network system in protecting against the development of spinal cord injury (SCI) after aortic procedures. We strongly believe that these two lines of research are complementary and are both equally important for a better understanding of the pathophysiology of spinal cord ischemia and how to prevent it.

Please note that the order of presentation in this chapter as well as the order in which the authors are listed does not reflect any partiality for one line of research over the other.

35.1 Introduction

A precise preoperative knowledge of the spinal cord (SC) blood supply is an important aid for preventing spinal ischemic complications after procedures involving the thoracic and thoracoabdominal aorta [1].

Unfortunately, *in vivo* studies of the SC vasculature are complex and difficult to perform for several reasons. The SC vasculature consists of very small vessels [2] (Table 35.1) running in intricate, three-dimensional planes with substantial regional and inter-individual variability. Comparative anatomy studies are of limited use: due to the significant anatomical differences between species, gross anatomical studies are arduous because of the relative inaccessibility of the SC within the spinal column [2]. *In vivo* angiography [3] fails to adequately image the entire spinal circulation due to competitive flow from several feeding arteries. Selective angiography before thoracoabdominal aortic surgery is technically demanding and invasive in this clinical setting and in spite of the initial interesting results it is currently employed only in selected centers [4-7].

Information about the SC circulation has for the most part been gained from post-mortem studies after microinjections of staining fluids and micro-radiological assessments [2]. Anatomy handbooks, on the other hand, are sometimes vague and imprecise concerning SC angio-architecture. Teaching is often based purely on anatomical sketches which are not al-

---

Germano Melissano (melissano.germano@hsr.it)
Vita-Salute San Raffaele University,
Scientific Institute Ospedale San Raffaele, Milan, Italy

G. Melissano - R. Chiesa (eds), Aortic Dissection patients true stories and the innovations that saved their lives

Table 35.1 Inner vessel diameter of the main arteries supplying the spinal cord according to Thron's post-mortem study (1988) on a total of 66 human specimens [2]

	Upper thoracic region (mm)	Thoracolumbar region (mm)
Anterior radicular artery	≤ 0.5	0.5-0.8
Posterior radicular artery	≤ 0.2	0.2-0.5
Anterior spinal artery	0.2-0.4	0.5-0.8
Posterolateral spinal artery	0.1-0.25	0.1-0.4
Arteria radicularis magna		0.55-1.2

ways accurate and, moreover, confusion can arise from inconsistent nomenclature among different authors.

Recently, imaging methods such as magnetic resonance (MR) angiography and computed tomography (CT) angiography [8, 9] have opened up new possibilities for the non-invasive evaluation of SC vasculature in individual patients, particularly for determining the presence and location of the artery of Adamkiewicz. The ability of MR and CT to detect the SC feeders was recently analyzed in a review involving 1196 patients [9]. Although MR angiography has shown brilliant results in this field, we have concentrated our efforts on CT angiography which also offers excellent imaging capabilities, particularly with the use of state-of-the-art multidetector scanners. 64-Row CT scans are now available at many institutions, and are widely used for the diagnosis and therapeutic planning of thoracic and thoracoabdominal disease. Hence, for our study of the SC anatomy in patients with aortic disease, the data set we need is, in fact, already available.

35.2 Vascular imaging

Nowadays, a data set of standard contrast-enhanced CT scans obtained with a multidetector 64-row scanner can be easily and inexpensively navigated and elaborated at the physician's own desktop with the use of dedicated software. The ability to scroll through an image set, magnify an image, adjust its intensity and contrast, and measure lengths, angles, or volumes are useful basic features of a workstation. However, rendering tools for the display and manipulation of the data such as reformatting axial images in coronal and sagittal planes are necessary, and a variety of such tools is available. A specific tool allows simultaneous viewing of data reformatted in three orthogonal or oblique planes (multiplanar reformatting, MPR). Curved MPR allows the user to manually draw a curved path to generate a curved plane through the three-dimensional (3D) data set. This is useful, for instance, in following tortuous arteries. Three-dimensional maximum intensity projection (MIP) allows "flattening" of a volume and is useful for reconstructions of vascular detail. One of the most impressive features is 3D volume rendering, which assigns different colors and transparency to different intensity values in the data set, producing highly realistic images. While different reformatting software products are available today, all the CT reconstructions presented in this paper were obtained using OsiriX [10] software (Pixmeo srl, Geneva, Switzerland) applied to standard CT scan data sets in patients with thoracic or thoracoabdominal pathology.

35.3 Vascular anatomy

As surgeons, in the past we generally did not have a gross visualization of the vessels that contribute to SC vascularization much beyond the origin of the intercostal or lumbar arteries. CT analysis has allowed us to fill this gap, at least in the virtual world of medical images,

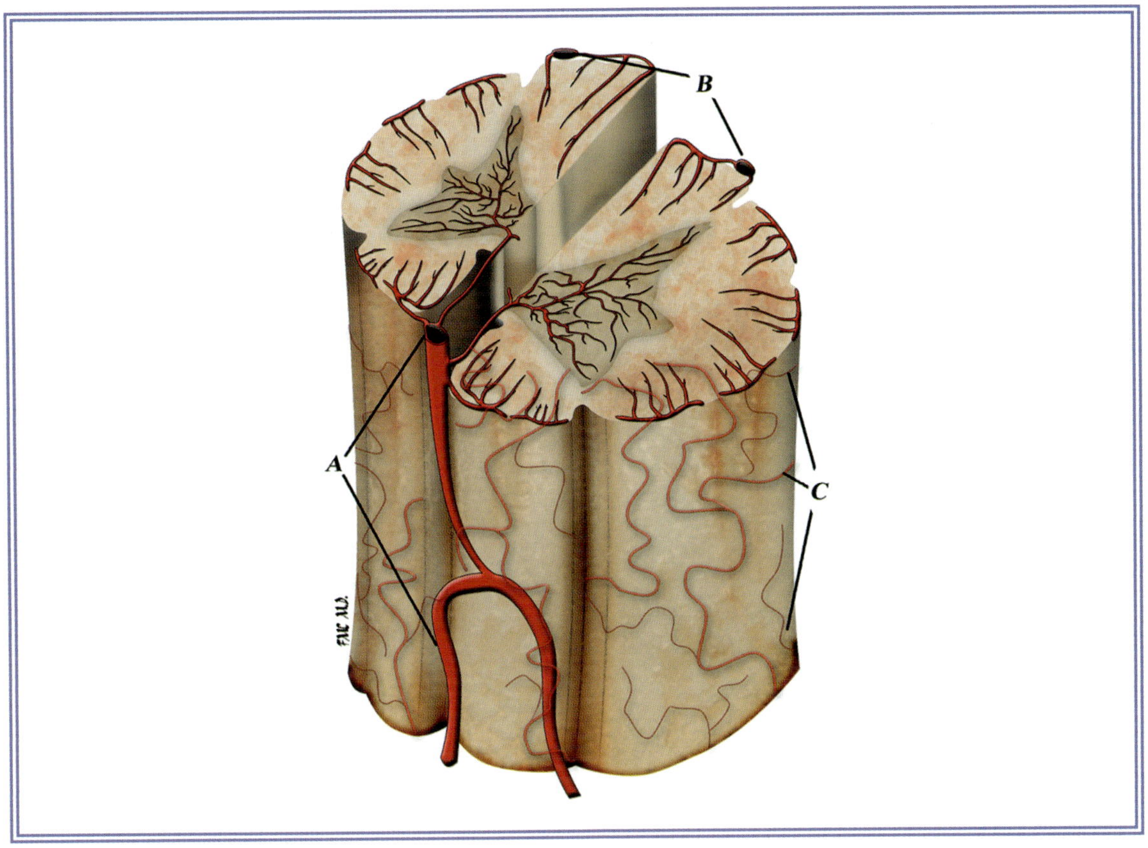

Fig. 35.1 The spinal cord is covered by a net-like anastomosing vascular system in which the anterior spinal artery (A) and the two posterolateral spinal arteries (B) can be considered the most constant longitudinal anastomotic trunks. The network is supplemented by a system of closely meshed longitudinal and transverse anastomoses of second and third degree. However, as far as acute demands are concerned, the anastomotic capacity of the anterior spinal artery may not be sufficient because of narrowing or interruptions at different levels. The pial network (C) and intra-medullary anastomoses may only be important for slower circulatory adjustments since their calibers are inadequate for a sudden intake of larger volumes of blood. This concept may be crucial for understanding the pathogenesis of SC ischemia after surgical or endovascular procedures involving the thoracoabdominal aorta. Reproduced from [25], with permission.

in many individual patients, producing interesting and pictorially fascinating results. These images obtained with 2D MPR and 3D volume rendering techniques have enabled us now to follow the SC blood supply from the aorta to the anterior spinal artery (ASA), offering a complete visualization of the branching pattern (refer to Fig. 35.3 legend for further detail).

Spinal cord vessels have remarkably efficient collateral pathways that make spontaneous spinal stroke very rare, even when the origin of most intercostal and lumbar arteries is chronically obstructed. Remarkably, the first accurate anatomical descriptions were provided in 1881 by Adamkiewicz and Kady [11]. They used a clearing method with clove oil (mentioned by Virchow in 1857) that produces transparent tissue sections so that the stained vessels can be studied under the microscope. They described the vascular system of the SC as consisting of one anterior and two posterolateral anastomotic trunks running longitudinally (Fig. 35.1).

Inflow vessels to the SC include: the subclavian artery through the vertebral artery, the thyrocervical trunk, and the costocervical trunk; several segmental feeders from the intercostal and lumbar arteries; and the hypogastric arteries through the lateral sacral and iliolumbar arteries. Arteries directly nourishing the SC (intrinsic arterial system) are divided into two different systems: a central (centrifugal) system fed by the sulcal arteries; and a peripheral (centripetal) system, the pial plexus (or pial network), which gives origin to perforating branches (Fig. 35.2). The pial network forms an impressive secondary anastomotic system along the entire length of the SC between the anterior and posterolateral longitudinal vessels. Intraparenchymal anastomoses have been rarely documented.

In order to reach the ASA, which supplies blood to the spinal gray matter, the intercostal arteries divide three times:

1) the first branch of the intercostal artery is the nervo-medullary artery;
2) the latter divides into an anterior and posterior radicular artery;
3) the anterior radicular artery then divides into a descending and an ascending branch.

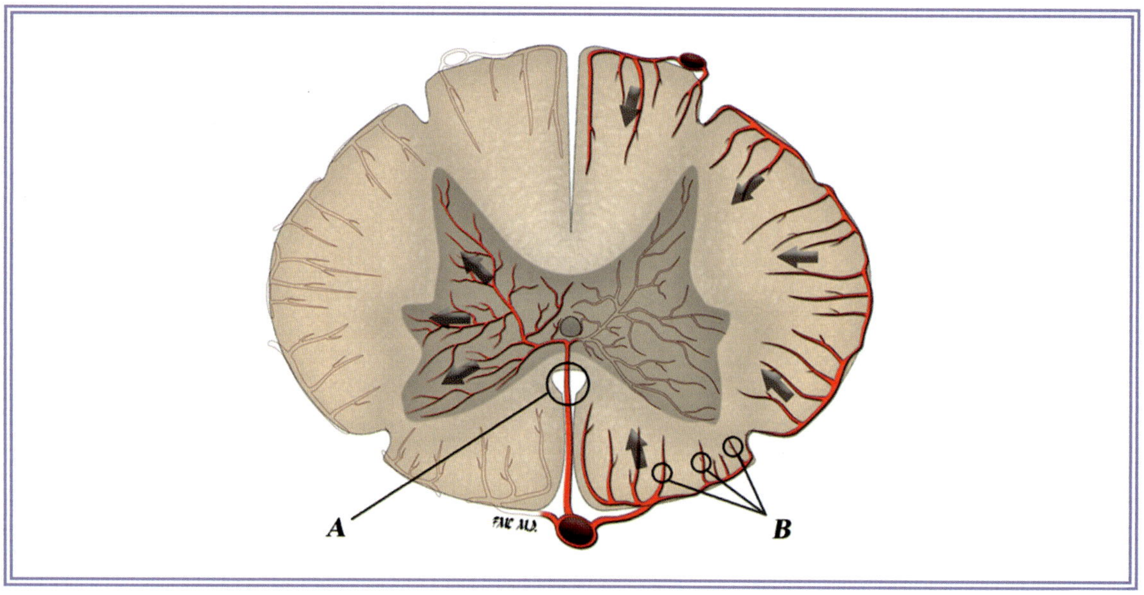

Fig. 35.2 The intrinsic arterial system of the spinal cord is divided into a central (centrifugal) system and a peripheral (centripetal) system. The central system (highlighted on the left side of the figure) is represented by the sulcal arteries, which approach from the anterior arterial tract, pass into the anterior median fissures (A), penetrate into the medulla on the left or right, and branch out, tree-like, mainly in the gray matter. The peripheral system (highlighted on the right side of the figure) consists of numerous small arteries denominated "rami perforantes" (B) which originate in the pial network covering the spinal cord and pass through the white matter in a radial course. Reproduced from [25], with permission.

The ASA is ultimately an anastomotic channel between ascending and descending branches of neighboring anterior radicular arteries.

This branching pattern is schematically shown in Figure 35.3; it should be noted that this simplification has a misleading aspect because all the arteries are shown on the same plane; this is certainly not the case *in vivo*, where vessel tortuosity, combined with the narrow diameter, often make imaging difficult. Figure 35.3 depicts images of these arteries obtained from actual patients' CT data sets and rendered with different algorithms (refer to Figure 35.3 legend for further detail).

It is notable that the nervo-medullary artery division is a constant supplying vessel of the anterior and posterior part of the vertebral canal, the nerve roots, and the dura; however, at only a few levels do the anterior and posterior radicular arteries cross the dura together with the anterior and posterior nerve roots to reach the surface of the medulla. Phylogenetic embryological studies have shown that by the 16th week, development of the ASA is followed by regression of most of the original 31 bilateral segmental feeders (Fig. 35.4). In fact only a few (2-14, on average 6) of these segmental branches remain in the adult: a mean of 2-3 at the cervical level (left = right), 2-3 at the thoracic level (left > right), and 0-1 at the lumbosacral level (left > right) (Fig. 35.4). The statistical frequency of vaso-afference, i.e. anterior radicular artery feeders to the anterior spinal artery, in the different vertebral regions according to Thron's topographical analysis [2] is described in Table 35.2. In the thoracolumbar region, one (occasionally 2 or 3) anterior radicular artery is always distinctly dominant in caliber and is therefore called the great radicular artery or arteria radicularis magna (ARM) or the artery of Adamkiewicz.

The division of the ARM is, anatomically speaking, highly characteristic (Figs. 35.5-35.7): the radicular artery has a steep cranially-directed course in the thoracolumbar region due to the ontogenetical "ascent" of the SC. Branching takes place lateral to the midline, where a smaller ascending branch is issued before reaching the midline, while the main artery con-

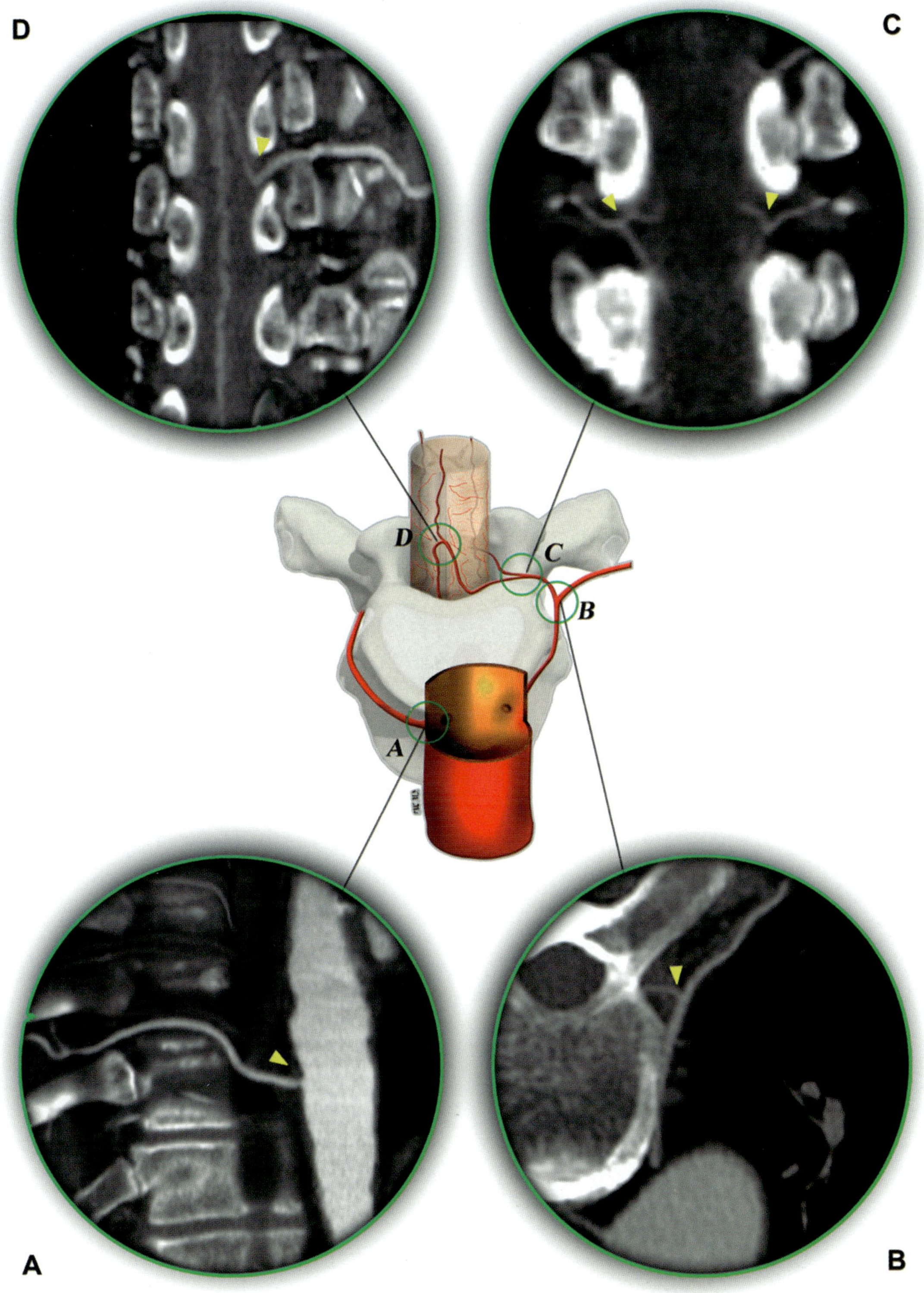

Fig. 35.3 Schematic depiction of the spinal cord extrinsic arterial system. **A**, Origin of the intercostal arteries from the aorta [insert: CT curved multiplanar reformatting (MPR)]. **B**, Origin of the nervo-medullary artery (or radiculomedullary artery) from the intercostal artery [insert: CT maximum intensity projection (MIP) of an axial view]. **C**, The nervo-medullary artery divides into constant branches, the anterior and posterior radicular artery [insert: CT MIP of a coronal view]. **D**, One anterior radicular artery is always dominant in caliber in the thoracic region and is therefore called the great radicular artery (or the artery of Adamkiewicz) [insert: CT curved MPR]. Reproduced from [25], with permission.

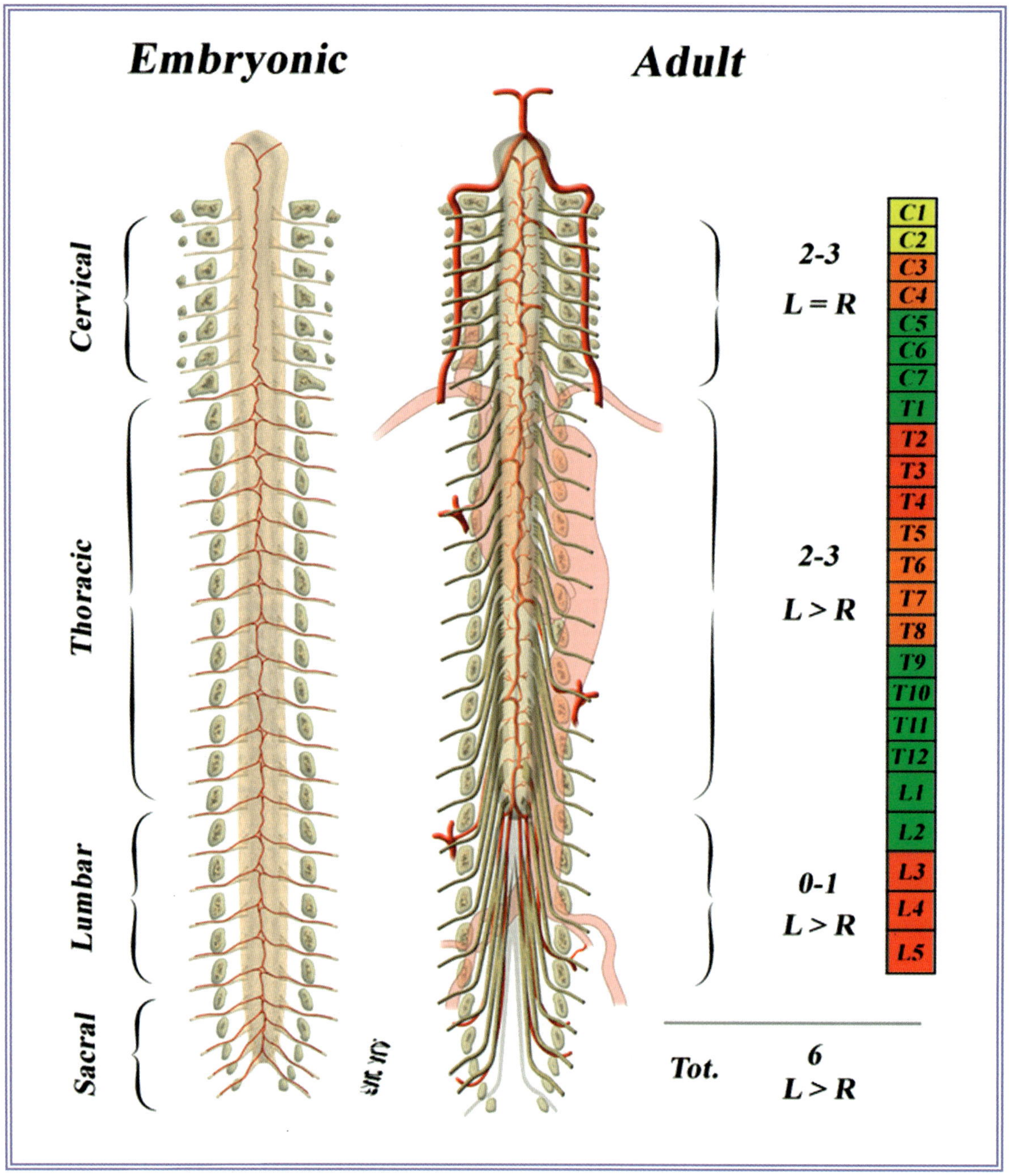

Fig. 35.4 Artistic depiction of embryological development (16th week) of the anterior spinal artery from 31 bilateral segmental feeders. The anterior spinal artery develops from the anastomosis of ascending and descending branches of each segmental anterior radicular artery. In the adult, most of the segmental feeders of the anterior spinal artery (ASA) regress. Only a few (2-14, mean 6) of these feeders are left in the adult. A mean of 2-3 at the cervical level (left = right), 2-3 at the thoracic level (left > right) and 0-1 at the lumbosacral level (left > right). The frequency of segmental feeders varies according to vertebral topography. The differences of the vaso-afference in the vertebral regions are depicted in different colors (obligatory = green, deficient = red, facultative = orange, and variable = yellow); see also Table 35.2. Reproduced from [25], with permission.

Table 35.2 Regions of vaso-afference: statistical frequency of anterior radicular artery feeders to the anterior spinal artery, according to vertebral topography as described by Thron [2]

Vertebral regions			
Obligatory	C5-C8	T9-L2	
Facultative	C3-C4	T4-T6	
Deficient		T1-T3	L3-L5
Variable	C1-C2		

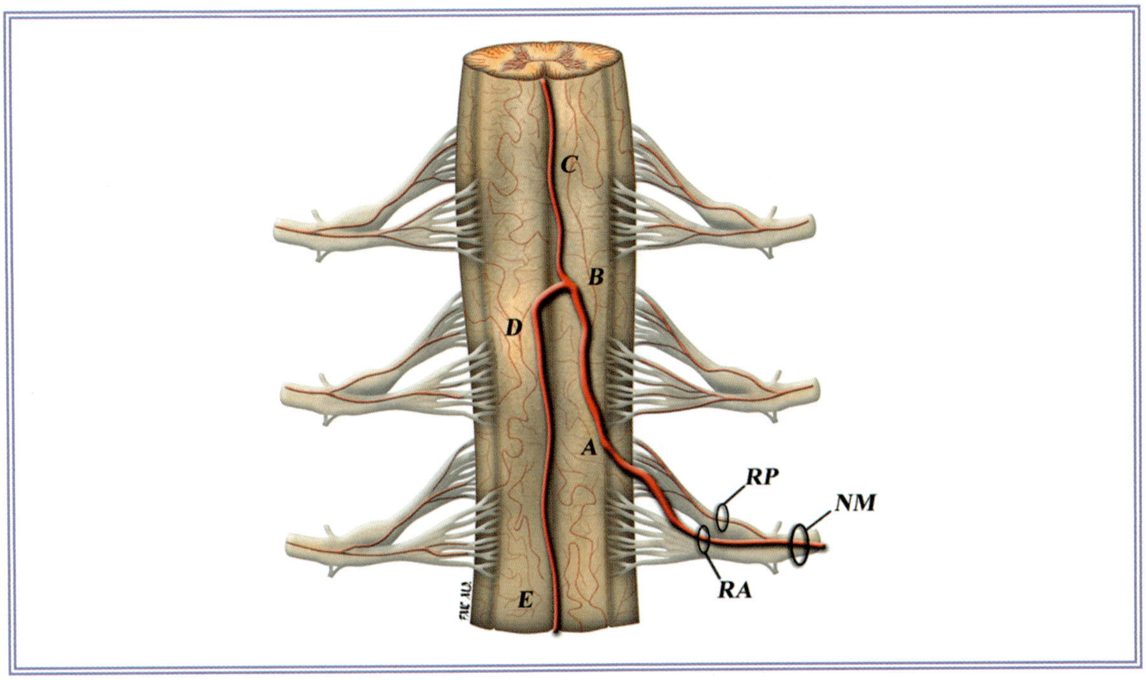

Fig. 35.5 Schematic view of the great radicular artery or arteria radicularis magna (the artery of Adamkiewicz). The nervo-medullary (NM) artery divides into an anterior (RA) and posterior radicular (RP) artery. However, few arteries cross the dura and only a few anterior radicular arteries feed directly into the anterior spinal artery (see also Fig. 35.2 and Table 35.2). The artery of Adamkiewicz division has a steep cranially directed course (A); branching takes place lateral to the midline (B), and a smaller ascending branch (C) is issued before reaching the midline; the main artery continues its vertical course, and then bends sharply in a typical "hairpin" curve (D) into the larger descending branch (E). Reproduced from [25], with permission.

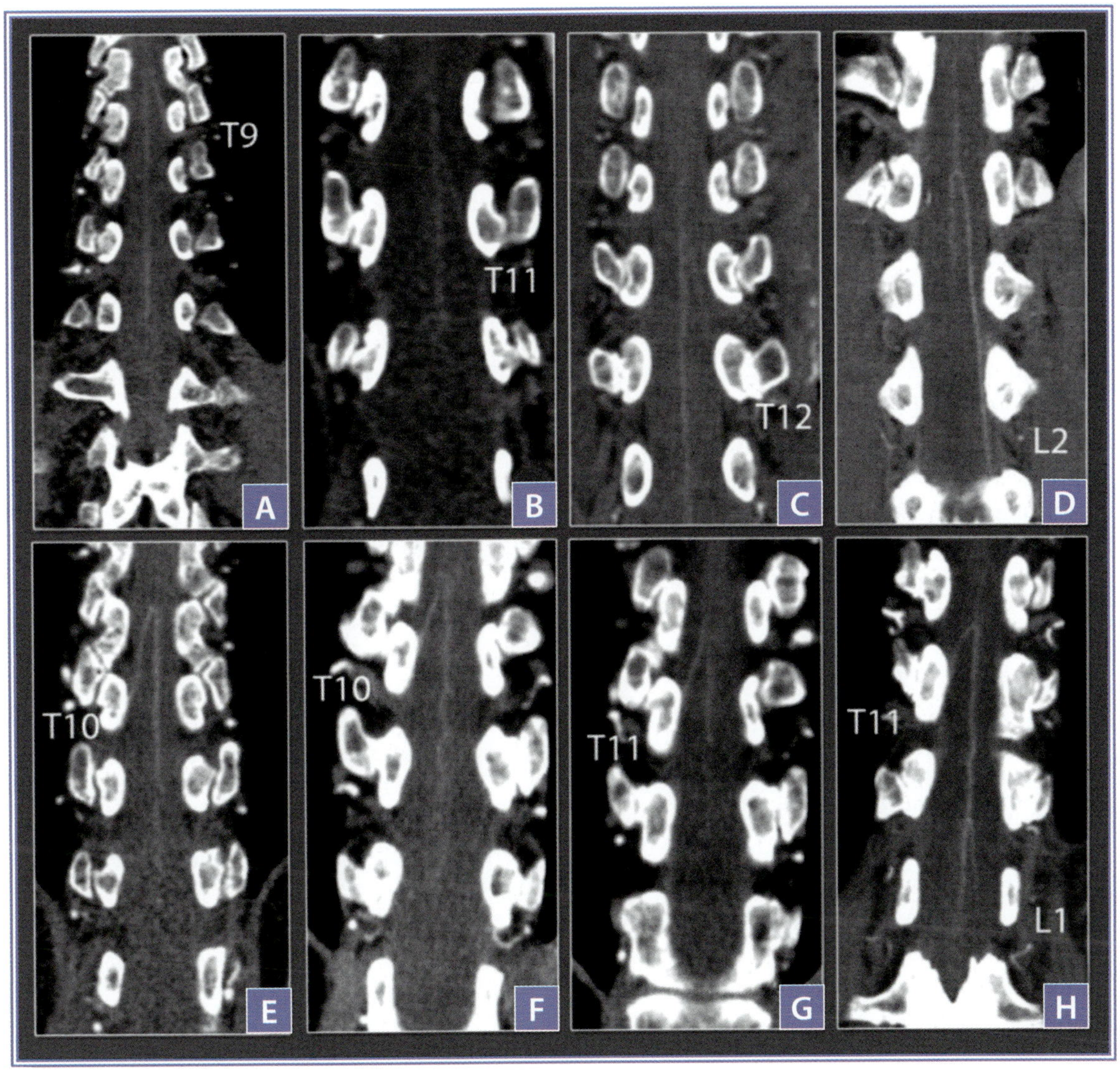

Fig. 35.6 CT MPR of different cases of patients with thoracoabdominal pathology. Note from **A** to **D** the different patterns of left branching of the arteria radicularis magna (ARM), or artery of Adamkiewicz, arising from T9 to L2. Moreover, from **E** to **G** it is possible to observe different patterns of right branching of the ARM, and in **H** a double ARM, fed respectively from T11 and L1.

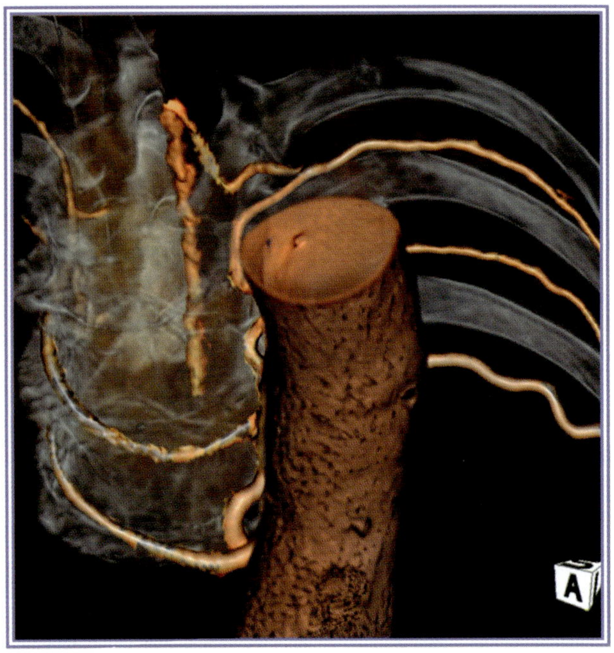

Fig. 35.7 CT 3D volume rendering, performed with the OsiriX software and the Fovia plug-in, in which the soft tissues were removed and the bone rendered transparent to enhance visibility of the Adamkiewicz artery and its typical conformation in a left anterolateral view. Reproduced from [25], with permission.

tinues its vertical course, bending sharply in a typical "hairpin" curve into the descending branch. In the upper thoracic region, on the other hand, branching is more often T-shaped.

In the cervical region, the ASA continuity is less constant and sometimes duplication is present. The course of the ASA often deviates in a zigzag from the midline and varies in caliber with typical narrowing.

35.4 Discussion

SC vasculature was originally visualized with routine contrast-enhanced CT scanning in 1994 [12]. Only in the last decade, however, have improvements in CT scanners and post processing techniques made it possible to systematically detect the ARM. Multi-detector row helical CT enables examination over an extensive range in the cranio-caudal direction with thin collimation in a short time interval (excellent temporal and spatial resolution). Millimeter sized arteries are nowadays well within the detection capabilities of this technique; however, the ARM detection rate reported in the literature has reached 100% or near 100% in only a minority of studies [9]. CT angiography performed with intra-aortic contrast media injection offers outstanding images and 100% detection of the ARM, but this is not the standard method used in most centers [13]. Recent advancement of CT scan techniques has made it possible to obtain higher rates of visualization of the ARM also with 64-slice intravenous CT angiography [14].

With CT angiography, however, some degree of uncertainty can exist concerning the differential diagnosis between artery (ARM) and vein, because the anterior median vein draining to a radicular vein presents a similar shape to that of the ARM. The differentiation is especially difficult for the anterior SC vasculature, since the draining vein usually has a larger diameter and is more easily detected. To help identify a radicular vessel such as the artery, several criteria may be applied:

1. simultaneous visualization of ARM and ASA as two enhanced spots in the ventral aspect of the SC in consecutive transverse scans;
2. characteristic anatomic relation of the two vessels (hairpin shape);
3. continuity of the ARM traceable to vessels of certain arterial nature (e.g. intercostal-lumbar artery, aorta);

4. failure of enhancement and visualization of the posterior spinal vein and of other veins surrounding the spine (e.g. intercostal, lumbar, and azygos veins).

Continuity with a vessel that is definitely an artery is clearly pathognomonic; since this is not always possible, judgment will have to rely on the other criteria which are less certain.

Knowledge about the venous anatomy and overall SC circulatory physiology is even less clear than that about the arteries. Intrinsic medullary veins lie within the dura mater, which is relatively inextensible, and drain to the extra-dural venous plexus via the anterior and posterior radicular veins that cross the dura with the nerve roots. Obstruction of venous outflow secondary to cerebrospinal fluid (CSF) hypertension during thoracic aortic cross-clamping could play a role in reduced SC perfusion, sustaining a vicious cycle of edema, CSF hypertension, venous obstruction, and malperfusion. This possibility supports the use of CSF drainage to prevent or treat peri-procedural SC ischemia [15].

The circulatory physiology at the level of the complex anatomical network previously described is also not fully clear. The ASA can narrow or even be interrupted at different locations, supporting the concept of a "circulatory partial system". Since anterior radicular feeders, reaching the medullary surface, join the ASA branching cranially and caudally, the blood stream should also divide into two partial streams, one running superiorly and one inferiorly. Therefore, opposing partial flows should approach each other in the longitudinally running spinal arteries at least for a portion of the cardiac cycle. While a complete anatomo-functional continuity of the ASA or of the pial plexus as anastomotic pathways is proposed by some authors [16, 17], a key characteristic of SC blood supply is the extreme inter-individual anatomical variability. Therefore, studies based on only a small number of cases will fail to obtain a clear general picture of this complex system. Moreover, the low but consistent incidence of paraplegia after thoracic stent-grafting [18-22], which does not necessitate aortic cross-clamping but may reduce the intercostal segmental supply to the ASA, demonstrates that, in an acute setting, the anastomotic capability of the SC blood supply is not unlimited.

Knowing the principal anatomical features of SC blood supply of individual patients undergoing thoracoabdominal interventions, whether open or endovascular, has several potential benefits [23, 24]. This is especially true if the information can be gathered from an exam that is already part of the diagnostic workup of these patients (namely, CT angiography). For open surgery, analysis of SC vasculature could tell us about the aortic region feeding the ARM, and thus requiring reimplantation, although the benefits and drawbacks of segmental artery reimplantation are still heavily debated in the scientific community. For endovascular procedures, knowledge about the SC vasculature could tell us whether the ARM will be covered by the stent graft and so make it possible to avoid unnecessary coverage. It can also be used to stratify patients according to risk of ischemic SC events, possibly guiding the selective use of CSF drainage.

35.5 New concepts in spinal cord vascularization: the paraspinal collateral network

Despite various techniques to avoid spinal cord injury, the incidence of paraplegia and paraparesis after open and endovascular interventions of extensive thoracic and thoracoabdominal aneurysms remains unacceptably high. Therefore, over the past decade, efforts have been made by dedicated research groups to reevaluate not only the anatomy but also the physiology of the spinal cord circulation [26-28]. Through systematic exploration and description of pressure and perfusion characteristics in large animal models as well as in clinical studies [26, 29], the existence of an extensive network of vessels supplying the spinal cord and the adjacent paraspinal muscles has been demonstrated (Fig. 35.8). The ASA is richly interconnected within this network, which in turn has multiple connections at each level allowing for an overarching horizontal and longitudinal collateralization across segments [27, 30]. Moreover,

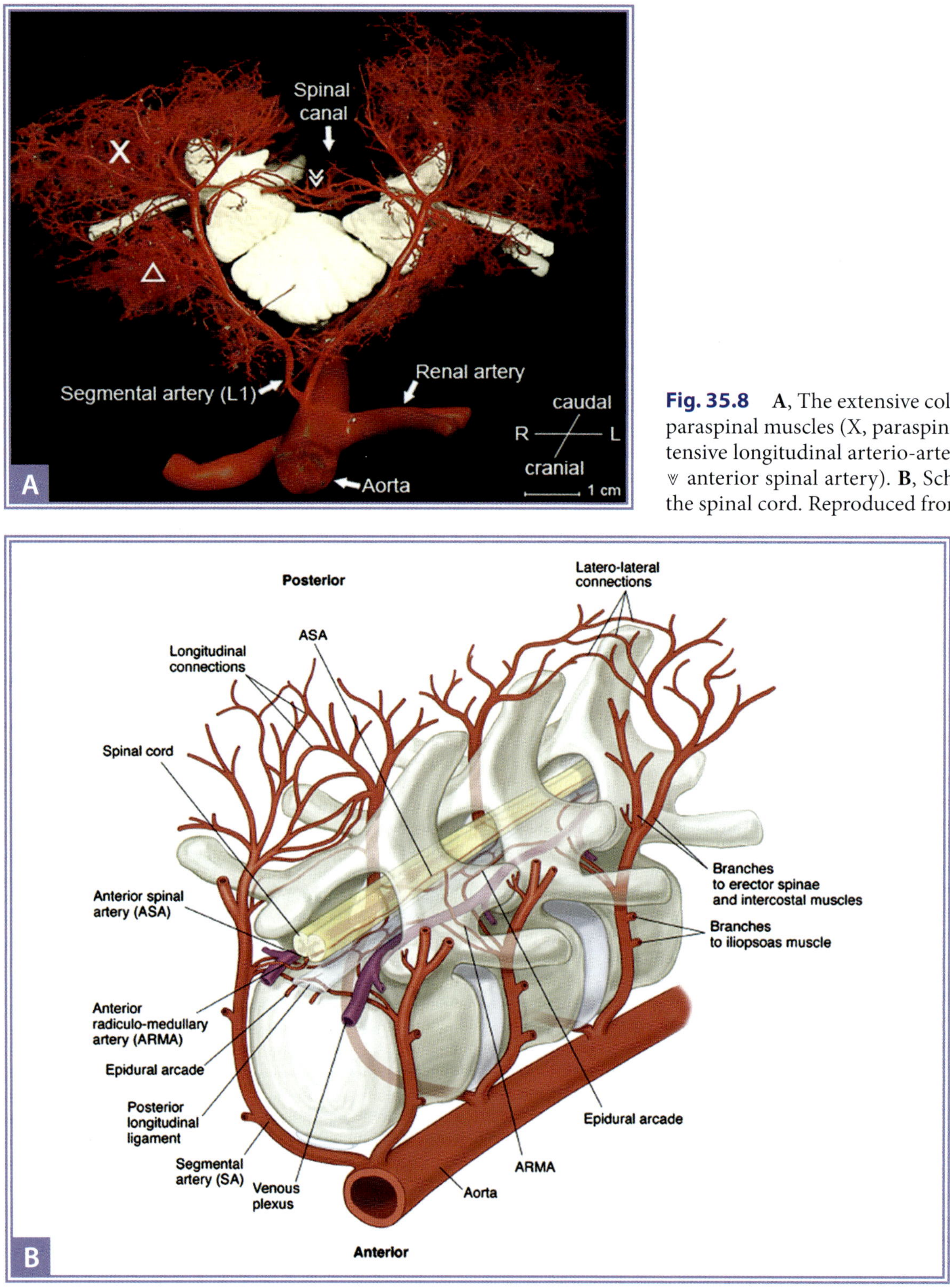

Fig. 35.8 **A**, The extensive collateral network that can be found in the paraspinal muscles (X, paraspinous muscular vasculature providing extensive longitudinal arterio-arterioral connections; Δ, iliopsoas muscle; ⩔ anterior spinal artery). **B**, Schematic diagram of the blood supply to the spinal cord. Reproduced from [27], with permission.

the paraspinal network possesses the ability to adapt to the loss of direct perfusion input from aortic segmental arteries (SA), as has been shown in experimental studies after consecutive SA sacrifice. Through vascular remodeling – by means of arteriogenesis, vessel parallelization and caliber expansion – the paraspinal collateral network (PCN) maintains spinal cord viability to guard against the development of subsequent spinal cord injury (SCI) (Fig. 35.9).

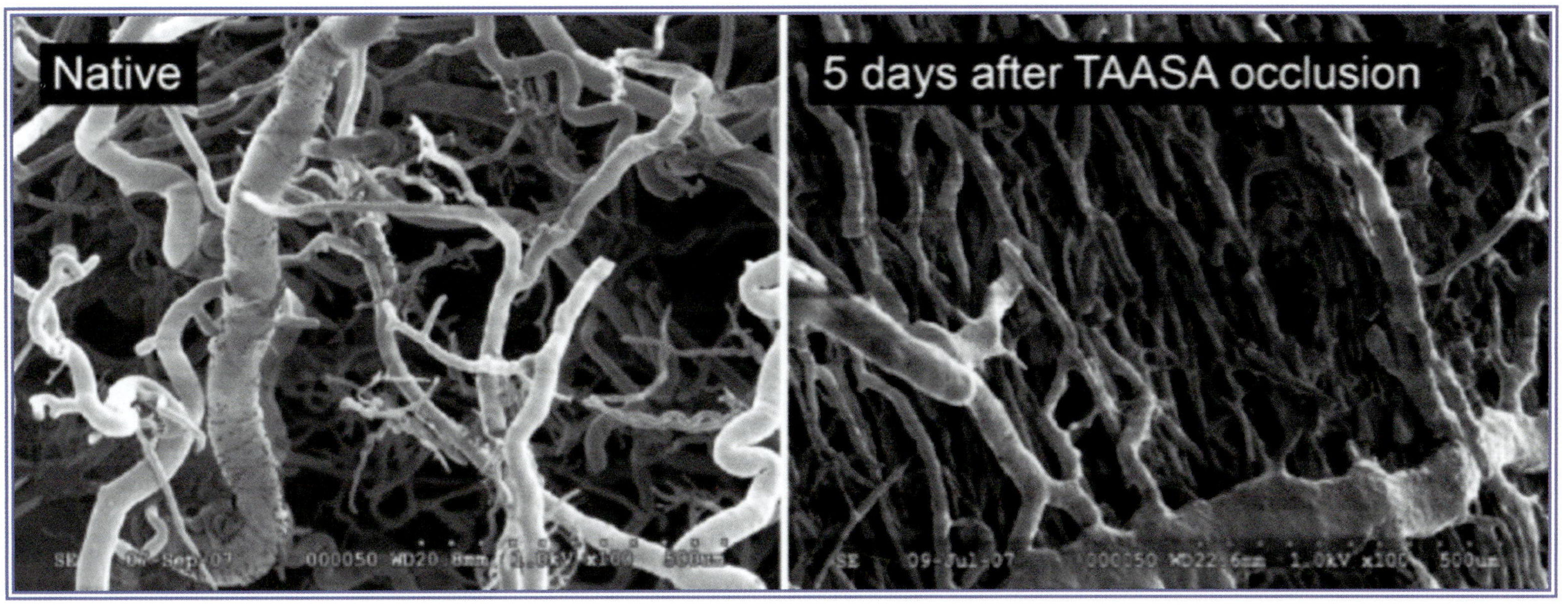

Fig. 35.9 Vascular remodelling by means of arteriogenesis vessel parallelization and caliber expansion (modified from [26]).

The implications of the role played by the PCN have now, for the first time, provided the basis for understanding the reasons for a staged approach in treatment of extensive thoracoabdominal aneurysms [30, 31]. It has been shown that "staged repair" significantly reduces SCI compared to a conventional one-stage approach [31, 32], paving the way for a holistic preconditioning concept in SCI prevention prior to thoracic and thoracoabdominal aortic repair [33-35]. Based on the concept of a collateral network, and the new principle of "staged-repair" proposed by Etz et al., a trial involving an international consortium of world-renowned aortic centers funded by the European Research Commission has been set up and will be launched in 2017: "Paraplegia Prevention in Aortic Aneurysm Repair by Thoracoabdominal staging with 'Minimally-Invasive Segmental Artery Coil-Embolization' (MISACE): A Randomized Controlled Multicenter Trial (PAPA_ARTiS)".

35.6 Conclusions

In the past when surgeons operated on the aorta, the variable anatomy of the SC-feeding arteries required them to make a "leap of faith". This leap is no longer necessary given recent breakthroughs in imaging technologies and post-processing software. It is, in fact, now possible to visualize the SC vascularization from the aorta to the ASA, in many cases.

For this to be clinically relevant, however, additional clinical studies are needed in subjects with and without aortic disease, both before and after operative procedures. Large numbers of patients will need to be studied in order to compensate for the inter-individual variability of the SC blood supply. While this task may seem overwhelming, substantial and rapid technological improvements have now made this type of study easy to perform, and able to provide significant clinical benefit in the management of patients with aortic disease.

Acknowledgments

The Authors gratefully acknowledge for their contribution to this chapter and to the underlying research in the past years: Drs. Luca Bertoglio, Andrea Kahlberg and Enrico Rinaldi.

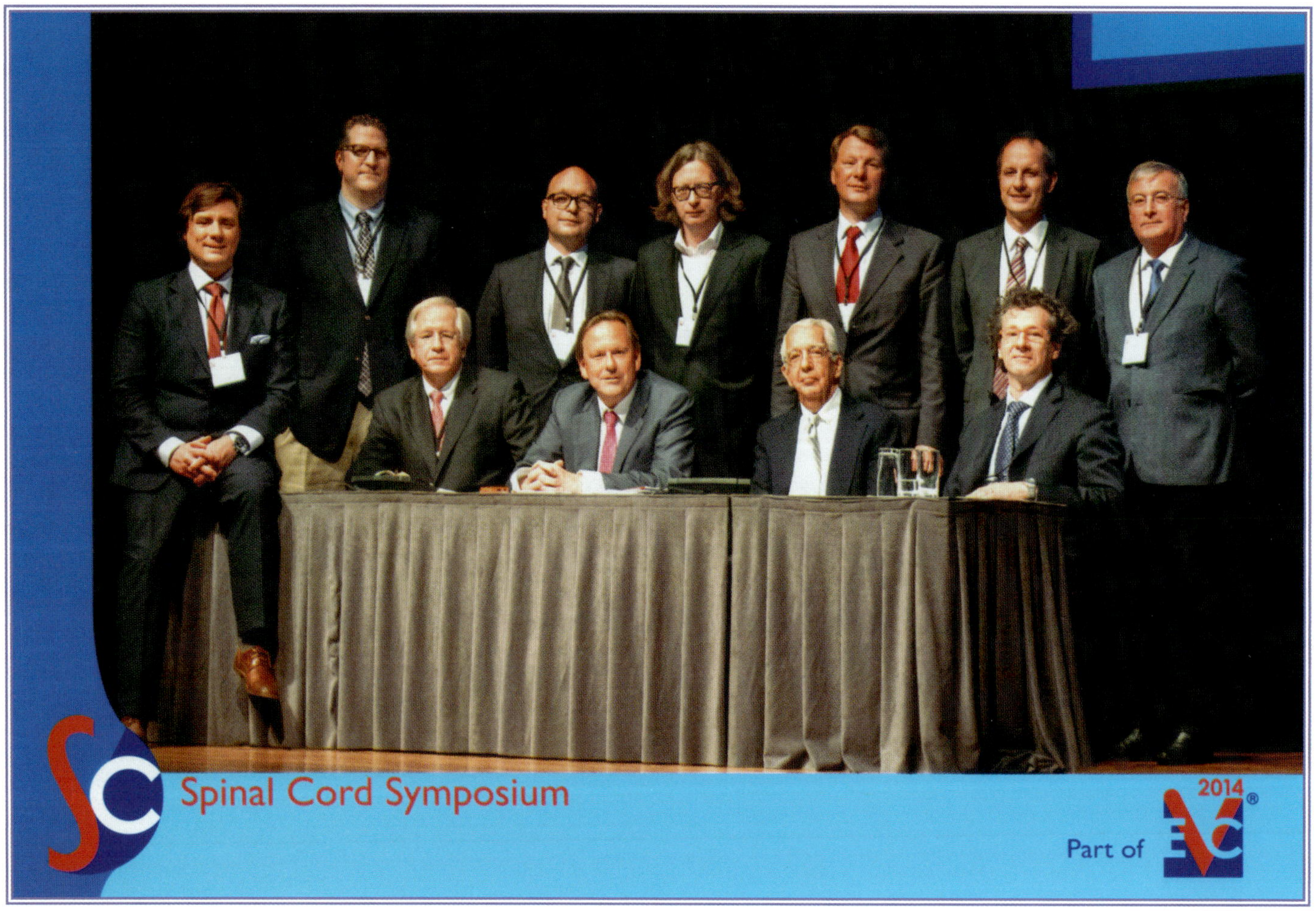

Advancements in this highly specialized field rely also on meetings and symposia where experts can share their recent research. This picture portrays some of the authors of this book gathered at the Spinal Cord Symposium during the 2014 EVC in Maastricht. Seated from left to right are: Profs. Etz, Coselli, Jacobs, Griepp and Melissano.

REFERENCES

1) Hershberger R, Cho JS. Neurologic complications of aortic diseases and aortic surgery. Handb Clin Neurol 2014; 119: 223-38.
2) Thron AK. Vascular anatomy of the spinal cord: neuroradiological investigations and clinical syndromes. New York: Springer-Verlag; 1989.
3) Di Chiro G, Fried LC, Doppman JL. Experimental angiography of the spinal cord. Fortschr Geb Rontgenstr Nuklearmed 1970; 112: 380-1.
4) Williams GM, Perler BA, Burdick JF, et al. Angiographic localization of spinal cord blood supply and its relationship to postoperative paraplegia. J Vasc Surg 1991; 13: 23-35.
5) Heinemann MK, Brassel F, Herzog T, et al. The role of spinal angiography in operations on the thoracic aorta: myth or reality? Ann Thorac Surg 1998; 65: 346-51.
6) Kieffer E, Fukui S, Chiras J, et al. Spinal cord arteriography: a safe adjunct before descending thoracic or thoracoabdominal aortic aneurysmectomy. J Vasc Surg 2002; 35: 262-8.
7) Minatoya K, Karck M, Hagl C, et al. The impact of spinal angiography on the neurological outcome after surgery on the descending thoracic and thoracoabdominal aorta. Ann Thorac Surg 2002; 74: S1870-2.
8) Melissano G, Bertoglio L, Civelli V, et al. Demonstration of the Adamkiewicz artery by multidetector computed tomography angiography analysed with the open-source software OsiriX. Eur J Vasc Endovasc Surg 2009; 37: 395-400.
9) Melissano G, Chiesa R. Advances in imaging of the spinal cord vascular supply, and its relationship with paraplegia after aortic interventions. A review. Eur J Vasc Endovasc Surg 2009; 38: 567-77.

10) Setacci F, Sirignano P, Cappelli A, Setacci C. The wonders of a newly available post-analysis CT software in the hands of vascular surgeons. Eur J Vasc Endovasc Surg 2012; 43: 404-6.
11) Skalski PJ. Albert Wojciech Adamkiewicz (1850-1921). J Neurol 2007; 254: 818-9.
12) Sakai O, Furuse M, Nakashima N, et al. Visualization of the spinal vessels on routine abdominal CT. Eur Radiol 1994; 4: 545-8.
13) Uotani K, Yamada N, Kono AK, et al. Preoperative visualization of the artery of Adamkiewicz by intra-arterial CT angiography. Am J Neuroradiol 2008; 29: 314-8.
14) Nishii T, Kono AK, Negi N, et al. The feasibility of a 64-slice MDCT for detection of the Adamkiewicz artery: comparison of the detection rate of intravenous injection CT angiography using a 64-slice MDCT versus intra-arterial and intravenous injection CT angiography using a 16-slice MDCT. Int J Cardiovasc Imaging 2013; 29 Suppl 2:127-33.
15) Cinà CS, Abouzahr L, Arena GO, et al. Cerebrospinal fluid drainage to prevent paraplegia during thoracic and thoracoabdominal aortic aneurysm surgery: a systematic review and meta-analysis. J Vasc Surg 2004; 40: 36-44.
16) Griepp RB, Griepp EB. Spinal cord perfusion and protection during descending thoracic and thoracoabdominal aortic surgery: the collateral network concept. Ann Thorac Surg 2007; 83: S865-9.
17) Biglioli P, Roberto M, Cannata A, et al. Upper and lower spinal cord blood supply: the continuity of the anterior spinal artery and the relevance of the lumbar arteries. J Thorac Cardiovasc Surg 2004; 127: 1188-92.
18) Makaroun MS, Dillavou ED, Kee ST, et al. Endovascular treatment of thoracic aortic aneurysms: results of the phase II multicenter trial of the GORE TAG thoracic endoprosthesis. J Vasc Surg 2005; 41: 1-9.
19) Fairman RM, Criado F, Farber M, et al. VALOR Investigators. Pivotal results of the Medtronic Vascular Talent Thoracic Stent Graft System: the VALOR trial. J Vasc Surg 2008; 48: 546-54.
20) Matsumura JS, Cambria RP, Dake MD, et al.; TX2 Clinical Trial Investigators. International controlled clinical trial of thoracic endovascular aneurysm repair with the Zenith TX2 endovascular graft: 1-year results. J Vasc Surg 2008; 47: 247-57.
21) Chiesa R, Melissano G, Marrocco-Trischitta MM, Civilini E, Setacci F. Spinal cord ischemia after elective stent-graft repair of the thoracic aorta. J Vasc Surg 2005; 42: 11-7.
22) Chiesa R, Melissano G, Bertoglio L, et al. The risk of spinal cord ischemia during thoracic aorta endografting. Acta Chir Belg 2008; 108: 492-502.
23) Furukawa K, Kamohara K, Nojiri J, et al. Operative strategy for descending and thoracoabdominal aneurysm repair with preoperative demonstration of the Adamkiewicz artery. Ann Thorac Surg 2010; 90: 1840-6.
24) Shimizu H, Yozu R. Current strategies for spinal cord protection during thoracic and thoracoabdominal aortic aneurysm repair. Gen Thorac Cardiovasc Surg 2011; 59: 155-63.
25) Melissano G, Civilini E, Bertoglio L, et al. Angio-CT imaging of the spinal cord vascularisation: a pictorial essay. Eur J Vasc Endovasc Surg 2010; 39: 436-40.
26) Etz CD, Kari FA, Mueller CS, et al. The collateral network concept: remodeling of the arterial collateral network after experimental segmental artery sacrifice. J Thorac Cardiovasc Surg 2011; 141(4): 1029-36.
27) Etz CD, Kari FA, Mueller CS, et al. The collateral network concept: a reassessment of the anatomy of spinal cord perfusion. J Thorac Cardiovasc Surg 2011; 141(4): 1020-8.
28) Griepp EB, Griepp RB. The collateral network concept: minimizing paraplegia secondary to thoracoabdominal aortic aneurysm resection. Tex Heart Inst J 2010; 37(6): 672-4.
29) Etz CD, Zoli S, Bischoff MS, et al. Measuring the collateral network pressure to minimize paraplegia risk in thoracoabdominal aneurysm resection. J Thorac Cardiovasc Surg 2010; 140 (6 Suppl): S125-30.
30) Griepp RB, Griepp EB. Spinal cord protection in surgical and endovascular repair of thoracoabdominal aortic disease. J Thorac Cardiovasc Surg 2015; 149(2 Suppl): S86-90.
31) Etz CD, Zoli S, Mueller CS, et al. Staged repair significantly reduces paraplegia rate after extensive thoracoabdominal aortic aneurysm repair. J Thorac Cardiovasc Surg 2010; 139(6): 1464-72.
32) Maurel B, Delclaux N, Sobocinski J, et al. The impact of early pelvic and lower limb reperfusion and attentive peri-operative management on the incidence of spinal cord ischemia during thoracoabdominal aortic aneurysm endovascular repair. Eur J Vasc Endovasc Surg 2015; 49(3): 248-54.
33) Etz CD, Debus ES, Mohr FW, Kölbel T. First-in-man endovascular preconditioning of the paraspinal collateral network by segmental artery coil embolization to prevent ischemic spinal cord injury. J Thorac Cardiovasc Surg 2015; 149(4): 1074-9.
34) Geisbüsch S, Stefanovic A, Koruth JS, et al. Endovascular coil embolization of segmental arteries prevents paraplegia after subsequent thoracoabdominal aneurysm repair: an experimental model. J Thorac Cardiovasc Surg 2014; 147(1): 220-6.
35) von Aspern K, Luehr M, Mohr FW, Etz CD. Spinal cord protection in open- and endovascular thoracoabdominal aortic aneurysm repair: critical review of current concepts and future perspectives. J Cardiovasc Surg (Torino) 2015; 56(5): 745-9.

36

Anesthetic management of patients undergoing operation for Type A aortic dissection

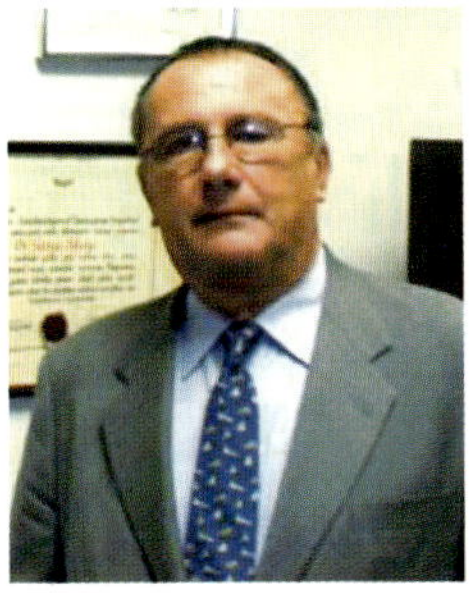

George Silvay and John G. Augoustides

36.1 Introduction

Type A aortic dissection (AD) is defined in the Stanford classification as dissection of the ascending aorta, regardless of distal extent [1]. Furthermore, acute Type A AD is defined as presentation within 2 weeks of clinical onset of the dissection process. Clinical presentation after 2 weeks of onset is defined as chronic Type A AD. Acute Type A AD is part of the spectrum of acute aortic syndromes that include intramural hematoma and penetrating ulcer [1]. Please refer to the relevant chapters in this textbook for a detailed overview of Type A AD, including the clinical presentations, diagnosis, and therapeutic considerations.

As described in this textbook, the etiologies for Type A AD include hypertension, atherosclerosis, connective tissue disorders, infection, trauma, and previous cardiac surgery. The inherited disorders associated with Type A AD include the aortopathies associated with Marfan syndrome, Ehlers-Danlos syndrome, Loeys-Dietz syndrome and the bicuspid aortic valve [1]. The management of acute Type A AD is emergent surgery after initial medical stabilization, including strict control of hypertension [1]. The management of chronic Type A AD is initially medical with surgery reserved for management of complications such as large aneurysm [1, 2].

36.2 Historical perspectives

One of the first observed diseases of the cardiovascular system – dilation of arteries – was observed in ancient Egypt dating back to 1550 BC [2]. Galen in the second century AD introduced the term "aneurysm" [2]. At a later date, aneurysms were divided into degenerative and traumatic [2]. Although aortic diseases including dissection were recognized long ago, the new era for surgical approaches to Type A AD was launched with the introduction of cardiopulmonary bypass (CPB) by Gibbon in 1953 and Kirklin in 1956 [3, 4]. Subsequent major milestones in the development towards the contemporary clinical paradigm included hemodilution, hypothermia, hypothermic circulatory arrest, antegrade and retrograde cere-

George Silvay (george.silvay@mountsinai.org)
Icahn School of Medicine, Mount Sinai Medical Center,
New York, NY, USA

G. Melissano - R. Chiesa (eds), Aortic Dissection patients true stories and the innovations that saved their lives

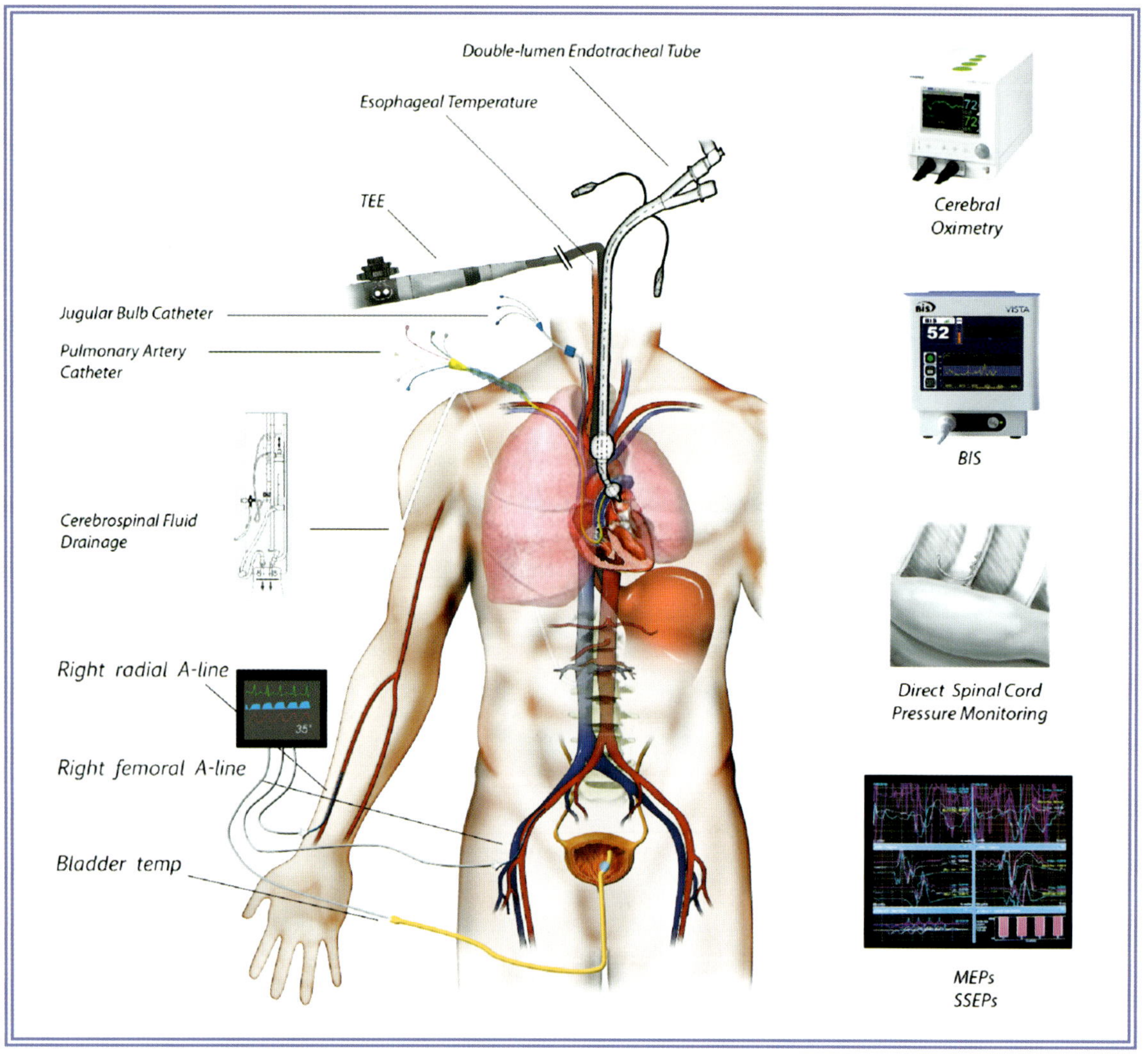

Fig. 36.1 Anesthetic approach and monitoring options in Type A AD. Adapted from [5].

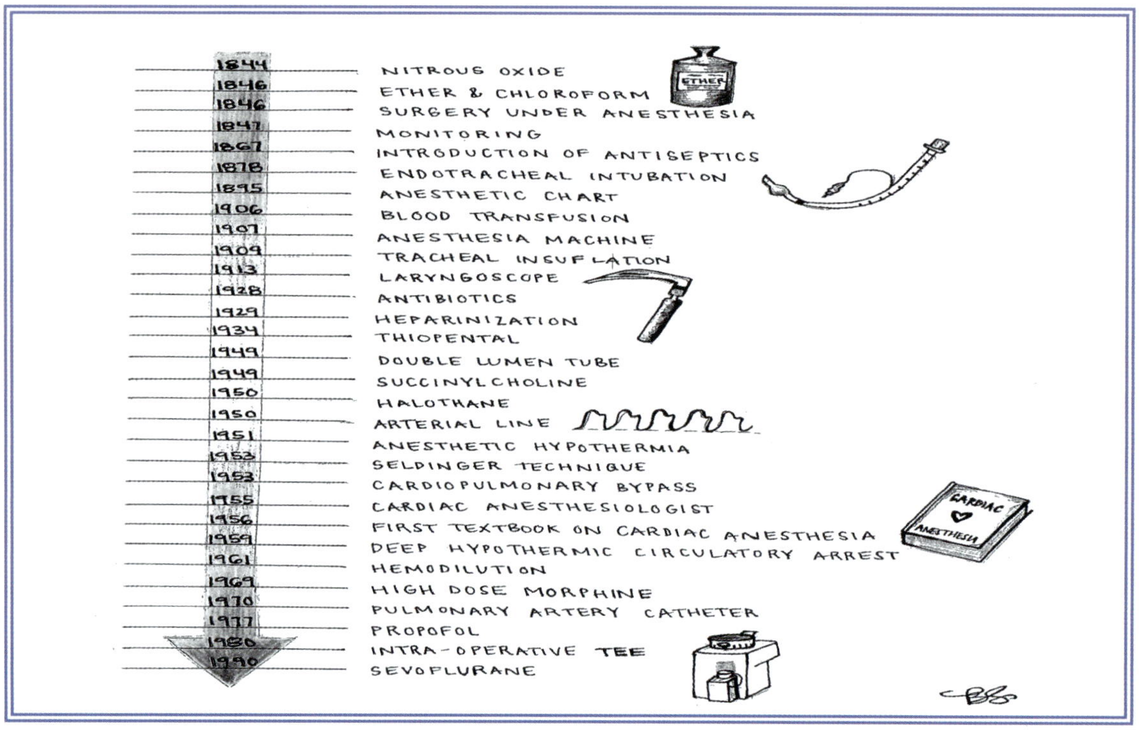
1844 NITROUS OXIDE
1846 ETHER & CHLOROFORM
1846 SURGERY UNDER ANESTHESIA
1847 MONITORING
1867 INTRODUCTION OF ANTISEPTICS
1878 ENDOTRACHEAL INTUBATION
1895 ANESTHETIC CHART
1906 BLOOD TRANSFUSION
1907 ANESTHESIA MACHINE
1909 TRACHEAL INSUFLATION
1913 LARYNGOSCOPE
1928 ANTIBIOTICS
1929 HEPARINIZATION
1934 THIOPENTAL
1949 DOUBLE LUMEN TUBE
1949 SUCCINYLCHOLINE
1950 HALOTHANE
1950 ARTERIAL LINE
1951 ANESTHETIC HYPOTHERMIA
1953 SELDINGER TECHNIQUE
1953 CARDIOPULMONARY BYPASS
1955 CARDIAC ANESTHESIOLOGIST
1956 FIRST TEXTBOOK ON CARDIAC ANESTHESIA
1959 DEEP HYPOTHERMIC CIRCULATORY ARREST
1961 HEMODILUTION
1969 HIGH DOSE MORPHINE
1970 PULMONARY ARTERY CATHETER
1977 PROPOFOL
1980 INTRA-OPERATIVE TEE
1990 SEVOFLURANE
ETHER
CARDIAC ANESTHESIA

Fig. 36.2 Historic timeline with relevant discoveries in cardiovascular anesthesia. Adapted from [5].

bral perfusion, as well as advances in anesthetic pharmacology and monitoring, including echocardiography (Figs. 36.1, 36.2) [5].

These multiple clinical advances in anesthesia and surgery facilitated the development and dissemination of techniques for reconstruction of the ascending aorta and aortic arch for diseases such as Type A AD [1-5].

36.2.1 Aortic perspective from the Mount Sinai Hospital

The Mount Sinai Hospital opened in Manhattan on 5 June 1852 with 45 beds and rapidly achieved a fully functioning status, including admitting all types of emergency cases [6]. In 1872, the hospital moved to a second location, expanding to 120 beds. Further growth in the surgical program prompted a third move in 1904 to the present location between Madison and Fifth Avenues on 100th Street [6]. The new facilities offered 450 beds with multiple medical and surgical specialities. The cardiothoracic surgery program was initiated in 1962 under the leadership of Robert Litwak and Howard Gadboys. The clinical program rapidly expanded and included an active research laboratory [7]. Dr Silvay was appointed in 1967 as their first cardiac surgical fellow. In 1970 Dr Litwak opened the Cardiothoracic Intensive Care Unit.

In 1985 Dr Griepp was recruited as chair of the cardiothoracic surgery at Mount Sinai. Dr Griepp championed the technique of deep hypothermic circulatory arrest (DHCA) for surgical repair of the aortic arch [8, 9]. Over a period of 20 years, Dr Griepp remained a leader in thoracic aortic surgery, including Type A AD [9]. He was the founding director of the Aortic Symposium, a leading aortic surgery conference that is held biennially in New York City [10]. Following the retirement of Dr Griepp, Dr DiLuozzo was appointed to continue the leadership of aortic surgery at Mount Sinai. In 2013, Dr Allan Stewart was appointed as the director of the thoracic aortic surgical program and continues in this role to the present day [11].

36.2.2 Aortic perspective from the University of Pennsylvania

The University of Pennsylvania was founded in 1751 by Benjamin Franklin in the city of Philadelphia [12]. In 1765, John Morgan organized a medical faculty for the school of medicine at the University of Pennsylvania. This was the first medical school in the American colonies at the time and is consequently the oldest medical school in the United States of America [12]. In 1872, the University moved out of center city to its present location in University City west of the Schuykill River [12]. The chief of cardiothoracic surgery at Penn before World War II was Dr George Muller who had a special interest in the surgical management of lung diseases and also served as a president of the American Association for Thoracic Surgery (AATS) [13]. During the 1930's at Penn, John H. Gibbon conducted his animal experiments in the development of CPB before his move to Thomas Jefferson University where he successfully introduced CPB for cardiac surgery in 1953 [3, 14].

Dr Julian Johnson succeeded Dr Muller as chief of cardiothoracic surgery in 1938 [13]. During his long tenure that lasted till 1972, he championed open-heart surgery at Penn, including aortic valve procedures [13]. He was an early adopter of CPB, served as a president of the AATS, and was an editor for the first edition of a leading thoracic surgical textbook, *Surgery of the Chest* [13]. Dr L. Henry Edmunds succeeded Dr Johnson in 1973 and served as chief till 1992, making seminal contributions in areas such as blood surface interactions, the coagulation cascade, and the effects of CPB on blood [13]. He was also the editor for another leading thoracic surgical textbook, *Cardiac Surgery in the Adult* [13]. Dr Timothy Gardner took the helm as chief of cardiothoracic surgery at Penn in 1993 and served in this capacity till 2003, whereafter he was succeeded by Dr Michael Acker who continues to direct the division to the present day [13].

In the 1990's during the tenure of Dr Gardner, Dr Joseph Bavaria founded the thoracic aortic surgery program at Penn, introducing a systematic multidisciplinary approach to complex aortic diseases such as acute Type A AD that has continued under his leadership till today [13, 15]. This multidisciplinary collaboration has included neurologists, cardiologists and cardiothoracic anesthesiologists. Further aortic milestones at Penn include the role of the electroencephalogram (EEG) in DHCA [16, 17], the application of endovascular stent grafts in the thoracic aorta [18], refinements in the classification of Type A AD [19], ascending aortic cannulation in Type A AD [20], and the surgical techniques for aortic valve repair, including valve resuspension in Type A AD [21]. Dr Bavaria and his team have also launched an annual focus on the techniques of aortic valve repair with the North American Aortic Valve Repair Symposium, currently in its second year. Dr Bavaria also currently serves as the president of the Society of Thoracic Surgeons [13].

36.2.3 Further aortic perspectives pertinent to Type A aortic dissection

The International Aortic Arch Study Group

Despite the pioneering work of Dr Griepp from Mount Sinai and Dr Bavaria from Penn, further advances in Type A AD and aortic arch reconstruction has been hampered by factors such as clinical trials with limited power, a paucity of uniform definitions for clinical end-points, and multiple technical strategies [22]. In an effort to address this evidence vacuum, the International Aortic Arch Surgery Study Group (IAASSG) was recently organized with 41 surgeons from 10 countries, including both Mount Sinai and Penn [23]. This multicenter IAASSG plans to expand the current evidence base for adult aortic arch procedures through consensus development, large multicenter database development, and adequately powered randomized controlled clinical trials [23]. This international consortium has also recently published their expert consensus for definitions of clinical end-points, including hypothermia in aortic arch surgery (Table 36.1) [23, 24]. The collaborative effort from the IAASSG is a turning point in the surgical management of aortic arch pathologies, including Type A AD. Their consensus, data analyses and prospective trials will likely advance and disseminate the science and conduct of these complex procedures globally in a systematic fashion for further improvements in clinical outcomes [22-24].

Programmatic approach to the operative management of Type A aortic dissection

An integrated and programmatic approach to Type A AD at Penn has been demonstrated to reduce mortality from a 15-30% baseline published in the literature to below 10% (no. = 163: 1994-2002: in-hospital mortality 9.8%) [25]. This concept was further highlighted in a second single medical center series from Duke University (no. = 128: 1999-2011) where the

Table 36.1 Classification consensus for levels of hypothermia in aortic arch surgery

Level of hypothermia	Patient temperature (°C)
Mild	28.1-34.0
Moderate	20.1-28.0
Deep	14.1-20.0
Profound	14.0 or less

Adapted from [24].

implementation of a multidisciplinary thoracic aortic program significantly reduced operative mortality from 18.2 to 2.8% (observed-to-expected mortality ratio 0.15; p = 0.005) and improved long-term survival at 5 years from 55 to 85% (p = 0.002) [26]. The components of a thoracic surgical program both at Penn and Duke include dedicated high-volume aortic surgeons, a standardized protocol for Type A AD repair, and a multidisciplinary approach to management in the perioperative period and beyond [25, 26].

Despite these important advances, 2 analyses of operative mortality across the United States demonstrate that Type A AD still has a high mortality [27, 28]. In the first analysis (N = 3,013: 1995-2003: mean age 62±14 years), in-hospital mortality significantly decreased from 27% in 1996 to 23% in 2003 (p = 0.03) [27]. High-volume centers were associated with a significant reduction in mortality (p <0.0001). Independent predictors of mortality in this first nationwide analysis included advanced age (p <0.0001) and surgery at a non-teaching hospital (p = 0.002) [27]. In the second analysis (N = 5,184: 2003-2008: mean age 60.3 years), low-volume surgeons as compared to high-volume surgeons had a significantly mean operative mortality (27.5 vs. 17.0%; odds ratio 1.78; 95% confidence interval 1.39-2.29; p <0.001) [28]. A similar relationship was observed for mortality at low-volume versus high-volume institutions (27.4 vs. 16.4%; p <0.001) [28]. Taken all together, the cumulative evidence base strongly suggests that surgery for Type A AD undertaken by experienced teams as a routine is an important strategy to reduce mortality and major morbidity in this important aortic syndrome [25-28].

Brief history of cardiovascular anesthesia

The Association of Cardiac Anesthesiologists (ACA) was founded in 1970 in Boston when Brian Dalton from Massachusetts General Hospital invited 50 anesthesiologists to discuss major topics in the subspecialty of cardiac anesthesiology [5, 29]. Although the ACA was the first professional society dedicated to the emerging specialty of cardiac anesthesiology, its membership has always been limited to a maximum of 50 [5, 29]. The restrictive membership of the ACA resulted in the creation of a parallel professional organization in 1979 that was called the Society of Cardiovascular Anesthesiologists (SCA). The founding members were George Burgess, Robert Marino and Martin Peuler [29]. Since then, the membership of the SCA has grown substantially to surpass 7,500 physicians from all over the world [29]. Similar stimuli resulted in the creation of professional societies for cardiac anesthesiologists around the world: the European Association of Cardiothoracic Anesthesiologists in 1985, the Indian Association of Cardiovascular Thoracic Anesthesiologists in 1997, and more recently in 2010 the Cardiothoracic Anesthesia Society of South Africa. The creation of these professional societies around the world has confirmed cardiac anesthesiology as a rapidly developing subspecialty. This subspecialty had its own dedicated journals such as the *Journal of Cardiothoracic and Vascular Anesthesia* founded in 1986 by Joel A. Kaplan [30]. The journal has a strong thoracic aortic focus.

36.3 Preoperative anesthetic considerations for Type A aortic dissection

The spectrum of Type A AD involves five classes of aortic pathology (Fig. 36.3) [1, 31]. Class I is defined as classic aortic dissection with true and false lumens. Class II is defined as intramural hematoma. Class III is defined as discrete localized dissection with bulging of the aortic wall. Class IV is defined as a penetrating aortic ulcer. Class V is defined as traumatic or iatrogenic dissection [1, 31]. Acute Type A AD is a term that describes an acute aortic syndrome due to the life-threatening presentations from the spectrum of aortic dissection (classes I-V) [1, 31].

Recent advances in imaging have emphasized the importance of early diagnosis since the

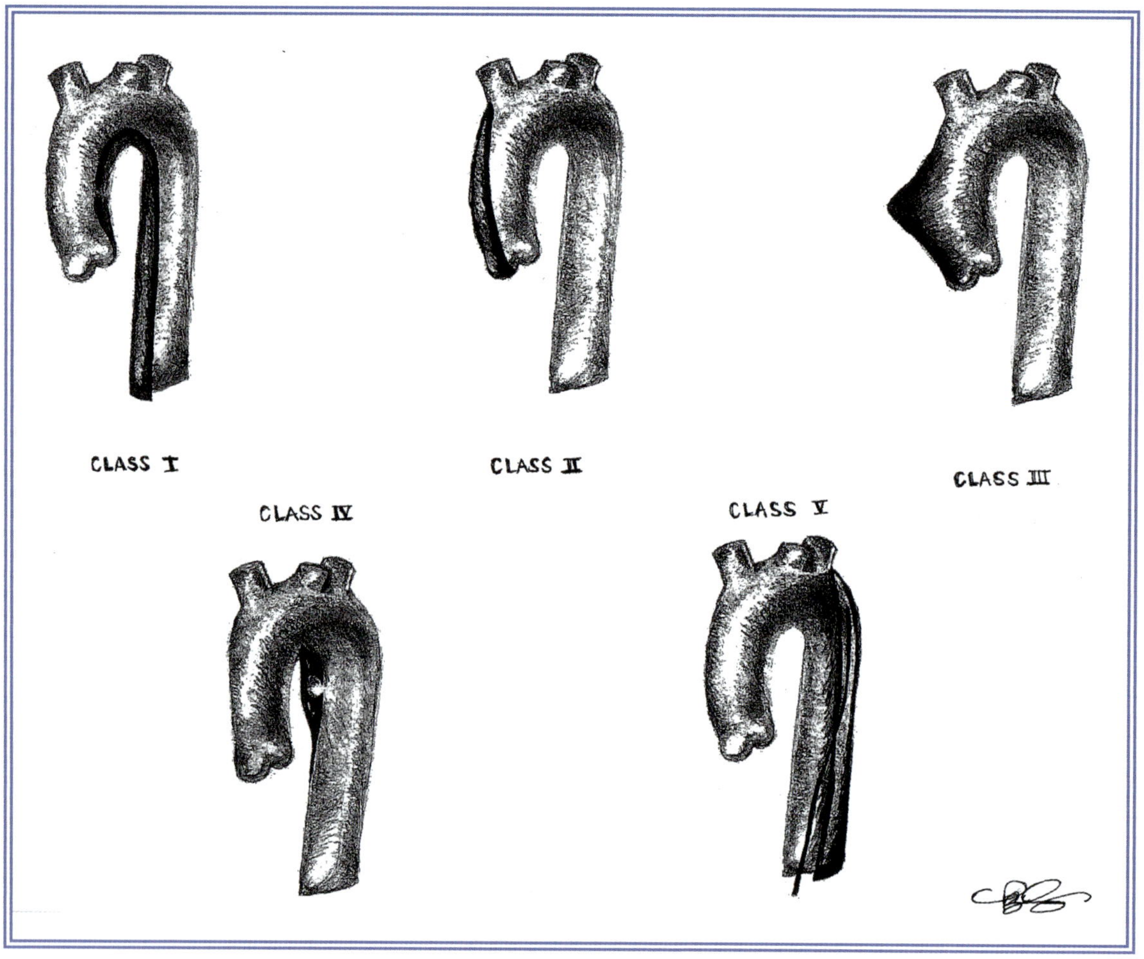

Fig. 36.3 Classification of acute aortic syndromes in AD spectrum. Class I is defined as classic aortic dissection with true and false lumens that may or may not be in communication. Class II is intramural hematoma. Class III is defined as discrete aortic dissection with bulging of the aortic wall. Class IV is penetrating aortic ulcer. Class V is defined as iatrogenic or traumatic aortic dissection as illustrated here with a catheter-induced dissection. Adapted from [1] and [31].

definitive management for Type A AD after initial stabilization involves prompt surgical intervention [1, 32, 33]. Since acute Type A AD is a life-threatening surgical emergency, time is of the essence, given that the mortality rate is 50% if surgery is delayed beyond 24-48 hours with an average mortality rate of 1-2% per hour in this critical period [1, 32, 33]. Early diagnosis and stabilization, prompt referral to an aortic center, and direct transportation to operating room for further team-based management significantly reduce mortality, as highlighted in the published Penn and Duke experiences [15, 25, 26].

High-quality communication between the entire intraoperative team (anesthesia, nursing, perfusion, and surgery) is very important to develop an overall strategy for optimization of the unstable patient with Type A AD in the preoperative phase. The preoperative phase should be appropriately abbreviated given that the patients can succumb from aortic rupture in the setting of unnecessary delays. The role of the anesthesia team in this scenario is to stabilize the patient on admission to the operating room including taking accurate report from the transport team, informed consent when possible, analgesia, hemodynamic control, as well as securing intravenous and arterial access [34, 35]. The operating room is in this setting both a diagnostic and therapeutic suite [34-36]. The anesthesia team must ensure that compatible blood is rapidly available and that all preparations for major resuscitation are arranged, given that critical presentations of Type A AD may be characterized by major hemodynamic instability despite aggressive therapy [34-36].

The preoperative approach to Type A AD thus depends on the clinical scenario and whether emergency surgery is planned. Patients with acute Type A AD require urgent team-based intervention with little time for a focused preoperative evaluation as outlined [1, 25, 26]. If the patient is scheduled for elective surgery for chronic Type A AD, then there is ample time for a more structured and detailed preoperative evaluation including patient interview, physical examination, dental clearance and detailed review of all laboratory tests and imaging studies [37].

36.4 Intraoperative anesthetic considerations for Type A aortic dissection

36.4.1 Anesthetic plan and induction

The anesthetic plan for operative management of Type A AD is balanced general endotracheal anesthesia with extensive monitoring that will be discussed in detail in subsequent dedicated sections. As outlined in this textbook, the unstable clinical presentations of acute Type A AD include acute aortic regurgitation, coronary ischemia, cardiac tamponade, aortic rupture, and vasoplegia [1, 19]. These challenging clinical presentations are often accompanied by hemodynamic instability that can significantly complicate the induction of general anesthesia. Careful anesthetic planning can typically accommodate these hemodynamic perturbations (Table 36.2). Although a single-lumen endotracheal tube is typically the airway of choice, a double-lumen endotracheal tube may be required to facilitate selective lung ventilation for enhanced surgical exposure (see Fig. 36.1).

The intraoperative team (anesthesia, nursing, perfusion, and surgery) must be ready for immediate surgery with rapid institution of CPB in these scenarios, given the lack of hemodynamic reserve due to Type A AD. The goals of anesthetic induction in this setting include hemodynamic control with particular care to maintain an acceptable degree of deliberate hypotension so as to avoid aortic rupture due to excessive wall stress from hypertension. In the setting of chronic Type A AD, these acute presentations are typically absent. The goals of the anesthetic induction in operative management for chronic Type A AD include the maintenance of hemodynamic stability, taking into account concomitant aortic regurgitation and avoiding hypertension to relieve wall stress in the aneurysmal aortic segments. Furthermore, thoracic aortic aneurysm can cause compression of vital mediastinal structures such as the tracheobronchial tree, esophagus, pulmonary artery and right ventricular outflow tract. This anatomic compression may complicate anesthetic induction, endotracheal intubation, and

Table 36.2 Clinical presentations in Type A aortic dissection that complicate anesthetic induction

Clinical presentation	Anesthetic plan to maintain cardiac output
Aortic regurgitation (multiple mechanisms)	Sinus tachycardia; systemic vasodilation: titrated propofol is very suitable
Coronary ischemia (coronary dissection)	Avoid increased myocardial oxygen demand due to tachycardia and hypertension: titrated etomidate is very suitable. Inotropic support may be required.
Cardiac tamponade (contained aortic rupture)	Sinus tachycardia; systemic vasoconstriction: titrated ketamine is very suitable
Hypovolemia (uncontained aortic rupture)	Volume resuscitation: titrated ketamine or etomidate are very suitable
Vasoplegia (severe metabolic acidosis; spinal ischemia)	Restore vascular tone with titrated pressor and sodium bicarbonate: titrated ketamine or ketamine are very suitable

Adapted from [1].

placement of the transesophageal echocardiography probe. In the setting of tracheobronchial compression, a right-sided double-lumen endotracheal tube may be indicated to avoid left mainstem intubation with possible aortic trauma. Although a bronchial blocker may offer selective lung ventilation, it does not allow reliable suctioning of the collapsed lung that is important in these long complex procedures.

36.4.2 Anesthetic maintenance

The anesthetic maintenance in these complex procedures is typically a balanced regimen titrated to achieve adequate analgesia (opioid such as fentanyl), amnesia (volatile inhalational anesthetic such as isoflurane and/or benzodiazepine such as midazolam), and immobility (neuromuscular blockade with agents such as pancuronium, vecuronium or rocuronium) [38]. The anesthetic regimen must be flexibly administered to accommodate modifying features such as patient variability, case length, degree of hypothermia, major blood loss and hemodilution, and neuromonitoring such as EEG [39]. The anesthetic maintenance must be titrated to facilitate optimal signal intensity for all neuromonitoring modalities such as EEG so that signal attenuation reflects important etiologies such as hypothermia and ischemia rather than anesthetic depth [16, 17, 38-40].

36.4.3 Anesthetic monitoring

Invasive blood pressure monitoring

The continuous accurate measurement of the blood pressure with invasive monitoring is essential throughout these cases due to factors such as hemodynamic instability, aortic fragility, and complex conduct of hypothermic CPB with non-pulsatile flow (see Fig. 36.1) [38, 39]. A second but equally important rationale for an indwelling arterial line is the requirement for frequent arterial blood gases to guide anesthetic management [38, 39]. The selection of the site for arterial cannulation for these purposes should take into account modifying factors such as the surgical plan, and the pattern of aortic branch dissection [1, 25, 26]. For example a right radial arterial line may not be suitable in the case of extensive innominate dissection with a cold right upper extremity. Although a right radial arterial line may be indicated in the case of planned right axillary artery cannulation to monitor right upper extremity perfusion and to guide the conduct of antegrade cerebral perfusion, it is not a reliable indicator of systemic perfusion and so a second arterial line elsewhere may be indicated for this purpose. High-quality communication between all team members will often smoothly facilitate these decisions [25, 26].

Invasive central pressure monitoring

The indications for central venous cannulation in this setting include large bore vascular access for volume resuscitation, reliable intravenous route for administration of vasoactive agents, and access for pulmonary artery catheterization [41]. An oximetric pulmonary arterial catheter is very useful in these challenging cases to monitor central pressures, cardiac output and systemic vascular resistance in real time not only in the operating room but also subsequently in the intensive care unit, given the abundant potential for hemodynamic instability before and after CPB (see Fig. 36.1 and Table 36.2) [41, 42].

A specialized indication for central venous pressure monitoring is for pressure monitoring to guide the conduct of retrograde cerebral perfusion during aortic arch repair [38, 39]. In this setting, the pressure is transduced at the level of the internal jugular vein above the tip of the perfusion cannula in the superior vena cava [41, 42]. The goal is to maintain the central venous pressure in the 15-20 mmHg range to avoid cerebral edema. Furthermore, this pressure can be continuously monitored during aortic arch reconstruction to allow meticulous titration of flow rate for optimal delivery of this cerebral perfusion adjunct [38, 39].

Temperature monitoring

Accurate temperature monitoring is essential to guide the management of hypothermic CPB for optimal neuroprotection during thoracic aortic reconstruction as outlined in the IAASSG consensus for hypothermia in aortic arch surgery (see Table 36.1) [24, 43]. While multiple sites for temperature monitoring such as the tympanum, the nasopharynx, the esophagus, the bladder and the rectum are possible, the pertinent question is which site best reflects brain temperature, given that the success of hypothermia for neuroprotection depends on metabolic suppression. Based on results from 2 studies, nasopharyngeal temperature provided very accurate approximations of brain temperature throughout the hypothermic spectrum as outlined in Table 36.1 [44, 45]. In these closed chest studies, the nasopharyngeal temperature had a mean difference of about 0.5 °C from brain temperature throughout cooling and rewarming (Fig. 36.4) [44, 45]. Although temperature monitoring in the distal esophagus was a little more accurate than in the nasopharynx, the distal esophagus is not recommended by the IAASSG since surgery for Type A AD is in the setting of an open chest with consequent heat loss from this site [24, 44, 45]. Temperature monitoring in the bladder and rectum does not accurately reflect brain temperature during hypothermic CPB. These temperatures often lag behind nasopharyngeal temperatures, being significantly warmer during the cooling phase and significantly colder during the rewarming phase [24, 44, 45]. In light of all these considerations, the IAASSG expert consensus has recommended the nasopharynx for temperature monitoring to guide the conduct of hypothermic CPB for aortic arch reconstruction, including Type A AD [24].

Besides the optimal site for brain temperature measurement, the expert consensus from the IAASSG has also recommended the axillary artery for the arterial inflow route during CPB

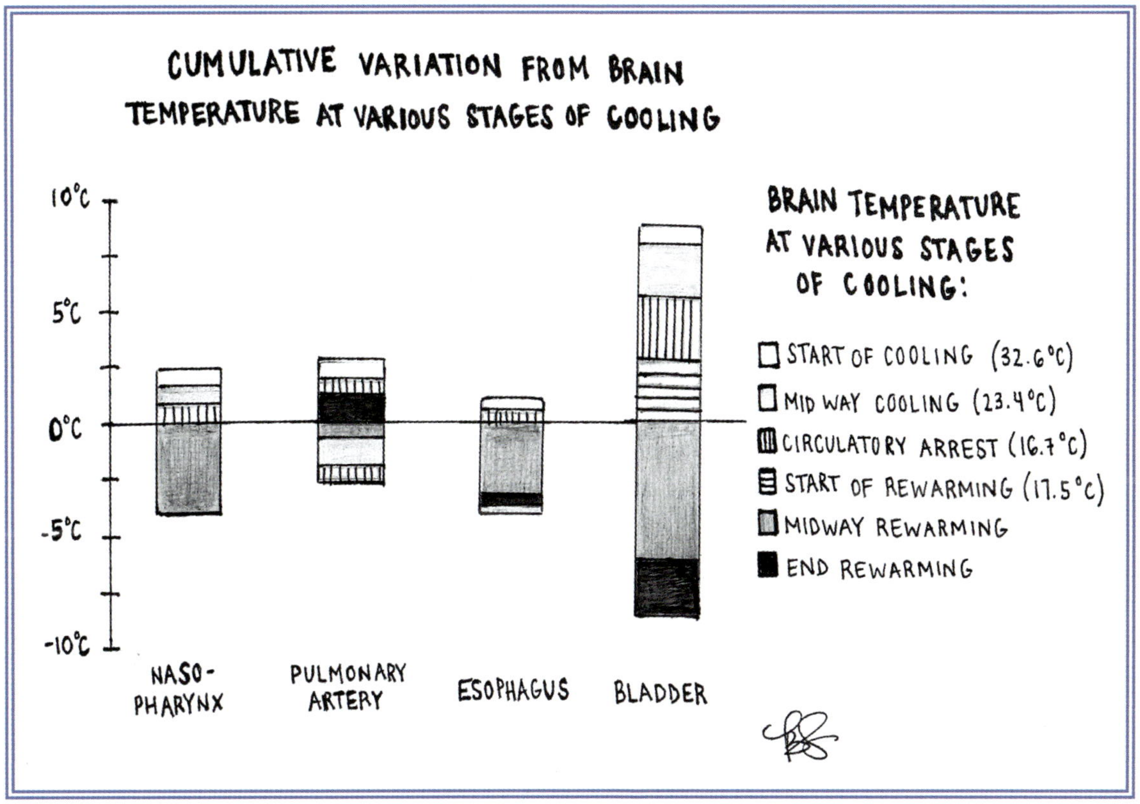

Fig. 36.4 Temperature variations at various sites compared to brain temperature during cerebral aneurysm repair. Each bar represents temperature change compared to brain temperature at various stages of systemic cooling and rewarming. In this closed chest setting, the esophagus temperature most closely follows cortical temperature, followed by pulmonary artery and nasopharyngeal temperatures. Adapted from [24] and [44].

Table 36.3 Clinical advantages of axillary artery cannulation in Type A aortic cannulation

Clinical advantage	Comment
Eliminates risk of retrograde cerebral embolization from distal aorta	Blood flow is antegrade
Reduces risk of retrograde aortic dissection	Blood flow is antegrade
Reduces risk of cerebral atheroembolism	Axillary artery is typically free from atherosclerotic disease
Often allows antegrade blood flow in true lumen to decompress false lumen	Caution in innominate artery dissection
May reduce risk of malperfusion and subsequent regional hypoperfusion	Caution in innominate artery dissection
Provides access for subsequent unilateral antegrade cerebral perfusion	Monitor adequacy of contralateral cerebral perfusion

Adapted from [24].

for induction of hypothermia [24]. The multiple advantages of this arterial cannulation route have been summarized in Table 36.3 [24]. Furthermore, if this arterial approach is chosen, the experts have recommended that it be conducted via an anastomosed graft to minimize local complications such as dissection, hematoma, and compartment syndrome [24]. Two recent meta-analyses have provided high-quality data to support this recommendation even more [46, 47]. The first meta-analysis (cumulative N = 715: 9 observational trials: 1992-2011) found that axillary artery as compared to femoral artery cannulation significantly reduced short-term mortality in Type A AD (odds ratio 0.25; 95% confidence interval 0.15-0.42; $p < 0.01$) [46]. The second meta-analysis (cumulative N = 4,476) demonstrated that central cannulation arterial techniques (including axillary artery) as compared to femoral cannulation significantly reduced in-hospital mortality (risk ratio 0.59; 95% confidence interval 0.48-0.70; $p < 0.001$) and permanent neurologic deficit (risk ratio 0.71; 95% confidence interval 0.55-0.90; $p = 0.005$) [47]. The mortality reduction was further enhanced in the setting of axillary artery cannulation (risk ratio 0.35; 95% confidence interval 0.22-0.55; $p < 0.001$) [47].

In summary, the cumulative evidence base favors the nasopharynx for temperature monitoring to track hypothermia and axillary artery cannulation for induction of hypothermia during the operative management of Type A AD.

Transesophageal echocardiography

Transesophageal echocardiography (TEE) is a major imaging modality for perioperative evaluation of the thoracic aorta [32, 33]. The major advantages of comprehensive TEE in the diagnosis and management of Type A AD are summarized in Table 36.4 [1, 32, 33, 48-50]. Given this immense clinical utility, TEE has become a standard component of the programmatic perioperative approach to Type A AD at experienced aortic centers such as Penn, Mount Sinai and Duke [15, 25, 26, 32, 33]. In strong support of this TEE application, a recent single center observational trial (N = 64) documented that TEE confirmed the diagnosis in 97% of patients, reliably detected and quantified the associated cardiac complications, demonstrated new imaging findings in 64% of patients, and significantly altered the surgical plan in 39% of patients [48].

A major limitation with TEE is the blind spot, namely its inability to image the distal ascending aorta and proximal aortic arch due to the air-filled tracheobronchial tree that lies between the esophagus and thoracic aorta at this level [32, 33]. Modified TEE can overcome this limitation with placement of fluid-filled balloon in the trachea that permits accurate visualization of the entire aortic arch including the brachiocephalic vessels [32, 33, 50]. An alter-

Table 36.4 Clinical advantages of transesophageal echocardiography in Type A aortic dissection

Clinical advantage	Comment
Readily available in operating room	Routine imaging modality of choice at high-volume aortic centers
Lack of iodinated contrast	No risks of anaphylaxis or acute kidney injury
Lack of ionizing radiation	No exposure risks
Safety	Extremely safe but has small risks of upper gastrointestinal injury including perforation and bleeding
Cost	Already accounted for at high volume aortic centers
Sensitivity	Close to 100%
Specificity	Close to 100%
Intimal flap imaging	Precise characterization of intimal extent, morphology, fenestrations and dynamics
Valvular assessment	Standard of care – precise analysis of aortic valve dysfunction including severity and mechanism
Ventricular assessment	Standard of care – precise analysis of global and regional biventricular function; detection and full characterization of coronary dissection
Pericardial assessment	Standard of care – precise analysis of pericardial tamponade
Branch vessel assessment	Limited utility in the aortic arch due to the blind spot (air-filled tracheobronchial tree between esophagus and aorta)
Guide cannulation for cardiopulmonary bypass	Can confirm wire and cannula placement in the ascending aorta, aortic arch, great veins, left ventricle (vent) and coronary sinus (retrograde cardioplegia)
Guide separation from cardiopulmonary bypass	Standard of care – can assess deairing maneuvers; can diagnose valvular dysfunction; can diagnose extent and severity of ventricular dysfunction

Adapted from [1], [32], [33].

nate option to modified TEE for imaging this blind spot and the entire aortic arch is epiaortic imaging in the setting of an open chest [32, 33].

Enhanced imaging of these thoracic aortic segments can significantly guide cannulation of true lumen in the dissected ascending aorta for CPB, a technique that is gaining traction at leading aortic centers as an alternative route to harness the advantages of central arterial cannulation in Type A AD [20]. Another alternative for central arterial cannulation for CPB in Type A AD is the innominate artery [51, 52]. It is readily accessible in the surgical field after sternotomy, avoids the requirement for an anastomosed graft, and yet offers all the advantages of axillary cannulation (see Table 36.3) [51, 52].

A major role for TEE in Type A AD is the comprehensive analysis of the aortic valve to quantify the severity and mechanism of aortic regurgitation (Table 36.5) [32, 33, 49]. The mechanisms of aortic regurgitation can be classified from an aortic valve repair perspective utilizing the El Khoury approach (see Table 36.5) [49]. The main interventional question in this setting is whether the native valve can be repaired. Careful echocardiographic analysis can precisely delineate the El Khoury mechanisms to guide decision-making about whether to repair or replace the aortic valve [32, 33, 49]. The integrity of the aortic valve repair can also be rigorously assessed after separation from CPB according to the standard criteria [49].

Although TEE is a gold standard in the operative management for Type A AD, the echocar-

Table 36.5 Mechanisms of aortic regurgitation in Type A dissection

Clinical mechanism	Comment
Dilation of the sinotubular junction (El Khoury Type IA)	Central jet – native valve preservation likely
Dilation of the sinus segment (El Khoury Type IB)	Central jet – native valve preservation likely unless aortic root is extensively dissected
Disruption of commissural attachments (El Khoury Type II)	Eccentric jet – native valve preservation likely unless aortic root is extensively dissected
Diastolic prolapse of intimal flap through aortic valve into left ventricle (El Khoury Type III)	Central jet – native valve preservation likely unless aortic root is extensively dissected

Adapted from [1], [32], [33], [49].

diographer must remain vigilant for false-positive presentations [34, 53]. Benign conditions can at times mimic aortic dissection to put the patient at risk for a major misdiagnosis [53]. The list of these conditions includes aortitis, atheromatous plaque, pericardial recess, the innominate vein, perioaortic fat; the hemiazygos sheath, congenital remnants such as a patent ductus arteriosus, motion and streak artifacts in computed tomography, and reverberation artifacts in the ascending aorta during TEE [1, 32, 33]. The imaging findings must always be integrated in multiple planes and reconciled to the clinical presentation to facilitate the correct interpretation of false positives for Type A AD [53].

Scanning of the carotid arteries during operative repair for Type A AD can monitor the adequacy of cerebral perfusion during critical phases of the procedure when the kinetics of the intimal flap may precipitate cerebral malperfusion, including initiation of CPB, clamping of the ascending aorta, and during antegrade cerebral perfusion [54, 55]. This imaging of the carotid arteries can be achieved by withdrawal of the TEE probe into the pharynx or by transcutaneous scanning with a handheld probe [54, 55]. Detection of cerebral malperfusion in these phases may be corrected by maneuvers such as adjusting the site of arterial cannulation (e.g. axillary artery instead of femoral artery), surgical fenestration of the intimal flap to restore perfusion to both the true and false lumina, adjustment of the arterial cannula, external carotid compression and/or initiation of bilateral antegrade cerebral perfusion [56-59]. Team vigilance and communication during these critical phases of the operative procedure are of major importance to detect and correct these complications. An alternative monitor for detection of cerebral malperfusion in these setting is cerebral oximetry that will be discussed in the following section [56, 57].

Cerebral oximetry for neuroprotection in Type A aortic dissection

Cerebral oximetry via bilateral sensors on the forehead can be measured noninvasively by near-infrared spectroscopy (NIRS) [56]. The emission of near-infrared light in this setting allows the analysis of the reflected light to measure oxygenated and deoxygenated hemoglobin [56, 57]. The regional oxygen saturation (rSO_2) is calculated as the ratio of oxygenated hemoglobin to total hemoglobin, defined as oxygenated hemoglobin divided by the sum of oxygenated and deoxygenated hemoglobin [56, 57]. The determination of rSO_2 is not only noninvasive but also continuous as it is updated very few seconds to monitor of the balance between cerebral oxygen delivery and consumption in a local section of the brain [56]. Although there is a spectrum of commercial NIRS devices, the evidence base to guide device selection and utilization of NIRS is still limited [57]. Despite this limitation, NIRS has gradually been adopted as a monitor of cerebral perfusion during Type A AD surgery to facilitate detection of cerebral malperfusion and restoration of cerebral perfusion [56-59]. The adoption of NIRS has been particularly widespread in aortic centers where unilateral antegrade cerebral perfusion is the routine perfusion adjunct during aortic arch reconstruction [60]. In this setting, a fall in rSO_2 from the contralateral cerebral hemisphere would alert the intraoperative team to intervene systematically to correct cerebral perfusion, including maneuvers such as correction of cannula malposition, augmentation of perfusion pressure, and/or switching to bilateral antegrade cerebral perfusion [57-60].

The clinical utility of rSO_2 determination by NIRS was highlighted in a large clinical trial (N = 1,178) of adult cardiac surgical patients undergoing CPB. In this observational trial, multivariate analysis demonstrated that rSO_2 values <50% independently predicted mortality both at 30 days and 1 year [61]. Further trials are underway to evaluate whether interventions guided by rSO_2 monitoring can improve clinical outcome in high-risk cardiac surgery [62]. These high-quality trials will considerably strengthen the evidence base to guide the rational application of this monitoring technology in high-risk cardiac surgery, including Type A AD.

Electroencephalography

The role of EEG monitoring in the conduct of hypothermia for Type A AD has been well-established [16, 17, 40, 63]. The goal of hypothermia is to achieve suppression of brain metabolism and hence a degree of ischemic tolerance is a dose-related fashion [24]. The degree of hypothermia confers an increasing level of neuroprotection through greater suppression of cerebral metabolic rate to extend the safe duration of hypothermic circulatory arrest for aortic arch reconstruction (Fig. 36.5) [25, 64]. The clinical end-point for maximal degree of cerebral metabolic suppression is electrocerebral silence indicated as an isoelectric EEG [16, 17]. Since the temperature at which this end-point is reached in a given individual varies, EEG monitoring during cooling on CPB offers precise determination of that temperature for the patient in question (Figs. 36.6, 36.7) [16, 17]. In this setting, EEG monitoring can guide the conduct of hypothermia for neuroprotection before circulatory arrest in an accurate and reliable fashion

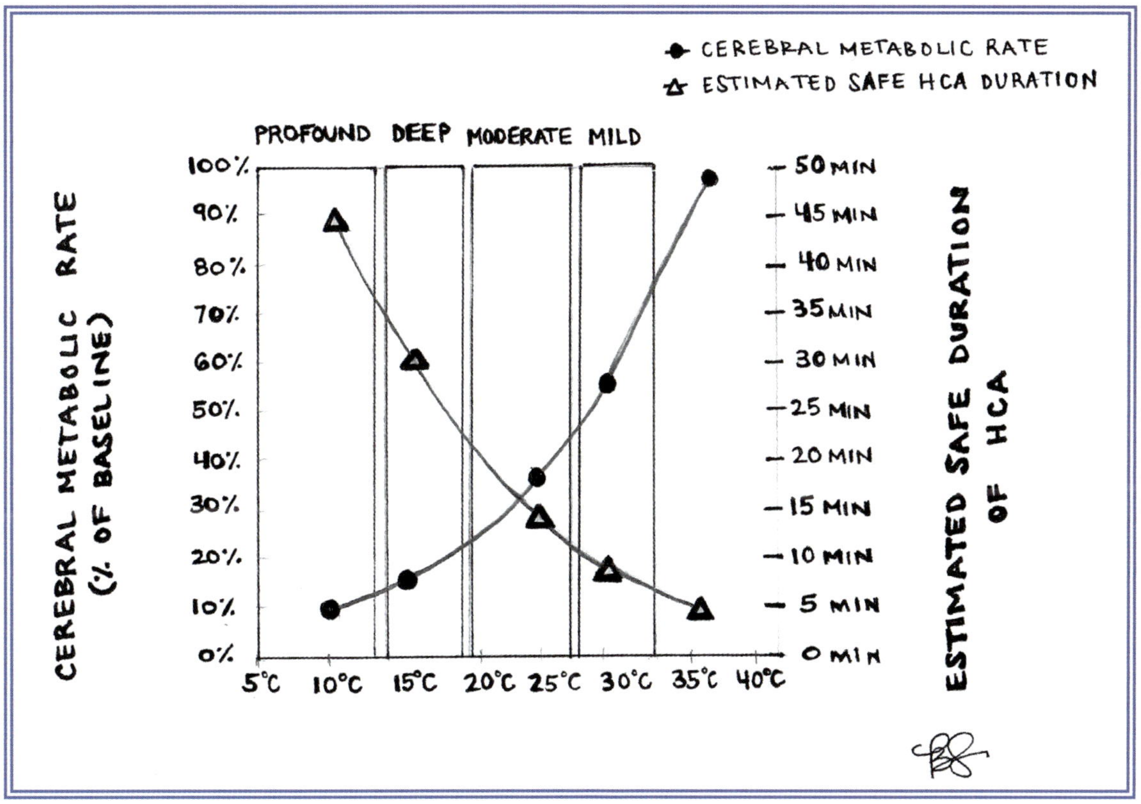

Fig. 36.5 The relationship between suppression of cerebral metabolic rate due to hypothermia and the estimated safe duration for hypothermic circulatory arrest (HCA). The indicated levels of hypothermia have been defined by expert consensus (see Table 36.1). Adapted from [24] and [64].

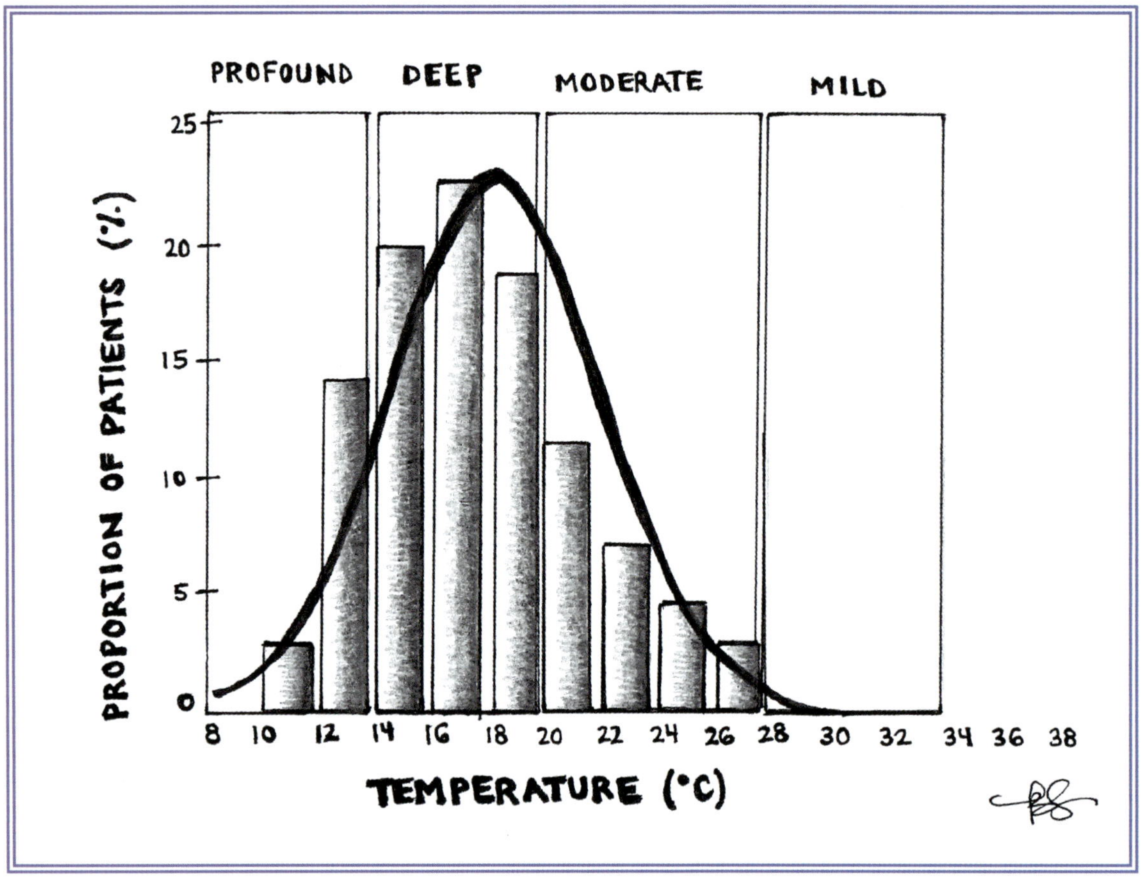

Fig. 36.6 The relationship between nasopharyngeal temperature and the electrocerebral silence during cooling on cardiopulmonary bypass. The indicated levels of hypothermia have been defined by expert consensus (see Table 36.1). Adapted from [24] and [16].

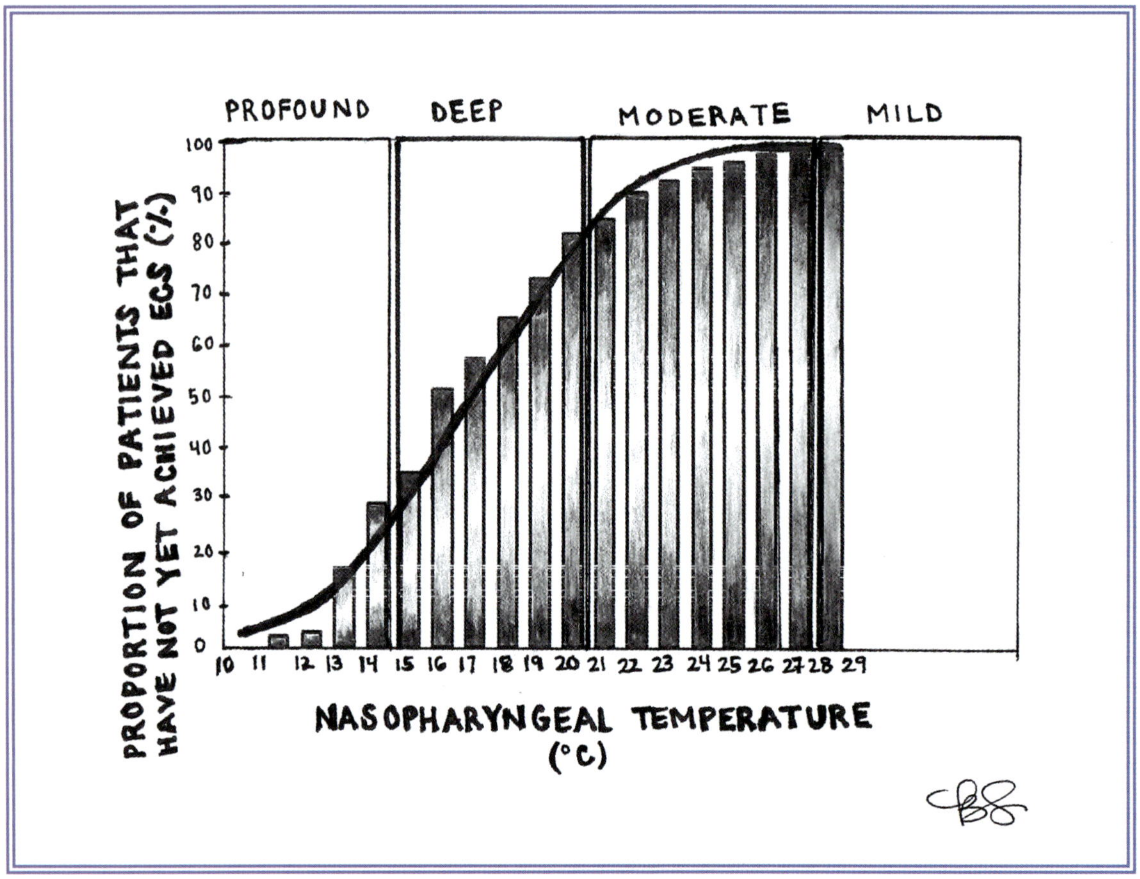

Fig. 36.7 The relationship between nasopharyngeal temperature and the probability of electrocerebral silence during cooling on cardiopulmonary bypass. The indicated levels of hypothermia have been defined by expert consensus (see Table 36.1). At 14 degrees Celsius, about 15% of patients have not achieved electrocerebral silence. At 20 °C, about 75% of patients have not achieved electrocerebral silence. At 28 °C, about 100% of patients have not achieved electrocerebral silence. Adapted from [24] and [16].

for each patient, despite the variation in brain sensitivity to hypothermic suppression of metabolic rate [16, 17, 65]. In the absence of EEG monitoring as it may occur in emergency settings such as acute Type A AD, cooling to profound hypothermia or longer than a hour will typically achieve electrocerebral silence in more than 80-90% of patients [16, 17, 65]. This clinical utility of EEG explains its adoption in experienced aortic centers such as Penn and Duke [16, 17, 65].

In the contemporary era, there has a clinical drift away from DHCA towards moderate hypothermic circulatory arrest (MHCA) with routine antegrade cerebral perfusion for aortic arch reconstruction in Type A AD [60, 66]. This MHCA paradigm offers equivalent clinical outcomes with significant reductions in operative times and blood transfusion without compromise of distal organ protection [67-69]. In this setting of MHCA with routine unilateral antegrade cerebral perfusion, EEG monitoring remains valuable to identify patients with cerebral ischemia to guide interventions such as bilateral antegrade cerebral perfusion and/or further systemic cooling [70].

36.4.4 Neuroprotective pharmacology

Neuroprotective drugs such as steroids, thiopental and lidocaine have been administered in Type A AD during the conduct of CPB in an effort to minimize the risks of delirium, stroke and coma [41-43, 63]. Although multiple agents have entered clinical practice for this purpose in this clinical setting, the evidence base supporting this application is limited [71]. Lidocaine administered as an intravenous bolus for neuroprotection may precipitate intraoperative seizures that can be detected during EEG monitoring [72]. A recent evidence review concluded that thiopental as part of a multimodal neuroprotective protocol was likely beneficial in adult thoracic aortic surgery with DHCA such as Type A AD repair [73]. In a large German Type A AD registry analysis (N = 2,137), intraoperative steroid administration was associated with improved neurological outcome (odds ratio 0.5; 95% confidence interval 0.24-0.96; p = 0.0049) [74]. Overall, further trials are required to strengthen the evidence base to guide the choice of perioperative pharmacology for neuroprotection in Type A AD.

36.4.5 Management of coagulopathy

Significant coagulopathy is common after operative repair for Type A AD due to multiple factors such as preoperative consumption of clotting factors, mesenteric ischemia, hemodilution, prolonged CPB, and hypothermia [75, 76]. The profound perioperative systemic activation of coagulation, fibrinolysis and platelets in Type A AD may require aggressive hemostatic therapy to restore fibrin, clotting factor, and platelet homeostasis in a multimodal fashion [38, 39, 75, 77]. An individualized, goal-directed hemostatic therapy may be the appropriate clinical approach in this complex clinical setting [78]. This "theranostic" multimodal approach may include point-of-care viscoelastic testing with thromboelastometry or thromboelastography, point-of-care platelet function testing such as aggregometry, transfusion algorithms, antifibrinolytics, and a low clinical thresholds for titrated fibrinogen, prothrombin complex concentrates and recombinant activated factor VII [38, 39, 75, 78, 79]. An integrated team-based approach significantly contributes to highly effective intervention in these complex scenarios [38, 39].

36.5 Postoperative anesthetic considerations for Type A aortic dissection

After operative repair for Type A AD, patients are admitted for further management to the intensive care unit (ICU) with structured handoff of care [38, 39, 80]. The early postoperative care is focused on serial clinical assessment, hemodynamic resuscitation and stabilization, analgesia, and gradual weaning from mechanical ventilation [80]. Prolonged stay in the ICU in this setting has been defined as greater than 5 days [81, 82]. The incidence of prolonged ICU stay at experienced aortic centers is in the range of 20-25% and has been significantly associated with major organ dysfunction such as stroke, low cardiac output syndrome, acute respiratory failure, and renal failure [81, 82].

Acute respiratory failure is relatively common after surgery for Type A AD [83, 84]. In a large single center clinical trial (N = 276: 1994-2008), acute respiratory failure was defined as an arterial oxygen/inspired oxygen ratio <150 within the first 72 hours after surgery [83]. According to this definition, the incidence of acute respiratory failure was 13% [83]. An independent predictor for this complication was preoperative malperfusion (odds ratio 3.2; 95% confidence interval 2.2-4.9; $p < 0.05$) [83]. Prone positioning ventilation significantly improved oxygenation ($p < 0.001$) with a tendency to both a shorter duration of mechanical ventilation ($p < 0.2$) and ICU stay ($p < 0.2$) [83]. The risk of acute respiratory failure also appears to be related to the extent of the dissection process and its accompanying systemic inflammatory reaction (odds ratio 1.32; 95% confidence interval 1.04-1.69; $p = 0.03$) [84].

36.6 Future considerations for Type A aortic dissection

Advanced age has been presented as a significant risk factor for mortality and morbidity after surgery for Type A AD, prompting debate about whether this complex surgery is indicted in octogenarians [85]. On the other hand, this intervention in octogenarians with Type A AD may be associated with significant clinical benefits beyond the perioperative period [85, 86]. The unresolved and important question in this setting is: what does age really mean [86, 87]? Advanced age by itself does not provide an objective measure of a patient's physiologic reserve and ability to tolerate major thoracic aortic surgery [87]. An octogenarian may exhibit sound physical and mental fitness with a high quality of life. A guiding principle in this setting may be to focus on frailty rather than advanced age as a marker of limited reserve and resilience [88]. A validated scoring system for frailty has been developed from the following 5 domains: weight loss; grip strength; exhaustion; low physical activity; and walking speed [88]. Although this quantified approach to frailty significantly predicts outcomes after surgery, further trials are required to better clarify the role of frailty in outcomes after operative repair for Type A AD [87, 88].

A second evolving trend in Type A AD is the growing role of endovascular intervention [85]. A reasonable indication for aortic stenting in this setting is the frozen elephant trunk for distal aortic stabilization [1, 85]. A second role for endovascular therapy in Type A AD is for hybrid arch repair that has the potential to offer a safe and efficient option for total arch therapy in this complex setting [1, 18, 85]. A third role for endovascular therapy in Type A AD is proximal thoracic aortic repair in patients deemed too high-risk for conventional surgery with CPB such as may be the case in the frail elderly [85, 88, 89]. It is highly likely that these roles for thoracic endovascular aortic repair in Type A AD will expand in a steady fashion as has already happened for aortic diseases distal to the aortic arch [1, 85].

A third aspect of management in Type A AD is the optimal approach to high-risk patients presenting with malperfusion, given their high perioperative mortality and the limited role of classic thoracic aortic reconstruction in this setting [1, 11, 19, 36, 90]. The clinical presentation of malperfusion in Type A AD may merit an organ-specific multidisciplinary therapeutic approach beyond the classic "tube graft" including options such as the hybrid operating room, aortic branch stenting, and intimal fenestration [36, 76, 90]. This theranostic approach requires further evaluation in high-volume aortic centers with specialized aortic teams to advance the treatment paradigm for this challenging disease [36]. Due to this increasing appreciation of the protean presentations of Type A AD and their relevance to clinical outcome, the management approach is undergoing a paradigm shift to account for this presentation spectrum [36, 76, 90]. The Penn classification of clinical presentations in Type A AD offers a principle-based framework for these advances [19, 39].

36.7 Conclusions

Acute Type A AD involves the ascending aorta and is a surgical emergency. The anesthesia team must regard the operating room in this setting both as a diagnostic and therapeutic suite. Anesthetic priorities include securing the airway, achieving hemodynamic control, establishing invasive monitoring, and completing a comprehensive echocardiography examination to facilitate the operative plan. Thereafter, a team-based initiation of CPB should include TEE guidance of cannulation where appropriate.

The anesthesia team must retain vigilance during CPB. This vigilance must include management of the following aspects: the metabolic milieu, anesthetic maintenance to include minimal interference with neuromonitoring, accurate temperature measurement for conduct of hypothermia, and appropriate monitoring of antegrade and retrograde cerebral perfusion. Intermittent echocardiographic scanning for surveillance is helpful for detection of complications. Preparation for separation from CPB should also be comprehensive.

During separation from CPB, the anesthesia team must titrate mechanical ventilation and vasopressor support to restore and maintain systemic hemodynamics. Comprehensive TEE at this juncture should guide deairing procedures and assess the operative repair, including the aortic valve, the aortic root and the aortic arch. The restoration of adequate hemostasis after protamine administration should proceed in a systematic protocol-based fashion with titrated transfusion, point-of-care testing, and a low threshold for specialized factor administration in refractory cases. The handover of care to the ICU team should be conducted in a structured and systematic fashion.

Acknowledgements

The authors thank Dr Toby Steinberg in the Department of Anesthesiology and Critical Care at the University of Pennsylvania for her expert artistic assistance with all the figures in this chapter.

REFERENCES

1) Erbel R, Aboyans V, Boileau C, et al. 2014 ESC guidelines on the diagnosis and treatment of aortic diseases: document covering acute and chronic aortic diseases of the thoracic and abdominal aorta of the adult. Eur Heart J 2014; 35: 2873-926.
2) Stehbens WE. History of aneurysm. Med Hist 1958; 2: 274-80.
3) Gibbon JH Jr. Application of the mechanical heart and lung apparatus to the cardiac surgery. Minn Med 1954; 37: 171-85.
4) Kirklin JW, Donald DE, Harshbarger HG, et al. Studies in extracorporeal circulation I. Applicability of Gibbon-type pump-oxygenator to human intra-cardiac surgery: 40 cases. Ann Surg 1956; 144: 2-8.
5) Silvay G, Castillo JG. History of anesthesia for aortic surgery. In: Chiesa R, Melissano G, Setacci C, Argenteri A, eds. History of aortic surgery in the world. Torino: Edizioni Minerva Medica; 2015: 58-69.
6) Aufses A. The house of noble deeds: The Mount Sinai Hospital, 1852-2002. New York and London: New York University Press; 2002.
7) Litwak RS, Lev R, Baron M, Silvay G, Gadboys H. The surgical treatment of aortic aneurysms. Geriatrics 1967; 22: 105-21.
8) Griepp RB, Stinson EB, Hollingsworth JF, Buehler D. Prosthetic replacement of the aortic arch. J Thorac Cardiovasc Surg 1975; 70: 1051-63.
9) Griepp RB, Di Luozzo G. Hypothermia for aortic surgery. J Thorac Cardiovasc Surg 2013; 145(3 Suppl): S56-8.

10) Lansman S. The Randall B. Griepp Honorary Paper. J Thorac Cardiovasc Surg 2015; 149(2 Suppl): S1-2.
11) Goldfinger JZ, Halperin JL, Marin ML, Stewart AS, Eagle KA, Fuster V. Thoracic aortic aneurysm and dissection. J Am Coll Cardiol 2014; 21: 1725-39.
12) Friedman SM. A brief history of the University of Pennsylvania. The University of Pennsylvania Archives and Records Center – available at www.archives.upenn.edu (last accessed August 8th 2016).
13) Acker MA, Bavaria JE, Barker CF. History and current status of cardiovascular surgery at the University of Pennsylvania. Semin Thorac Cardiovasc Surg 2015; 27: 370-3.
14) Castillo JG, Silvay G. John H. Gibbon Jr and the 60th anniversary of the first successful heart-lung machine. J Cardiothorac Vasc Anesth 2013; 27: 203-7.
15) Bavaria JE, Pochettino A, Brinster DR, et al. New paradigms and improved results for the surgical treatment of acute type A dissection. Ann Surg 2001; 234: 336-42.
16) Stecker MM, Cheung AT, Pochettino A, et al. Deep hypothermic circulatory arrest I: effects of cooling on electroencephalogram and evoked potentials. Ann Thorac Surg 2001; 71: 14-21.
17) Stecker MM, Cheung AT, Pochettino A, et al. Deep hypothermic circulatory arrest II: changes in electroencephalogram and evoked potentials during rewarming. Ann Thorac Surg 2001; 71: 22-8.
18) Vallabhajosyula P, Szeto W, Desai N, Bavaria JE. Type I and Type II hybrid aortic arch replacement: postoperative and midterm outcome analysis. Ann Cardiothorac Surg 2013; 2: 280-7.
19) Augoustides JG, Szeto WY, Desai ND, et al. Classification of acute type A dissection: focus on clinical presentation and extent. Eur J Cardiothorac Surg 2011; 39: 519-22.
20) Frederick JR, Yang E, Trubelja A, et al. Ascending aortic cannulation in acute type A dissection repair. Ann Thorac Surg 2013; 95: 1808-11.
21) Rylski B, Siepe M, Beyersdorf F, et al. Bicuspid aortic valve resuspension in acute type A aortic dissection patients. Ann Thoracic Surg 2015; 100: 827-32.
22) Yan TD, Tian DH, LeMaire SA, et al. The ARCH Projects: design and rationale (IAASSG 001). Eur J Cardiothorac Surg 2014; 45: 10-6.
23) Yan TD, Tian DH, LeMaire SA, et al. Standardizing clinical end points in aortic arch surgery: a consensus statement from the International Aortic Arch Surgery Study Group. Circulation 2014; 129: 1610-6.
24) Yan TD, Bannon PG, Bavaria JE, et al. Consensus on hypothermia in aortic arch surgery. Ann Cardiothorac Surg 2013; 2: 163-8.
25) Bavaria JE, Brinster DR, Gorman RC, Woo YJ, Gleason T, Pochettino A. Advances in the treatment of acute type A dissection: an integrated approach. Ann Thoracic Surg 2002; 74(Suppl 1): S1848-52.
26) Andersen ND, Ganapathi AM, Hanna JM, Williams JB, Gaca JG, Hughes GC. Outcomes of acute type A dissection before and after implementation of a multidisciplinary thoracic aortic surgery program. J Am Coll Cardiol 2014; 63: 1796-1803.
27) Knipp JS, Deeb GM, Prager RL, Williams CY, Upchurch GR Jr, Patel HJ. A contemporary analysis of outcomes for operative repair of type A aortic dissection in the United States. Surgery 2007; 142: 524-8.
28) Chikwe J, Cavallero P, Itagaki S, Seigerman M, Diluozzo G, Adams DH. National outcomes in acute aortic dissection: influence of surgeon and institutional volume on operative mortality. Ann Thorac Surg 2013; 95: 1563-9.
29) Reves JG. An essay on 35 years of the Society of Cardiovascular Anesthesiologists. Anesth Analg 2014; 119: 255-65.
30) Kaplan JA. Twenty-five years old and only getting better. J Cardiothorac Vasc Anesth 2011; 25: 1-2.
31) Svensson LG, Labib SR, Eisenhauer AC, Butterly JR. Intimal tear without hematoma: an important variant of aortic dissection that can elude current imaging techniques. Circulation 1999; 99: 1331-6.
32) Goldstein SA, Evangelista A, Abbara S, et al. Multimodality imaging of diseases of the thoracic aorta in adults: from the American Society of Echocardiography and the European Association of Cardiovascular Imaging. J Am Soc Echocardiogr 2015; 119: 119-82.
33) MacKnight BM, Maldonado Y, Augoustides JG, et al. Advances in imaging for the management of acute aortic syndromes: focus on transesophageal echocardiography and type A aortic dissection for the perioperative echocardiographer. J Cardiothorac Vasc Anesth 2016; 30(4): 1129-41.
34) Augoustides JG, Floyd TF, Kolansky DM. Echocardiography in suspected acute type A aortic dissection: detection and management of a false positive presentation. J Cardiothorac Vasc Anesth 2006; 20: 912-4.
35) Denault A, Lamarche Y, Rochon A, et al. Innovative approaches to the perioperative care of the cardiac surgical patient in the operating room and intensive care unit. Can J Cardiol 2014; 30(12 Suppl): S459-77.
36) Augoustides JG, Patel PA, Savino JS, Bavaria JE. The heart team approach to acute type A dissection: a new paradigm in the era of the integrated Penn classification and the Essen concept. Eur J Cardiothorac Surg 2013; 43: 404-5.
37) Silvay G, Zafirova Z. Ten years experiences with preoperative evaluation clinic for day admission cardiac and major vascular surgical patients: model for 'perioperative anesthesia and surgical home'. Semin Cardiothorac Vasc Anesth 2016; 20: 120-32.

38) Appoo J, Augoustides JG, Pochettino A, et al. Perioperative outcome in adults undergoing elective deep hypothermic circulatory arrest with retrograde cerebral perfusion in proximal aortic arch repair: evaluation of protocol-based care. J Cardiothorac Vasc Anesth 2006; 20: 3-7.
39) Augoustides JG, Floyd TF, McGarvey ML, et al. Major clinical outcomes in adults undergoing thoracic aortic surgery requiring deep hypothermic circulatory arrest: quantification of organ-based perioperative outcome and detection of opportunities for perioperative intervention. J Cardiothorac Vasc Anesth 2005; 19: 446-52.
40) Sloan TB, Edmonds HL, Koht A. Intraoperative electrophysiologic monitoring in aortic surgery. J Cardiothorac Vasc Anesth 2013; 27: 1364-73.
41) Augoustides JG, Pochettino A, Ochroch EA, et al. Renal dysfunction after thoracic aortic surgery requiring deep hypothermic circulatory arrest: definition, incidence, and clinical predictors. J Cardiothorac Vasc Anesth 2006; 20: 673-7.
42) Augoustides JG, Pochettino A, McGarvey ML, et al. Clinical predictors for mortality in adults undergoing thoracic aortic surgery requiring deep hypothermic circulatory arrest. Ann Card Anaesth 2006; 9: 114-9.
43) Augoustides JG, Patel P, Ghadimi K, Choi J, Yue Y, Silvay G. Current conduct of deep hypothermic circulatory arrest in China. HSR Proc Intensive Care Cardiovasc Anesth 2013; 5: 25-32.
44) Stone JG, Young WL, Smith CR, et al. Do standard monitoring sites reflect true brain temperature when profound hypothermia is rapidly induced and reversed? Anesthesiology 1995; 82: 344-51.
45) Whitby JD, Dunkin LJ. Cerebral, esophageal, and nasopharyngeal temperatures. Br J Anaesth 1971; 43: 673-6.
46) Ren Z, Wang Z, Hu R, et al. Which cannulation (axillary cannulation or femoral cannulation) is better for acute type A aortic dissection repair? A meta-analysis of 9 clinical studies. Eur J Cardiotorac Surg 2015; 47: 408-15.
47) Benedetto U, Raja SG, Amrani M, et al. The impact of arterial cannulation strategy on operative outcomes in aortic surgery: evidence from a comprehensive meta-analysis of comparative studies on 4476 patients. J Thorac Cardiovasc Surg 2014; 148: 2936-43.
48) Thorsguard ME, Mornissette GJ, Sun B, et al. Impact of intraoperative transesophageal echocardiography on acute type A aortic dissection. J Cardiothorac Vasc Anesth 2014; 28: 1203-7.
49) Augoustides JG, Szeto WY, Bavaria JE. Advances in aortic valve repair: focus on functional approach, clinical outcomes, and central role of echocardiography. J Cardiothorac Vasc Anesth 2010; 24: 1016-20.
50) Jansen Klomp WW, Peelen LM, Brandon Bravo Bruinisma GJ, Van't Hof AW, Grandjean JG, Nierich AP. Modified transesophageal echocardiography of the dissected thoracic aorta: a novel diagnostic approach. Cardiovasc Ultrasound 2016; 14: 28.
51) Augoustides JG, Haris H, Pochettino A. Direct innominate artery cannulation in type A dissection and severe aortic atheroma. J Cardiothor Vasc Anesth 2007; 21: 727-8.
52) Augoustides JG, Desai ND, Szeto WY, Bavaria JE. Innominate artery cannulation: the Toronto technique for antegrade cerebral perfusion in aortic arch reconstruction – a clinical trial opportunity for the International Aortic Arch Surgery Study Group. J Thorac Cardiovasc Surg 2014; 148: 2924-6.
53) Lanigan MJ, Chaney MA, Gologorsky E, Chavanon O, Augoustides JG. Case 2--2014: Aortic dissection: real or artifact? J Cardiothorac Vasc Anesth 2014; 28: 398-407.
54) Augoustides JG, Kohl BA, Harris H, Pochettino A. Color-flow Doppler recognition of intraoperative brachocephalic malperfusion during operative repair of acute type A aortic dissection: utility of transcutaneous carotid artery ultrasound scanning. J Cardiothorac Vasc Anesth 2007; 21: 81-4.
55) Pulido JN, Pallohusky BS, Park SJ, Cook DJ. Transcutaneous ultrasound measurements of carotid flow to monitor for cerebral malperfusion during type A aortic dissection repair. J Cardiothoracic Vasc Anesth 2013; 27: 728-30.
56) Orihashi K. Cerebral malperfusion in acute aortic dissection. Surg Today 2016; 46(12): 1353-61.
57) Douds MT, Straub EJ, Kent AC, Bistrick CH, Sistino JJ. A systematic review of cerebral oxygenation-monitoring devices in cardiac surgery. Perfusion 2014; 29: 545-52.
58) Chan SK, Underwood MJ, Ho Am, So JM, Wan IY, Wong RH. Cannula malposition during antegrade cerebral perfusion for aortic surgery: role of cerebral oximetry. Can J Anesth 2014; 61: 736-40.
59) Grocott HP, Ambrose E, Moon W. External carotid compression: a novel technique to improve cerebral perfusion during selective antegrade cerebral perfusion for aortic arch surgery. Can J Anesth 2016; 63(10): 1179-83.
60) Gutsche JT, Feinamn J, Silvay G, et al. Practice variations in the conduct of hypothermic circulatory arrest for adult aortic arch repair: focus on an emerging European paradigm. Heart Lung Vessel 2014; 6: 43-51.
61) Heringlake M, Garbers C, Kabler JH, et al. Preoperative cerebral oxygen saturation and clinical outcome in cardiac surgery. Anesthesiology 2011; 114: 58-69.
62) Deschamps A, Hall R, Grocott H, et al. Cerebral oximetry monitoring to maintain normal cerebral oxygen saturation during high-risk cardiac surgery: a randomized controlled feasibility trial. Anesthesiology 2016; 124: 826-36.

63) Silvay G, Weinrich A, Owitz S, Mindich B, Litwak RS. The cerebral function monitor during open-heart surgery. Herz 1978; 3: 270-5.
64) McCullough JN, Zhang N, Reich DL, et al. Cerebral metabolic rate during hypothermic circulatory arrest. Ann Thoracic Surg 1999; 67: 1895-9.
65) Janes ML, Andersen ND, Swaminathan M, et al. Predictors of electrocerebral silence inactivity with deep hypothermia. J Thorac Cardiovasc Surg 2014; 147: 1002-7.
66) Gutsche JT, Ghadimi K, Patel PA, et al. New frontiers in aortic therapy: focus on deep hypothermic circulatory arrest. J Cardiothorac Vasc Anesth 2014; 28: 1159-63.
67) Vallbhajosyula P, Jassar AG, Menon RS, et al. Moderate versus deep hypothermic circulatory arrest for elective aortic transverse hemiarch reconstruction. Ann Thorac Surg 2015; 99: 1511-7.
68) Conas GM, Leshnower BG, Halkos ME, et al. Acute type A dissection: impact of antegrade cerebral perfusion under moderate hypothermia. Ann Thorac Surg 2013; 96: 2135-41.
69) Arnaoutakis GJ, Vallaghajosyula P, Bavaria JE, et al. The impact of deep versus moderate hypothermia on postoperative kidney function after elective aortic hemiarch repair. Ann Thorac Surg 2016 102(4): 1313-21.
70) Keenan JE, Wang H, Ganapathi AM, et al. Electroencephalography during hemiarch replacement with moderate hypothermic circulatory arrest. Ann Thorac Surg 2016; 101: 631-7.
71) Dewhurst AT, Moore SJ, Liban JB. Pharmacological agents as cerebral protectants during deep hypothermic circulatory arrest in adult thoracic aortic surgery: a survey of current practice. Anaesthesia 2002; 57: 1016-21.
72) Cheung AT, Weiss SJ, Kent G, Pochettino A, Bavaria JE, Stecker MM. Intraoperative seizures in cardiac surgical patients undergoing deep hypothermic circulatory arrest monitored with EEG. Anesthesiology 2001; 94: 1143-7.
73) Al-Hashimi S, Zaman M, Waterworth P, Bilal H. Does the use of thiopental provide added cerebral protection during deep hypothermic circulatory arrest? Interact Cardiovasc Thorac Surg 2013; 17: 392-7.
74) Kruger T, Hoffmann I, Blether M, et al. Intraoperative neuroprotective drugs without beneficial effects? Results of the German Registry for Acute Aortic Dissection Type A (GERAADA). Eur J Cardiothorac Surg 2013; 44: 939-46.
75) Guan XL, Wang XL, Liu YY, et al. Changes in the hemostatic system of patients with acute aortic dissection undergoing aortic arch surgery. Ann Thorac Surg 2016; 101: 945-51.
76) Czerny M, Schoenhoff P, Etz C, et al. The impact of preoperative malperfusion on outcome in acute type A aortic dissection: results from the GERAADA registry. J Am Coll Cardiol 2015; 65: 2628-35.
77) Paparella D, Rotunmo C, Guida P, et al. Hemostasis alterations in patients with acute aortic dissection. Ann Thorac Surg 2011; 91: 1364-9.
78) Gorlinger K, Shore-Lesserson L, Dirkmann D, Hanke AA, Rahe-Meyer N, Tanaka KA. Management of hemorrhage in cardiothoracic surgery. J Cardiothorac Vasc Anesth 2013; 27(4 Suppl): S20-S34.
79) Brase J, Finger B, He J, et al. Analysis of outcomes using low-dose and early administration of recombinant activated factor VII in cardiac surgery. Ann Thorac Surg 2016; 102: 35-40.
80) Tolis G, Sundt TM. Contemporary insights into the management of type A aortic dissection. Exp Rev Cardiovasc Ther 2016; 14(10): 1189-96.
81) Augoustides JG, Pochettino A, Ochroch EA, et al. Clinical predictors for prolonged intensive care unit stay in adults undergoing thoracic aortic surgery requiring deep hypothermic circulatory arrest. J Cardiothorac Vasc Anesth 2006; 20: 8-13.
82) Lei Q, Chen L, Jin M, et al. Preoperative and intraoperative risk factors for prolonged intensive care unit stay after aortic arch surgery. J Cardiothorac Vasc Anesth 2009; 23: 789-94.
83) Girdauskas E, Kuntze T, Borger MA, et al. Acute respiratory dysfunction after surgery for acute type A aortic dissection. Eur J Cardiothoracic Surg 2010; 37: 691-6.
84) Kurabavashi M, Okishige K, Azegami K, et al. Reduction of the PaO2/FiO2 ratio in acute aortic dissection – relationship between the extent of dissection and inflammation. Circ J 2010; 74: 2066-73.
85) El-Hamamsy I, Ouzounian M, Demers P, et al. State-of-the-art surgical management of acute type A aortic dissection. Can J Cardiol 2016; 32: 100-9.
86) Kondoh H, Satoh H, Daimon T, et al. Outcomes of limited proximal aortic replacement for type A aortic dissection in octogenarians. J Thorac Cardiovasc Surg 2016; 152: 439-46.
87) Bachet J. Outcomes of limited proximal aortic replacement for type A aortic dissection in octogenarians: what does 'age' mean? J Thorac Cardiovasc Surg 2016; 152: 447.
88) Makary MA, Seger DL, Pronovost PI, et al. Frailty as a predictor of surgical outcomes in older patients. J Am Coll Cardiol 2010; 210: 901-8.
89) Ronchey S, Serrao E, Albert V, et al. Endovascular stenting of the ascending aorta for type A aortic dissections in patients at high risk for open surgery. Eur J Vasc Endovasc Surg 2013; 45: 475-80.
90) Stewart A, Chikwe J. Thinking beyond the tube graft: using malperfusion as a guide to define treatment of type A dissection. J Am Coll Cardiol 2015; 65: 2636-7.

37

Anesthetic management of patients undergoing open or endovascular procedures for Type B aortic dissection

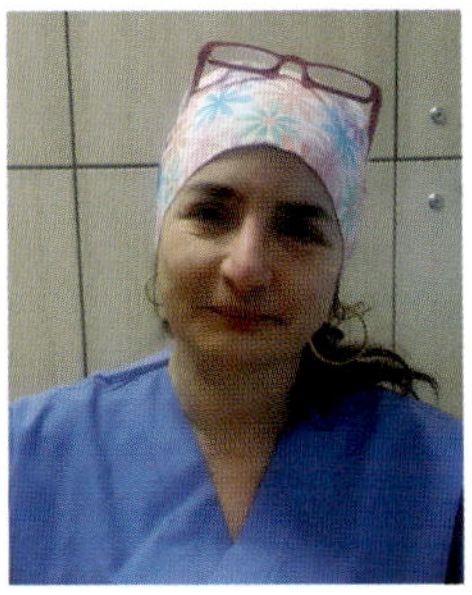

Monica De Luca, Fabrizio Monaco, Salvatore Sardo,
Marina Pieri, Silvio Magrin, Alberto Zangrillo

37.1 Introduction

Aortic dissection (AD) is the result of an aortic intimal wall tear leading to the separation of aortic wall layers driven by pulsatile blood flow [1]. The progression of the dissection distal to the left subclavian artery defines a Type B AD according to the Stanford classification [2]. The typical clinical presentation is characterized by sudden severe pain, signs and symptoms of organ ischemia, and/or shock [3, 4]. Three different therapeutic approaches to acute Type B AD are available (Fig. 37.1):

- medical management;
- endovascular repair (Thoracic EndoVascular Aortic Repair, TEVAR);
- open surgery [5].

37.2 Diagnostic workup

Although the clinical scenario of acute Type B AD may be initially stable, a sudden deterioration can occur at any time. Therefore, in the suspicion of acute Type B AD, two large-bore peripheral venous catheters and a full monitoring with invasive blood pressure, peripheral oxygen pulse oximetry, and 5-lead electrocardiogram (EKG) are strongly recommended. The type of diagnostic imaging to perform depends on the patient's clinical conditions and the local expertise, logistics and available equipment at the clinic. The goals of the diagnostic tools are to quickly detect or exclude: the presence of an intimal flap, principal and secondary tears, true lumen (TL) and false lumen (FL), aortic side branch involvement, aortic valve regurgitation, hemopericardium and hemothorax, myocardial ischemia, or infarction.

Transthoracic echocardiography (TTE) is usually the first diagnostic process in patients with thoracic pain and suspected Type B AD due to its minimal invasiveness, availability in

Monica De Luca (monica.deluca@libero.it)
Scientific Institute Ospedale San Raffaele,
Milan, Italy

G. Melissano - R. Chiesa (eds), Aortic Dissection patients true stories and the innovations that saved their lives

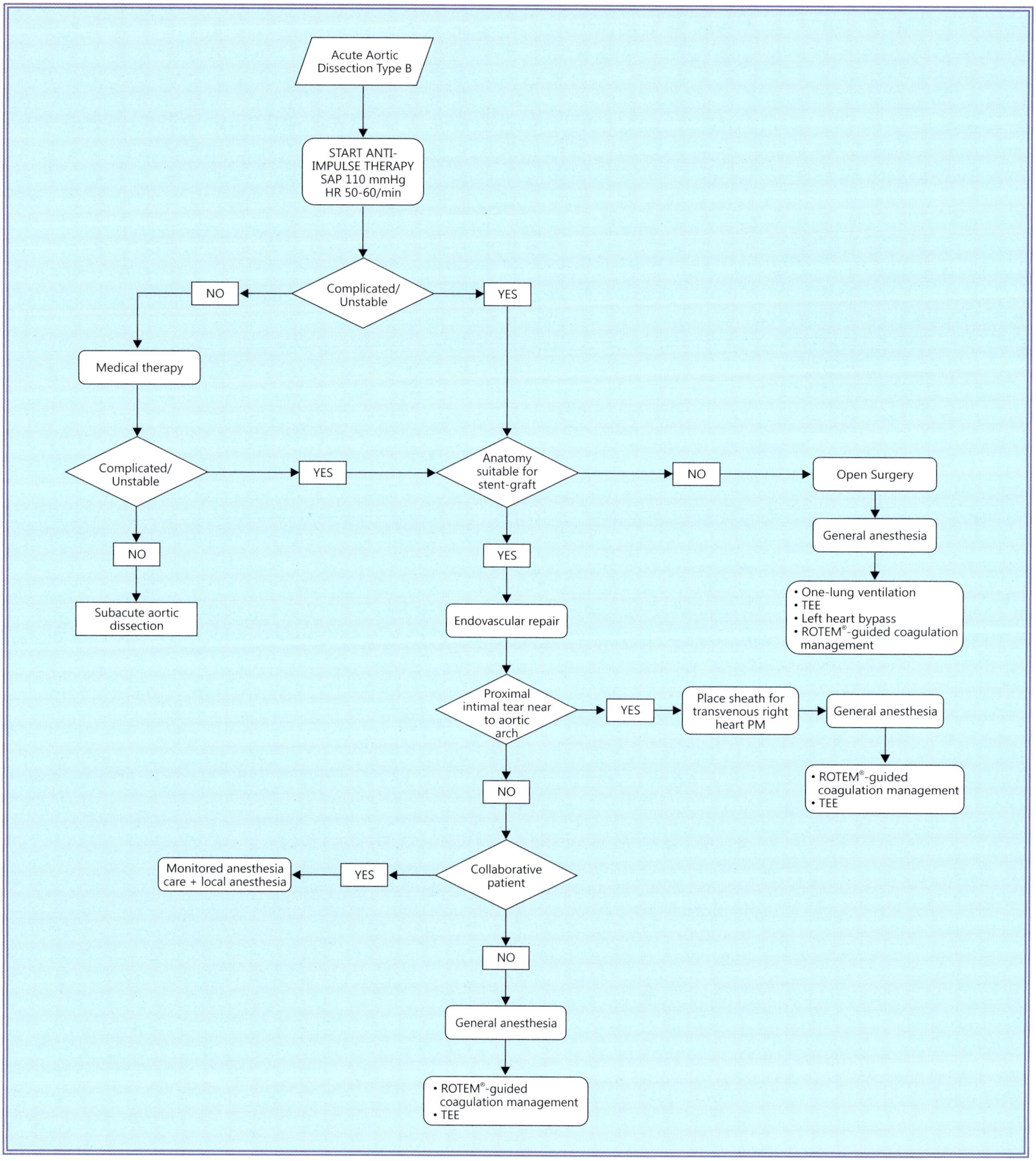

Fig. 37.1 Type B AD: therapeutic approache. PM, pacemaker; ROTEM, ROtation ThromboElastoMetry; TEE, TransEsophageal Echocardiography.

the emergency departments, and diagnostic efficacy and efficiency. Although TTE allows the differential diagnosis with other cardiac life-threatening complications, its sensitivity for acute Type B AD diagnosis is low, ranging between 31 and 55% [6]. Adequate imaging techniques are essential to establish a complete and correct diagnosis in patients with Type B AD. Computed tomography angiography (CTA) is used in 63% of cases, transesophageal echocardiography (TEE) in 32% and magnetic resonance angiography (MRA) in less than 1% [7]. As CTA, TEE and MRI have similar sensitivity (98-100%) and specificity (95-98%) the choice of the diagnostic tool should be driven by the patient's hemodynamic stability [6, 8, 9].

In patients with suspected Type B AD and hemodynamic stability, a CT angiography is the gold standard to investigate the entire aorta down to the iliac arteries, and the involvement of aortic side branches. For critically ill and unstable patients, TEE is recommended [8, 9] since it is available at the patient's bedside [8].

37.3 Medical management

As recommended by current guidelines, medical treatment is reserved to patients with stable and uncomplicated acute Type B AD [5], with the aim to reduce arterial blood pressure, provide adequate analgesia, prevent AD progression, detect complications, and stabilize the patient. Blood pressure management is the cornerstone of medical treatment since, as observed by Wheat et al., the rate of pressure rise (dP/dT) and arterial pressure are the driving forces of both FL extension and vascular ostia compression [10, 11]. Administration of beta-blocker is the first-line therapy for decreasing blood pressure and heart rate. Labetalol (a nonselective beta-blocker and alpha-blocker with intrinsic sympathomimetic activity) is administered to manage hypertension. Sodium nitroprusside, nitrates and calcium channel blockers can be added to maintain systolic arterial pressure around 100-120 mmHg. A heart rate of 50-60 beats/min can be achieved with esmolol or diltiazem. Morphine, titrated to the analgesic effect, is the drug of choice for pain management. Further details on pharmacological management can be found in Chapter 9.

After 10-15 days of medical treatment, the vascular tissues are expected to be less fragile and, therefore, in selected patients an elective TEVAR can be performed with reduced risks. Recently, some authors have shown that elective TEVAR is a therapeutic option also in uncomplicated patients, allowing the exclusion and the thrombosis of the false lumen, so preventing an adverse aortic remodelling, and improving the long term prognosis [12-14].

37.4 Thoracic endovascular aortic repair

Endovascular repair is indicated when acute AD is complicated by refractory hypertension, intractable pain, signs/symptoms of impaired perfusion with tissue ischemia (i.e. malperfusion syndrome), signs of impending rupture, rapid growth, and hemodynamic instability and when the anatomy of the lesion is suitable for stenting. The role of TEVAR in the complicated acute Type B AD is highlighted by a class IC recommendation of the European Society of Cardiology [5].

The choice of the anesthetic technique depends on patient characteristics and the site of the lesion. In the case of proximal entry flap near the emergence of the left subclavian artery, to decrease the risk of stent-graft misplacement and supra-aortic vessels occlusion due to the patient's involuntary movements, a general anesthesia is recommended. However, collaborative or extremely ill patients can be managed with local anesthesia and propofol-based total intravenous anesthesia (TIVA)/target controlled infusion (TCI) for the modulation of the level of consciousness. Locoregional anesthesia should be avoided in order to permit an early eventual detection of spinal cord ischemia.

37.4.1 Preoperative evaluation

Even in an emergency setting it is important to obtain a brief medical history (e.g. previous surgeries, comorbidities, prescribed medications, allergies) and standard blood tests including: electrolytes, creatinine, blood urea nitrogen (BUN), complete blood count, and coagulation type and screen (prothrombin time, activated partial thromboplastin time, antithrombin III activity, d-dimer). Preoperative aggregometry and a viscoelastic test may play a role in patients on dual antiplatelet therapy (DAPT) or new generation anticoagulant drugs, respectively. In order to balance hemorrhagic and thrombotic risks in patients on DAPT, aspirin should be continued and P2Y12 inhibitors stopped, in accordance with guideline recommendations [15]. After the discontinuation of adenosine diphosphate (ADP)-receptor inhibitors, the bridging with tirofiban or eptifibatide should start 72 hours before surgery and be discontinued 6-8 hours prior to surgery. In patients with renal impairment (creatinine clearance <50 mL/min) a dose adjustment and a longer suspension before surgery (8-12 hours) is required.

Pulmonary function and difficulty of intubation must be carefully evaluated. In fact, most of the young patients affected by acute AD are also affected by Marfan syndrome or other connective tissue disorders. These conditions require extreme caution with regard to difficult airway management (micrognathia, cervical spine instability, tracheomalacia), pulmonary comorbidities (restrictive disorder, emphysema, higher risk for spontaneous pneumothorax), cardiac comorbidities (aortic and/or mitral regurgitation), and difficult positioning (kyphoscoliosis and joint hyperlaxity) [16].

37.4.2 Monitoring

A right radial artery for invasive arterial pressure (IAP) monitoring is obtained because the left radial arterial line would be compromised in the event of stent-graft placement covering the left subclavian artery. The procedure requires an additional access in the right femoral artery, offering the anesthesiologist another site for IAP monitoring (otherwise a side line of the sheaths used for the endovascular procedure may be used). The hemodynamic management has to ensure a controlled blood pressure to guarantee adequate tissue perfusion, avoiding stent-graft misplacement during deployment. Electrocardiogram with 5 leads and continuous visualization through DII and V5 derivations are used to detect signs of myocardial ischemia. Seriate arterial blood gas analysis guides the mechanical ventilation strategy in intubated patients, and monitors gas exchange, and lactate and hemoglobin concentrations. Urine output has to be assessed carefully. In fact, a diuresis less than 0.5 mL/kg/h may promptly reveal signs of renal ischemia (with the need for additional endovascular procedures to the renal arteries), or a border-line cardiac function. Core temperature is recorded at the bladder or nasopharyngeal site, and warm fluids and a circulating water mattress are used in order to maintain normothermia.

37.4.3 Venous access

A large-bore peripheral venous access (16-14 G) and central venous catheterization are required for fluids resuscitation, transfusions and vasopressors. A high-flow 8.5-Fr multilumen access and, in selected patients with known high-risk cardiac comorbidities, an 8.5-Fr pulmonary artery catheter introducer sheath are placed in the right jugular vein using a "double stick" technique. The Trendelenburg position, fluid infusion and ultrasound guidance decrease the risk of accidental carotid puncture and right pneumothorax. The use of a pulmonary artery catheter may be optional if real-time TEE monitoring is available. In fact, the latter provides, amongst other things, information regarding the cardiac function and hemodynamics, allowing a differential diagnosis (see Chapter 39). If the proximal entry tear is located near the aortic arch, a right heart pacemaker catheter with a transvenous femoral approach can be used for rapid pacing.

37.4.4 Airways

A single lumen tracheal tube is appropriate for the TEVAR procedure. To avoid hypertensive peaks which may lead to progression or rupture of the AD, an intravenous fentanyl bolus (3 μg/kg) is administered or a remifentanil infusion (0.5-1 μg/kg/min) is started 5 min before attempting laryngoscopy.

37.4.5 Coagulation

Heparin anticoagulation reversal is accomplished through the administration of intravenous protamine at a 1:1 ratio with the heparin dose. An activated clotting time (ACT) ranging above 220 s is required throughout the procedure. Administration of fresh frozen plasma (FFP), fibrinogen and platelets usage should be driven by viscoelastic tests, whenever possible.

37.4.6 Transesophageal echocardiography

In patients undergoing general anesthesia, TEE allows the evaluation of left and right ventricular systolic function, new regional wall motion abnormalities, diastolic function, the anatomy of the ascending aorta, aortic arch, and descending thoracic aorta, and fluid status. After stent grafting deployment, TEE has shown high sensitivity and specificity in detecting endoleaks [17]. The role of TEE in the management of acute Type B AD is further discussed in Chapter 39.

37.4.7 Intraoperative evaluation

The main goals of anesthetic management during TEVAR are:
- hemodynamic stability;
- the patient's immobility during stent-graft deployment.

During aortographies and stent-graft deployment, the mechanical ventilation (or spontaneous breathing in the sedated patient) is stopped to prevent imaging artifacts due to intrathoracic structure movements. Arterial blood pressure is reduced to prevent stent-graft misplacement. In particular, when the proximal entry tear is located in the aortic arch, a rapid pacing (160-180 bpm) leads to a reversible reduction (7-15 s) of arterial blood pressure offering the perfect conditions for stent-graft deployment. This approach is safer and more effective than infusion of vasodilator drugs (e.g. nitroprusside), or occlusion of the inferior vena cava with an inflated balloon and adenosine [18-21]. It should be noted that rapid pacing may not be effective in young patients with healthy hearts.

37.4.8 Emergence from anesthesia and postoperative care

After an uneventful TEVAR, the patient can be safely transferred to the post-anesthesia care unit. At the end of the procedure, a neurological window may help to detect the onset of spinal cord injury. In the case of paraplegia/paresis, placement of a cerebral-spinal fluid drainage and the maintenance of a mean arterial pressure (MAP) above 90 mmHg with or without vasopressor administration are recommended. In the ward, a strict monitoring of blood pressure, EKG, and diuresis along with serial neurological assessment of motor function is needed.

37.5 Open surgical repair

The indication for open surgical repair is: hemodynamically unstable and/or complicated Type B AD which is not anatomically suitable for endovascular repair. Surgical repair of acute Type B AD closely resembles the surgical repair of a thoracoabdominal aortic aneurysm (TAAA) in terms of the surgical trauma, risk of massive hemorrhage, and risk of visceral ischemia and spinal injury, along with the adoption of left heart bypass as a hemodynamic support.

37.5.1 Preoperative evaluation

Given the potential risks and complications associated with open surgery for Type B AD, a full perioperative evaluation of cardiac, respiratory, renal, neurological function is performed whenever possible. During aortic cross-clamping the heart is at high risk of developing myocardial ischemia and infarction. Thus, the presence of coronary artery disease, valvular dysfunction, and systolic and diastolic dysfunction should be investigated in accordance with current guideline recommendations [22]. Pulmonary function has to be fully evaluated due to the need for single lung ventilation (SLV) and the high rate of postoperative respiratory failure associated with diaphragmatic dysfunction. A decreased renal function is common in patients undergoing Type B AD surgery; therefore, in order to avoid contrast-related renal dysfunction, the radiologic studies requiring iodinated contrast medium should be performed as far away from the procedure as possible, using the smallest possible amount of contrast medium. Preoperative administration of N-acetylcysteine with the aim to reduce the risk of contrast-related nephropathy and progressive renal failure has been investigated, but without conclusive results [23].

In the vast majority of cases a preoperative CT scan angiography allows the evaluation of the aortic anatomy, supra-aortic vessels, Adamkiewicz artery, major branches, conditioning surgical workup and level of the aortic cross-clamping. In fact, if the entry tear is close to the aortic arch the aorta has to be cross-clamped between the left carotid and subclavian arteries, further impairing cerebral perfusion.

37.5.2 Monitoring

A 20-G catheter is placed in the right radial artery because of the possibility of left subclavian artery exclusion during aortic cross-clamping. Invasive arterial pressure is also monitored at the right femoral artery because during left heart bypass (LHB) the MAP distal to cross-clamping affects spinal and visceral perfusion pressure. The two reading sites may also display a pressure gradient, before aortic cross-clamping, due to extension of the dissection to the femoral artery and the proximity of intimal flap. MAP should be maintained above 80 mmHg throughout the procedure to ensure organ perfusion.

Ischemic spinal cord injury with subsequent paraplegia is a devastating complication following acute Type B AD surgical repair. The estimated incidence of paraplegia after TAAA open repair and elective TEVAR may be as high as 22 and 13%, respectively (Chapter 31) [24, 25]. Spinal cord ischemia is a consequence of the interruption of intercostal arteries perfusion due to the dissection or complicated surgical repair [26, 27]. Motor (MEP) and somatosensory evoked potentials (SSEP) may detect early signs of spinal cord hypoperfusion and ischemia during the procedure. To assure the validity and reproducibility of the evoked potentials (EPs), a stable anesthesiological plan without volatile agents should be adopted. Similarly, the neuromuscular blockade affects the EPs and, therefore, the administration of a single dose of a neuromuscular blocking agent (i.e. rocuronium) prior to intubation has to be reversed before the acquisition of a baseline recording. The grade of residual neuromuscular blockade can be assessed by the train-of-four stimulation. Further administration of neuromuscular blockade agents throughout the procedure should be avoided.

Keyhani et al. have reported that, for intraoperative EPs, the alterations overestimate the incidence of immediate postoperative neurologic dysfunction while persistent pathological changes are significantly associated with clinically evident spinal injury. However, the sensitivity and the positive predictive power of EPs remain low (37 and 33% for SSEP; 22 and 45% for MEP, respectively) [28]. Intraoperatively, in the event of SSEP/MEP alterations it is recommended to increase the MAP to 80-100 mmHg and decrease the cerebrospinal fluid (CSF) pressure below 10 mmHg in order to improve the spinal cord perfusion pressure.

Spinal near-infrared spectroscopy (NIRS) has also been proposed as a method for monitoring spinal cord vascularization. Theoretically, the measure of hemoglobin saturation fluctuations is associated with spinal cord region tissue perfusion and oxygenation during aortic surgery. However, larger trials are required to confirm the potential usefulness of this technique [29].

In a large randomized controlled clinical trial on CSF drainage strategy in patients undergoing TAAA open surgery, CSF drainage has shown an 80% decrease of postoperative paraplegia rate (class Ia European Society of Cardiology guidelines) [5, 30]. In elective surgery for chronic aortic dissection and TAAA, percutaneous placement of a CSF drainage catheter is routinely used. In particular, maintaining a CSF pressure around 10 mmHg increases the spinal cord perfusion pressure. In an emergency context, the placement of a lumbar intrathecal drainage catheter is often unfeasible. Therefore, it may be used as rescue therapy in the event of postoperative signs of spinal cord ischemia.

Core temperature monitoring is required to prevent severe hypothermia. A mild hypothermia (33-34 °C) is auspicable for neurological and renal protection during the aortic clamping time. A temperature above 35 °C should be achieved at the end of the procedure to avoid hemostasis impairment. Hot fluids and a circulating water mattress can be used to manipulate the temperature during the surgery.

37.5.3 Venous access

The ability to quickly respond to a volume shift is crucial during open surgery for Type B AD. Two large-bore peripheral venous access (16-14 G) are obtained before the induction. Compared to TEVAR, to the 8.5-Fr four-lumen central venous catheter a 12.5-Fr high flow 3 lumen is added in the right jugular vein. Cannulation of the right jugular vein under ultrasound (US) guidance and sparing of the right subclavian vein are measures able to decrease the risk of right-sided pneumothorax, which may impair the mechanical ventilation during surgery. The left jugular vein cannulation is an alternative approach, although the right lateral decubitus may decrease the maximum flow rate through the venous access.

37.5.4 Induction and maintenance of anesthesia

The priority during induction and airway management is to ensure a stable hemodynamic status and an adequate analgesia during laryngoscopy and airway stimulation. High dose opioid administration (fentanyl bolus 5 µg/kg) guarantees a good hemodynamic stability. Cefazolin 2 g is administered as antibiotic prophylaxis 30 min prior to skin incision. Methylprednisolone (30 mg/kg) and mannitol (0.5 g/kg) are administered before aortic cross-clamping for renal protection with the aim to decrease the ischemic reperfusion injury [31]. A propofol and remifentanil TIVA or TCI is suggested for both a constant level of anesthesia and hemodynamic stability.

37.5.5 Airways

Acute Type B AD open surgery requires SLV of the right lung. A left side double lumen Robertshaw-type tube is the first choice, reducing the rate of intraoperative dislocations. In the case of unfavorable anatomy such as an advantageous angle between the trachea and the right main bronchus, airway distortion, or compression of a left-sided main bronchus, a right-sided double lumen tube or a left endobronchial excluder should be considered (Fig. 37.2). A fiberoptic bronchoscopy verifies the correct tube placement.

The series of images illustrates dislocation of the trachea and left main bronchus of increasing severity. In order to obtain single lung ventilation, a right Robertshaw double lumen tube may be employed or, alternatively, a single lumen tube with an occluder for the left bronchus can be used; bronchoscopy is useful during intubation. Careful examination of the chest X-ray and CT scan allows a correct preoperative diagnosis and the choice of the best strategy for intubation. Interestingly, the aerogram of the left lung in the case of a large aneurysm shows a significant reduction of the ventilated parenchyma; pleural adhesions are also common in these cases.

37.5.6 Coagulation and blood products

Leading causes of bleeding during open repair are: hyperfibrinolysis, surgical bleeding, aortic friability, patent intercostal/lumbar arteries, dilution and consumption coagulopathy, visceral ischemic reperfusion injury, and chronic therapy with long-acting antiplatelet or anticoagulant drugs when not promptly suspended. An intraoperative strategy with antifibrinolytic drugs (tranexamic acid 1 g as loading dose, 2 g as a 300 mg/h infusion), intraoperative red cell salvage for autologous transfusion, hemodilution and viscoelastic tests reduces the need for allogeneic blood product transfusions. Massive bleeding in patients undergoing Type B AD surgery is usually managed with a pre-emptive transfusion approach in which blood products are transfused before the results of the laboratory tests became available. However, as suggested by a recent review, the approach to vascular hemostasis should be scientific, rational, monitored and goal-directed because transfusions are associated with noninfectious serious hazards of transfusion (NISHOT) [32, 33].

Viscoelastic tests answer to these requirements, distinguishing between surgical bleeding, which should be managed with a more accurate surgical hemostasis avoiding unnecessary transfusions, and microvascular bleeding, which should be managed with blood products administration [34]. During bleeding, fibrinogen and platelets typically reach a critical low value before the coagulation factors, and thus “the substrates” should be reintegrated before FFP administration [15, 16]. Moreover, hemostatic agents, such as fibrinogen and prothrombin concentrate complex, are now available and allow a more effective and targeted hemostasis when associated with point of care testing. With this strategy, several authors have shown a significant decrease of allogeneic blood product transfusions [35]. Even so, at least 5 packed red blood cell and FFP units have to be available in case of uncontrolled bleeding.

There is no agreement on which hemoglobin trigger is better in vascular surgery. Fominskiy et al. in a recent meta-analysis of randomized control trials showed that, during surgery,

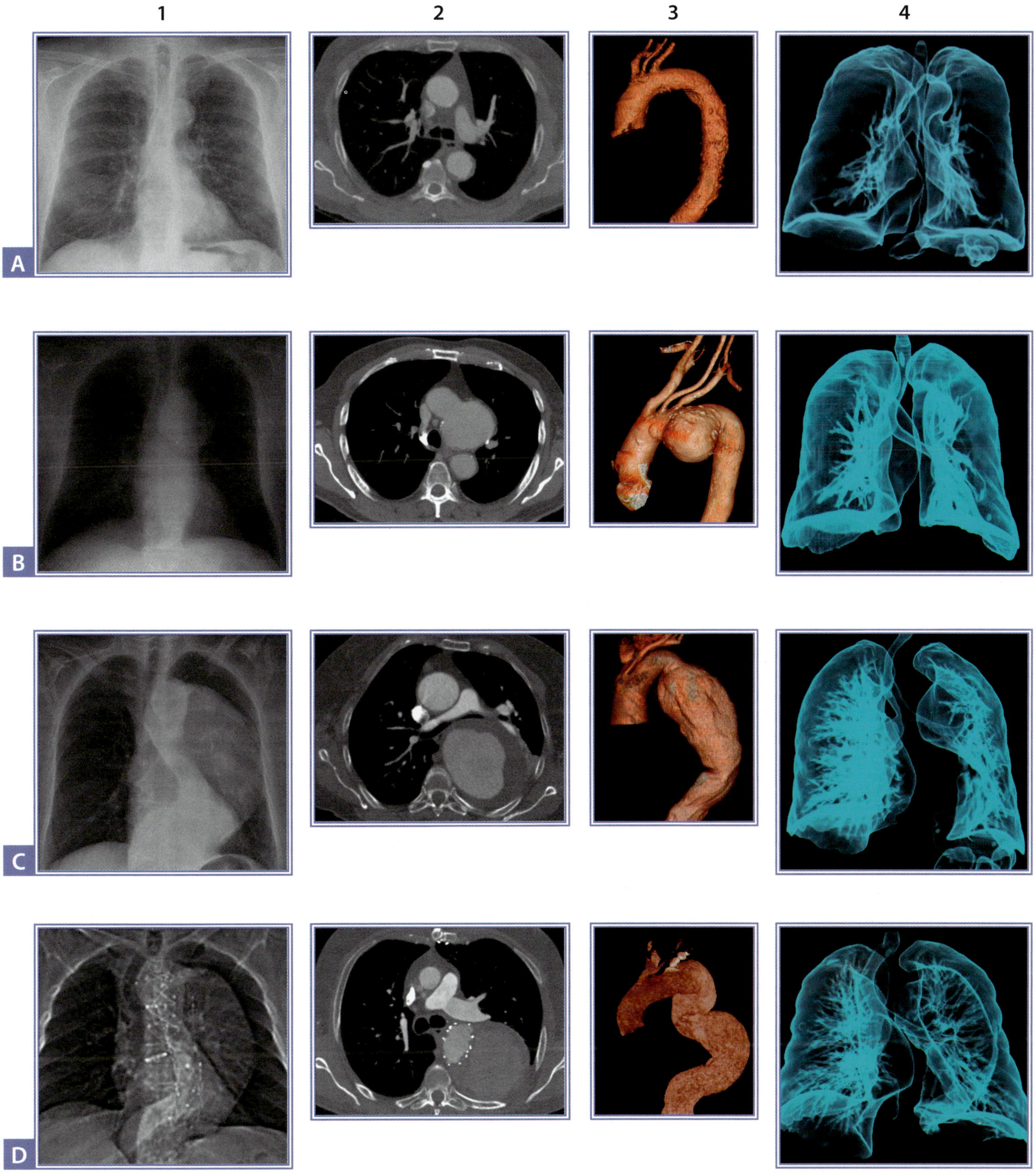

Fig. 37.2 Shows four cases with: **A**) normal aorta, **B**) aortic arch aneurysm, **C**) descending thoracic aneurysm and **D**) thoracoabdominal aneurysm, with four different imaging modalities: 1) chest X-ray, 2) angio-CT scan at the level of the carina, 3) 3D reconstruction of the aorta from an angio-CT scan, 4) 3D broncho-aerogram of the airways and the lungs obtained from the CT scan.

a liberal transfusion strategy (threshold hematocrit >29%) leads to a better outcome when compared to a more restrictive approach because intraoperative anemia is synonymous with active bleeding [36]. However, the hemoglobin transfusion trigger depends on the patient's comorbidities and cardiovascular reserve.

37.5.7 Left heart bypass

Although several strategies have been proposed for Type B AD surgery, LHB, with the outflow cannula in the left atrium and the inflow cannula in the left femoral artery or distal aorta, is probably the best option for reducing preload to the left ventricle and maintaining spinal cord, renal, mesenteric, and lower extremity perfusion during proximal aortic clamping. LHB requires a mild systemic anticoagulation (ACT 200-250 s), achieved with a small amount of unfractionated heparin.

37.5.8 Emergence from anesthesia and postoperative care

At the end of the procedure, the patient is transferred to the ICU. At arrival, mechanical ventilation is resumed and a 12-lead electrocardiogram, chest X-ray, blood chemistry, complete blood count and coagulation tests are performed. Invasive arterial pressure, central venous pressure, diuresis, and temperature are continuously monitored. As in the operating theatre, also in the ICU the hemodynamic goals are maintenance of hemodynamic stability, urine output, and adequate end-organ perfusion. When the patient is stable and normothermic, sedation is interrupted and weaning from cardiovascular support and mechanical ventilation can be accomplished. After emergence from sedation, it is mandatory to serially assess the neurological function in order to detect early signs of spinal cord injury. If paraparesis or paraplegia become evident, the augmentation of MAP above 90 mmHg and increase of CSF drainage (or the placement of a CSF drainage catheter, if not already inserted) may revert spinal cord ischemia, decreasing the neurological impairment.

37.6 Conclusions

Although significant progress has been achieved in decreasing the morbidity and mortality, the management of Type B AD patients remains a significant clinical challenge. Type B AD is a complex disease that places the patient at high risk of developing cardiovascular, respiratory, renal and neurological complications and requires a detailed anesthesiological and surgical workup. Therefore, an adequate preoperative assessment and risk stratification, when possible, and a skillful anesthetic technique, meticulous intraoperative monitoring and postoperative course are all necessary measures to guarantee an uneventful procedure.

REFERENCES

1) Vilacosta I, San Román J. Acute aortic syndrome. Heart 2001; 85: 365-8.
2) Daily PO, Trueblood HW, Stinson EB, Wuerflein RD, Shumway NE. Management of acute aortic dissections. Ann Thorac Surg 1970; 10: 237-47.
3) Patel AY, Eagle KA, Vaishnava P. Acute type B aortic dissection: insights from the International Registry of Acute Aortic Dissection. Ann Cardiothorac Surg 2014; 3: 368-74.
4) Pape LA, Awais M, Woznicki EM, et al. Presentation, diagnosis, and outcomes of acute aortic dissection: 17-year trends from the International Registry of Acute Aortic Dissection. J Am Coll Cardiol 2015; 66: 350-8.

5) Erbel R, Aboyans V, Boileau C, et al. 2014 ESC Guidelines on the diagnosis and treatment of aortic diseases. Eur Heart J 2014; 35: 2873-926.
6) Baliga RR, Nienaber CA, Bossone E, et al. The role of imaging in aortic dissection and related syndromes. JACC Cardiovasc Imaging 2014; 7: 406-24.
7) Moore A, Eagle K, Bruckman D, et al. Choice of computed tomography, transesophageal echocardiography, magnetic resonance imaging, and aortography in acute aortic dissection: International Registry of Acute Aortic Dissection (IRAD). Am J Cardiol 2002; 89: 1235-8.
8) Shiga T, Wajima Z, Apfel C, Inoue T, Ohe Y. Diagnostic accuracy of transesophageal echocardiography, helical computed tomography, and magnetic resonance imaging for suspected thoracic aortic dissection. Arch Intern Med 2006; 166: 1350-6.
9) Evangelista A, Flachskampf F, Erbel R, et al. Echocardiography in aortic diseases: EAE recommendations for clinical practice. Eur J Echocardiogr 2010; 11: 645-58.
10) Prokop EK, Palmer RF, Wheat MW. Hydrodynamic forces in dissecting aneurysms: in-vitro studies in a tygon model and in dog aortas. Circ Res 1970; 27: 121-7.
11) Wheat M, Palmer R, Bartley T, Seelman R. Treatment of dissecting aneurysms of the aorta without surgery. J Thorac Cardiovasc Surg 1965; 50: 364-73.
12) Nienaber CA, Rousseau H, Eggebrecht H, et al; INSTEAD Trial. Randomized comparison of strategies for type B aortic dissection: the INvestigation of STEnt Grafts in Aortic Dissection (INSTEAD) trial. Circulation 2009; 120: 2519-28.
13) Nienaber CA, Kische S, Rousseau H, et al. Endovascular repair of type B aortic dissection: long-term results of the randomized investigation of stent grafts in aortic dissection Trial. Circ Cardiovasc Interv 2013; 6: 407-16.
14) Brunkwall J, Kasprzak P, Verhoeven E, et al. Endovascular repair of acute uncomplicated aortic type B dissection promotes aortic remodelling: 1 year results of the ADSORB trial. Eur J Vasc Endovasc Surg 2014; 48: 285-91.
15) Fleisher LA, Beckman JA, Brown KA, et al. ACC/AHA 2007 guidelines on perioperative cardiovascular evaluation and care for noncardiac surgery: a report of the American College of Cardiology/American Heart Association Task Force on Practice Guidelines (Writing Committee to Revise the 2002 Guideline). J Am Coll Cardiol 2007; 50: e159-241.
16) Monaco F, De Luca M, Sala A. Anesthesia in Marfan patients. Ital J Vasc Endovasc Surg 2015; 22: 37-41.
17) Rocchi G, Lofiego C, Biagini E, et al. Transesophageal echocardiography-guided algorithm for stent-graft implantation in aortic dissection. J Vasc Surg 2004; 40: 880-5.
18) Pornratanarangsi S, Webster MWI, Alison P, Nand P. Rapid ventricular pacing to lower blood pressure during endograft deployment in the thoracic aorta. Ann Thorac Surg 2006, 81(5): e21-3.
19) Nienaber CA, Kische S, Rehders TC, et al. Rapid pacing for better placing: comparison of techniques for precise deployment of endografts in the thoracic aorta. J Endovasc Ther 2007; 14: 506-12.
20) Chen J, Huang W, Luo S, et al. Application of rapid artificial cardiac pacing in thoracic endovascular aortic repair in aged patients. Clin Interv Aging 2014; 9: 73-8.
21) Lhommet P, Espitalier F, Merlini T, et al. Tolerance of rapid right ventricular pacing during thoracic endovascular aortic repair. Ann Vasc Surg 2015; 29: 578-85.
22) Fleisher L, Fleischmann K, Auerbach A, et al. 2014 ACC/AHA guideline on perioperative cardiovascular evaluation and management of patients undergoing noncardiac surgery: executive summary: a report of the American College of Cardiology/American Heart Association Task Force on Practice Guidelines. Circulation 2014; 130: 2215-45.
23) Oldemeyer JB, Biddle WP, Wurdeman RL, et al. Acetylcysteine in the prevention of contrast-induced nephropathy after coronary angiography. Am Heart J 2003; 146: E23.
24) Bicknell CD, Riga CV, Wolfe JHN. Prevention of paraplegia during thoracoabdominal aortic aneurysm repair. Eur J Vasc Endovasc Surg 2009; 37: 654-60.
25) Bobadilla JL, Wynn M, Tefera G, Acher CW. Low incidence of paraplegia after thoracic endovascular aneurysm repair with proactive spinal cord protective protocols. J Vasc Surg 2013; 57: 1537-42.
26) Gaul C, Dietrich W, Erbguth FJ. Neurological symptoms in aortic dissection: a challenge for neurologists 2008; 26: 1-8.
27) Kato M, Motoki M, Isaji T, et al. Spinal cord injury after endovascular treatment for thoracoabdominal aneurysm or dissection. Eur J Cardiothorac Surg 2015; 48: 571-7.
28) Keyhani K, Miller CC, Estrera AL, et al. Analysis of motor and somatosensory evoked potentials during thoracic and thoracoabdominal aortic aneurysm repair. J Vasc Surg 2009; 49: 36-41.
29) Bozeman R, van Dongen E, Morshuis W, et al. Spinal near-infrared spectroscopy measurements during and after thoracoabdominal aortic aneurysm repair: a pilot study. Ann Thorac Surg 2015; 99: 1267-74.
30) Coselli JS, LeMaire SA, Köksoy C, Schmittling ZC, Curling PE. Cerebrospinal fluid drainage reduces paraplegia after thoracoabdominal aortic aneurysm repair: results of a randomized clinical trial. J Vasc Surg 2002; 35: 631-9.

31) Laschinger JC, Cunningham JN, Cooper MM, et al. Prevention of ischemic spinal cord injury following aortic cross-clamping: use of corticosteroids. Ann Thorac Surg 1984; 38: 500-7.
32) Hendrickson JE, Hillyer CD. Noninfectious serious hazards of transfusion. Anesth Analg 2009; 108: 759-69.
33) Chee Y, Liu S, Irwin M. Management of bleeding in vascular surgery. Br J Anaesth 2016: ii85-ii94.
34) Rahe-Meyer N, Hanke A, Schmidt DS, Hagl C, Pichlmaier M. Fibrinogen concentrate reduces intraoperative bleeding when used as first-line hemostatic therapy during major aortic replacement surgery: results from a randomized, placebo-controlled trial. J Thorac Cardiovasc Surg 2013; 145: S178-85.
35) Rahe-Meyer N, Solomon C, Hanke A, et al. Effects of fibrinogen concentrate as first-line therapy during major aortic replacement surgery: a randomized, placebo-controlled trial. Anesthesiology 2013; 118: 40-50.
36) Fominskiy E, Putzu A, Monaco F, et al. Liberal transfusion strategy improves survival in perioperative but not in critically ill patients. A meta-analysis of randomised trials. Br J Anaesth 2015; 115: 511-9.

38

Intravascular ultrasound is essential for the endovascular management of aortic dissection

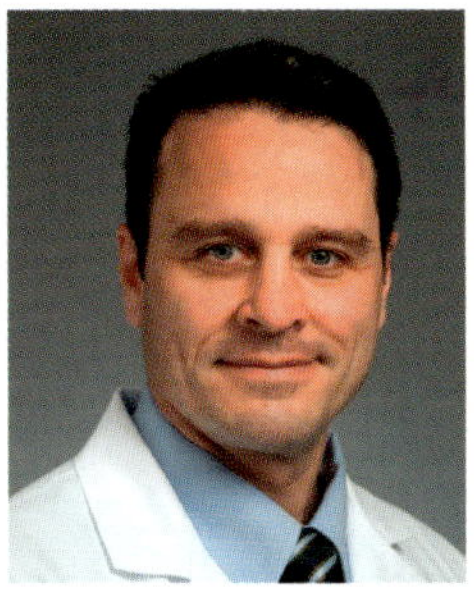

Benjamin W. Starnes

38.1 Introduction

The mainstay of therapy for complicated acute Type B aortic dissection (AD) with evidence of visceral or lower extremity malperfusion is central endovascular aortic repair and sealing of the primary entry tear with an endoluminal graft [1]. Considerable debate remains regarding the management of uncomplicated or chronic Type B AD with aneurysmal degeneration. AD is a lethal disease entity, particularly when associated with end-organ malperfusion.

Approximately 25% of patients presenting with acute Type B AD have complicated AD which carries an attendant high mortality risk [2, 3].

In a recent IRAD (International Registry of Acute Aortic Dissection) review, the in-hospital mortality for patients requiring surgical treatment for acute Type B dissection was nearly 30% [4]. Preoperative malperfusion was present in 30% of patients, which included half of patients with mesenteric ischemia or bowel infarction, and half with limb ischemia. Surgical intervention was indicated for aortic rupture in 23.1% of patients, for visceral ischemia in 23.9%, and for limb ischemia in 15.5%. Patients with severe hypotension and shock on admission or at the time of surgery had a mortality of greater than 50%. Another independent predictor of surgical mortality was age greater than 70 years. Factors associated with favorable outcomes included: radiating pain, normal blood pressure at the time of surgery, and reduced hypothermic circulatory arrest time [4].

In a more recent IRAD review, patients with visceral malperfusion had a 30-day mortality of 31% despite visceral patency after Thoracic EndoVascular Repair (TEVAR), compared to 9.1% in those without visceral malperfusion [5].

Thus timely diagnosis and swift and efficient repair are absolutely paramount to successful outcomes.

Benjamin W. Starnes (starnes@uw.edu)
University of Washington,
Seattle, WA, USA

G. Melissano - R. Chiesa (eds), Aortic Dissection patients true stories and the innovations that saved their lives

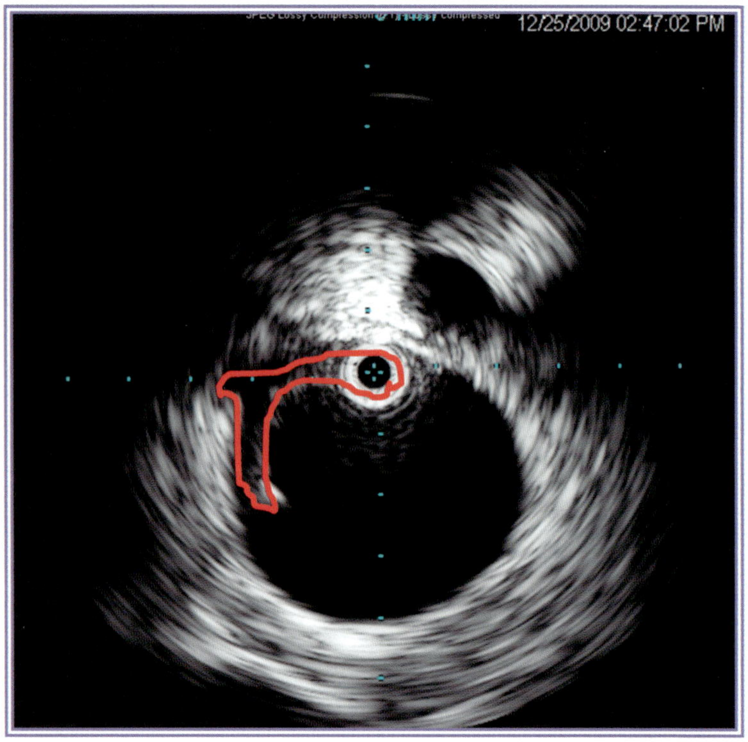

Fig. 38.1 Intravascular ultrasound (IVUS) image at the level of the superior mesenteric artery with catheter in the true lumen (red outline), demonstrating severe static obstruction of blood flow into this vessel.

38.2 The case for intravascular ultrasound

The pathophysiology of AD involves cystic medial degeneration and the sudden development of an entry tear and two separate channels for blood flow: a true lumen and false lumen (Figs. 38.1, 38.2).

Navigating between or within these lumens can be difficult if not impossible using stan-

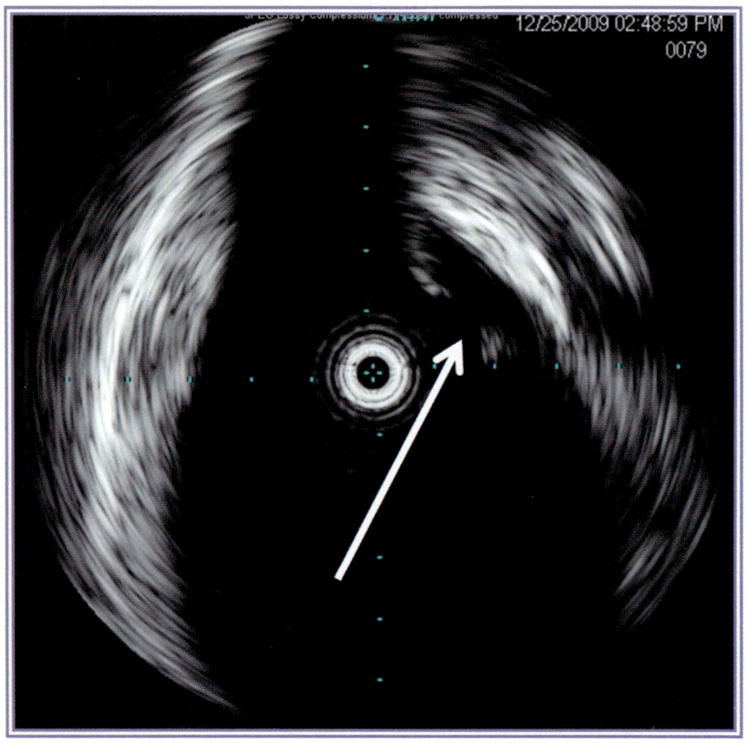

Fig. 38.2 Intravascular ultrasound (IVUS) image demonstrating proximal entry tear (white arrow) at the level of the left subclavian artery.

dard two dimensional imaging with fluoroscopy and angiography. Essential to the successful repair of any AD is the placement of a guidewire in the true lumen of the dissection both above and below the entry tear.

38.3 Techniques of endovascular repair

Access into the true lumen is usually achieved via the femoral artery with either cutdown or a percutaneous technique. Occasionally, iliac artery access with a conduit is required if the diameters of the access vessels are too small for device delivery. Transesophageal echocardiography and intravascular ultrasound (IVUS) can be used to verify placement of the guidewire in the true lumen and localize the location of the entry tear. Depending on which endovascular device is being used, sheath placement in the aortic arch may be required before endograft positioning. A flush catheter is placed into the ascending aorta through contralateral femoral or brachial access. A 260-cm stiff guidewire is then positioned in the ascending aorta and the endograft is advanced to the level of desired deployment. Ideally, 2 cm of seal zone proximal to the entry tear is required to minimize type I endoleak. Balloon molding of the endograft is generally avoided, especially in patients with acute dissection because the risk of retrograde dissection or rupture is thought to be high in these patients. Adequate device size should be based on the diameter of the aorta proximal to the dissected segment. Device oversizing should be no more than 0-10% as oversizing is associated with stent graft-induced new entry tears, retrograde Type A dissection, and proximal neck dilatation with subsequent stent-graft migration [6].

If coverage of the left subclavian artery is required, carotid-subclavian bypass prior to thoracic endovascular repair is performed in the presence of a dominant left vertebral artery, a patent left internal mammary artery to coronary artery bypass graft, or in patients with a history of arm ischemia. In the emergency setting, left carotid-subclavian bypass is not routinely required and can be performed postoperatively in symptomatic patients [7].

Literature supporting the mandatory use of IVUS in AD is scant. In a prospective cohort study comparing TEVAR with IVUS-assisted TEVAR versus angiography alone in 47 patients, technical success was 100% in both groups and outcomes were no different. However, IVUS-assisted TEVAR was associated with significantly lower operative times and contrast usage [8]. Many sources cite the use of TEVAR without any contrast whatsoever when using IVUS-assisted TEVAR [9]. IVUS provides for all of the information necessary for device selection, target site identification as well as safe deployment of the endograft into the true lumen [10]. In addition, many of these terribly moribund patients have renal malperfusion at the time of presentation and IVUS allows for reduced contrast administration in this situation. Table 38.1 lists advantages of IVUS for use in AD cases.

Table 38.1 Advantages and disadvantages of intravascular ultrasound in the treatment of aortic dissection

Advantages of IVUS	Disadvantages of IVUS
Reduced operative time	Additional cost of catheter
Reduced contrast dosage	Sheath size 8.5 Fr minimum
Reduced radiation exposure to patient and staff	
Precise diameter and length measurements	
Accurate visualization of vital branch origins	
Dynamic post-treatment assessment	

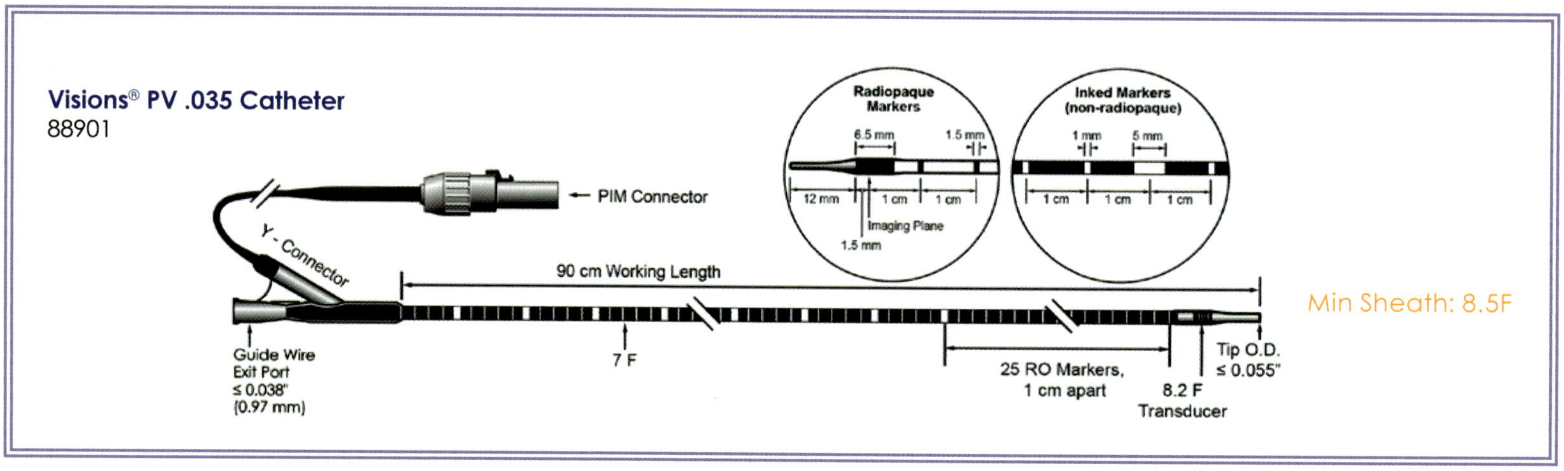

Fig. 38.3 Visions® PV .035 catheter (Philips Volcano, San Diego, CA).

Table 38.2 Visions® PV .035 Digital IVUS Catheter

Characteristic	Value
Frequency	10 MHz
Maximum guidewire	0.038"
Platform	OTW
PIM connector length	100 cm
Minimum sheath size	9 Fr
Maximum image diameter	60 mm

PIM, passive intermodulation.

Our institution prefers the use of the Philips Volcano (San Diego, CA) intravascular ultrasound platform (Fig. 38.3). The Visions® PV .035 8.2 Fr catheter is a 10 MHz, 90-cm over-the-wire catheter with 25 radio-opaque markers spaced at 1-cm intervals to allow for accurate length measurement. Table 38.2 demonstrates IVUS catheter specifications.

38.4 Conclusions

Intravascular ultrasound is an essential tool for the management of acute AD. It allows for proven reductions in operative time, fluoroscopy time, radiation exposure and contrast usage. Advantages of IVUS in managing AD far outweigh the disadvantages. In a disease entity where rapid diagnosis and efficient treatment is associated with improved outcomes, it would be foolish for any provider to manage AD without the use of intravascular ultrasound.

REFERENCES

1) Szeto WY, McGarvey M, Pochettino A, et al. Results of a new surgical paradigm: endovascular repair for acute complicated type B aortic dissection. Ann Thorac Surg 2008; 86(1): 87-93; discussion 93-4.
2) Fattori R, Cao P, De Rango P, et al. Interdisciplinary expert consensus document on management of type B aortic dissection. J Am Coll Cardiol 2013; 61(16): 1661-78.
3) Erbel R, Aboyans V, Boileau C, et al. 2014 ESC Guidelines on the diagnosis and treatment of aortic dis-

eases: document covering acute and chronic aortic diseases of the thoracic and abdominal aorta of the adult. The Task Force for the Diagnosis and Treatment of Aortic Diseases of the European Society of Cardiology (ESC). Eur Heart J 2014; 35(41): 2873-926.

4) Trimarchi S, Nienaber CA, Rampoldi V, et al. Role and results of surgery in acute type B aortic dissection: insights from the International Registry of Acute Aortic Dissection (IRAD). Circulation 2006; 114(1 Suppl): I357-64.
5) Jonker FH, Patel HJ, Upchurch GR, et al. Acute type B aortic dissection complicated by visceral ischemia. J Thorac Cardiovasc Surg 2015; 149(4): 1081-6.
6) Eggebrecht H, Thompson M, Rousseau H, et al. Retrograde ascending aortic dissection during or after thoracic aortic stent graft placement: insight from the European registry on endovascular aortic repair complications. Circulation 2009; 120(11 Suppl): S276-S281.
7) Woo EY, Carpenter JP, Jackson BM, et al. Left subclavian artery coverage during thoracic endovascular aortic repair: a single-center experience. J Vasc Surg 2008; 48(3): 555-60.
8) Guo BL, Shi ZY, Guo DQ, et al. Effect of intravascular ultrasound-assisted thoracic endovascular aortic repair for "complicated" type B aortic dissection. Chin Med J (Engl) 2015; 128(17): 2322-9.
9) Starnes BW, O'Donnell SD, Gillespie DL, Goff JM, Rosa P, Rich NM. Endovascular management of renal ischemia in a patient with acute aortic dissection and renovascular hypertension. Ann Vasc Surg 2002; 16(3): 368-74.
10) Tozzi P, Marty B, Ruchat P, Ferrari E, Siniscalchi G, von Segesser LK. Endovascular thoracic aortic aneurysm repair without angiography. Innovations (Phila) 2009; 4(1): 32-5.

39

Transesophageal echocardiography in the management of patients undergoing procedures for Type B aortic dissection

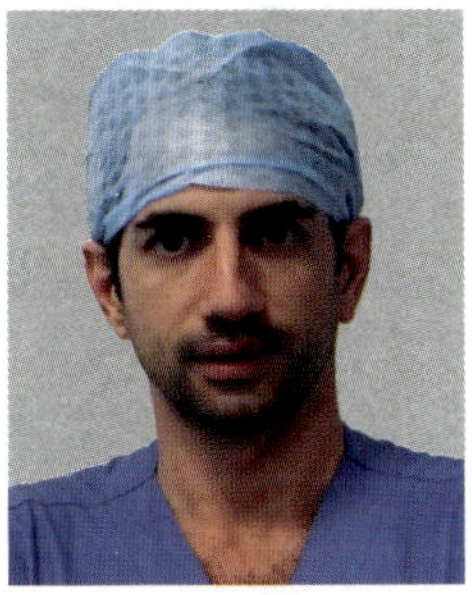

Fabrizio Monaco, Monica De Luca, Salvatore Sardo, Guglielmo Cornero, Cristina Mattioli, Alberto Zangrillo

39.1 Introduction

Two-dimensional transesophageal echocardiography (TEE) is an essential noninvasive diagnostic tool for both open and endovascular aortic repair of thoracic aortic dissection [1]. In open surgery for type B aortic dissection repair, TEE is helpful in detecting aortic insufficiency, pericardial effusion, pleural effusions, coronary artery involvement, and left and right ventricular systolic and diastolic dysfunction. In Thoracic Endovascular Aortic Repair (TEVAR), TEE plays an even more pivotal role and can change the surgical plan initially defined by computed tomography (CT) scan in up to 60% of cases [2]. In particular, as observed by Rapezzi et al., TEE modified the site of stent deployment in 33% of patients due to the detection of misdiagnosed protruding atherosclerotic plaque, it showed a higher sensitivity compared to angiography in the detection of endoleaks after stent-graft placement and, finally, it had a sensitivity as high as 100% in the location of the principal intimal tear entry site within the descending thoracic aorta [2].

39.2 Aortic anatomy

Understanding the position of the esophagus with respect to the surrounding anatomic structures is of paramount importance for the echographer. The ascending aorta courses from the aortic annulus to the brachiocephalic artery passing to the right over the origin of the right pulmonary artery. The distal part of the ascending aorta and the proximal portion of the aortic arch are invisible with TEE due to the interposition of the trachea and left main bronchus which prevents ultrasound transmission (blind-spot). To overcome this limitation, recently, Jansen Klomp et al. have reported a modified approach of TEE which allows the visualization of the distal ascending aorta, aortic arch and branching vessels by inflating a balloon with 20-50 mL of saline in the trachea [3]. The descending aorta lies on the left side of the esophagus in its proximal part

Fabrizio Monaco (monaco.fabrizio@hsr.it)
Scientific Institute Ospedale San Raffaele,
Milan, Italy

G. Melissano - R. Chiesa (eds), Aortic Dissection patients true stories and the innovations that saved their lives

and then follows a rightward trajectory as it approaches the diaphragm. Below the diaphragmatic hiatus, the aorta is posterior to the stomach with a variable position. Therefore the visceral arteries have a significant interpatient variability and are only occasionally visible with TEE.

39.3 Echocardiographic evaluation

The transesophageal probe should be inserted gently avoiding to force it through areas of resistance especially in the presence of aneurysmal dilatation and an anamnesis of dysphagia, stridor or hoarseness. As intubation of the esophagus with TEE can lead to hypertension, increasing the risk of further tearing or rupture of the dissection, TEE should be inserted under general anesthesia.

As the descending aorta is adjacent to the esophagus and in normal subjects has a diameter of 3-4 cm at this level, the spatial and temporal resolutions of the view can be improved by reducing the scan depth to 6-8 cm. For the color flow Doppler (CFD), a Niquist limit set at 50

Table 39.1 Recommended views for the thoracic aorta

Views	Depth from the teeth (cm)	Multiplane angle (grade)	Structures	Assessment
UE aortic arch LAX	20-25	0	Aortic arch	• Atheromatous plaque • Calcification • Vessel dimensions • Aneurysm • Dissection
UE aortic arch SAX	20-25	90	Aortic arch, RVOT, MPA	
ME ascending aorta SAX	30-45	0	Asc Ao, MPA, RPA, SVC	
ME ascending aorta LAX	30-45	110-150	Asc Ao, PA	
Descending aorta SAX	30-45	0	Desc Ao, left pleural space	
Descending aorta LAX	30-45	90	Desc Ao, left pleural space	

Asc Ao, ascending aorta; Desc Ao, descending aorta; LAX, long axis; ME, midesophageal; MPA, main pulmonary artery; PA, pulmonary artery; RPA, right pulmonar artery; RVOT, right ventricle outflow tract; SAX, short axis; SVC, superior vena cava; UE, upper esophageal.

Table 39.2 Echocardiographic evaluation of cardiac structures and thoracic aorta

Structure	Views	Evaluation
Left ventricle	ME4C, ME mitral commissural, ME2C, MELAX, TG2C, TG basal SAX, TG mid-papillary, TG2C, TG apical SAX	FAC, EF, RWMA, chamber dimensions, pericardial effusion, LVH
Mitral valve	ME4C, ME mitral commissural, ME2C, MELAX, TGLAX, TG basal SAX	Mitral regurgitation, stenosis, transmitral pattern
LVOT aortic valve, aortic root, ascending aorta	MELAX, ME aortic SAX, TG LAX, deep TG LAX, ME ascending aorta SAX, ME ascending aorta LAX	Aortic valve morphology, aortic stenosis and regurgitation, LVOT/aortic root/ascending aorta dimensions, SAM
Atrial septum, left pulmonary veins	Bicaval, ME2C	ASD, correct position of the left bypass inflow cannula
Right ventricle, tricuspid and pulmonary valve	ME4C, RV inflow and outflow, TG SAX, RV inflow, UE aortic arch SAX	Chamber dimensions, contractility, tricuspid valve regurgitation, stenosis, pulmonary valve pathology
Aortic arch, descending thoracic aorta	UE aortic arch SAX, UE aortic arch LAX, ME descending aorta SAX, ME descending aorta LAX	Atheromatous plaque, calcifications, aortic arch and descending aorta dimensions, aneurysm, dissection

ASD, atrial septum defects; EF, ejection fraction; FAC, fractional area change; LAX, long axis; LVH, left ventricular hypertrophy; LVOT, left ventricle outflow tract; ME, midesophageal; MELAX, midesophageal long axis; ME2C, midesophageal 2-chamber; ME4C, midesophageal 4-chamber; RV, right ventricular; RWMA, regional wall motion abnormalities; SAM, systolic anterior motion; TG, transgastric; TG2C, transgastric 2-chamber; SAX, short axis; UE, upper esophageal.

cm/s improves the visualization of the left subclavian and carotid arteries in the upper esophageal aortic arch long axis view. Finally, to complete the standard echocardiographic exam, the superimposition of pulse-wave Doppler (PWD), continuous-wave Doppler (CWD), and grey-scale and color M-Mode makes it possible to detect most aortic pathologies.

After probe insertion, a systematic evaluation of the whole thoracic aorta according to SCA/ASE guidelines [4] is recommended (Table 39.1).

39.4 Role of transesophageal echocardiography in open aortic repair surgery for type B aortic dissection

A comprehensive echocardiographic evaluation of the heart and aorta is performed in patients undergoing open repair surgery of Type B aortic dissection (AD). As suggested by the American Society of Echocardiography (ASE) and the Society of Cardiovascular Anesthesiologists (SCA), a complete examination should include 20 standard views [5].

The sequence should start with midesophageal views, then transgastric views and end with the upper esophageal views. Due to anatomic variations and the surgical context it is not always possible to get the whole sequence, but it is mandatory to at least get sufficient views to be able to rule out coexisting cardiac disease, the presence of wall motion abnormalities, and pericardial or pleural effusion. The following structures should be evaluated in two-dimensional (2D) imaging, adding PWD or CWD and CFD when required (Table 39.2):

- left ventricle and mitral valve
- aortic valve, aortic root and ascending aorta
- atrial septum, left pulmonary veins
- right ventricle, tricuspid and pulmonary valve
- aortic arch and descending thoracic aorta.

39.4.1 Left ventricular function

The initial assessment of the left ventricle starts from the evaluation of the linear dimensions. The major long axis is best acquired in midesophageal 4-chamber (ME4C) view from the apical endocardium to the mitral annulus in diastole. The anterior posterior diameter is made in transgastric (TG) mid-papillary short axis (SAX) (Fig. 39.1) or long axis (LAX) view. A diameter in end diastole above 5.4 cm is considered enlarged. A left ventricle wall thickness above 1.1 cm in TG LAX or mid-papillary SAX is considered increased and indicative of hypertrophy.

The evaluation of cardiac output with the Doppler method provides an alternative to the thermo-dilution method. The echocardiographic approach is based on the concept that the blood flow is equal in all parts at a given time in the absence of significant valve dysfunction (continuity equation). The stroke volume is the product of the velocity time integral (VTI) recorded in the deep TG view or TG LAX and the left ventricular outflow tract (LVOT) diameter recorded in midesophageal long axis (MELAX) view (Fig. 39.2). Another way to assess the systolic volume (SV) is the difference between the left ventricle (LV) end diastolic volume and the LV end systolic volume. Multiplying the SV by the heart rate one can obtain the cardiac output.

The ejection phase indices are the fractional shortening and the fractional area change (FAC). Both are recorded in TG mid-papillary SAX view and provide a sense of global LV function in the case of absence of regional wall dysfunction. Values above 25% and 60% for fractional shortening and FAC, respectively, are normal. In the dynamic setting of thoracoabdominal surgery, FAC is the most reliable and quickest method to assess the LV systolic performance.

The modified Simpson's rule is the currently recommended method to evaluate ventricular volume and ejection fraction (EF). The need of adequate ME4C and ME2C views with defined

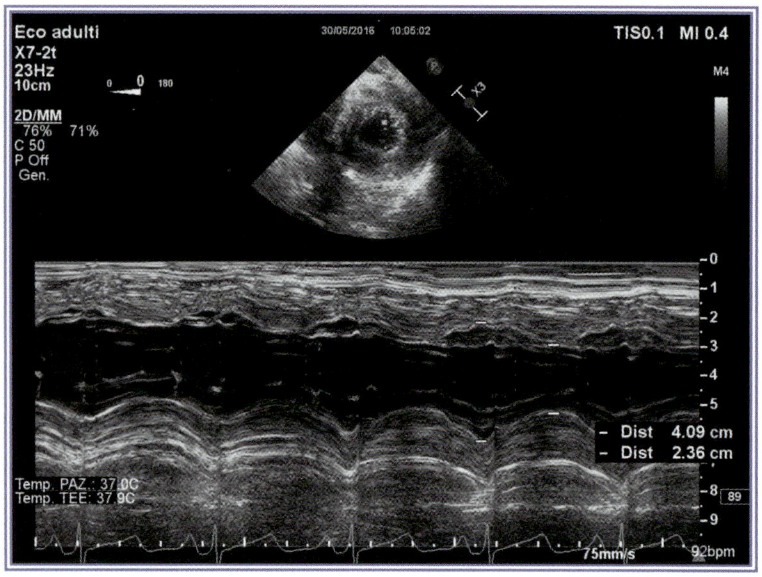

Fig. 39.1 Transgastric mid-papillary short axis view. M-mode of left ventricular end diastolic and end systolic diameter.

endocardium in systole and diastole with no apex-base foreshortening limits the use of this method in a dynamic surgical setting (Fig. 39.3).

Regional wall motion abnormalities (RWMA) can be preoperative or develop during the surgery. A wall thickness in systole above 30% compared to diastole is considered normal, between 10 and 30% mildly reduced, below 10% severely impaired [6]. The excursion is assessed semi-quantitatively and described as hypokinesia, akinesia or dyskinesia. In the clinical practice, a segment normally contracting can be used as a reference, improving the recognition of adjacent RWMA.

Diastolic function evaluation usually completes the assessment of the LV [7]. Transmitral flow pattern, pulmonary flow pattern and tissue Doppler imaging of the lateral mitral annulus distinguish a normal diastolic function from impaired relaxation, pseudonormal diastolic dysfunction and restrictive filling (Table 39.3).

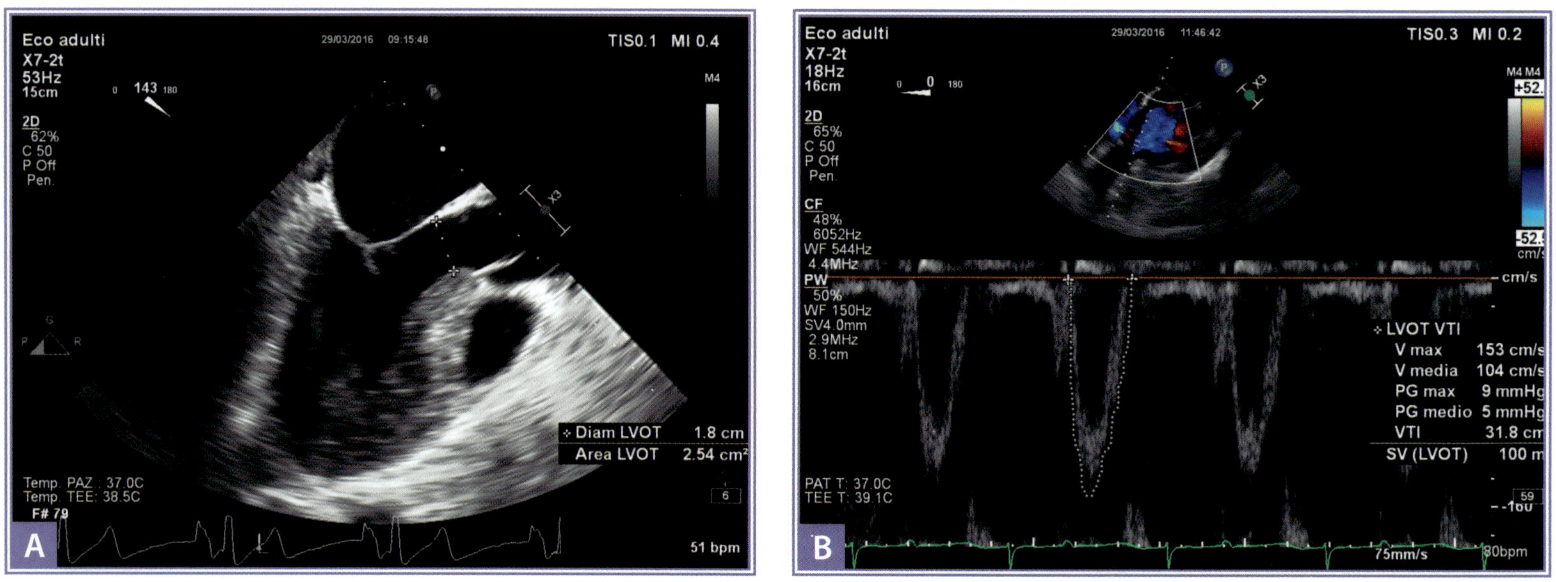

Fig. 39.2 Calculation of the cardiac output. **A**, Left ventricular outflow tract diameter measured in midesophageal long axis view. **B**, Velocity time integral of the pulse-wave Doppler recorded in deep transgastric long axis view.

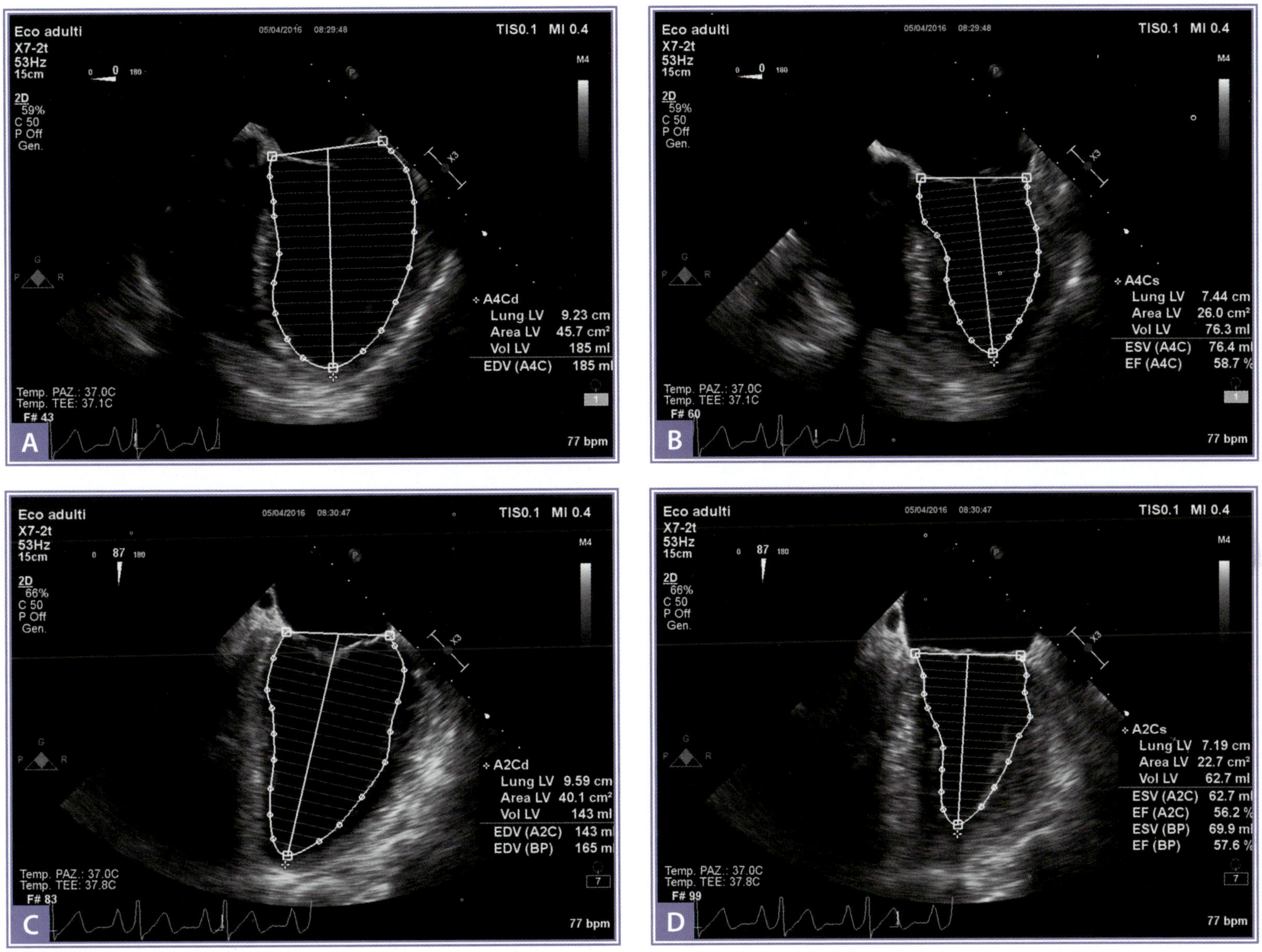

Fig. 39.3 Simpson's method biplane ejection fraction. **A**, End diastolic volume in midesophageal 4-chamber view. **B**, End systolic volume in midesophageal 4-chamber view. **C**, End diastolic volume in midesophageal 2-chamber view. **D**, End systolic volume in midesophageal 2-chamber view.

Table 39.3 Diastolic dysfunction classification

Parameter	Grade I Impaired relaxation	Grade II Pseudonormal	Grade III Restrictive filling
E′	<10 cm/s	<10 cm/s	<10 cm/s
E/A	0.8	0.8-1.5	≥2
DT	>200 ms	160-200 ms	<160 ms
E/E′	≤8	9-12	≥13
Ar-A	<0 ms	≥30 ms	≥30 ms
Vals ΔE/A	<0.5	≥0.5	≥0.5

A, transmitral late filling peak velocity; Ar-A, duration of the pulmonary flow atrial reversal flow minus duration of the transmitral A wave; DT, deceleration time; E′, peak tissue Doppler velocity in the early diastole; E, transmitral early filling peak velocity; Vals, Valsalva maneuver.

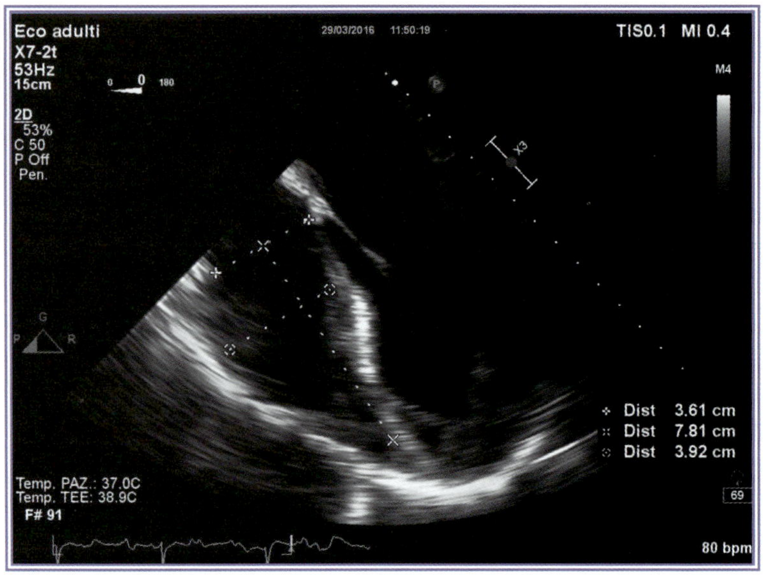

Fig. 39.4 Right ventricle dimensions. Midesophageal 4-chamber view

39.4.2 Right ventricular function

The open repair surgical technique of Type B AD with left ventricular bypass fails to support the right ventricle (RV) which is at high risk of intraoperative failure due to fluid overload, transfusions, hemodynamic instability and ischemia. A prompt diagnosis of ongoing RV failure with TEE makes it possible to commence the most appropriate treatment, decreasing the rate of serious complications. Similarly as for the LV, the evaluation of the RV should begin from the assessment of the linear dimensions in ME4C view (Fig. 39.4). A mid-diameter above 4.2 cm is a sign of RV dilatation and it exposes the patient undergoing open surgery to additional risks. An RV free wall thicker than 0.5 cm is associated to RV hypertrophy and should raise the suspicion of long-standing pulmonary hypertension [8]. In the TG mid-papillary SAX view, the RV has a triangular shape. In the case of dilatation/dysfunction, the RV is more circular while the LV assumes a D-shape due to the flattening of the interventricular septum. In particular, a D-shape LV in diastole occurs in the case of RV volume overload, while a D-shape LV in systole is a sign of RV pressure overload [9]. The most common indices of RV systolic performance are listed in Table 39.4.

Each method carries its own set of limitations. Tricuspid annular systolic excursion is dependent on the angle of interrogation, load conditions and ventricular interdependence [10]. Tissue Doppler imaging is sensitive to technical pitfalls such as alignment, tethering,

Table 39.4 Right ventricular systolic function indices

Index	Normal range	View
TAPSE	15-20 mm	RV inflow, deep TG LAX
S'TDI	>10 cm/s	TG RV inflow, deep TG LAX
FAC	>30%	ME4C
Tei index	0.3-0.5	TG RV outflow, ME4C

FAC, fractional area change; LAX, long axis view; ME4C, midesophageal 4-chamber; RV, right ventricle; TAPSE, tricuspid annular plane systolic excursion; Tei index (pulsed-wave Doppler), ratio between the two isovolumic intervals (isovolumic contraction time + isovolumic relaxation time) and the ejection time; S'TDI, peak systolic wave velocity with tissue Doppler imaging; TG, transgastric.

and spectral broadening. Although the Tei index is free of geometrical assumptions, it needs regular R-R intervals and is not load independent. In fact, when the atrial pressure is high the Tei index is pseudonormalized due to a shortened isovolumic relaxation time. The right ventricular fractional area change (RVFAC) is not recommended due to heterogeneity of the methods and numerous geometric assumptions [11].

To complete the RV evaluation a diastolic function should be considered [12]. The approach is similar to that of the LV although the Doppler interpretation is still unclear. The views most often used for the tricuspid inflow are the ME4C view and the modified bicaval view in which the ultrasound beam is parallel to the RV inflow. The E and A waves show a lower velocity compared to the transmitral pattern due to a larger tricuspid annulus. An estimate of the right atrial (RA) pressure can be derived from the assessment of the diameter of the inferior vena cava (IVC) 1-2 cm before the point of insertion in the right atrium. An IVC diameter below 2 cm is associated to an estimated central venous pressure (CVP) lower than 10 mmHg. On the contrary an IVC diameter above 2 cm is associated to a CVP higher than 10 mmHg [13].

The afterload of the RV can be estimated in the case of tricuspid regurgitation. In fact, the peak velocity of the tricuspid regurgitation sampled by CWD reflects the pressure gradient between RA and RV. Then, by adding the CVP a reliable estimation of the systolic pulmonary pressure can be obtained. A cut-off of 50 mmHg distinguishes severe from moderate pulmonary hypertension. A systolic pulmonary pressure below 30 mmHg is considered normal.

39.5 Transesophageal echocardiography and thoracic endovascular aortic repair

39.5.1 Endovascular stent-graft procedure

In the endovascular setting, TEE is fundamental for: 1) verifying the aortic pathology, 2) guiding the endograft placement, 3) detecting endoleaks after endograft release, and 4) monitoring cardiac performance [14].

Verifying aortic pathology

Patients undergoing TEVAR are usually assessed with contrast-enhanced spiral CT or magnetic resonance imaging (MRI) before the procedure. Therefore TEE has a lesser role in the definition of the primary diagnosis although a sensitivity of 98% and a specificity of 97% has been reported for the diagnosis of acute AD [15]. On the other hand, TEE can provide supplemental information on the aortic anatomy and, with its high sensitivity in detecting atherosclerotic plaques or calcification, it may potentially alter the surgical plan. The presence of atheromatous disease in the thoracic aorta is graded according to Katz's classification [16] (Table 39.5).

Before stent-graft implantation TEE allows the evaluation of the true lumen (TL) and false lumen (FL) along with the primary and secondary entry tears [17] (Fig. 39.5). The presence

Table 39.5 Katz's classification of atheroma

Grade	Description
1	Normal aorta
2	Severe intimal thickening
3	Atheroma protruding <5 mm into the lumen
4	Atheroma protruding >5 mm into the lumen
5	Mobile atheroma

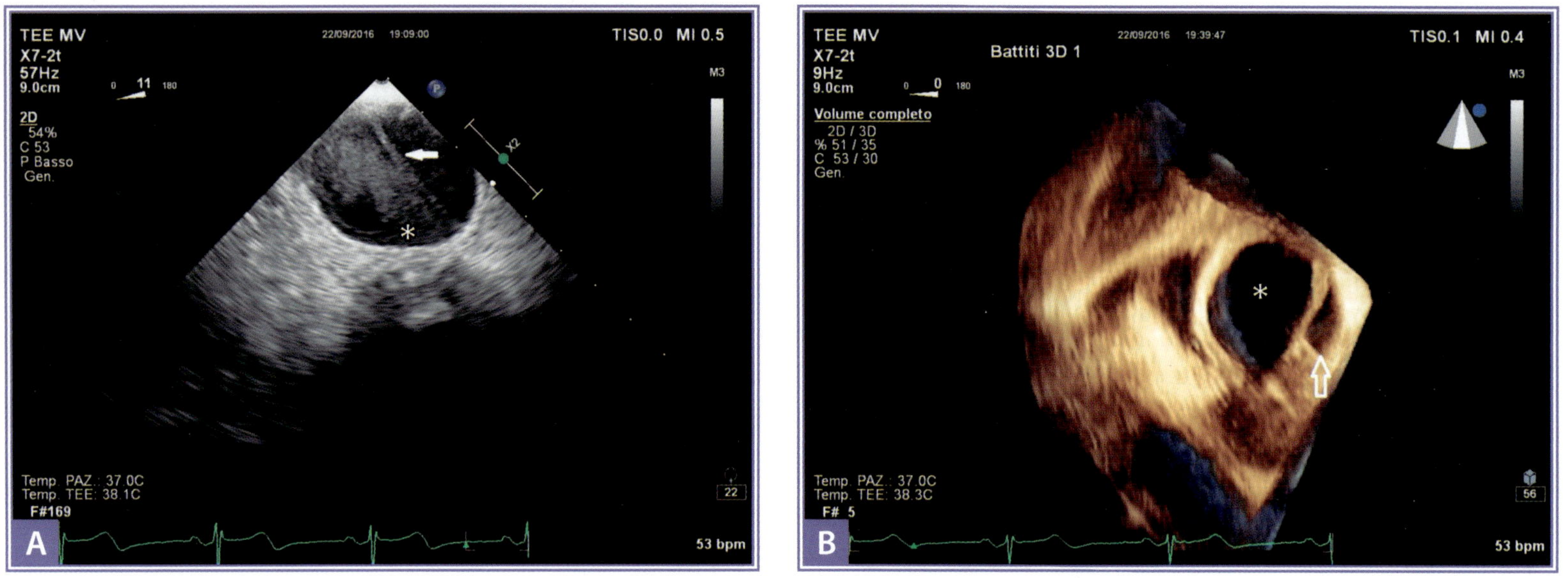

Fig. 39.5 Type B aortic dissection. **A**, Descending thoracic aorta short axis view. Asterisk shows spontaneous echo contrast within the false lumen. Arrow shows the intimal flap. **B**, Descending thoracic aorta short axis view 3D zoom. Asterisk shows the false lumen and arrow shows the true lumen.

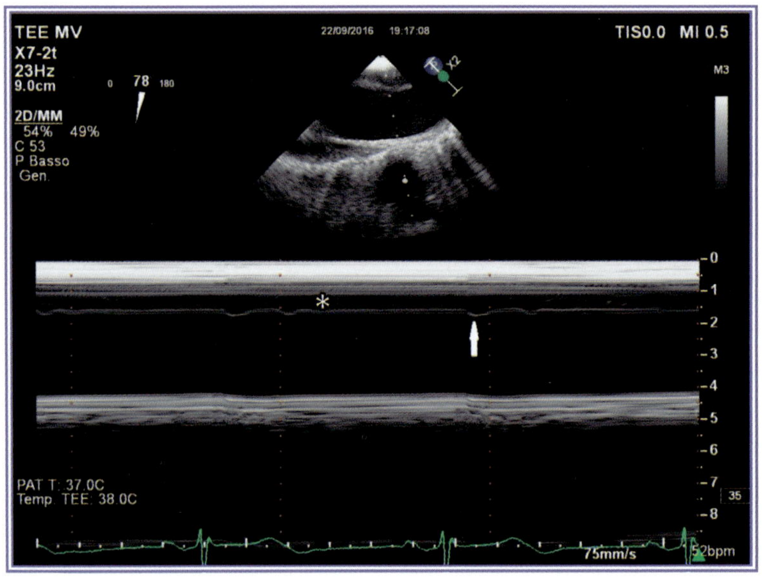

Fig. 39.6 M-mode. Descending thoracic aorta long axis view. Asterisk shows the true lumen. Arrow demonstrates systolic expansion toward the false lumen during the cardiac cycle.

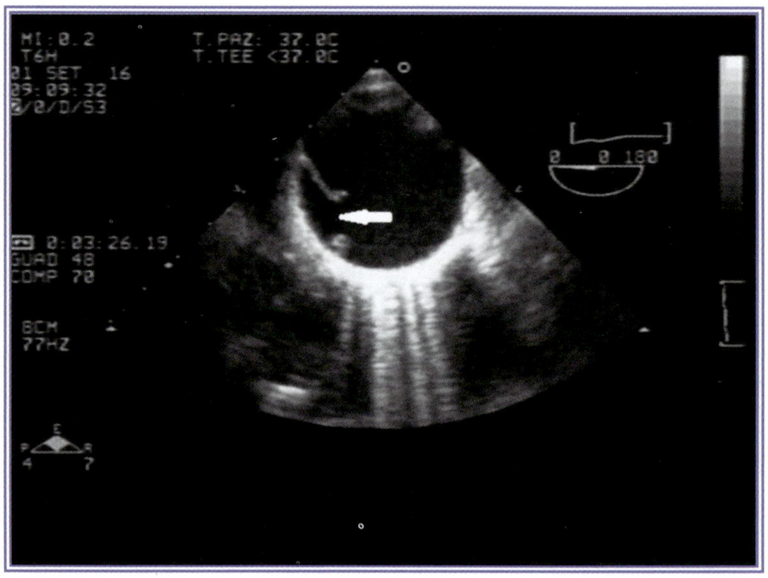

Fig. 39.7 Descending thoracic aorta short axis view. Arrow show the principal entry tear.

of an intimal flap, appearing as a thin mobile echogenic membrane bulging in the aortic lumen, is a distinctive sign of AD. The addition of CFD with a scale set at 50 cm/s increases the chance to detect intimal tears. The TL is usual circular, smaller in size than the FL, with a systolic expansion and normal CFD and PWD profiles. M-Mode, showing the direction of the intimal flap during the cardiac cycle, may help to identify the TL (Fig. 39.6). The FL typically is larger than the TL, with echo contrast inside due to low blood flow. Sometimes the difference between the lamina may be not straightforward. For instance, in the event of acute dissection the FL may not be dilated. Similarly, a collapsed TL may assume a crescent shape with diastolic collapse due to higher diastolic pressure in the FL [11, 18].

The goal of TEVAR for AD is to close the primary entry tear with the stent graft to avoid further dilatation and rupture of the aorta [19] (Fig. 39.7). Moreover, intraoperative TEE confirms both the correct stent size and the most favorable aortic segment in which to deploy the stent graft (landing zone).

Guidance of endograft placement

Transesophageal echocardiography offers valuable information for the stent-graft implantation [2]. It is superior to angiography in checking the position of the guidewire in the TL (Fig. 39.8). The guidewire is visible in the aortic lumen as a bright echo-dense image while the sheath of the delivery system can be distinguished from the wire based on the thickness (Fig. 39.9) . TEE provides a better image of the primary entry tear than angiography. The probe itself, which is radio-opaque, can be used as a marker of the aortic level on the fluoroscope without need for further contrast administration. The appearance of spontaneous echo-contrast in the FL after stent implantation is a marker of complete exclusion. The appearance of a static smoke effect in the FL is a sign of a complete exclusion (Fig. 39.10). On the other hand, a swirling smoke effect in the FL suggests the presence of endoleaks or the occurrence of new intimal tears. Additional intimal tears can be pre-existent but visible only after stent-graft implantation, due to an increased pressure gradient between the TL and FL after closure of the primary entry tear, or they can be induced by the stent graft itself (stent graft-induced new entry, SINE) due to the fragility of the aortic wall. Marfan's patients, for example, are at higher risk of developing SINE [20]. With the aim to improve the evaluation of Type B AD morphology some authors have proposed the use of intravascular ultrasound (IVUS), which is discussed in Chapter 38, or intraluminal phased-array imaging (IPAI). Table 39.6 lists the technical differences between TEE, IVUS and IPAI [21].

Table 39.6 Characteristics of ultrasound tools

	TEE	IVUS	IPAI
Transducer frequency	3.5-7 Mhz	10-20 Mhz	5-10 Mhz
Sector	90 degrees	360 degrees	90 degrees
Depth	20 cm	5 cm	12 cm
M-mode	yes	no	yes
Color flow Doppler	yes	no	yes
Pulse-wave Doppler	yes	no	yes
Continuous-wave Doppler	yes	no	yes
Tissue Doppler	yes	no	yes
Guidewire	No	yes	no
Catheter dimension		8 F	10 F

IPAI, intraluminal phased-array imaging; IVUS, intravascular ultrasound; TEE, transesophageal echocardiography.

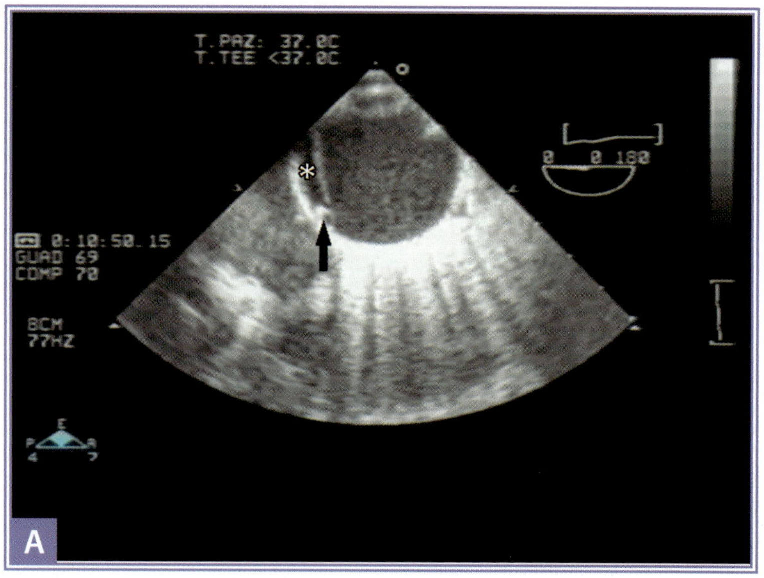

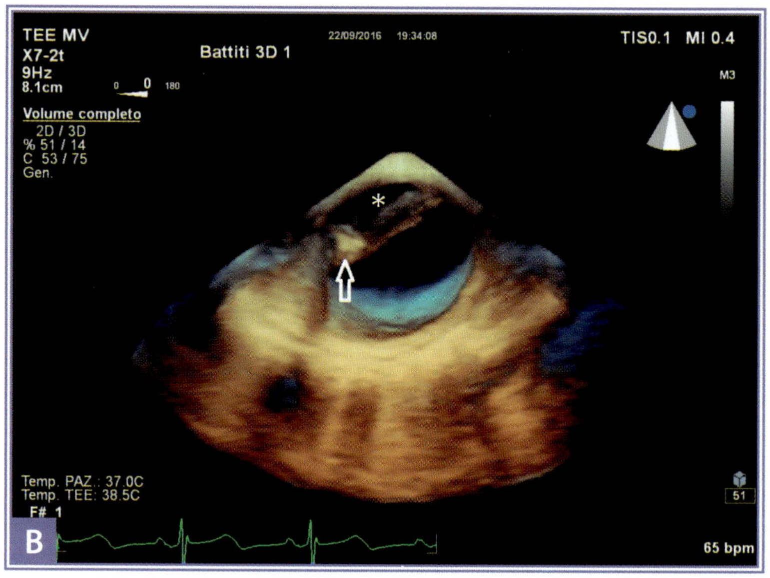

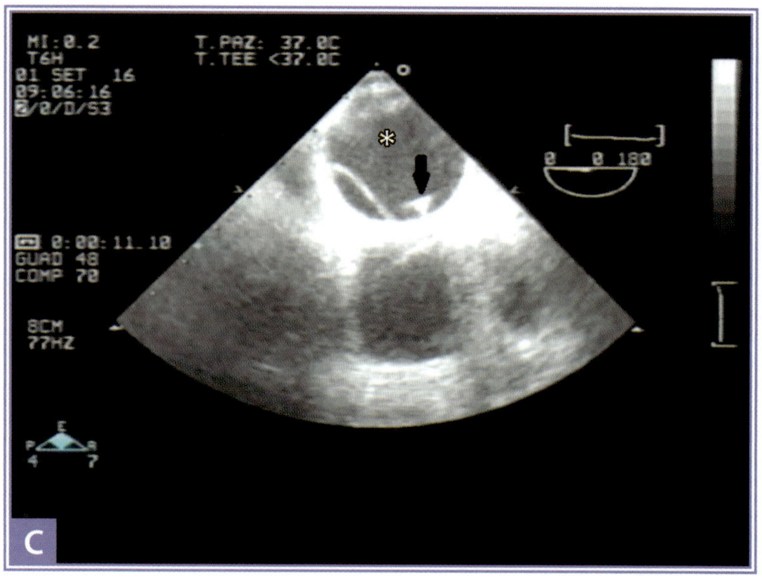

Fig. 39.8 **A**, Descending thoracic aorta short axis view. Asterisk shows the true lumen. Arrow demonstrates the guidewire in the true lumen. **B**, Descending thoracic aorta short axis view 3D zoom. Asterisk shows the true lumen. Arrow demonstrates the guidewire in the true lumen. **C**, Descending thoracic aorta short axis view. Asterisk shows the false lumen. Arrow demonstrates the guidewire in the false lumen.

Koschyk et al. compared the usefulness and capabilities of angiography, TEE and IVUS in guiding aortic stent-graft implantation in 42 patients undergoing TEVAR for acute and chronic Type B AD [22]. IVUS performed better than TEE and angiography in detecting multiple entries, in diagnosing both slow flow in the FL after stent-graft implantation and incomplete stent apposition. Angiography alone was inferior to IVUS and TEE in the localization of the guidewire in the FL or TL. TEE was superior to angiography and IVUS in the documentation of endoleaks. Recently Guo et al. reported that IVUS, used with angiography for guiding TEVAR in complicated Type B AD, was superior to angiography alone and TEE in the evaluation of acute Type B AD morphology, and in reducing the amount of contrast administered and total operating time [23, 24]. IVUS reduces the use of angiography and the amount of contrast medium needed to discern the TL and FL on cross-section images, detecting size and location of the entries, and depicting the origins of visceral branches from the TL or FL. A reduced amount of contrast medium is significant in patients with renal dysfunction [25]. Blasco et al. reported that IVUS provides measurements of the aorta comparable to three-dimensional CT scan [26]. Other authors observed a systematic overestimation of the aortic measurements

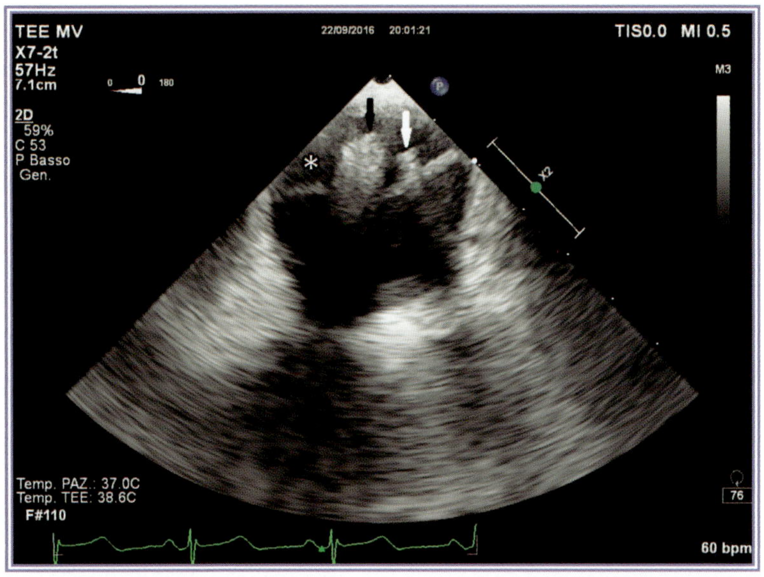

Fig. 39.9 Descending thoracic aorta short axis view. Asterisk shows the true lumen. Guidewire, white arrow; delivery system, black arrow.

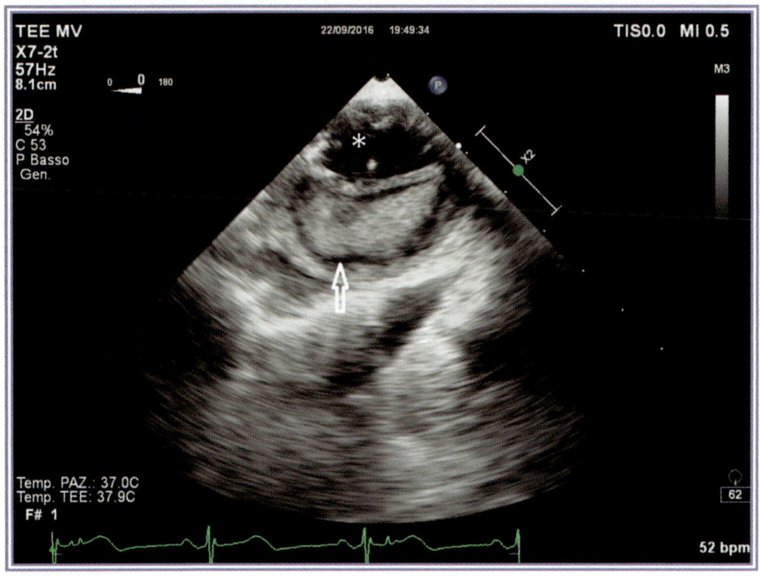

Fig. 39.10 Descending thoracic aorta short axis view. Stent graft in aortic dissection (asterisk). Static smoke effect in the false lumen after stent-graft deployment (arrow).

with IVUS, especially for those not centered along the aortic arch or in twisted aortic parts [27]. Therefore, CT scan still remains the gold standard for the choice of the stent graft.

The technical advance of IVUS has led to IPAI. Unlike IVUS, IPAI allows for Doppler quantification similarly to TEE. With respect to TEE, IPAI has a higher imaging resolution, requires femoral access and can investigate also the abdominal aorta. Bartel et al. tested IVUS, TEE and IPAI diagnostic capabilities in 23 patients with Type B AD [21]. The authors observed that IPAI was more sensitive than TEE in both detection of entries in the descending thoracic aorta and assessment of the effective systolic pressure separation (pressure gradient >20 mmHg) between the TL and FL evaluated with CWD. The difference in Doppler velocities between the two tools is related to a better alignment of the Doppler beam between ultrasounds and entry flow in IPAI compared to TEE. Correct quantification of the effective systolic separation is not negligible during the decision-making process of the interventional treatment. In fact, a higher interluminal gradient is associated to a lower flow and pressure in the FL which make thrombus formation more probable. In the same study, although both IVUS and IPAI were able to correctly identify the visceral arteries and

Table 39.7 Classification of endoleaks

Type 1	Persistent flow at the proximal (IA) or distal (IB) attachment sites
Type 2	Retrograde flow from collateral vessels
Type 3	Graft defects or inadequate sealing of overlapping graft joints
Type 4	Graft porosity
Type 5	No clear evidence of endoleak origin in the context of aneurysmal sac expansion

their origins from the TL or FL with a rate higher than angiography alone, only IPAI was capable of detecting flow in the visceral branches, distinguishing between perfused or non perfused abdominal arteries [21].

Moreover IPAI, when positioned in the inferior vena cava, may play a role in guiding emergency balloon fenestrations in the case of distal malperfusion syndrome, both identifying the optimal position of puncture for fluoroscopic imaging and working as a marker for a correct needle orientation [23]. Also IVUS may identify a collapsed TL during malperfusion syndrome but it does not provide a longitudinal view of the aorta and Brockenbrough needle.

Detection of endoleaks

Transesophageal echocardiography (TEE) is more sensitive than angiography in the detection of endoleaks. A CFD with a scale of 25 cm/s allows the depiction of peri-stent leaks in the vast majority of cases [17]. To discriminate between Dacron porosity (false positive) and true endoleak, the use of PWD is strongly recommended. In fact a CFD velocity below 50 cm/s is usually associated to Dacron porosity, while a higher velocity suggests a true endoleak. The recognition of false positive with TEE avoids unnecessary balloon expansion in the context of a fragile aortic wall.

The occurrence of peri-stent leakages needs to be addressed and treated in the operating theatre. In fact, Type 1 and 3 endoleaks significantly increase the rupture rates of degenerative aneurysms, negatively affecting the long-term results of TEVAR treatment of Type B AD [28]. Table 39.7 presents the classification of endoleaks.

Recently, to increase the the diagnostic power of TEE in detecting endoleaks, the use of contrast-enhanced TEE (cTEE) has been proposed. In particular, Agricola et al. have shown that cTEE is more accurate than TEE and angiography in detecting peri-stent leakages, incomplete stent expansion, and the need for a further balloon expansion or further stent implantation [29]. In detecting endoleaks, IVUS is inferior to TEE due to its limited Doppler capabilities, while IPAI, although promising, has not been extensively investigated.

Cardiac performance assessment

Although TEVAR for AD does not need aortic cross-clamping, an aortic balloon inflation, if performed, could be associated with myocardial ischemia. TEE is able to detect new regional wall motion abnormalities during hemodynamic instability of stent deployment, allowing prompt treatment. Finally, TEE is probably the only intraoperative technique useful for the assessment of diastolic function in real time. This is very important as diastolic dysfunction may be the only manifestation of an ongoing ischemia.

39.5.2 Transesophageal echocardiography limitations

As with other imaging modalities, TEE has several pitfalls. First, the distal abdominal aorta cannot be accurately visualized. Second, in the case of a tortuous aorta the interpretation of the imaging may be difficult due to the inability to view the aorta at crucial locations. Third, the echogenic characteristics of the stent grafts may make the imaging of the aorta poor. In particular, Dacron allows the visualization beyond the stent while other materials like expanded polytetrafluoroethylene (ePTFE) absorb and reflect the ultrasound significantly decreasing the quality of the echo views. Fourth, small entry tears can be difficult to detect when the Doppler beam is perpendicular to the flow. Fifth, reverberations, abrupt aortic dilatation and aortic kinking can create a barrel-like structure which can mimic a dissection flap. However, perpendicular views are very useful to sort out these cases.

39.5.3 Intravascular ultrasound and intraluminal phased-array imaging limitations

When IVUS and IPAI are adopted in clinical practice the following limitations have to be taken into account. First, requiring a vascular access, these tools are invasive procedures and may be associated to serious complications. Second, both the IVUS equipment and the disposable catheters may be extremely expensive. For IPAI the price of catheters is also expensive, although there are catheters which can be re-sterilized with gas. Third, during insertion of the catheter in the aortic lumen, inadvertent manipulation may cause new entry sites or progression of the AD. Finally, IVUS lacks Doppler capabilities and ultrasound penetration. These last two limitations have been overcome by IPAI.

39.5.4 Pitfalls

In the evaluation of the aortic arch and descending thoracic aorta, several artifacts make the diagnosis challenging. In fact, the echo-dense posterior aortic wall reflecting ultrasound produces multiple-path artifacts and introduces structures into the views that have no corresponding anatomic tissue structure. Appelbe et al. reported a rate of "mirror image" artifacts mimicking a double-barrel aorta in a percentage of patients as high as 80% [30]. However, normal anatomic variants differ from artifacts because they have the same echo-density of the adjacent structure, move synchronously with the rest of the heart and appear in multiple planes [31].

39.6 Conclusions

The close proximity of the aorta to the esophagus makes TEE the gold standard in the management of aortic disease both in TEVAR and in open aortic surgery. In fact TEE provides intraoperative information on RV and LV function, fluid volume status, flow detection in bypass grafts, placement of endografts and endoleaks detection, significantly affecting the patient outcome. The use of IPAI in the context of TEVAR for Type B AD is promising, but the lack of large studies along with the high cost of the catheters and the need for adequate training are major limitations to its widespread adoption.

REFERENCES

1) Flachskampf FA, Wouters PF, Edvardsen T, et al. Recommendations for transoesophageal echocardiography: EACVI update 2014. Eur Heart J Cardiovasc Imaging 2014; 15: 353-65.
2) Rapezzi C, Rocchi G, Fattori R, et al. Usefulness of transesophageal echocardiographic monitoring to improve the outcome of stent-graft treatment of thoracic aortic aneurysms. Am J Cardiol 2001; 87: 315-9.
3) Jansen Klomp WW, Peelen LM, Brandon Bravo Bruinsma GJ, et al. Modified transesophageal echocardiography of the dissected thoracic aorta; a novel diagnostic approach. Cardiovasc Ultrasound 2016; 14: 28.
4) Hiratzka LF, Bakris GL, Beckman JA, et al. 2010 ACCF/AHA/AATS/ACR/ASA/SCA/SCAI/SIR/STS/SVM guidelines for the diagnosis and management of patients with thoracic aortic disease: a report of the American College of Cardiology Foundation/American Heart Association Task Force on Practice Guidelines, American Association for Thoracic Surgery, American College of Radiology, American Stroke Association, Society of Cardiovascular Anesthesiologists, Society for Cardiovascular Angiography and Interventions, Society of Interventional Radiology, Society of Thoracic Surgeons, and Society for Vascular Medicine. Circulation 2010; 121: e266-e369.
5) Hahn RT, Abraham T, Adams MS, et al. Guidelines for performing a comprehensive transesophageal echocardiographic examination: recommendations from the American Society of Echocardiography and the Society of Cardiovascular Anesthesiologists. J Am Soc Echocardiogr 2013; 26: 921-64.
6) Jungwirth B, Mackensen GB. Real-time 3-dimensional echocardiography in the operating room. Semin Cardiothorac Vasc Anesth 2008; 12: 248-64.
7) Nagueh SF, Smiseth OA, Appleton CP, et al. Recommendations for the evaluation of left ventricular diastolic function by echocardiography: an update from the American Society of Echocardiography and the European Association of Cardiovascular Imaging. Eur Heart J Cardiovasc Imaging 2016; pii: jew082. [Epub ahead of print].
8) Lang RM, Bierig M, Devereux RB, et al. Recommendations for chamber quantification: a report from the American Society of Echocardiography's Guidelines and Standards Committee and the Chamber Quantification Writing Group, developed in conjunction with the European Association of Echocardiography, a branch of the European Society of Cardiology. J Am Soc Echocardiogr 2005; 18: 1440-63.
9) Louie EK, Lin SS, Reynertson SI, et al. Pressure and volume loading of the right ventricle have opposite effects on left ventricular ejection fraction. Circulation 1995; 92: 819-24.
10) Tamborini G, Muratori M, Brusoni D, et al. Is right ventricular systolic function reduced after cardiac surgery? A two- and three-dimensional echocardiographic study. Eur J Echocardiogr 2009; 10: 630-4.
11) Rudski LG, Lai WW, Afilalo J, et al. Guidelines for the echocardiographic assessment of the right heart in adults: a report from the American Society of Echocardiography endorsed by the European Association of Echocardiography, a registered branch of the European Society of Cardiology, and the Canadian Society of Echocardiography. J Am Soc Echocardiogr 2010; 23: 685-713.
12) Klein AL, Leung DY, Murray RD, et al. Effects of age and physiologic variables on right ventricular filling dynamics in normal subjects. Am J Cardiol 1999; 84: 440-8.
13) Ciozda W, Kedan I, Kehl DW, et al. The efficacy of sonographic measurement of inferior vena cava diameter as an estimate of central venous pressure. Cardiovasc Ultrasound 2016; 14: 33.
14) Gonzalez-Fajardo JA, Gutierrez V, San Roman JA, et al. Utility of intraoperative transesophageal echocardiography during endovascular stent-graft repair of acute thoracic aortic dissection. Ann Vasc Surg 2002; 16: 297-303.
15) Ballal RS, Nanda NC, Gatewood R, et al. Usefulness of transesophageal echocardiography in assessment of aortic dissection. Circulation 1991; 84: 1903-14.
16) Katz ES, Tunick PA, Rusinek H, et al. Protruding aortic atheromas predict stroke in elderly patients undergoing cardiopulmonary bypass: experience with intraoperative transesophageal echocardiography. J Am Coll Cardiol 1992; 20: 70-7.
17) Rocchi G, Lofiego C, Biagini E, et al. Transesophageal echocardiography-guided algorithm for stent-graft implantation in aortic dissection. J Vasc Surg 2004; 40: 880-5.
18) Rudenick PA, Bijnens BH, Garcia-Dorado D, Evangelista A. An in vitro phantom study on the influence of tear size and configuration on the hemodynamics of the lumina in chronic type B aortic dissections. J Vasc Surg 2013; 57: 464-74.
19) Sampaio SM, Shin SH, Panneton JM, et al. Intraoperative endoleak during EVAR: frequency, nature, and significance. Vasc Endovascular Surg 2009; 43: 352-9.
20) Monaco F, Sala A, De Luca M. Anesthesia in Marfan patient. Italian Journal of Vascular and Endovascular Surgery 2015; 22 (Suppl 3/3): 37-41.
21) Bartel T, Eggebrecht H, Muller S, et al. Comparison of diagnostic and therapeutic value of transesophageal echocardiography, intravascular ultrasonic imaging, and intraluminal phased-array imaging in aortic dissection with tear in the descending thoracic aorta (type B). Am J Cardiol 2007; 99: 270-4.

22) Koschyk DH, Nienaber CA, Knap M, et al. How to guide stent-graft implantation in type B aortic dissection? Comparison of angiography, transesophageal echocardiography, and intravascular ultrasound. Circulation 2005; 112: 1260-4.
23) Guo BL, Shi ZY, Guo DQ, et al. Effect of intravascular ultrasound-assisted thoracic endovascular aortic repair for "complicated" type B aortic dissection. Chin Med J (Engl) 2015; 128: 2322-9.
24) Kpodonu J, Ramaiah VG, Diethrich EB. Intravascular ultrasound imaging as applied to the aorta: a new tool for the cardiovascular surgeon. Ann Thorac Surg 2008; 86: 1391-8.
25) Hoshina K, Kato M, Miyahara T, et al. A retrospective study of intravascular ultrasound use in patients undergoing endovascular aneurysm repair: its usefulness and a description of the procedure. Eur J Vasc Endovasc Surg 2010; 40: 559-63.
26) Blasco A, Piazza A, Goicolea J, et al. Intravascular ultrasound measurement of the aortic lumen. Rev Esp Cardiol 2010; 63: 598-601.
27) Fernandez JD, Donovan S, Garrett HE Jr, Burgar S. Endovascular thoracic aortic aneurysm repair: evaluating the utility of intravascular ultrasound measurements. J Endovasc Ther 2008; 15: 68-72.
28) Jonker FH, Verhagen HJ, Heijmen RH, Lin PH, Trimarchi S, Lee WA et al. Endovascular repair of ruptured thoracic aortic aneurysms: predictors of procedure-related stroke. Ann Vasc Surg 2011; 25: 3-8.
29) Agricola E, Slavich M, Rinaldi E, et al. Usefulness of contrast-enhanced transoesophageal echocardiography to guide thoracic endovascular aortic repair procedure. Eur Heart J Cardiovasc Imaging 2016; 17: 67-75.
30) Appelbe AF, Walker PG, Yeoh JK, et al. Clinical significance and origin of artifacts in transesophageal echocardiography of the thoracic aorta. J Am Coll Cardiol 1993; 21: 754-60.
31) Bertrand PB, Levine RA, Isselbacher EM, Vandervoort PM. Fact or artifact in two-dimensional echocardiography: avoiding misdiagnosis and missed diagnosis. J Am Soc Echocardiogr 2016; 29: 381-91.

40

Experimental and clinical evidence supporting septectomy in the primary treatment of acute Type B thoracic aortic dissection

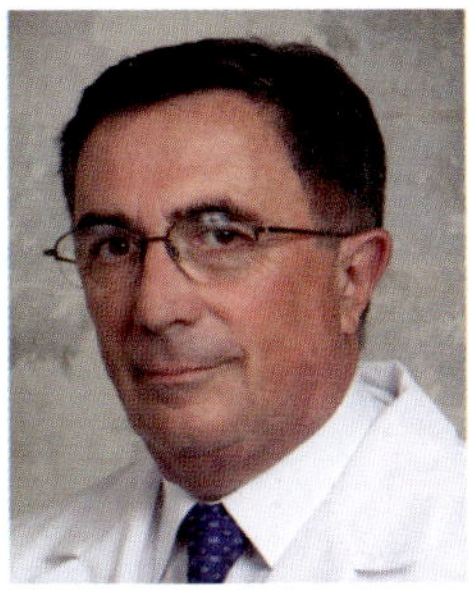

Juan Carlos Parodi and Ramon Berguer

40.1 Introduction

To discuss the mechanics of aortic dissection (AD), the aorta should be considered a coaxial tube of two layers: inner and outer (Fig. 40.1). The inner layer is made of intima, internal elastic membrane and a variable thickness of tunica media, and this inner layer makes up the septum. The outer layer contains a variable thickness of tunica media, the external elastic membrane and the adventitia. The description of the AD septum as an "intimal" flap is a misnomer inasmuch as layers other than the intima are involved.

40.1.1 Mechanics of restricted outflow of the false lumen

A review of data [1, 2] from the International Registry of Acute Aortic Dissection (IRAD) found that among patients with chronic Type B AD those with partial thrombosis of the false lumen (FL) had worse outcomes than those with either fully thrombosed or fully patent FL. To explain the mechanics of this seemingly paradoxical clinical outcome, we assumed that a tortuous and partially thrombosed FL is a conduit parallel to the true lumen (TL) that is pressurized simultaneously with it but has a restricted outflow in diastole. This construct is similar to the one we used to explain the continuous expansion of the aneurysmal sac in a Type I endoleak following EndoVascular Aneurysm Repair (EVAR) [3].

To test this assumption we had constructed a bench-top model of a chronically dissected aorta [4, 5]. The model (Fig. 40.2) was cast with a polydimethylsiloxane polymer (PDMS) to which we could assign elastic values similar to those measured in human specimens of chronic Type B dissections [6]. In this bench-top model of chronic dissection, a small communication (representing a small tear) between the false and true lumina resulted in the former displaying a higher diastolic pressure than the latter [4, 5]. This differential of pressure favoring the false lumen was held to be the mechanism for the more frequent development and eventual rup-

Juan Carlos Parodi (Parodijc@yandex.com)
Trinidad Hospital, Buenos Aires, Argentina
University of Michigan, Ann Arbor, MI, USA

G. Melissano - R. Chiesa (eds), Aortic Dissection patients true stories and the innovations that saved their lives

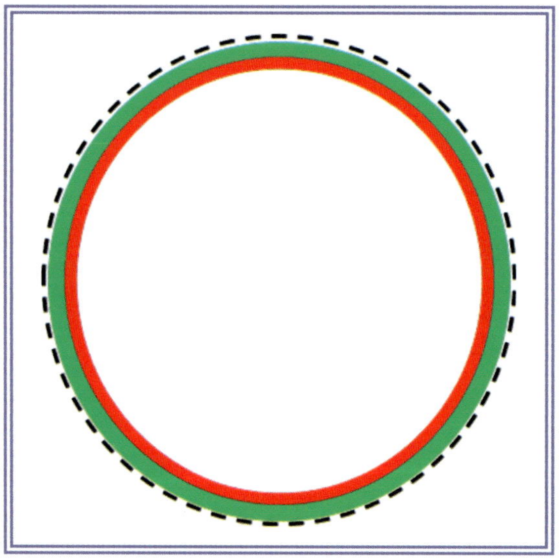

Fig. 40.1 Schematic representation of the two coaxial layers in a normal and dissected aorta. Green: outer layer; red: inner layer; dotted line: outer aortic diameter. Reproduced from [20], with permission.

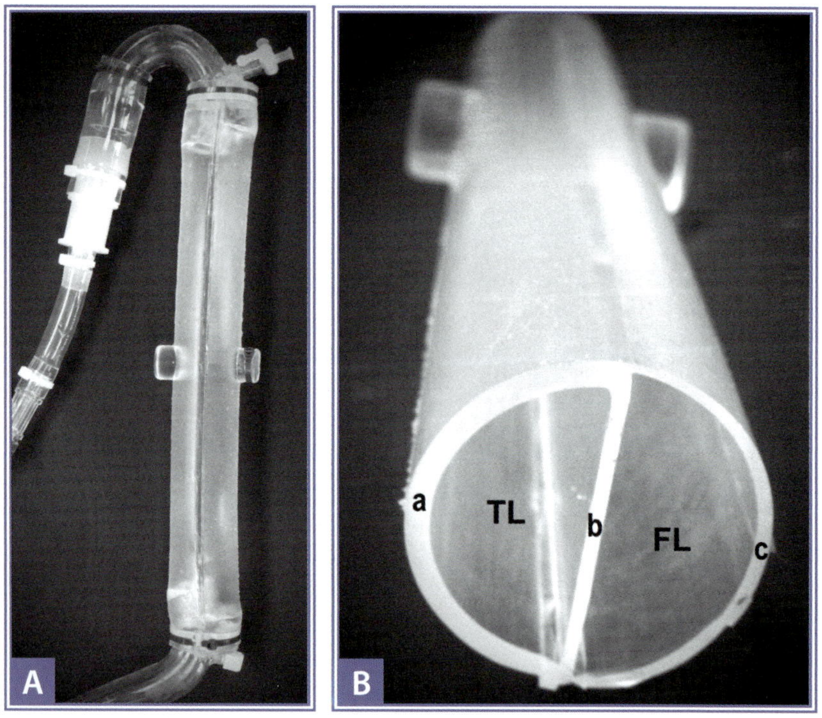

Fig. 40.2 **A**, Cast model of chronic dissection of the descending thoracic aorta. **B**, Transverse section shows: **a**, inner e outer layer; **b**, septum; **c**, outer layer. FL, false lumen; TL, true lumen. Reproduced from [20], with permission.

ture of aneurysms in patients with a chronic dissection and partially thrombosed FL. Patients with a fully patent FL have equally thinned outer wall but do not have a pressure differential because the outflow of the FL is not restricted.

40.1.2 Clinical reports of isolated behavior of the outer wall of the aorta

It is generally thought that the stress imposed by the blood pressure on the thinned out, and hence weaker, wall of the FL causes it to dilate into an aneurysm. But this however does not explain why patients with a fully patent FL have a lower tendency to develop aneurysms than those that have a partially thrombosed FL. If the thinned wall of the FL is responsible for the development of an aneurysm we need to explain why patients who underwent aorto-iliac

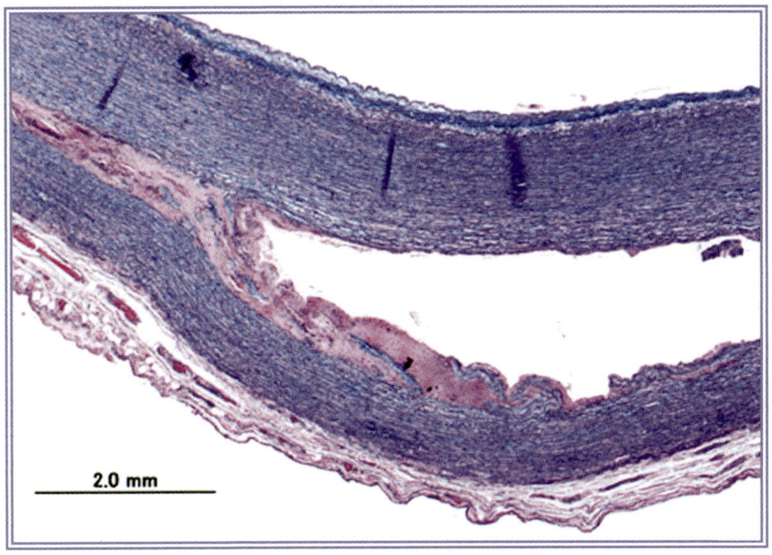

Fig. 40.3 The plane of AD. Reproduced from [20], with permission.

endarterectomy did not develop aneurysms at the endarterectomy sites. After all, the plane of acute AD (Fig. 40.3) is the same as the plane exposed by endarterectomy as has been noted by surgeons doing septectomy for acute dissection of the abdominal aorta [7].

A meta-analysis review [8] of 1,940 patients who underwent aorto-iliac endarterectomy did not show any aneurysm of the infrarenal aorta on long-term follow-up. Stoney [9] did not see any postoperative aneurysms at the site of transaortic visceral endarterectomies in the aortic segment containing the visceral branches. Carlson [10] reported on innominate endarterectomies prolonged into part of the ascending aorta where no aneurysm was observed on follow-up. In the transverse aortic arch, Thevenet (personal communication, April 2014) did not encounter aneurysmal dilatation in any of the 14 patients in whom, under deep hypothermic arrest, he did an endarterectomy of the entire aortic arch through a longitudinal incision. He followed these patients for up to 25 years [11].

Common to all these endarterectomies of different segments of the aorta is the fact that they were all closed primarily and longitudinally, resulting in a conduit of a diameter smaller than its original dimension (Fig. 40.4). It may be argued that the thin wall that results from a dissection may very well have the same thickness as the one that follows endarterectomy but has different elastic properties given that the former has the altered elastic parameters [12] and increased expression of matrix metalloproteases associated with Type B AD [13]. We searched the literature for reports of surgical fenestration (or septectomy) in dissected aortas because in these patients the FL wall, along which the aorta is closed, has the elastic abnormalities peculiar to acutely dissected aortas. In chronically dissected aortas, Webb and Williams [7] did excision of the dissection flap and primary closure with "tailoring" – meaning slight narrowing – of the infrarenal aorta in 18 patients. Only 2 of 18 patients developed dilatation of the tailored aorta on long-term follow-up and both patients had Marfan disease. The other 16 patients with atherosclerotic disease did not dilate. This information on the stability of the operated aorta was confirmed after 14 years post operation (personal communication, February 2014). There were 5 additional reports [7, 14-17], totaling 62 patients with acutely dissected aortas, in whom a segmental resection of the septum was done. None of these patients developed an aneurysm at the site of septectomy on follow-up. Noticing that the fenestrated aortas showed no evidence of enlargement on follow-up, Elefteriades [18] suggested a possible "protective effect of fenestration". From these clinical data it can be concluded that the outer aortic layer, whether from an atherosclerotic or a dissected aorta, is capable of withstanding blood pressure stresses without experiencing dilatation as long as the repaired aorta has a diameter slightly smaller than it had before.

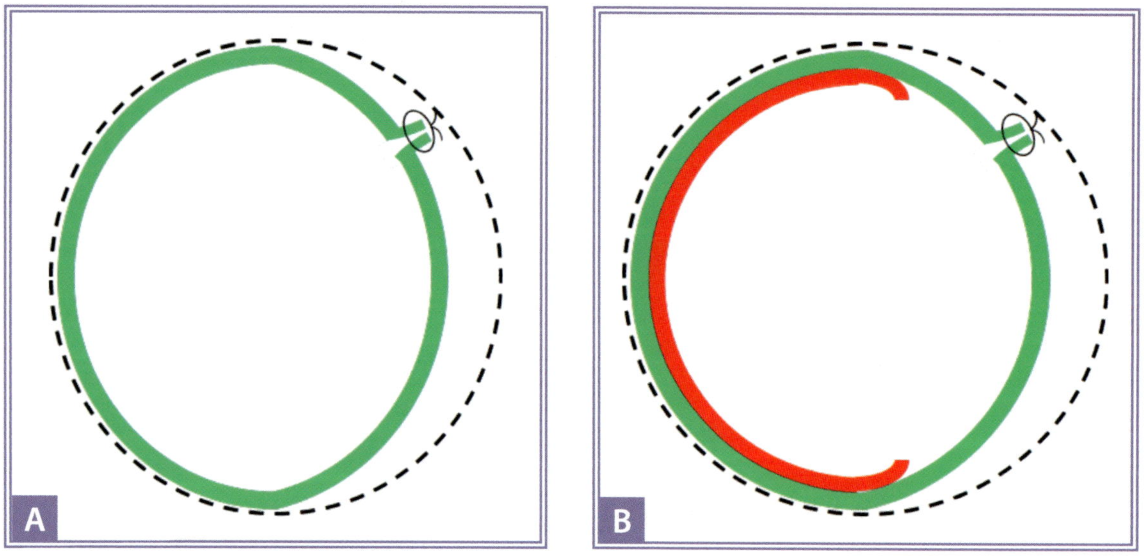

Fig. 40.4 Reduced aortic diameter after closure of endarterectomy (**A**) and open longitudinal septectomy (**B**). Reproduced from [20], with permission.

40.1.3 Pressure mechanics in acute dissection of the thoracic aorta

In acute AD the thinner outer wall of the FL undergoes a slight dilatation (~12%) because its tension rises as its wall thickness (h) decreases and the product P×r/h increases (Fig. 40.5). The FL has two walls each covering similar sectors: an inner wall, which is the septum, and an outer wall which is the outer layer of aorta. The stresses on the two walls of the FL are different: on the inner wall, the septum, the stress is minimal given that the intraluminal pressure in the FL is opposed by an approximately equal pressure across the septum from the TL. In acute dissection intravascular ultrasound (IVUS) images show the septum to be thicker than the outer wall of the FL [19]. This is the result of elastic contraction: there is no pressure stress exerted on it as the FL and TL bear equivalent pressure on its two surfaces. On the other hand, the flap is thinner than the outer wall of the FL when its thickness is measured on an acute dissection specimen (depressurized). As the dissection becomes chronic, the septum not only does not stretch but actually shortens and thickens. In the FL the stress is borne by the thinned outer wall that has already stretched by ~12% to accommodate its decrease in thickness (assuming a mean pressure of 90 mmHg, a 10% increase in radius and a 50% decrease in wall thickness,

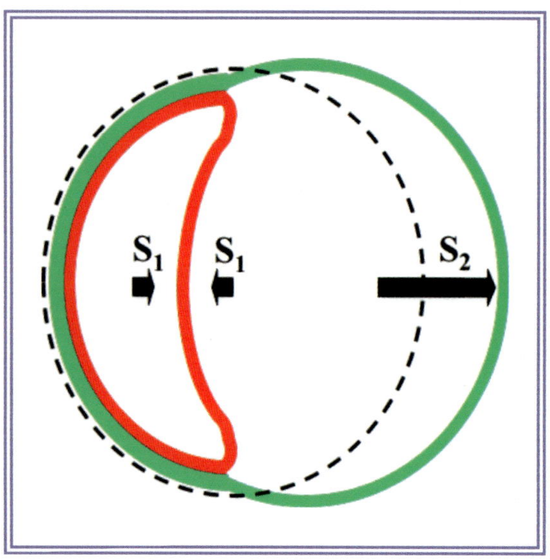

Fig. 40.5 Changes in geometry and wall stress in acute AD. S1, stress bearing on inner wall; S2, stress bearing on outer wall. Reproduced from [20], with permission.

the tension in the FL wall would more than double from 11.0 kPa to 26.3 kPa immediately after an acute dissection). In these circumstances, any increase in the pressure of the FL (as it happens when it has a reduced outflow) will bear on the thinned outer wall of the false lumen and may result in its aneurysmal dilatation.

With regards to whether the septectomy should be carried out antegrade, starting at the proximal tear, or retrograde from the distal tear, it is anticipated that a septectomy that begins at the proximal tear may cause sudden distention of the FL with extension of the dissection and collapse of the TL. A retrograde septectomy involving the visceral segment of the aorta will also correct an existing visceral malperfusion.

40.2 Method

If the differential of pressure between FL and TL is responsible for the aneurysmal dilatation of the latter we proposed to ascertain how extensive a septectomy should be in order to equalize the pressure in both lumina. We built a model of Type B AD connected to a circulatory pump (Harvard Apparatus®, Holliston, MA) (Fig. 40.6). The bench-top model was built using a combination of glass for the true wall of the aorta and polytetrafluoroethylene (PTFE) for the FL outer wall and septum.

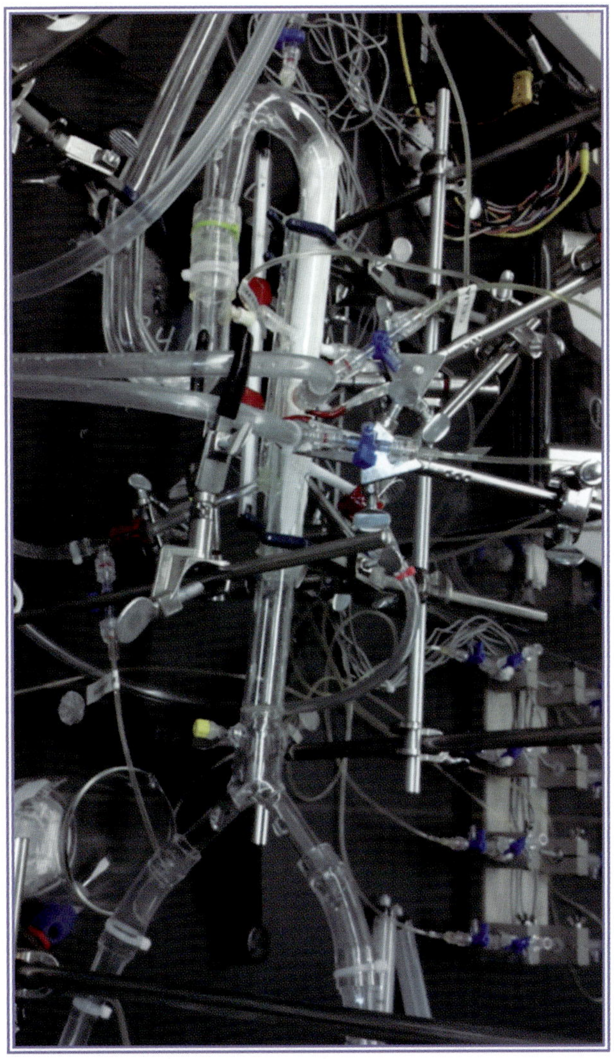

Fig. 40.6 Acute Type B AD model built with glass and PTFE. Reproduced from [20], with permission.

Table 40.1 Correlation between size of tear(s) and pressure difference between false and true lumen [20]

Model (proximal area-distal area in mm²)	Pressure difference (false-true) in mmHg		
	Mean	Peak systole	End diastole
65-0	6.77	9.86	5.44
65-20	3.67	5.64	2.35
65-40	1.33	1.98	1.17
145-40	1.58	2.52	1.31
145-90	0.44	0.8	0.01

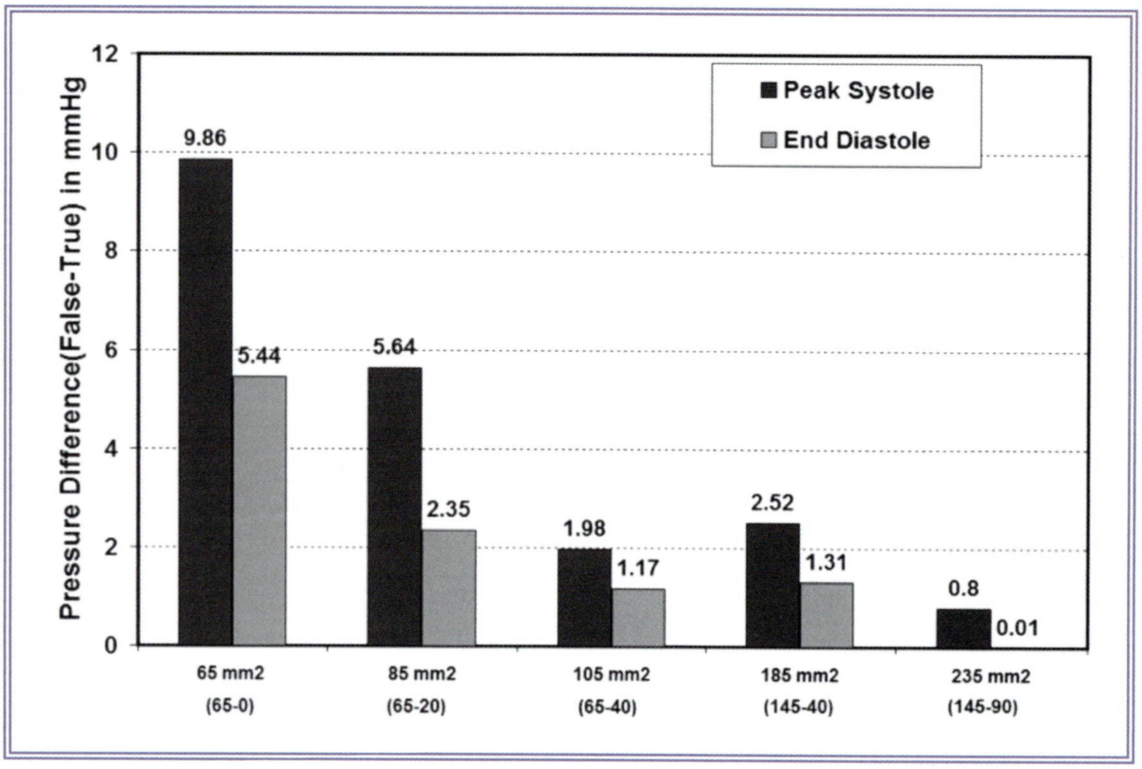

Fig. 40.7 Pressure difference between false and true lumina vs. total area of the tear sizes. Reproduced from [20], with permission.

40.3 Results

Different numbers and arrangements of tears were tested (Table 40.1). The cross sectional area of the proximal tear opening varied from 65 to 145 mm^2; the distal tear varied from 0 to 90 mm^2. The greater the distal tear opening the lower the differential of pressure between FL and TL. Once the sum of the area of the tears approaches 250 mm^2 pressure equalization is achieved (Fig. 40.7). This then should be the minimum area created by a septectomy that will equalize the pressure in both lumina.

40.4 Conclusions

Primary treatment of acute Type B AD should include an endovascular septectomy creating at least a 250 mm^2 communication between FL and TL. The septectomy should be carried from distal to proximal. Obliteration of the proximal tear with a bare stent or a stent graft should also be part of the management of acute Type B AD, because the proximal tear may have caused additionally a short retrograde dissection into the arch or create a funnel-shaped preferential inflow into the FL.

We are in the process of creating a septotomy percutaneous catheter guided by two guidewires placed one in the true lumen and the second in the false lumen. We are testing devices using radio-frequency or laser energy to cut the septum from the distal end of the dissection, directing the cutter towards the entry site.

Acknowledgments

This work was supported by the Frankel Vascular Research Fund.

REFERENCES

1) Hagan PG, Nienaber CA, Isselbacher EM, et al. The International Registry of Acute Aortic Dissection (IRAD): new insights into an old disease. JAMA 2000; 283: 897-903.
2) Tsai TT, Evagelista A, Nienaber CA, et al. Partial thrombosis of the false lumen in patients with acute type B aortic dissection. N Engl J Med 2007; 357: 349-59.
3) Parodi JC, Berguer R, Ferreira LM, La Mura R, Schermerhorn ML. Intra-aneurysmal pressure after incomplete endovascular exclusion. J Vasc Surg 2001; 34: 909-14.
4) Tsai TT, Schlicht M, Khanafer K, et al. Tear size and location impacts false lumen pressure in an ex-vivo model of chronic type B aortic dissection. J Am Coll Cardiol 2007; 49(9): 383a.
5) Tsai TT, Schlicht MS, Khanafer K et al. Tear size and location impacts false lumen pressure in an ex vivo model of chronic type B aortic dissection. J Vasc Surg 2008; 47(4): 844-51.
6) Khanafer K, Duprey A, Schlicht M, Berguer R. Effects of strain rate, mixing ratio, and stress-strain definition on the mechanical behavior of the polydimethylsiloxane (PDMS) material as related to its biological applications. Biomed Microdevices 2009; 11(2): 503-8.
7) Webb TH, Williams GM. Abdominal aortic tailoring for renal, visceral, and lower extremity malperfusion resulting from acute aortic dissection. J Vasc Surg 1997; 26: 474-81.
8) Chiu KW, Davies RSM, Nightingale PG, et al. Review of direct anatomical open surgical management of atherosclerotic aorto-iliac occlusive disease. Euro J Endovasc Surg 2010; 39: 460-71.
9) Stoney RJ, Ehrenfeld WK, Wylie EJ. Revascularization methods in chronic visceral ischemia caused by atherosclerosis. Ann Surg 1977; 4: 468-75.
10) Carlson RE, Ehrenfeld WK, Stoney RJ, Wylie EJ. Innominate artery endarterectomy. A 16-year experience. Arch Surg 1977; 112: 1389-93.
11) Thevenet A. Personal communication, April 2014.
12) Duprey A, Khanafer K, Schlicht M, Avril S, Williams D, Berguer R. In vitro characterisation of physiological and maximum elastic modulus of ascending thoracic aortic aneurysms using uniaxial tensile testing. Eur J Vasc Endovasc 2010; 39(6): 700-7.
13) Sokolis DP, Iliopoulos DC. Impaired mechanics and matrix metalloproteinases/inhibitors expression in female ascending thoracic aortic aneurysms. J Mech Behav Biomed Mater 2014; 34: 154-64.
14) Williams GM. Personal communication, February 2014.
15) Trimarchi S, Jonker FH, Muhs BE, et al. Long-term outcomes of surgical aortic fenestration for complicated acute type B aortic dissections. J Vasc Surg 2010; 52(2): 261-6.
16) Atkins M, Black JH III, Cambria RC. Acute dissection. Perspectives in the era of stent-graft repair. J Vasc Surg 2006; 42(2 suppl): A30-A43.
17) Panneton JM, The SH, Cherry KJ, et al. Aortic fenestration for acute or chronic aortic dissection: an uncommon but effective procedure. J Vasc Surg 2000; 32(4): 711-21.
18) Elefteriades JA, Hartelroad J, Gusberg RJ, et al. Long-term experience with descending aortic dissection: the complication-specific approach. Ann Thorac Surg 1992; 53: 11-21.
19) Williams DM, LePage MA, Lee DY. The dissected aorta: part I. Early anatomic changes in an in vitro model. Radiology 1997; 203: 23-31.
20) Berguer R, Parodi JC, Schlicht M, Khanafer K. Experimental and clinical evidence supporting septectomy in the primary treatment of acute type B thoracic aortic dissection. Ann Vasc Surg 2015; 29(2): 167-73.